Handbuch der experimentellen Pharmakologie
Handbook of Experimental Pharmacology

Heffter Heubner New Series

XXXIV

Add: JORPES, J E and MUTT, V. editors

Secretin, Cholecystokinin, Pancreozymin and Gastrin

By

M. Bodanszky, R. Carratù, D. A. Dreiling, R. Fussgänger,
H. D. Janowitz, J. D. Jamieson, J. E. Jorpes, V. Mutt, E. F. Pfeiffer,
J. Plessier, M. L. Ramorino, S. Raptis, A. Torsoli,
M. Zimmerman

Editors
J. E. Jorpes and V. Mutt

With 135 Figures

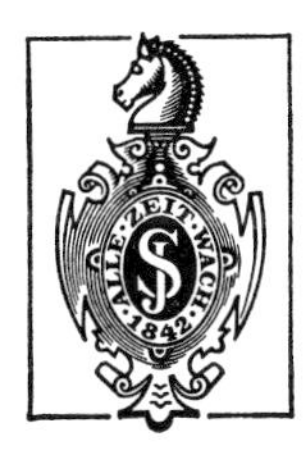

Springer-Verlag Berlin · Heidelberg · New York 1973

J. E. JORPES and V. MUTT
Karolinska Institutet
Kemiska Institutionen II
S-10401 Stockholm/Sweden

ISBN 3-540-05952-0 Springer-Verlag Berlin · Heidelberg · New York
ISBN 0-387-05952-0 Springer-Verlag New York · Heidelberg · Berlin

Type-setting, printing and binding: Konrad Triltsch, Graphischer Betrieb, Würzburg

List of Contributors

BODANSZKY, M., Case Western Reserve University, Dept. of Chemistry
Cleveland, Ohio 44106/USA

JAMIESON, J. D., The Rockefeller University, New York, N.Y. 10021/USA

JORPES, J. E., Karolinska Institutet, Kemiska Institutionen II,
S-10401 Stockholm/Sweden

MUTT, V., Karolinska Institutet, Kemiska Institutionen II,
S-10401 Stockholm/Sweden

PFEIFFER, E. F., Zentrum für Innere Medizin und Kinderheilkunde
7900 Ulm, Steinhövelstraße 9/Deutschland

PLESSIER, J., Médecin Attaché de L'Hopital St.-Antoine,
23, Rue Bertrand, Paris VIIE/France

TORSOLI, A., Divisone Gastroenterologica, II. Clinica Medica,
Università, 00100 Roma/Italy

ZIMMERMAN, M. J., 755 Park Avenue, New York, N.Y. 10021/USA

Foreword

In the beginning of this century physiology witnessed the creation of a new concept, the hormonal regulation of the work of the digestive organs. It was found that such essential functions as the flow of pancreatic juice and emptying of bile into the intestine were regulated by two hormones, secretin and cholecystokinin, respectively. Already in 1925 French authors attempted to measure the functional capacity of the exocrine pancreas by means of stimulation with secretin. The usefulness of the secretin test in this connection was definitely established by Scandinavian workers in the 1930's. In spite of the difficulties in obtaining secretin American authors succeeded in keeping the interest in the secretin test alive.

The development in the 1950's of counter-current, ion exchange and chromatographic techniques offered new possibilities in this field. The intestinal hormones were known to be relatively low molecular peptides and these could now be isolated in pure form. Thus secretin was isolated in 1961, and cholecystokinin in 1964. The newly developed methods for peptide analysis likewise soon brought us full information about the primary structure of the peptides. Gastrin, the specific stimulant of the gastric acid secretion, which was discovered in 1905 and acknowledged as a hormone in 1938, was the first of the gastrointestinal hormones for which the structure became known. This was in 1964. Synthesis soon followed.

These developments are reviewed in the first chapter of the present volume. The chemistry of the gastrointestinal hormones unexpectedly revealed close interrelationships between them. Thus secretin was found to have 14 of its 27 amino acid units in the same position as in the molecule of pancreatic glucagon and the C-terminal pentapeptide of gastrin, involving the active center, is identical to that of cholecystokinin. Two other polypeptides recently extracted from the upper intestinal mucosa show similarities to glucagon and secretin both in structure and in biological actions. Here we consequently have an analogy with the group of enzymes: trypsin, chymotrypsin, elastase and thrombin, deriving from the pancreas and the liver, with extensive similarities in structure.

Since the secretin test now could be performed with pure secretin of standard potency the interest in the pancreatic function test was revived. Furthermore a highly purified preparation of cholecystokinin with pancreozymin activity proved useful not only as a supplement to the secretin test but in particular as an aid in cholecystography, cholangiography and in the roentgenological examination of the small intestine. A separate chapter of this volume deals with the pancreatic function test, another with the physiology and a third with the clinical application of cholecystokinin.

The purification of cholecystokinin resulted in the unforeseen finding that it is responsible for the pancreozymin effect of the English authors i.e. it is a strong stimulator of the enzyme secretion from the pancreas as secretin is for the water and electrolyte secretion. A separate chapter is devoted to the studies on the subcellular level of the action of cholecystokinin on the acinar cells of the pancreas. Recently new questions as to the function of the two hormones have been actualized. They cause both in *in vitro* and in *in vivo* experiments a release of insulin from the islet tissue of the pancreas. The development in this field has been followed up in a separate chapter.

J. E. Jorpes · V. Mutt

Contents

Chapter I

Chapter IV

Chapter V

Chapter VI

Chapter VII

Chapter I

Secretin and Cholecystokinin (CCK)

J. ERIK JORPES and VIKTOR MUTT

With 42 Figures

I. Secretin

1. The Exocrine Function of the Pancreas and the Discovery of Secretin

In the history of our knowledge about the pancreas and its function, two names are particularly outstanding: those of CLAUDE BERNARD and IVAN PAVLOV. But even BERNARD, working in the middle of the 19th century, had his forerunners. About two hundred years earlier, WIRSUNGIUS had demonstrated that the pancreas has an excretory duct, and is by no means only a cushion of flesh ($\pi\alpha\nu$ = all, $\varkappa\varrho\varepsilon\alpha\sigma$ = flesh) on which the stomach rests. The Russian name for the pancreas, *Поджелудочная железá*, means the gland under the stomach. In the 1660's REGNIER DE GRAAF had cannulated the duct with a goose quill, and ascribed some importance for digestion to the juice collected from it. He found the name pancreas "minime conveniens" because "pancreatis substantia tota glandulosa est". In 1828 LEURET and LASSAIGNE in France made a fundamental discovery. Upon finding that acetic acid, introduced into the duodenum, led to the secretion of pancreatic juice and bile, with dilation of the orifices of the pancreatic and bile ducts in the duodenum, they came to the following conclusion: "Since a weak acid is able to elicit secretion to the duodenum and to dilate the secretory ducts from the liver and the pancreas, the acid chyme ought to have the same property. It is acidic and it is emptied into the intestine when the digestive juices are needed."

a) CLAUDE BERNARD and the Pancreatic Secretion

The clinician MAGENDIE, who was BERNARD's teacher and coworker, showed that pancreatic juice, in contrast to bile coagulates like egg white on boiling, and in 1844 their compatriot VALENTIN demonstrated its ability to split starch. But it was CLAUDE BERNARD who elucidated the role that pancreatic juice plays in the digestion and absorption of fat.

"In the winter of 1846, I made a comparative study of the digestion of various substances in carnivora and herbivora. After administering fatty material orally to dogs and rabbits, I followed the physical and chemical changes which this material underwent in order to be digested and absorbed by the chyle vessels. I then discovered, when I opened the gut of these animals, that in the dog the fat was emulsified and absorbed by the chyle vessels in the upper part of the small intestine, just beyond the pylorus, whereas in the rabbit this phenomenon was not distinct until much further down, at a distance of 30—40 cm from the pylorus. Surprised by this difference, I carefully investigated whether it had any

Acknowledgement: Research project supported by grants from U.S. Public Health Service, National Institutes of Health (No. Am 06410-01-09), The Squibb Institute for Medical Research. New Brunswick, N. J., U. S. A., Torsten och Ragnar Söderbergs Stiftelser, The Swedish Cancer Society, The Swedish Medical Research Council, and Magnus Bergvalls Stiftelse.

anatomic cause. I then found that in the dog the two pancreatic ducts emptied very high up in the duodenum, in the vicinity of the choledochus, whereas the pancreatic duct in the rabbit opened much further down than the bile duct, exactly where I had seen the absorption of fat to start with great intensity.

After having observed the connection between the position of the chyle-containing lymph vessels and the outflow of pancreatic juice, I was naturally inclined to believe that it is to this fluid that we must ascribe the ability to alter fats so that they can be absorbed."

It was in these words that BERNARD described the observations which led to his discovery of the role of the pancreas in normal digestion. He considered this observation to be the most important that he had made with respect to the function of this gland. In his work "Mémoires sur le Pancréas" (BERNARD, 1856b), he gave an exceedingly good description of the situation in the rabbit, in which the pancreatic duct empties into the intestine considerably distal to the pylorus. Emulsification and absorption of fat as seen in the chyle vessels of the mesentery does not occur until well below the papilla of Vater.

BERNARD also tried to extirpate the pancreas in the dog, but was of course unsuccessful with the technique in use at that time. However, he did succeed in destroying the gland by filling its duct with melted, hardening tallow, which resulted in the dog's death in cachexia. He did not have the privilege of discovering the relationship between the pancreas and the diabetic state. VON MERING and MINKOWSKI, in 1889, were the first to observe diabetic symptoms in pancreatectomized dogs (MINKOWSKI, 1893). But it was BERNARD who, in connection with the discovery of glycogen in 1857, coined the term "sécrétion interne" (BERNARD, 1859, II, pp. 411, 412), by which he meant the passage of sugar from the stores of glycogen in the liver cells into the blood.

BERNARD's work has been described at some length because he was a direct predecessor of the Russian scientist PAVLOV (See OLMSTED & OLMSTED: CLAUDE BERNARD, 1952). An American physician who attended BERNARD's lectures at the Collège de France in 1851 described his surprise at seeing dogs and rabbits running around in the lecture hall with five or six fistula openings in the abdomen and neck, through which digestive juice from the salivary glands, stomach, liver or pancreas could be caused to flow at will. BERNARD was thus a worthy predecessor of PAVLOV, the most prominent personality in this field in the late 1890's (see BABKIN, 1949).

b) IVAN P. PAVLOV and the Double Mechanism of the Exocrine Pancreatic Secretion

PAVLOV observed in his famous fistula dogs that pancreatic secretion is controlled by a double mechanism, in part by the vagus nerve, and in part by a stimulus originating in the duodenal mucosa when acid material from the stomach comes in contact with it. PAVLOV obtained a vagal effect in unanesthetized pancreatic fistula dogs by electrical stimulation of the peripheral end of the cut thoracic vagus nerves. The effect could also be produced in dogs with the spinal cord cut below the medulla oblongata (PAVLOV, 1888; BABKIN, 1914, p. 297). The other mechanism has been observed as early as 1825 by LEURET and LASSAIGNE on introducing acetic acid into the duodenum. It could be provoked by carbon dioxide in the duodenum (BECKER, 1893). Pancreatic secretion could be provoked by acidification of the gastric juice preferably with hydrochloric acid (DOLINSKI, 1894). The stimulation of the pancreas, however, occurred at first, when the chymus or the acidified gastric contents entered the duodenum (POPIELSKI, 1896, p. 97, 1901).

The secretions elicited by these two means were very different in composition (BABKIN and SAVICH, 1908). That obtained on stimulation of the vagus nerve was thick, viscous and rich in enzymes (METT, 1889; KUDREWECKI, 1890), whereas that following stimulation of the duodenal mucosa with acid was copious but poor in enzymes. It was alkaline, due to the presence of sodium bicarbonate, and yielded a considerable amount of ash (WALTHER, 1897).

The studies of the Russian school were extended to include the microscopic changes taking place in the pancreatic gland under the influence of the different stimuli. Highly characteristic changes were described, distinctly specific for nervous and humoral stimulation respectively (BABKIN, RUBASHKIN and SAVICH, 1909). Stimulation of the vagal nerve of the cat gave rise to extensive extrusion of secretory granules, whereas, although the introduction of hydrochloric acid into the duodenum induced copious secretion, the glandular cells remained full of granules.

c) Enterokinase, the First Enzyme Activator

At this early date, PAVLOV's group was engaged in quantitative analyses of the various enzymes in the pancreatic juice. In 1899, in the course of this work, SHEPOVALNIKOV at PAVLOV's laboratory discovered the *enterokinase* of the intestinal juice, which activates trypsinogen, and was the first enzyme activator to be recognized. PAVLOV (1900, 1901) gave it its name and referred to it as "an enzyme of the enzymes". In his Nobel lecture in Stockholm in 1904, he stressed the fact that the proteolytic enzymes, which could be dangerous to their enzyme neighbours in the pancreatic juice, are present in an inactive form, whereas amylase and lipase are already activated.

Enterokinase was purified by KUNITZ (1939a, b). In 1956 YAMASHINA obtained in our laboratory a preparation which was uniform electrophoretically and had a specific activity 70 times that of the KUNITZ preparation. Chemically it is a glycoprotein, containing about 41 per cent carbohydrate. The neutral sugars: mannose, galactose and fucose, together make up 22.9 per cent, glucosamine 8.8 per cent, galactosamine 3.9 per cent, and sialic acid 5.5 per cent (YAMASHINA, 1955, 1956a, b, c). Enterokinase is resistant to proteolytic enzymes, probably because of its high content of sugar components. Russian workers, SHLYGIN (1956) and MICHLIN et al. (1958), have shown that it is destroyed only in the colon by the action of bacterial enzymes.

d) The Discovery of Secretin by BAYLISS and STARLING

The work of PAVLOV's group on the double secretory mechanism of the pancreas gave the impetus for the discovery of secretin in 1902 by BAYLISS and STARLING at the Physiological Laboratory, University College, London. The Russian school, like other physiologists of that time, were traditionally bound to the concept of reflex excitation. Therefore, when PAVLOV's coworker POPIELSKI (1896, 1901) found that pancreatic secretion was still elicited by hydrochloric acid in the duodenum when the vagal and splanchnic fibres to the pancreas and the duodenum were cut and the solar plexus and the spinal cord extirpated, the Pavlov school (PAVLOV, 1897, 1898) thought that a peripheral reflex passed directly from the duodenal mucosa to the pancreas, where a large collection of ganglion cells could be seen in the head of the pancreas close to the upper border of the hepato-gastro-duodenal ligament (POPIELSKI, 1901).

WERTHEIMER (1902a, b), WERTHEIMER and LEPAGE (1901a–d, 1902) extended the experiments and showed that pancreatic secretion is stimulated if dilute hydrochloric acid, chloroform or mustard oil is introduced, not only into the duodenum, but into intestinal loops of the upper third of the jejuno-ileum as well, in similarly treated dogs with the vagi and the splanchnics cut, the spinal cord excised and the coeliac and the superior mesenteric ganglia severed. They nevertheless envisioned a peripheral reflex of some kind from the intestine to the pancreas. The English workers, however, concluded from the experiments of Wertheimer and Lepage that a reflex mechanism was highly unlikely. To prove this they cut both vagi and removed the nervous masses around the superior mesenteric artery and the coeliac axis in the dog. A loop of jejunum was tied at both ends and the mesenteric nerves cut. The introduction of 0.4% hydrochloric acid into this loop produced a marked effect on the pancreas. The next step was to cut out the loop of jejunum, scrape off the mucous membrane, rub it up with sand and 0.4% hydrochloric acid in a mortar, heat to boiling and inject the neutralized and filtered extract intravenously. This crucial experiment on the cause of the so-called peripheral reflex secretion of the pancreas was performed on January 16th, 1902. The stimulating agent from the intestinal mucosa, carried to the pancreas by the blood, was named *secretin*. Three years later the term *hormone* was suggested (Starling, 1905a, p. 340, 1906, p. 90), for this type of chemical messenger, produced in one organ and carried by the blood stream to another organ, on which its effect is manifested. In his textbook, Principles of General Physiology, Bayliss (1915, 1920, 1924) characterized the hormones as substances which "enable a chemical correlation of the functions of the organism to be brought about by the blood, side by side with that which is the function of the nervous system". It was suggested that the term "should not be applied to any kind of substance which excites activity", in which case "a name of such very wide application would be of comparatively little value". To consider the secretin only as a product of an "internal secretion", a term introduced by Claude Bernard, seemed to the authors less adequate. When, according to Bayliss (1924, p. 112), Mr W. B. Hardy proposed the name "hormone", derived from ὁρμάω ("I arouse to activity"), it was accepted although the property of messenger was not suggested by it. The question of the chemical messengers had, as pointed out by Friedman in a lecture in 1954, become a topic of great general interest among the physiologists of that time through the discovery by Oliver and Schäfer (1895) of epinephrine in the adrenals and the pressor-active principle of the pituitary gland. It was also in these early days that Tigerstedt and Bergman (1898) discovered renin.

The first communication by Bayliss and Starling (1902a) on the discovery of secretin was made on January 23 to the Royal Society. The experimental details were published later in the year (Bayliss and Starling, 1902b).

Instead of making a decoction of the mucosa, Wertheimer (1902a), Wertheimer and Lepage (1902) filled an intestinal loop of a dog with dilute hydrochloric acid for half an hour and injected the neutralized fluid. By applying either of these methods Bayliss and Starling (1903) were then able to show, that a secretin mechanism is common to all types of vertebrates, to man, monkey, dog, cat, rabbit, ox, sheep, pig, squirrel, goose, tortoise, frog, salmon, dogfish and skate, a list which was enlarged by a number of contemporary authors. The specific activity was extractable only from the upper part of the duodeno-jejunum. Hallion and Lequeux (1906) extracted secretin from the corresponding parts of the intestine of two newborn infants and of a five months' foetus. The effect of secretin was unaltered by previous injection of atropine.

The findings of Bayliss and Starling were soon confirmed by other authors. Thus Wertheimer and Lepage (1902), Enriquez and Hallion (1903) and

FLEIG (1904) led the blood from the intestinal veins or the carotid artery of one dog into the jugular vein of another dog and found that injection of dilute acid into the intestine of the first dog evoked secretion of pancreatic juice in the second.

In his Croonian Lectures I—III of 1905 STARLING (1905a, b, c) reviewed the prevailing ideas about the nervous stimulation of the secretory glands, paying due tribute to the contributions of Pavlov and his school with the following statement: "Previous to the publication of PAVLOV's results no physiologist had succeeded in obtaining an invariable secretion of either gastric or pancreatic juice as the result of stimulation of any nerves" (STARLING, 1905b, p. 423). However, he was not convinced that the double mechanism of stimulation suggested by PAVLOV need be considered under normal circumstances. PAVLOV's results could as easily be explained by the purely chemical mechanism discovered by BAYLISS and STARLING, if electrical stimulation of the vagus and splanchnic nerves evokes movements of the stomach, squeezing some of its acid contents into the first part of the small intestine. The same view was expressed in a subsequent paper of BAYLISS and STARLING (1906, p. 675). Future developments, however, fully confirmed PAVLOV's observations and the conclusions he drew from them concerning the double secretory mechanism of the pancreas. The correctness of the conclusions drawn from his original experiments of 1888 could easily be confirmed by using animals with gastric, duodenal and pancreatic fistulas and with the stomach anatomically separated from the duodenum according to the technique of TONKICH (1924).

e) The Contemporary Reactions to the Discovery of Secretin

The new concepts introduced by the findings of BAYLISS and STARLING were too revolutionary to be generally accepted at once. The German physiologist EDUARD PFLÜGER in Bonn, known, according to MINKOWSKI (1905), for his tendency "die Untersuchungen anderer Autoren einer strengen Kritik zu unterziehen" was not convinced by the first communication of BAYLISS and STARLING, that they had succeeded in cutting all the nervous connections between the pancreas and the intestine. The action of the extracts on the pancreas could have been a toxic effect similar to that of tissue extracts on glands in general. Although PAVLOV soon accepted the new idea, his former pupil, POPIELSKI, did not. For years he continued to present evidence to the contrary (POPIELSKI, 1906, 1907, 1907/1908). He seriously questioned the specific nature of the active agent in the extracts of BAYLISS and STARLING. Extracts of WITTE peptone, when injected intravenously, had the same effect as duodenal extracts on the blood pressure and on the pancreatic and salivary secretions. To this BAYLISS and STARLING (1906) answered by pointing out the specific localization of the activity exclusively to the duodenum and the upper jejuno-ileum, the strong activity and the easy destructibility of the active agent as compared to peptone. Furthermore, CARLSON and coworkers (1916) of the Hull Physiological Laboratory, University of Chicago, showed that the secretory effect of secretin preparations is independent of blood pressure changes and that the secretagogue activity of the extracts is destroyed by digestion with gastric juice, whereas the vasodilating agent is not. As to the further evidence for the existence of the specific secretagogue principle in the duodenal mucosa brought forward by the Chicago University group, see LUCKHARDT and BLONDER (1924), WEAVER, LUCKHARDT and KOCH (1926).

By this time the experimental physiologists had presented quite convincing evidence for the existence of a humoral mechanism participating in the stimulation of pancreatic secretion. Further cross-circulation experiments were performed by MATSUO (1912—1913). In 1926 IVY and FARRELL performed auto-transplantation of the tail of the pancreas in the dog (IVY and FARRELL, 1926; FARRELL and IVY, 1926b) and in 1927 IVY, FARRELL and LUETH did auto-transplants of both the tail of the pancreas and of a jejunal loop. Application of 0.1 N HCl to the transplanted loop evoked secretion in the pancreatic transplant. Atropine decreased the response to hydrochloric acid only slightly or not at all. In the same year HOUSSAY and MOLINELLI (1927) performed a similar experiment with a transplanted pancreatico-duodenal region.

DELEZENNE, HALLION and GAYET (1927) perfused the duodenum and the adherent pancreas of a dog with blood from the neck vessels of another dog. Filling either one of the duodenal lumina, that *in situ* or the perfused one, with 0.4% hydrochloric acid elicited pancreatic secretion in both animals. NECHELES and LIM showed in 1928 that a concentrated vivo-dialysate of blood was active in stimulating pancreatic secretion in the dog, particularly a dialysate of the portal blood or of blood after a meal.

In his detailed review of the older physiological literature on the gastro-intestinal hormones, IVY (1930) stated that "secretin after going through the vicissitudes of pharmacological and physiological investigation, according to the evidence at hand appears to be quite specific for the pancreatic secretion".

2. Purification and Isolation of Secretin

a) Early Attempts

In 1912 DALE and LAIDLAW introduced a new rather cumbersome technique of denaturating inert proteins by mixing the minced intestinal mucosa of dogs and cats to a paste with one fifth of its weight of corrosive sublimate and heating. Secretin activity was extracted from the cake with 2% acetic acid containing 1% mercuric chloride, and precipitated on alkalinization. The mercuric ions were removed with hydrogen sulphide. After further purification 10 mg of the preparation produced 3.2 ml of pancreatic juice in a poorly responsive dog.

MELLANBY *(1928, 1932) of St. Thomas' Hospital, London,* extracted the duodenal mucosa with 4 volumes of absolute alcohol at room temperature. The alcohol was evaporated *in vacuo,* fats and soaps were removed with $CaCl_2$ and the activity was finally adsorbed on bile acids. The quality and composition of the bile salts were critical and frequent failures in using this technique were later reported (HAMMARSTEN and JORPES, 1928; MORTIMER and IVY, 1929; STILL, 1930; LEGGE et al., 1957). 0.017 mg of MELLANBY's purest preparation produced 2.5 ml of pancreatic juice in the cat, corresponding to 70 clin. u./mg.

Going back to an observation made by WERTHEIMER (1902a), WERTHEIMER and LEPAGE (1902) as confirmed by WERTHEIMER and DUVILLIER (1910) and by MATSUO (1912—1913), that acid washings of the lumen of the upper portion of the small intestine of a living dog when neutralized and injected intravenously stimulated the secretion of pancreatic juice, LUCKHARDT, BARLOW and WEAVER (1926) and WEAVER, LUCKHARDT *and* KOCH *(1926) from the Hull Laboratories of Physiology and Physiological Chemistry, University of Chicago,* modified the procedure of extracting secretin. After the intestinal contents had been washed out, 0.4% HCl was placed in an excised duodeno-jejunal loop of dog intestine clamped at one end. The loop was clamped at both ends and left at room temperature for 10 to 30 minutes. The admixture of a number of impurities including vasodilating agents, usually extracted from the ground mucosa, was thereby avoided. By saturating the filtered extract with NaCl and reprecipitating several times with NaCl, WEAVER, LUCKHARDT and KOCH (1926) obtained a practically vasodilatin-free "new secretin". The smallest amount of vasodilatin was found in the preparation made by perfusing the duodenum of the dog *in vivo*.

IVY, KLOSTER, DREWYER *and* LUETH *(1930b) at the Department of Physiology and Pharmacology, Northwestern University Medical School, Chicago,* took up work on secretin with the hope that they "by obtaining a 'purified' product might be able by its use to devise a human pancreatic function test". In fact, such a test had been introduced as early as 1926 by CHIRAY, SALMON and MERCIER in France, using secretin prepared by PENAU and SIMONNET (1925).

The "new secretin" of WEAVER, LUCKHARDT and KOCH (1926) and a sodium chloride precipitate prepared according to IVY, KLOSTER, LUETH and DREWYER (1929) were purified by IVY et al. (1930b). Impurities were removed by reprecipitating twice from 70 to 80% ethanol. The filtrate was concentrated by evaporation to dryness and the residue dissolved in water. On neutralization to pH 5.3—5.7 flocculation took place, the activity being found both in the mother liquor, S_I, and in the precipitate, from which it was eluted with 0.4% HCl, S_{II}. To both fractions trichloroacetic acid was added to 5% and the precipitates collected and dried with acetone and ether.

The average dose per dog was 0.7 mg for S_I and 0.64 mg for S_{II}. The smallest per kilogram dosage was 0.01 mg and the largest 0.1 mg. The easy solubility of secretin in 99% methanol was pointed out.

In 1930 STILL *of the Department of Physiology, University of Chicago,* used the extraction procedure of LUCKHARDT, BARLOV and WEAVER (1926) for the preparation of the crude sodium chloride precipitate. After removal of some denaturated material the activity was precipitated with trichloroacetic acid to 5% and dissolved in acidified 90% ethanol. Further impurities were removed by means of brucine and pyridine and the active fraction precipitated with acetone and ether. From this precipitate the activity was taken up in 99% methanol in a modified Soxhlet extractor. Thereby cholecystokinin and vasoactive and blood sugar lowering substances insoluble in methanol were removed.

In the early days numerous properties were ascribed to the crude secretin. It was believed by various authors to augment nitrogen metabolism, respiratory exchange and the secretion of urine, to stimulate the hematopoietic tissue, to mobilize carbohydrates and to cause hypoglycemia (See MELLANBY, 1928; STILL, 1931). As found by STILL, and by ZUNZ and LA BARRE (1928), MELLANBY's secretin preparations of 1928 still contained vasodilatin and hypoglycemic substances. As a consequence of the interest the physiologists took in the secretin suggestions appeared in the literature as to its use in medicine. It had been recommended for all kinds of digestive disturbances, frequently for oral intake. Particular attention had been paid to the possibility to use it as an antidiabetic. CARLSON, LEBENSOHN and PERLMAN (1916) summarized the literature dealing with this topic and in 1918 CARLSON, KANTES and TUMPOWSKY definitely demonstrated its uselessness when taken by mouth. Nevertheless ZUNZ and LA BARRE of Brussels during the years 1928 and 1929 contributed no fewer than 9 publications on the hypoglycemic action of secretin (See STILL, 1931, pp. 345—348). TAKACS (1927, 1928a, b) described secretin preparations, which, like those of PENAU and SIMONNET (1925) lowered the blood sugar in animals and in diabetic patients without, however, producing other hypoglycemic symptoms. Nor did they stimulate the flow of bile. The statements of TAKACS need not, however, to be taken more seriously than his claim (TAKACS, 1928c) that he had increased the strength of a Dale-Laidlaw preparation a thousandfold without any loss of activity.

Through the preparative procedure elaborated by STILL all these side reactions given by the earlier secretin preparations were eliminated. Likewise the discussion about the hypoglycemic properties of secretin died away when LA BARRE, on visiting the Chicago laboratory, was unable to demonstrate any hypoglycemic effect in STILL's secretin preparations, put at his disposal. As an explanation for the hypoglycemic activity found in secretin, IVY and FISHER (1924) suggested that it might have been due to insulin extracted from duodenal insular tissue, which does occur in a number of animals, particularly abundantly in the rabbit intestinal wall.

The activity of the Still preparation was also very high. Doses of 0.02 to 0.1 mg/kg caused secretion during 20 minutes of 6—10 ml of pancreatic juice in a 10 kg anesthetized pancreatic fistula dog.

In 1928 the HAMMARSTEN *group of Karolinska Institutet, Stockholm,* initiated a series of studies on secretin, its preparation, chemistry and clinical application. To begin with, a modification of the DALE and LAIDLAW method for the extraction and purification of secretin was applied (HAMMARSTEN and JORPES, 1928). The secretin accumulated in the "cake" formed in the interphase on centrifugation after shaking an aqueous solution with chloroform (HAMMARSTEN, WILANDER and ÅGREN, 1928). This material was subjected to electrodialysis (ÅGREN and WILANDER, 1933). Between pH 3.2 and 9.1 the secretin rapidly dialyzed into the cathode compartment. The activity of the preparations corresponded to one HAMMARSTEN cat unit per 0.006 mg substance or 166 cat units and 8.3 clinical units per mg (WILANDER and ÅGREN, 1932).

The authors soon went on to extract everted hog intestines on a large scale with dilute sulfuric acid. Mercuric sulfate was added to the extract, followed by sodium hydroxide to a slightly acid reaction. The precipitate was extracted with 80% ethanol and hydrogen sulfide bubbled in. The filtrate was concentrated *in vacuo* and the secretin precipitated with picric acid (HAMMARSTEN, JORPES and ÅGREN, 1933). Thereby a salt-free preparation suitable for electrodialysis could be obtained in good yield.

The electrodialyzed material, collected on salicylic acid, was converted into a phosphate and this into a picrolonate. The picrolonate was dissolved in water-free pyridine. On concentrating the solution *in vacuo* a crystalline product was obtained (HAMMARSTEN et al., 1933). The crystalline material was converted into a phosphate which was no longer crystalline. The activity of the crystalline material was 250 cat units or 12.5 clin.u./mg (HAMMARSTEN, 1939). ÅGREN (1934) improved the technique of making the crystalline picrolonate on a large scale and studied the pharmacological and chemical properties of the secretin purified over the crystalline picrolonate.

HAMMARSTEN and ÅGREN worked out a method for the preparation of non-toxic secretin preparations with an activity about 20% of that of the crystalline material, which found an extensive application for clinical trials (ÅGREN, LAGERLÖF and BERGLUND, 1936; HAMMARSTEN, ÅGREN and LAGERLÖF, 1937; LAGERLÖF, 1939, 1942). For the first time a pancreatic function test with secretin could be performed in larger series of patients and controls — up to 450 cases (HAMMARSTEN, 1939).

In 1938 GREENGARD and IVY prepared a crystalline secretin picrolonate similar to that of HAMMARSTEN and coworkers from 1933. Starting with the S I preparation of IVY, KLOSTER, LUETH and DREWYER (1930) impurities were removed with aniline and butyl alcohol extraction. The product was recrystallized from pyridine without loss of activity. The biological activity was the same as that of the HAMMARSTEN picrolonate, 250 cat units per mg. In their paper IVY and GREENGARD presented evidence for the relative strengths of the cat unit of HAMMARSTEN and the dog unit of IVY. Twenty units of the former were found to correspond to one unit of the latter, whereas the cat unit of IVY equalled 0.5 Ivy dog unit. There was one serious discrepancy in the composition of the two crystalline picrolonates, that of the IVY group consisted to 80% of picrolonic acid, that of ÅGREN and HAMMARSTEN to only 20%. Hence the activity of the peptide component of the former preparation ought to be four times higher than that of the latter.

Preparation of the crystalline picrolonates of secretin, assumed to be the final stage on the way to its isolation in a pure form, soon proved to be an illusory achievement. In 1947 GREENGARD, WOLFROM and NESS succeeded in dividing the crystalline material into two fractions, an easily crystallizable pyridine picrolonate, soluble in nitroethane, and an insoluble amorphous protein fraction with secretin activity. If crystallization had taken place in aniline an aniline pricrolonate came out. Further experience showed that less than one per cent of the amorphous fraction consisted of secretin. The numerous investigations on the chemical and physiological properties of secretin made during this period (See GREENGARD, 1948 and GROSSMAN, 1950, pp. 52—55) are therefore of only limited value. All the preparations, except possibly some of STILL's and HAMMARSTEN's preparations, contained cholecystokinin, even when claims to the contrary were made.

Along the same lines, FRIEDMAN *and* THOMAS *(1950a) of the Jefferson Medical College, Philadelphia, and* GERSHBEIN *and* KRUP *(1952) of Chicago made preparations with 6—8 and 75—100 Ivy dog units of secretin per mg, respectively.* The everted intestines had been soaked in ice-cold 0.13 N HCl for ½ h. The sodium chloride cake was either pressed as dry as possible and the secretin eluted with 5 parts of methanol, or it was dried with acetone and extracted with 95% ethanol. Stable fractions were obtained from the extracts by precipitation with acetone or ether. By precipitation with trichloroacetic acid, aniline or picric acid and removal of the precipitant GERSHBEIN and KRUP obtained samples with potencies of 20, 60 and 100 units per mg, respectively. Impurities causing side reactions were removed by treating the final product with n-butanol at 40°C in a water bath. The preparation of FRIEDMAN and THOMAS was, as Secretin WYETH, given intravenously to man.

b) The Isolation of Pure Secretin

In the 1950's four groups of workers took advantage of the possibilities the newly developed electrophoretic, ion exchange chromatographic and countercurrent distribution techniques offered for preparative peptide chemistry.

In 1957 LEGGE, MORIESON, ROGERS and MARGINSON in Melbourne, Australia, purified the GREENGARD and IVY preparations S_{I} and S_{II} and the picrolonate with an activity of 34 cat threshold units per mg (1 c.t.u. = 10 drops of pancreatic juice within 10 min) up to 300 c.t.u./mg by means of adsorption chromatography on silica gel and up to 3300 c.t.u., 500—750 clin.u., per mg by means of countercurrent distribution in a system prepared by equilibrating 2.12 l of water, 1.82 l 2-butanol, 41 ml glacial acetic acid and 17.1 ml of dichloroacetic acid. The appearance in the distribution curve of two active peaks in widely varying proportions in different preparations indicated that enzymatic transformations had taken place. In accordance with this, the yield of secretin activity per length of intestine was twice as high when the intestines had been heated before extraction. No better results were obtained with crude preparations made according to FRIEDMAN and THOMAS or GERSHBEIN and KRUP.

Similar difficulties were encountered by FISHMAN, New York, (1957, 1959), in his very serious attempts to purify a material supplied by ELI LILLY, Indianapolis. By means of electrophoresis on a column of polyvinyl chloride he obtained a highly purified product from which all tryptophan-, proline-, cystine- and methionine-containing impurities had been removed. Lysine, isoleucine and tyrosine were still present. The biological activity was almost totally lost during the purification procedure with only 55 clin. units per mg remaining.

Using the same starting material of crude secretin as the previous authors, NEWTON, LOVE, HEATLEY and ABRAHAM, Oxford (1959) increased the strength of the preparations up to 1000 rat units per mg (1 rat unit = 4.4 Hammarsten cat units and 0.1 Ivy dog unit) by converting the hydrochloride to an acetate and taking up the material on a CMC column, pH 4.0, washing the column with 0.02 N acetic acid and eluting with 0.1 N acetic acid. Subsequent counter-current distribution in the same system as used by LEGGE et al. and in a system of phenol-water-acetic acid (50:100:5) resolved the material after 95 transfers into two major active components with 4000 and 200 r.u. per mg, respectively.

Past experience had fully demonstrated the difficulties in purifying the salt cake, obtained after extracting the intestinal mucosa, whether minced or not, with 0.4% hydrochloric acid. In order to avoid the bulk of inert material extracted by the hydrochloric acid, the present authors (JORPES and MUTT, 1953a) at first used ethanol acidified with acetic acid for the extraction and then went over to denaturing the starting material, the upper first meter of the hog intestine, by boiling for 5—8 minutes, as we did earlier in our attempts to extract gastrin from the pyloric region of hog stomach (JORPES, JALLING and MUTT, 1952). Boiling the intestine destroyed enzymes otherwise deleterious to the peptide hormones.

Extraction of the minced frozen material was performed with 0.5 N acetic acid, in which heat-denaturated proteins are rather insoluble. For the recovery of the active material from the extract we applied the then recently introduced principle of adsorbing proteins on cation exchangers, in the case of the adrenocorticotropic hormone on oxycel (ASTWOOD et al., 1951) or on IRC 50 (DIXON et al., 1951). From the ethanol extract the activity was adsorbed on pectic acid or suitably treated lemon peel. In the large scale procedure alginic acid proved highly suitable for the quantitative uptake not only of secretin but also of cholecystokinin and pancreozymin from the dilute acetic acid extract (JORPES and MUTT, 1954, 1955; MUTT, 1959d, pp. 88—89). The activity was eluted with 0.2 N hydrochloric acid and precipitated by saturating with sodium chloride. The precipitate thus obtained contained twice as much secretin in a 30 times smaller amount of material as the most commonly used starting material in the past, the salt cake of WEAVER et al. (1926). This proved to be a prerequisite for successful further purification (JORPES and MUTT, 1956).

The rigorous adherence by the previous workers to the original salt cake of WEAVER, LUCKHARDT and KOCH as starting material thus led to results quite unlike those envisaged by WEAVER et al. when they in 1926 said that the sodium chloride precipitate "offers an excellent starting point for the ultimate isolation of the active principle in pure form".

The ethanol-pectic acid procedure had given preparations which after removal of impurities in 95% methanol at —20°C had an activity of 75 clin.u./mg (JORPES and MUTT, 1953b), or, if removal of impurities with n-propanol from an aqueous solution had been interposed, 300 clin.u./mg. The ordinary heat coagulation and extraction procedure yielded, after removal of impurities with 2 volumes of ethanol, uptake of the secretin from the mother liquor on alginic acid, and elution and precipitation with sodium chloride, a product which after precipitation with ether from methanol, contained 180 clin.u./mg (MUTT, 1959a).

The activity of these preparations could be adsorbed on stearic acid from a 0.1 M phosphate buffer, pH 7.1, leaving the bulk of the inert material including salts unadsorbed. After elution with 1 per cent acetic acid and lyophilization, the substance had an activity of 24,000 Hammarsten cat units (1200 clin.u.) per mg (JORPES and MUTT, 1955, MUTT, 1959d, p. 91). The high level of activity of this material was confirmed by IVY and JANECEK (1959), who in fact, using 16 dogs and 10 cats, found a potency of 3,300 Ivy dog units and 6,000 Ivy cat units per mg as compared with the highest activity, 500 Ivy dog units per mg, they ever had assayed in their laboratory. The preparation of GERSHBEIN and KRUP (1952) usually assayed to 100 dog units per mg. It was by now clear that all the secretin preparations earlier reported in the literature must have been grossly impure.

On subjecting a material with 800 clin.u. per mg to zone electrophoresis for 48 h at 6 m A (150 V) on a column of cellulose powder equilibrated with 0.1 M ammonium bicarbonate, pH 7.6—7.8, the bulk of impurities migrated in the front to the cathode leaving a fraction which after lyophilization assayed to 4000 clin.u. per mg (MUTT, 1959a).

Chromatography on a carboxymethyl cellulose column, already successfully applied by NEWTON et al. (1959) for the purification of secretin, turned out to be a more practical procedure in the purification process (MUTT, 1959b, c). The chromatography was performed in 0.02 M ammonium bicarbonate, pH 8.0. If elution with 0.02 M bicarbonate was continued for a sufficiently long time the secretin emerged from the column in good yield and in a high state of purity. Large quantities of impurities were both eluted from the column before, and left on it after, the secretin. The potency had now reached the level of 7,500 clin.u. per mg.

The final purification was achieved in a 60-transfer counter-current distribution system, 0.1 M phosphate buffer/n butanol, pH 7.0, phase volume 10 ml (JORPES and MUTT, 1961b). The activity was found in tubes 18—30 and the bulk of the proteinaceous impurities were in the first four tubes. The active fractions were combined and 15 volumes of water added. The activity was adsorbed on alginic acid (0.5 g dry weight), eluted with 10 ml of 0.2 M HCl and the chloride exchanged for acetate on a column of DEAE-Sephadex in acetate form. The

Table 1. *Isolation of porcine secretin* (MUTT and JORPES, 1968a)

	Weight	Activity in clinical units per mg
Starting material:		
Upper first meter of intestine from 10,000 hogs. Boiled, frozen, minced	ca. 700 kg	
Extracted with 0.5 N AcOH. Activity adsorbed on alginic acid, eluted with 0.2 M HCl. Precipitated with NaCl at saturation	1 kg	1.5—3.0
Fractionation of aqueous solution with ethanol. Recovery in water, precipitation with NaCl and reprecipitation at pH 4	150 g	5—15
Extraction of secretin into methanol	4 g	150—300
Chromatography on carboxymethyl cellulose	100 mg	1000
Countercurrent distribution in 0.1 M phosphate buffer/n-butanol	10 mg	4000

yield of lyophilized material was 3 mg out of 60 mg starting material. The potency was about 20,000 clin.u. per mg.

When the distribution was carried through 200 transfers in an all-glass automatic distribution apparatus during 70 hours in an argon atmosphere the bulk of peptide material was found in the first fifteen tubes and the secretin activity in tubes 60 through 100 (JORPES, MUTT, MAGNUSSON and STEELE, 1962).

In applying the described technique to a large scale extraction procedure (Table 1) the activities of the different fractions were irregular and consistently lower than those given above, down to a strength of 4,000 clin. units per mg in the final product. The approximate yields are given in Table 1.

The amino acid composition, however, was always the same as found earlier (JORPES et al., 1962).

The course of development as to the purification and analysis of the secretin and cholecystokinin preparations was followed up by JORPES and MUTT (1959, 1961a, 1964 and 1970a).

3. The Chemical Structure of Secretin

The pure hormone is a low molecular weight polypeptide composed of 27 amino acid residues and 11 different amino acids, with cystine, methionine, tyrosine, tryptophan, proline, isoleucine and lysine lacking (JORPES and MUTT, 1961b; JORPES, MUTT, MAGNUSSON and STEELE, 1962). The eleven amino acids are present in the proportions:

$$Ala_1\ Arg_4\ Asp_2\ Glu_3\ Gly_2\ His_1\ Leu_6\ Phe_1\ Ser_4\ Thr_2\ Val_1.$$

Using the phenylisothiocyanate method of EDMAN (ERIKSSON and SJÖQUIST, 1960) the N-terminal amino acid was found to be histidine. Qualitative and quantitative confirmation of the N-terminal histidyl residue was obtained by dinitrophenylation according to SANGER's method (FRAENKEL-CONRAT, HARRIS and LEVY, 1954). The N-terminal sequence was found to be histidyl-seryl-aspartyl — resembling the corresponding histidyl-seryl-glutaminyl-sequence in glucagon. Valine is carboxy-terminal in the form of its amide. In two of the glutamic acids the γ carboxyls are likewise amidated.

Complete tryptic hydrolysis with splitting of three -Arg.Leu-bonds and one -Arg.Asp-bond gave rise to five peptides, a to e, leads 1 and 5 in Fig. 1 and Table 2. Peptide b, containing histidine, is N-terminal, No. 1, and peptide e, lacking arginine, is C-terminal, No. 5. *Tryptic hydrolysis for a short time* left the -Arg.Asp-bond intact, resulting in a new peptide -Leu.Arg.Asp.Ser.Ala.Arg- (d + a) (Fig. 2).

Table 2. *The composition of the tryptic peptides of secretin* (MUTT and JORPES, 1967a)

1 (b)	His · Ser · Asp · Gly · Thr · Phe · Thr · Ser · Glu · Leu · Ser · Arg
2 (d)	Leu · Arg
3 (a)	Asp · Ser · Ala · Arg
4 (c)	Leu · Gln · Arg
5 (e)	Leu · Leu · Gln · Gly · Leu · Val · NH_2

Thrombin, however, attacked only the -Arg.Asp-linkage and split secretin into two large peptides, f and g, lead 3 in Fig. 1.

Since d, -Leu.Arg., is linked to the histidine-containing N-terminal peptide b, and peptide d is also linked to peptide a, -Asp.Ser.Ala.Arg.-, as found after a short time tryptic digestion, and peptide e with valine amide is C-terminal, the sequence of the five tryptic peptides in secretin is established (Fig. 2 and 3) (MUTT et al., 1965; MUTT and JORPES, 1966).

Conclusive evidence that valinamide is the C-terminal of peptide e, and therefore of the intact secretin, was obtained by electrophoretic isolation of valinamide as one of the products of degradation of peptide e with "Crystalline Bacterial Proteinase Novo". Its identity was established by co-chromatography with an authentic sample of valinamide.

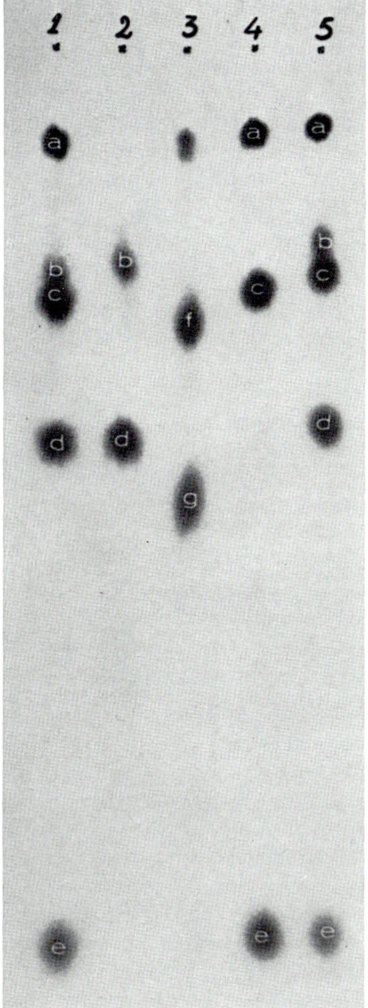

Fig. 1. Paper chromatography of split products of secretin. *Leads 1 and 5:* Descending chromatography of tryptic hydrolysate of secretin on Whatman No. 42 paper in the system 1-butanol-acetic acid-pyridine-water (30:6:10:24) (Waley and Watson, 1953). Peptides, are designated a to e, starting from the origin. Peptide e, which is C-terminal in secretin contains no arginine. Peptide b is N-terminal and the only one that contains histidine. *Lead 3:* Chromatogram of a thrombinic digest of secretin. If the thrombinic peptide f is digested with trypsin *(lead 2)* it splits into the tryptic peptide b, which is N-terminal in secretin, and peptide d, which therefore must be the second tryptic peptide from the N-terminus. Peptide d is known to be linked to peptide a, which consequently is the third in order of the tryptic peptides (Figure 2). The thrombinic peptide g is split by trypsin into the tryptic peptides a, c, and e *(lead 4)* (Mutt et al., 1965)

The γ-carboxylation of the two glutamic acid units in peptides 4 and 5 respectively was evidenced by the migration of the peptides on paper electrophoresis at pH 3.6 and 6.4.

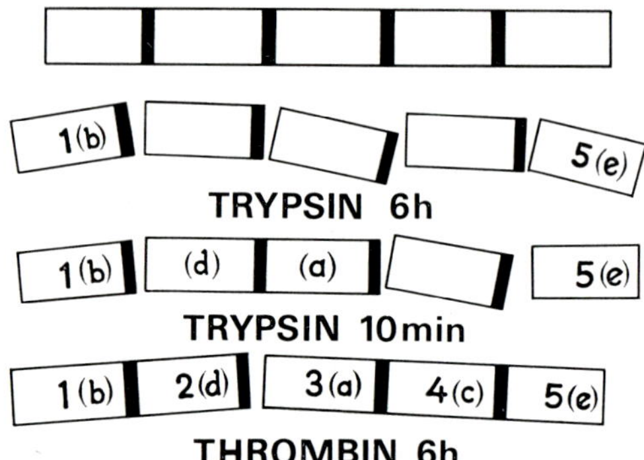

Fig. 2. Splitting of the secretin molecule with trypsin during 6 h and 10 min respectively and with thrombin during 6 h

1 (b) ↓ 2 (d) ↓ 3 (a) ↓
His-Ser-Asp-Gly-Thr-Phe-Thr-Ser-Glu-Leu-Ser-Arg-Leu-Arg-Asp-Ser-Ala-Arg
1 2 3 4 5 6 7 8 9 10 11 12 13 14 15 16 17 18

4 (c) ↓ 5 (e)
Leu-Gln-Arg-Leu-Leu-Gln-Gly-Leu-Val-NH_2
19 20 21 22 23 24 25 26 27

Fig. 3. The sequence of the tryptic peptides of secretin and the structure of the secretin molecule (Mutt and Jorpes, 1966)

Since the amino acid sequence of the tryptic peptides of the pure secretin had been determined only on eluates from paper after chromatography or electrophoresis, the analyses were repeated on the pure peptides, obtained through fractionation of the tryptic digest on short columns of Sephadex-based ion exchangers (Mutt, Jorpes and Magnusson, 1970). The tryptic peptide, Tr 1, was degraded with chymotrypsin into three fragments, and Tr 5 with subtilisin likewise into three fragments (Table 3). The analysis of these fragments, which could be performed with greater accuracy than the analysis of the whole peptides, confirmed the original findings as to the primary structure of the molecule of the porcine secretin. The corresponding molecular weight is 3055.

Table 3. *Splitting of the tryptic peptides, Tr 1 and Tr 5, with chymotrypsin and subtilisin respectively* (Mutt, Jorpes and Magnusson, 1970)

1. His · Ser · Asp · Gly · Thr · Phe ↓ Thr · Ser · Glu · Leu ↓ Ser · Arg
2. Leu · Arg
3. Asp · Ser · Ala · Arg
4. Leu · Gln · Arg
5. Leu · Leu · Gln ¦ Gly · Leu ¦ Val · NH_2

4. Synthesis of Secretin

The structure of secretin thus supposed to be known, attempts at synthesis were undertaken by Dr. MIKLOS BODANSZKY and his group at the Squibb Institute for Medical Research, New Brunswick, N.J., U.S.A. (BODANSZKY et al., 1966a, b; BODANSZKY and WILLIAMS, 1967; BODANSZKY et al., 1967; ONDETTI, 1967; ONDETTI et al., 1968a, b). (See Chapter II of this volume.)

To begin with, the C-terminal tetradecapeptide corresponding to the sequence 14 to 27 was synthesized by stepwise addition of the single amino acids starting from the C-terminal valine amide (BODANSZKY and WILLIAMS, 1967). The nitrophenyl ester method was used for the coupling steps, a principle introduced by BODANSZKY (1955) for the synthesis of oxytocin and vasopressin and applied by SCHWYZER and SIEBER (1966) in the synthesis of the C-terminal pentadecapeptide of ACTH. For threonine and arginine the dinitrophenyl ester was used. The protecting benzyloxycarbonyl group was removed in steps 17—27 by means of hydrogen bromide in acetic acid, but after introducing serine in position 16, the amino groups were protected by a tertiary butyloxycarbonyl group, which was removed by trifluoroacetic acid. Peptide 22—27 showed the same paper chromatographic behavior as the C-terminal tryptic peptide 5 (e) from natural secretin. The tridecapeptide 15—27 behaved like the thrombinic peptide g of the natural product. When the synthetic tridecapeptide was hydrolyzed with trypsin, the resulting three peptides (sequences 15—18, 19—21 and 22—27) showed the same mobility on paper chromatograms as the tryptic fragments from the natural compound.

The N-terminal half of the molecule was synthesized in two different ways. In one series the stepwise addition of the single amino acids was continued, in another the three peptides corresponding to the sequences 9—13, 5—8 and 1—4 were synthesized separately and added successively to the 14—27 tetradecapeptide. Irrespective of the route of synthesis the products, even before final purification, had marked specific biological activity, 500—1500 clinical units per mg.

Subsequent lots of the synthetic product showed the same potency, 4,000 U/mg, and the same spectrum of physiological actions as the pure natural porcine secretin (VAGNE, STENING, BROOKS and GROSSMAN, 1968).

In comparing in pancreatic fistula dogs different secretins for potency and spectrum of physiological actions VAGNE et al. (1968) found the natural and the synthetic porcine secretins fully identical both as stimulants of the liquid flow and bicarbonate output from the pancreas and the liver and as inhibitors of the gastric acid secretion and the spontaneous motility in innervated antral pouches in the dogs. Except for the potency of the synthetic preparation, which was somewhat lower, KONTUREK (1969) made similar findings in using the permanent pancreatic fistula cat with the major pancreatic duct cannulated, the bile diverted by a choledochoduodenostomy into the duodenum and a gastric fistula draining all of the gastric juice to the exterior.

The Secondary–Tertiary Structure of Secretin

The optical rotatory dispersion (ORD) and circular dichroism (CD) spectra of porcine secretin were found by BODANSZKY et al. (1969) to be strikingly similar to those of lysozyme, a protein the three dimensional structure of which was established by X-ray crystallography (BLAKE et al., 1965). The conclusions to be drawn from these findings as to the helical structure of part of the molecular chain of secretin were discussed by BODANSZKY (1972).

II. Cholecystokinin (CCK)

1. The Discovery of Cholecystokinin

It was early found that hydrochloric acid introduced into the duodenum causes a flow of bile (Bernard, 1856a, p. 429; Rutherford, 1880; Enriques and Hallion, 1903; Okada, 1914—1915). The response took place even after cutting the vagus and the thoracic sympathetic nerves (Wertheimer, 1903). Fleig (1903) demonstrated that blood from an isolated intestinal loop of a dog, into which acid had been introduced, increased the flow of bile, when injected into a second dog.

In his monographs Babkin (1927, pp. 784—791; 1928, table 145, pp. 664—665) summarized about 30 references from the older literature dealing with agents which on introduction into the stomach or the duodenum stimulated bile secretion. Bile acids were found to be the most active and evidently the physiological stimulant for bile formation. Great attention was paid by the Russian and the French physiologists to the action of fats, fatty acids and soaps on gastric, pancreatic and bile secretion (Babkin, 1928, pp. 510—519). When introduced into the stomach or the duodenum, fatty acids and soaps were almost as efficient stimuli for pancreatic and bile secretion as hydrochloric acid.

Based on the finding that in cats the gallbladder is almost completely empty a few hours after a meal of egg yolk and cream, whereas the ingestion of lean meat gives an incomplete emptying and carbohydrates an insignificant one (Boyden, 1923), Boyden's test meal in man, the egg yolk from five raw eggs and half a pint of cream taken by mouth, was developed (Boyden, 1925, 1926). It was fully confirmed that a fatty meal inevitably causes evacuation of a normal gallbladder, although no definite opinion was held as to the meal's mode of action (Whitaker, 1926; Higgins and Mann, 1926).

The discovery of secretin and its choleretic effect (see Chapter I, p. 87) raised the question of the mechanism of humoral stimulation. Fleig (1903) assumed there to be a dual secretory mechanism for the liver as well as for the pancreas, a humoral and a neural one. In 1904 he went one step further and claimed that soaps participate in the liberation of a specific "sapocrinine" acting in the same way as secretin.

The literature on the action of secretin preparations on the bile flow, which followed, was summarized by Ivy (1930), la Barre and Goffin (1937) and by Grossman (1950).

The humoral mechanism for the emptying of the gallbladder was at first a controversial subject. Boyden (1926) found that transfusion of blood from a fed or even from a starved cat into another cat caused partial evacuation of the latter's gallbladder. Brugsch and Horsters (1926a, b, c) observed contractions and rhythmic changes in the gallbladders of dogs after injection of a Dale and Laidlow (1912—1913) secretin preparation. They claimed that "Das physiologische Cholagogum der Gallenblase ist nach unseren Untersuchungen das Sekretin". Likewise Chiray, Jeandel and Salmon (1930) reported that since 1926 they had observed contractions of the gallbladder when performing the pancreatic function test in man with the Penau and Simonnet (1925) secretin. Their conclusion was: "Il semble donc que cet hormone, sécrétine, ait un puissant pouvoir cholecystokinetique." Other authors failed to see any effect of that kind on injecting crude secretin preparations (Ivy, 1930, p. 321).

The final proof of the existence of a humoral mechanism for the contraction and emptying of the gallbladder and for its non-identity with secretin was presented by IVY and coworkers. In connection with their experimental work on secretin, IVY and OLDBERG (1927) studied the action of the further purified "new secretin" of WEAVER, LUCKHARD and KOCH (1926) on the gallbladder. 1—3 mg of the preparation elicited pancreatic secretion in a 20 kg dog. 2 mg caused in the barbitalized cat a stepwise rise in the intra-gallbladder pressure from 180 to 240 mm water, which pressure began to decline after one-half to one hour. The emptying of the gallbladder of nonanesthetized dogs, filled with iodized oil according to WHITAKER and MILLIKEN (1925) and WHITAKER (1926), could be followed by fluoroscopy. The authors concluded that the active principle was secretin or some substance closely associated with it.

In further series (IVY and OLDBERG, 1928a, b) complete emptying of the gallbladder was observed in three out of ten dogs and in six of the dogs a reduction in volume of 50% or more. Introduction of 10—40 ml of 0.1 N hydrochloric acid into the duodenum caused, in every instance, contraction of the gallbladder when the cystic duct was clamped. In three out of four cross-circulation experiments, introduction of hydrochloric acid into the duodenum of the "first" dog caused a contraction of the gallbladder of the „second" dog as well. The humoral factor thus demonstrated caused no fall in blood pressure, nor was its action inhibited by atropine; therefore it could not be histamine or choline. "After some consideration we have decided", the authors said, "to name the substance in intestinal extracts which causes the gallbladder to contract, cholecystokinin." In some respects the gallbladder-contracting agent behaved differently from secretin.

A method for the preparation of cholecystokinin was described by IVY, KLOSTER, LUETH and DREWYER (1929). These authors found cholecystokinin to be less soluble in ethanol than secretin. Fractionation with 80—90% ethanol removed most of the secretin, as confirmed simultaneously by STILL (1930). Vasodilatin and much of the secretin present dissolved in 95% alcohol at room temperature. Secretin dissolved in absolute alcohol never gave a cholecystokinin effect. It was thus possible to prepare secretin free of cholecystokinin and cholecystokinin preparations without any significant secretin effect. Cholecystokinin was isolated from the upper intestine of the hog, dog, sheep and cattle.

Non-toxic preparations active in a dose of 1—3 mg or 0.2—0.1 mg/kg in the dog were likewise found to be active in man (IVY, DREWYER and ORNDOFF, 1930). 25—30 mg were injected intravenously at ten minute intervals in 5 normal subjects and 3 dispensary patients who volunteered for the experiment. Complete evacuation of the gallbladder occurred in one of the normal subjects and partial evacuation in three of them, as visualized in the roentgenogram with tetraiodophenolphthalein, according to GRAHAM and COLE (1924). After the experiment, which lasted one-half hour, two of the patients felt "light-headed" for the next one-half to one hour. At the time the authors could not visualize any future clinical use of the gallbladder-contracting principle. "This work", they said, "raises the question of the therapeutic value of cholecystokinin. Since it is well established that egg yolk and cream by mouth lead to evacuation of the gallbladder within several hours, the authors doubt the therapeutic value of this active principle, in that cholecystokinin must be given intravenously and will do nothing apparently that egg yolk and cream will not do."

Convincing evidence for the hormonal nature of the principle causing contraction of the gallbladder was also obtained at that time by HOUSSAY and RUBIO (1932) through viviperfusion of the gallbladder, its vascular system being anastomosed with the carotid artery and the external jugular vein of another dog, and by LA BARRE and GOFFIN (1937). The latter authors perfused the isolated dog duodenum and upper jejunum through the pancreatico-duodenal artery with blood from the carotid artery of another, cholecystectomized, dog with a biliary fistula. When the isolated intestine was filled with dilute hydrochloric acid the bile flow from the donor dog increased by 50%.

SANDBLOM (1933) demonstrated that the recipient's gallbladder contracts when blood is transfused from a person digesting a fat meal. Blood from a starving person had no similar effect.

Compared with the extraordinary interest in secretin on the part of physiologists all over the world, interest in CCK, although its hormonal nature had been convincingly demonstrated, was relatively slight. Only after a number of years did IVY himself (IVY, 1947) in his CALDWELL Lecture to the American Roentgen Ray Society 1946 express his conviction that "there is reason to hope that the isolation and use of cholecystokinin will assist in the solution of the roentgenological and clinical problems involved in the diagnosis of biliary dyskinesia". DENTON, GERSHBEIN and IVY (1950) then studied the effect on the human and canine gallbladder of preparations having a potency of 6 Ivy dog units of CCK per mg. Doses of 6 or 150 Ivy dog units given to 8 normal persons caused a 25—40% reduction in the shadow of the gallbladder. In 1951, IVY again called attention to the possibility of giving CCK intravenously as a substitute for the fatty meal, thereby avoiding the dependence upon the slow gastric emptying. Pictures showing complete emptying of the human gallbladder under the influence of CCK were presented (IVY, 1955) and preparations of CCK with a potency of 6 Ivy dog units per mg were shown to stimulate the motility of the intestine to a quite considerable degree.

In spite of IVY's repeated attempts to call attention to CCK and its possible clinical applications, up to 1954 the only publications dealing with this topic were one by ÅGREN (1939) on the purification of CCK and the writings of HARPER and his group (DUNCAN et al., 1950, 1952, 1953; HOWAT, 1952) about the gallbladder-contracting activity of their "pancreozymin" preparations, assumed to be contaminated with CCK.

2. The Isolation of Cholecystokinin

The CCK and the "pancreozymin" activities of the acetic acid extract of the boiled uppermost one meter of hog duodeno-jejunum were, like secretin, adsorbed on alginic acid and after elution with 0.2 N HCl precipitated with sodium chloride. The bulk of impurities were precipitated with 2 volumes 95% ethyl alcohol at pH 7.2 (MUTT, 1959c, d). The filtrate was diluted with an equal volume of 0.15% acetic acid and the active material taken up on alginic acid a second time and after elution reprecipitated with NaCl at saturation. On the subsequent elution of secretin from the NaCl-precipitate with methanol the CCK- and the "pancreozymin" activities remained in the salt cake. The yield of salt cake from 1000 hogs was 5 g air dried substance.

After removing impurities insoluble in water at pH 8.0 from a 5% solution and adjusting the reaction to pH 6.5, the solution was passed through a CMC column equilibrated with sodium phosphate buffer, pH 6.5, 0.02 molar in sodium (JORPES and MUTT, 1962). Impurities passed through on washing the column with the 0.02 molar equilibration solution and the activity was eluated with 0.2 molar NaCl and precipitated from the eluate by saturation with NaCl. The yield was about 2 g.

Vasoactive impurities were removed by precipitation with n-butanol from 70% ethanol. The salt cake was dissolved in 0.5% sodium chloride solution to a 3% solution. Three volumes of ethanol were added at room temperature and the precipitate that formed was filtered off and discarded. To the filtrate were added two volumes of n-butanol precooled to —15 C. The precipitate that formed was filtered off, washed on the funnel with butanol and ether, and then air-dried. The yield was about 1 g. The potency was 22 Ivy dog units of CCK per mg as assayed on one of our samples by IVY and JANECEK (1959). The pancreozymin activity was assayed by professor HARPER (HARPER et al., 1962) to be 100 times that of his original pancreozymin preparations, thus about 100—200 units, as defined by CRICK, HARPER and RAPER (1949), per milligram. The secretin content was 30 clinical units per 75 Ivy dog units of CCK.

Chromatography on a TEAE cellulose column then proved to be an important step of purification (JORPES and MUTT, 1962). The column was equilibrated with a sodium pyrophosphate-orthophosphoric acid buffer, containing N, N'dimethyl formamide. ($Na_4P_2O_7 \cdot 10\ H_2O$ 2.33 g + 1 ml 1 M H_3PO_4 in a volume of 1 liter).

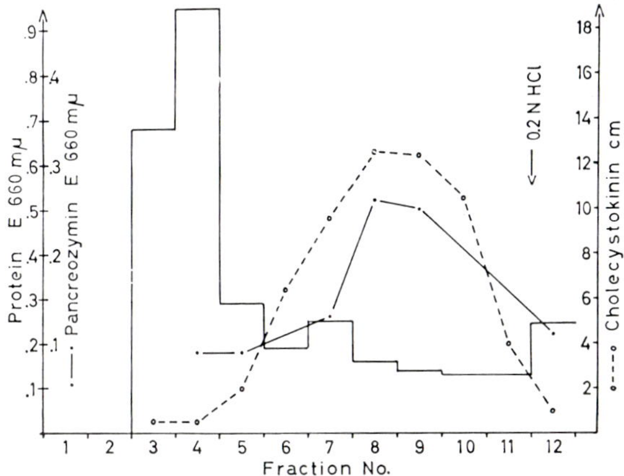

Fig. 4. Chromatographic purification of CCK on a TEAE cellulose column (JORPES and MUTT, 1962)

The pH was adjusted to 9.1. Nineteen parts by volume of this solution and one part N, N' dimethyl formamide were used. The precipitate formed on adding butanol was dissolved in the buffer to a 5% solution and the pH of the solution adjusted to 9.1 with a solution made by adding one part of dimethyl formamide to 19 parts 0.02 molar sodium hydroxide. A volume containing 0.5 g was passed into the TEAE cellulose-column (3 by 15 cm with 30 g of TEAE cellulose) and elution commenced with the buffer. Twenty-five milliliters fractional volumes were collected.

The distribution of protein and biological activity as regards cholecystokinin and pancreozymin is evident from Fig. 4. Working on a larger scale, 16 g of the butanol precipitate was taken for chromatography on a 14 cm high column, 10 cm in diameter, 500 ml fractions being collected. The active fractions 7—13 were combined, diluted with 1—2 volumes of distilled water and the activity taken up on 20 g alginic acid after adjusting the reaction to pH 2.6. After elution with 0.2 N HCl the activity was precipitated with NaCl at saturation. The chloride ions were removed either on a Sephadex G 25 column or on a column of DEAE cellulose in acetate form. The active fractions of the dilute acetic acid eluate were combined and lyophilized. The yield from 16 g of butanol precipitate was

0.5—0.8 g. The potency was about 250 Ivy dog units of CCK per mg. The secretin activity had been reduced to 6 clinical units per 75 Ivy dog units of CCK.

Starting with a raw material with a potency of about 20 Ivy dog units of CCK per mg, Dhariwal et al. (1963) obtained a fivefold purification with DEAE cellulose and a 20—30 fold purification after passage through first a Sephadex G-50 column and then a column of TEAE cellulose.

The material was purified further to an activity of about 3000 Ivy dog units of CCK per mg by chromatography in phosphate buffers, first on a Sephadex G-50 column in 0.25 M sodium orthophosphate, pH 8.0 (Fig. 5a), followed by chromatography on Amberlite XE-64 in 0.05 M phosphate, pH 7.5 (Fig. 5b) (Jorpes, Mutt and Toczko, 1964). In both instances the activity was taken up from the active fractions on alginic acid and after elution and precipitation with NaCl, chloride ions were removed from the salt cake on a column of DEAE

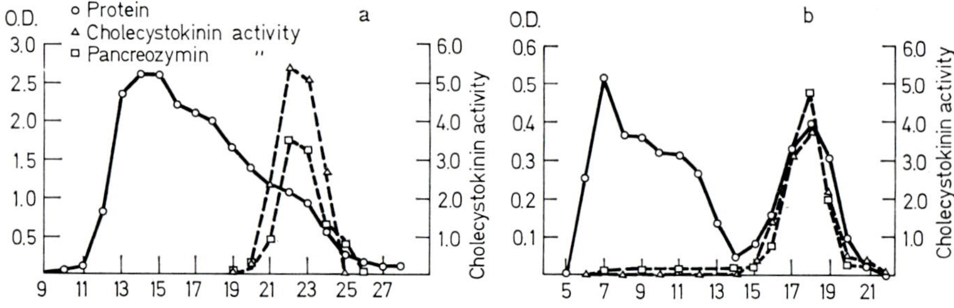

Fig. 5a. Column: Sephadex G-50, fine, 1.5×90 cm. Buffer: Sodium orthophosphate, 0.25 M, pH 8±0.1. Chromatographed material: 100 mg PC—TEAE—C. Fraction volume: 5 ml. Flow rate: ca. 8 min per fraction. ○, Optical density of fractions at 280 mμ. △, Cholecystokinin activity of fractions; Ljungberg method (relative values). □, Colour (Lowry) at 660 mμ of the pancreatic juice, diluted to 25 ml, of a cat after injection of equal aliquots of the fractions together with a basal dose of secretin

Fig. 5b. Column: Amberlite XE-64, 1×40 cm. Buffer: Sodium orthophosphate, 0.05 M, pH 7.5±0.1. Chromatographed material: 12 mg PC—SX. Fraction volume: 3 ml. Flow rate: ca. 14 minutes per fraction. ○, △ and □ the same as in Fig. 5a (Jorpes, Mutt and Toczko, 1964)

Table 4. *Purification of cholecystokinin* (Mutt and Jorpes, 1968a)

	Weight	Cholecystokinin (Ivy dog units) per mg	"Pancreozymin" activity (Crick, Harper and Raper units) per mg
Methanol-insoluble material after extracting the secretin (from 20,000 hogs)	100 g		
Adsorbed to CM cellulose at pH 6.5. Precipitated from eluate with NaCl	40 g		
Active material precipitated from 75% EtOH with n-BuOH	20 g	20	80
Chromatography on TEAE cellulose at pH 9.1	750 mg	250	1,000
Filtration through Sephadex G-50	60 mg	1,500	6,000
Chromatography at pH 7.5 on Amberlite XE-64	12 mg	3,000	12,000

cellulose in acetate form. *During these last purification steps secretin is completely removed, but the cholecystokinin and "pancreozymin" activities once again go parallel.* (Table 4).

3. Chemical Structure of CCK

The preliminary analysis of the CCK preparation with a potency of 3000 Ivy dog units per mg (MUTT and JORPES, 1967b) showed it to be an essentially homogeneous polypeptide with 33 amino acid units and the following amino acid composition, if amide groups were disregarded:

Ala_1, Arg_3, Asp_5, Glu_2, Gly_2, His_1, $Ileu_2$, Leu_2, Lys_2, Met_3, Phe_1, Pro_2, Ser_4, Tyr_1, Try_1, Val_1.

One of the two lysines was N-terminal. Cysteine, cystine and threonine were absent (JORPES, MUTT and TOCZKO, 1964).

On *treatment with cyanogen bromide* (MUTT and JORPES, 1967b) the dipeptide aspartylphenylalanine amide could be isolated from the reaction products, indicating that the polypeptide terminates in aspartyl-phenylalanine amide, and probably in methionyl-aspartyl-phenylalanine amide, a C-terminal sequence which is identical to that of gastrin (TRACY and GREGORY, 1964).

Another product of the cyanogen bromide degradation, the tripeptide · Gly · Try · Met ·, suggested that CCK and gastrin might have not only the sequence · Asp · Phe · NH_2 but the pentapeptide · Gly · Try · Met · Asp · Phe · NH_2 in common, as later proved to be the case.

When this material, as analyzed above, was subjected to chromatography on a CMC column, essentially as described for secretin (MUTT, 1959b), a further purification was achieved, which did not affect the previous findings, except that the quantitative amino acid analysis of the tryptic and thrombinic peptides indicated the presence of five serines instead of four and one glutamic acid unit instead of two (MUTT and JORPES, 1968a, b).

On *digestion of the final CMC-treated material with thrombin*, an inactive basic peptide, Th-1, with 6 amino acid units, Lys (Ala, Gly, Pro, Ser) Arg, was split off, leaving a well-defined neutral heptacosa peptide, Th-2, with 27 amino acid units and the following amino acid composition: Arg_2, Asp_5, Gly_1, Glu_1, His_1, Ile_2, Leu_2, Lys_1, Met_3, Phe_1, Pro_1, Ser_4, Tyr_1, Val_1. It had the full activity of the original preparation both on the gallbladder and on the enzyme secretion from the pancreas (MUTT and JORPES, 1968a, b) (Fig. 6).

Complete tryptic degradation was performed on 250 μg samples of CCK and Th-2 in 125 μl of 1% aqueous NH_4HCO_3. 2.5 μl of a 0.2% trypsin solution was added every two hours and the degradation was allowed to proceed at 21° for 6 hours, counted from the first addition of trypsin. The solution was then frozen and lyophilized. The residue was taken up in 125 μl of water and kept on a boiling water bath for 6 minutes. After cooling with tap water, undissolved material was spun down and discarded and the supernatant was lyophilized and then taken up in 125 μl of water. 10 μl aliquots of it were subjected to paper electrophoresis.

As is evident from Fig. 7 the thrombinic peptide Th-2 may be further degraded by trypsin into four peptides which are identical with peptides Tr-2 to Tr-5. On limited degradation of Th-2 with trypsin peptides Tr-4 and Tr-5 appear in very small quantities. Instead a peptide that is only weakly discernible between Tr-4 and Tr-5 in the electropherogram of the "completely" degraded material is now prominent.

The *partial tryptic degradation of Th-2* was carried out in the same way as the complete degradation except that the digestion was discontinued by freezing and lyophilization 20 minutes after the first and only addition of enzyme.

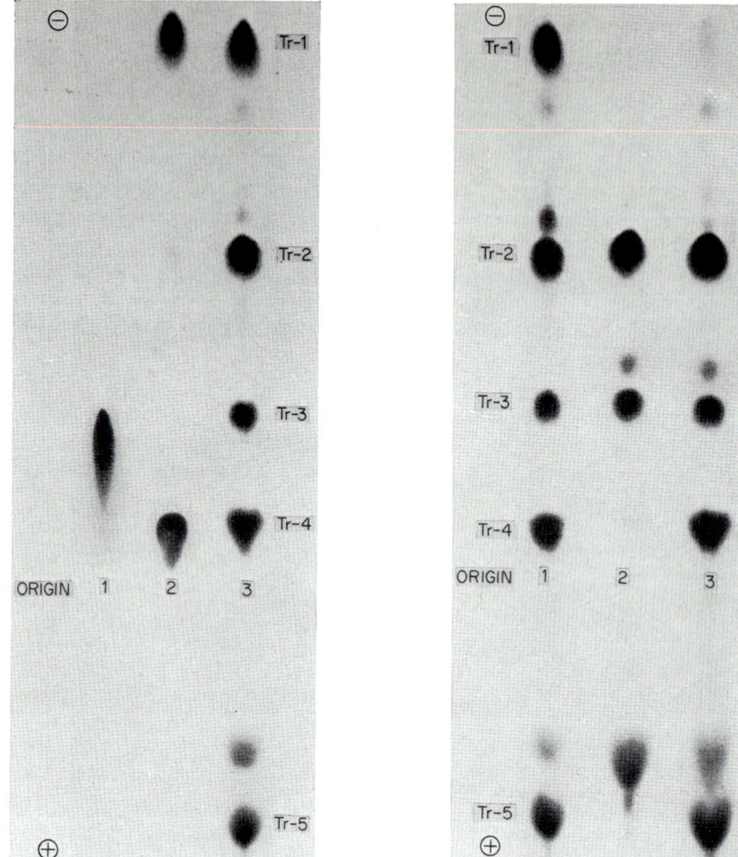

Fig. 6. Paper electrophoresis of cholecystokinin degraded with thrombin and trypsin. 1, 100 μg cholecystokinin; 2, 100 μg cholecystokinin degraded with thrombin; 3, 100 μg cholecystokinin degraded with trypsin. Electrophoresis was performed for 90 min at 50 V/cm in pyridine/acetic acid/water (300:11.5:2700, by vol.) at pH 6.4 using Whatman 3MM paper. Cholecystokinin is split by thrombin into the basic peptide Th-1, identical to the corresponding peptide Tr-1 of tryptic degradation, and the neutral Th-2 (Mutt and Jorpes, 1968b)

Fig. 7. Paper electrophoresis of cholecystokinin degraded with trypsin. 1, "complete" tryptic degradation of 100 μg cholecystokinin; 2, partial tryptic degradation of 100 μg Th-2; 3, "complete" tryptic degradation of 100 μg Th-2. Electrophoresis conditions were identical to those in Fig. 6. Peptide Tr-2 occurs in the same amount on "complete" and on partial tryptic degradation, as does peptide Tr-3. Peptides Tr-4 and Tr-5, however, are practically absent on partial degradation, which indicates that they are linked in Th-2 and in cholecystokinin itself (Mutt and Jorpes, 1968b)

The mixture of peptides obtained on degradation of CCK and Th-2 with trypsin was separated on paper electrophoresis at pH 6.4 into 5 components, designated Tr-1 to Tr-5, with Tr-1 the one that migrates most rapidly towards the cathode at this pH (Fig. 6 and 7).

Quantitative Amino Acid Analysis and N-Terminal Amino Acid Analysis of the Tryptic Peptides of CCK

The peptides were eluted from the lyophilized paper, Tr-5 with 0.05 M ammonia, the other three with 0.1 M acetic acid. The eluates were lyophilized.

Table 5. *Compositions of tryptic peptides of CCK* (Mutt and Jorpes, 1968b)

Peptide	Composition			N-terminal amino acid
	nmoles/sample (probable ratios)			
Tr-1	Ala 40 (1)	Arg 38 (1)	Gly 38 (1)	Lysine
	Lys 31 (1)	Pro 37 (1)	Ser 40 (1)	
Tr-2	Ile 19 (1)	Lys 20 (1)	Met 18 (1)	Valine
	Ser 22 (1)	Val 23 (1)		
Tr-3	Arg 12 (1)	Asp 31 (2)	Glu 16 (1)	Asparagine
	His 12 (1)	Leu 28 (2)	Pro 14 (1)	
	Ser 28 (2)			
Tr-4	Arg 37 (1)	Asp 40 (1)		Isoleucine
	Ile 35 (1)	Ser 38 (1)		
Tr-5	Asp 27 (2)	Gly 16 (1)		Aspartic acid
	Met 26 (2)	Phe 13 (1)	Trp 13 (1)	
	Tyr	(SO_3H) — (1)		

For amino acid analysis appropriate aliquots were hydrolyzed with either leucine amino peptidase (peptides Tr-2 and Tr-5) or 6 M HCl (peptides Tr-1, Tr-3 and Tr-4). The amino acid composition of the peptides and their N-terminal amino acids are given in Table 5. It seemed probable that the tyrosine was esterified with sulfuric acid in CCK as well as in gastrin and caerulein. This was confirmed by subjecting a leucine aminopeptidase hydrolysate of peptide Tr-5 to paper electrophoresis at pH 6.4, extracting an acidic substance with 0.05 M ammonia, and demonstrating that this substance migrates indistinguishably from synthetic tyrosine-0-sulfate.

The sequence of the tryptic peptides in CCK was determined as shown in Fig. 8. In accordance herewith the partial structure of CCK should be as follows (Mutt and Jorpes, 1968b):

Lys (Ala_1, Gly_1, Pro_1, Ser_1) Arg · Val · (Ile_1, Met_1, Ser_1) Lys · Asn (Asx_1, Glx_1, His_1, Leu_2, Pro_1, Ser_2) Arg · Ile · (Asp_1, Ser_1) Arg · Asp [Gly_1, Met_2, Try_1, Tyr $(SO_3H)_1$] Asp · Phe · NH_2.

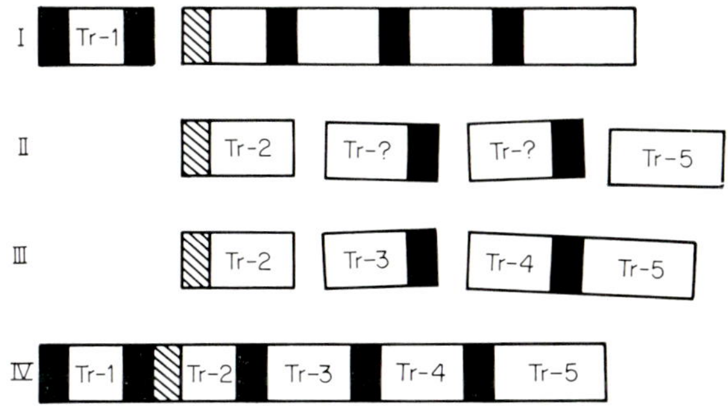

Fig. 8. Sequence of tryptic peptides in cholecystokinin. ■, arginine or lysine; ▨, valine. I, cholecystokinin degraded with thrombin into Th-1, identical to Tr-1, and Th-2; II, Th-2 completely degraded with trypsin; Tr-2 recognized by N-terminal valine. Tr-5 by absence of arginine and lysine; III, limited degradation of Th-2 with trypsin identifies Tr-4 through unbroken link to previously identified Tr-5; Tr-3 identified by exclusion of any other position; IV, cholecystokinin (Mutt and Jorpes, 1968b)

The Amino Acid Sequence of Cholecystokinin

One micromole of the pure CCK was completely degraded with trypsin and the peptides obtained were separated on columns of Sephadex-based ion-exchangers. Peptides 1, 2, 3 and 5 were split further, either enzymatically or with cyanogen bromide, or with a combination of both techniques as shown in Table 6.

Table 6. *Further splitting of the tryptic peptides of cholecystokinin* (Mutt and Jorpes, unpublished)

Tryptic peptide number	
	Elastase ↓ (between Ser and Gly)
1	Lys · Ala · Pro · Ser · Gly · Arg
	CNBr ↑ (between Met and Ile)
2	Val · Ser · Met · Ile · Lys
	Thermolysin (1) ↓ (between Ser and Leu); Subtilisin (2) ↓ (between Ser and His)
3	Asn · Leu · Gln · Ser · Leu · Asp · Pro · Ser · His · Arg
4	Ile · Ser · Asp · Arg ·
	CNBr (2) ↓ (between Met and Gly); Chymotrypsin(1) ↓ (between Trp and Met)
5	Asp · $Tyr(SO_3)$ · Met · Gly · Trp · Met · Asp · Phe · NH_2

When two fragmentation techniques were used on the same peptide the order in which they were applied is indicated by a number in parenthesis following the type of method.

The amino acid sequences of the sub-fragments, also given in the table, and of tryptic peptide number 4 were arrived at by the "dansyl-Edman" procedure (Gray, 1967). The amino acid sequence of cholecystokinin thus determined is given in Fig. 9. Molecular weight 3919.

Lys · Ala · Pro · Ser · Gly · Arg · Val · Ser · Met · Ile · Lys · Asn · Leu · Gln · Ser · Leu · Asp · Pro · Ser · His · Arg · Ile · Ser · Asp · Arg · Asp · $Tyr(SO_3)$ · Met · Gly · Trp · Met · Asp · Phe · NH_2

Fig. 9. The amino acid sequence of cholecystokinin (Mutt and Jorpes, 1971)

4. Urocholecystokinin

Because of the relatively low molecular weight of CCK and the potentiated activity of its C-terminal peptides, CCK or "pancreozymin" activity is to be expected in the urine. In fact the urine from both man and animals contains electrophoretically separated fractions which show such an activity (Svatos 1959, 1960; Svatos and Vokac, 1960; Svatos and Queisnerova, 1960).

5. The "Pancreozymin" Activity of Cholecystokinin

In Pavlov's laboratory it was observed on dogs that pancreatic juice with a high enzyme content could be obtained after a meal, even when the vagal and splanchnic branches to the gland were severed (BUCHSTAB, 1904). Similar experiments were performed by HARPER and VASS (1941) on anesthetized cats and by CRIDER and THOMAS (1944) on unanesthetized dogs. The same phenomenon was also observed by FARREL and IVY (1926a), and by WANG and GROSSMAN (1951), in a subcutaneously transplanted pancreas after adequate stimulation of the duodenal mucosa. In 1943, HARPER and RAPER succeeded in demonstrating an enzyme-mobilizing activity in extracts of the intestinal mucosa, assumed to be elicited by a specific hormone, named *pancreozymin (PZ)*. The findings of HARPER and RAPER were soon confirmed by GREENGARD et al. (1944).

HARPER and RAPER used their own method of preparing PZ. The intestinal mucosa was extracted with absolute alcohol and the extract concentrated. Secretin was precipitated by the addition of bile salts and acetic acid. The filtrate from this precipitate was saturated with NaCl and the NaCl precipitate extracted with absolute alcohol, in which the PZ was concentrated. Traces of secretin were removed by means of 80% acetone. Preparations active in animals in doses of a few milligrams were obtained. Equally active samples were obtained by GREENGARD and IVY (1945) after removal of the secretin by means of acid MeOH from S I.

Our preparations with 22 Ivy dog units of CCK per mg exerted a PZ activity corresponding to about 100—120 CRICK, HARPER and RAPER (1949) units per mg (HARPER et al., 1962, p. 171). When these samples were purified by chromatography on the basic TEAE cellulose up to a strength of 200—250 Ivy dog units of CCK per mg substance there was a corresponding increase in the PZ activity (Table 4).

At this stage of purity we determined the PZ activity of our CCK preparations, and the CCK:PZ ratio was compared with that in HARPER and RAPER's original PZ preparation, given to us by professor HARPER in 1969, as well as in a recent sample of a commercial PZ with 91 Crick, Harper and Raper units per ampoule and 1.1 PZ units per mg. The last two each had about 0.3 Ivy dog unit of CCK-activity per mg dry substance, as determined by the LJUNGBERG (1964) procedure, measuring the contraction of the gallbladder *in situ* in anesthetized guinea pigs against the CCK sample assayed by IVY and JANECEK (1959).

The PZ activity of the commercial sample, stated by the label to be 91 Crick, Harper and Raper units per ampoule, was then compared with that of a CCK preparation with 220 Ivy dog units of CCK per mg. For that purpose 1.5, 3.0 and 6.0 Ivy dog units of CCK of each of the two samples were injected in two anesthetized cats under continuous secretin stimulation with 3 clinical units of secretin every 30 minutes intravenously. Through a cannula in the pancreatic duct (MUTT and SÖDERBERG, 1959) the juice was collected during 15 minutes after injection. After another 15 minutes the next injection was made. The volume, usually 1.5—2 ml, was diluted to 25 ml with physiological saline solution and the protein content determined spectrophotometrically by means of the Lowry method, reading at 660 μm. The results are given in Table 7.

At the three different dilutions there was little, if any, difference in the PZ activity between the two preparations, and the ratio CCK:PZ is the same. The PZ activity was proportional to the amount of CCK injected, whether the degree of purity of the preparation was 0.3 or 220 Ivy dog units of CCK per mg. That is, on increasing the CCK activity of the preparation about 650 times there was an equal rise in the PZ activity (JORPES and MUTT, 1966a).

Again on increasing the strength of CCK from 220 to 3000 Ivy dog units per mg there was a proportional rise in the PZ activity. Both entities thus increased

Table 7. *PZ activity of a PZ preparation (A) with 0.3 Ivy dog units of CCK per mg as compared with that of a CCK preparation with 220 Ivy dog units of CCK per mg (B)* (JORPES and MUTT, 1966a)

Sample	Secretin Clin. units	CCK Ivy dog units	Spectrophotometric reading (660 μm) Cat No. 1	Cat No. 2	Mean
—	3.0	—	0.055	0.058	
A	3.0	1.5	0.155	0.126	0.140
B	3.0	1.5	0.140	0.186	0.163
A	3.0	3.0	0.227	0.212	0.220
B	3.0	3.0	0.245	0.195	0.220
A	3.0	6.0	0.292	0.290	0.291
—	3.0	—	0.046	0.034	
B	3.0	6.0	0.310	0.282	0.296

about equally, by a factor of 10,000 over the CCK and PZ activities of the commercial sample and HARPER's original PZ preparation.

The fact that the material in question had passed over an acidic ion exchanger, CM cellulose, a basic ion exchanger, TEAE cellulose, a Sephadex column and yet another acidic ion exchanger, Amberlite XE-64, resulting in a 10,000 fold increase in hormonal activity, without any detectable change in the ratio CCK:PZ favors the assumption that both activities are exerted by one and the same substance.

Strong support for this assumption was presented by MUTT (1964), who showed that CCK, which contains methionine, can, like the pituitary adreno-corticotropic hormone, the α- and β-melanocyte stimulating hormones and the parathyroid hormone, be oxidized by hydrogen peroxide with complete loss of activity and reactivated to practically full strength with cysteine. The PZ activity simultaneously underwent the same changes. Under similar conditions, pure secretin, which does not contain methionine, did not show any change in activity.

The C-terminal heptacosapeptide of CCK, Th 2, obtained after digestion with thrombin, and the C-terminal octa- and dodecapeptides resulting from the total and the partial tryptic splittings of CCK likewise showed full activity in both directions (MUTT and JORPES, 1968b). Even if the potency of the dry substance of the octa- and dodecapeptides, the synthetic and the natural ones alike, is 10 and 4 times higher than that of pure CCK, the PZ activity, expressed as light absorption of the pancreatic juice, begins to appear after injection of 1.5 Ivy dog units of CCK of any of the preparations and rises steadily on increasing the dose to 6 or 10 Ivy dog units (JORPES and MUTT, 1970b) (Table 8).

Further evidence for the identity of CCK and PZ accumulated when it was found that the decapeptide caerulein from the skin of the Australian frog, Hyla caerulea (ANASTASI et al., 1967), has an activity spectrum which covers those of both CCK and gastrin (ERSPAMER et al., 1967). In 7—8 times smaller doses than CCK, or 0.2 ng per kg, it causes the gallbladder to contract; it stimulates the enzyme output from the dog pancreas in a dose of 3 ng per kg, and acts like CCK on the sphincter of Oddi and on intestinal peristalsis. The C-terminal octapeptide of caerulein is identical with that of CCK, except for an exchange of Thr in caerulein for Met in CCK. Tyrosine ester sulfate occurs in both of them (Fig. 11). The similarity in structure and biological activity also extends to some extent to gastrin which has the C-terminal pentapeptide and the adjacent tyrosine sulfate in common with CCK and caerulein.

Table 8. *The PZ activity of the synthetic C-terminal octa- and dodecapeptides of CCK as compared with their CCK-activity*

Sample	Secretin Clin. units	CCK Ivy dog units	Direct spectrophotometric reading (280 μm) Cat No. 1	Cat No. 2
—	3	—	0.04	0.10
A	3	1.2	0.13	
B	3	1.2		0.14
A	3	2.4	0.35	
B	3	2.4		0.22
A	3	4.8	0.50	
B	3	4.8		0.32
A	3	9.6	0.65	
B	3	9.6		0.42
—	3	—	0.22	0.12

The potency of the synthetic octapeptide (A) was 30 Ivy dog units of CCK per μg and that of the synthetic dodecapeptide (B) 12 Ivy dog units per μg. Synthesis was performed by M. ONDETTI, The Squibb Institute for Medical Research, New Brunswick, N.J., U.S.A. (JORPES and MUTT, 1970b).

There is thus a series of chemically well defined compounds: CCK, its heptacosa-, dodeca- and octapeptides, caerulein and some of its synthetic analogues, and to a certain extent also gastrin, which, besides other actions, cause in adequate concentrations an emptying of the gallbladder at the same time as they exert a cholinergic action on the pancreas, resulting in enzyme secretion. The "pancreozymin" activity of the extracts of the duodeno-jejunal mucosa is thereby shown to be due to cholecystokinin.

6. Terminology, Cholecystokinin (CCK) or Cholecystokinin–Pancreozymin (CCK–PZ)

In their first communication on cholecystokinin IVY and OLDBERG (1928) used the designation CCK. GROSSMAN (1950) found the suggestion appropriate and used the term consistently in his review article in Physiological Reviews of that year. In accordance herewith Cecekin became the protected name of the first commercial brand of CCK available, supplied between the years 1955 and 1965 by Apoteksvarucentralen Vitrum, Stockholm, Sweden.

When it was shown (MUTT, 1964; JORPES and MUTT, 1966a) that both the CCK and the "pancreozymin" activities are exerted by one and the same substance, the concept of "pancreozymin" as an individual hormone still being deeply rooted in the general opinion, the term CCK-PZ was introduced (MUTT and JORPES, 1968a, b). It was also applied by GROSSMAN (1968).

This designation, CCK-PZ, however, proved to be quite unsuitable through the necessity to express the biological activity with two different unitages, Ivy dog units of CCK and Crick, Harper and Raper units of PZ, which differ widely in size. One Ivy dog unit of CCK was found to be equivalent to 4 Crick, Harper and Raper units of PZ. Considerable confusion then arose when authors communicated in terms of units only. Hence it became necessary to go back to the original terminology of IVY and OLDBERG and to use the term CCK and Ivy dog units exclusively (GROSSMAN, 1970, 1972a).

After all no serious objection can be raised against the use of the name cholecystokinin or CCK for the duodenal hormone. The effect of the hormone on the gallbladder was discovered fifteen years before the pancreozymin concept was created. The action of the hormone on enzyme secretion from the pancreas is no more specific than the effect on the sphincter of Oddi or intestinal peristalsis. The main application of this "hormone duodeno-cholecystocinétique" (Houssay and Rubio, 1932b) will also be that predicted by Ivy (1947) to "assist in the solution of the roentgenological and clinical problems involved in the diagnosis of biliary dyskinesia", namely in cholecystographies, cholangiographies, washing out small concrements from the biliary system and in X-ray examination of the intestine.

B. Common Aspects on the Gastrointestinal Hormones

I. Common Features in the Chemical Structure of the Gastrointestinal Hormones

1. Secretin–Glucagon

The preliminary analysis of pure porcine secretin (Jorpes et al., 1962) showed that the first three residues from the N-terminal end are his.ser.asp(NH_2) or his.ser.asp., a sequence which resembles the his.ser.glu. sequence at the N-terminal end of glucagon (Bromer, Sinn and Behrens, 1957). The final analysis (Mutt and Jorpes, 1967a) brought out the surprising fact that no less than 14 of the 27 amino acid units of secretin have the same position as in glucagon. The N-terminal nonapeptide of secretin, making up one third of the molecule, is identical with that of glucagon, except for two places where the dicarboxylic acids, aspartic and glutamic acid, replace each other, the latter being γ-carbamidated in glucagon. In four other places, arginine-lysine or leucine-tyrosine (phenylalanine) replace each other (Fig. 10).

The similarity in the primary structures of secretin and glucagon is an expression of the genetic relationship between the cells of the intestinal mucosa producing the hormones. The differentiation of synthesis on two separate lines, or the duplication of the common ancestral gene for the glucagon-secretin system is postulated to have taken place about $200 \cdot 10^6$ years ago, in the early Mesozoic or in the late Paleozoic era (Weinstein, 1968).

Secretin: *His* · *Ser* · Asp · *Gly* · *Thr* · *Phe* · *Thr* · *Ser* · Glu · Leu · *Ser* · Arg · Leu · Arg · *Asp* · *Ser* · Ala · *Arg* · Leu · *Gln* · Arg · Leu · Leu · *Gln* · Gly · *Leu* · Val · NH_2

Glucagon: *His* · *Ser* · Gln · *Gly* · *Thr* · *Phe* · *Thr* · *Ser* · Asp · Tyr · *Ser* · Lys · Tyr · Leu · *Asp* · *Ser* · Arg · *Arg* · Ala · *Gln* · Asp · Phe · Val · *Gln* · Try · *Leu* · Met · Asn · Thr.

Fig. 10. Amino acid sequences of secretin and glucagon (Mutt and Jorpes, 1968a)

2. Gastrin–Cholecystokinin–Caerulein

Applying the cyanogen bromide technique of Gross and Witkop (1961) to the pure CCK, Mutt and Jorpes (1967b) found that a dipeptide, aspartylphenylalanine amide, was split off. Because of the method used for fragmentation, a C-terminal sequence methionyl-aspartyl-phenylalanine amide, identical to that of gastrin, could be expected. Other evidence indicated a still greater similarity, making the C-terminal structure Met.Gly.Try.Met.Asp.Phe.NH_2 in CCK probable. In fact the C-terminal pentapeptide -Gly Try.Met.Asp.Phe.NH_2 is common to both gastrin and CCK. Furthermore, a sulfated tyrosine unit occurs next to the pentapeptide in gastrin II and in the subsequent position in CCK (Fig. 11).

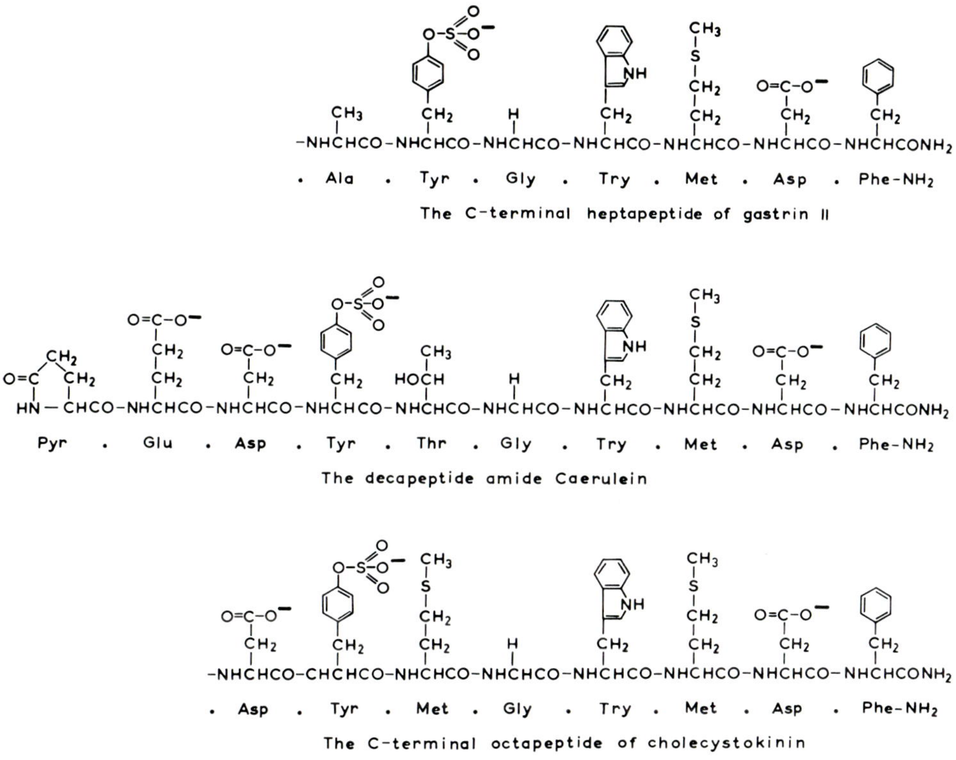

. Ala . Tyr . Gly . Try . Met . Asp . Phe-NH_2

The C-terminal heptapeptide of gastrin II

Pyr . Glu . Asp . Tyr . Thr . Gly . Try . Met . Asp . Phe-NH_2

The decapeptide amide Caerulein

. Asp . Tyr . Met . Gly . Try . Met . Asp . Phe-NH_2

The C-terminal octapeptide of cholecystokinin

Fig. 11. The similarities in structure between gastrin, cholecystokinin and caerulein

Highly unexpected and very surprising was the finding of Professor ERSPAMER and coworkers that substances with an analogous structure and biological activities similar to that of CCK occur in the animal kingdom outside of the digestive tract. In the decapeptide caerulein, Pyr.Gln.Asp.Tyr(SO_3H).Thr.Gly.Try.Met.Asp. Phe.NH_2, isolated from the skin of an Australian hylid frog, *Hyla caerulea*, by Professor ERSPAMER and coworkers (ANASTASI, ERSPAMER and ENDEAN, 1967; ERSPAMER and ANASTASI, 1966; ERSPAMER et al., 1966), the C-terminal octapeptide is identical to that of CCK, except for an exchange of Thr in caerulein for Met in CCK. Tyrosine ester sulfate in position 7 counting from the C-terminal is present in both of them (Fig. 10). Caerulein was shown by its discoverers to have all the activities listed for both gastrin and cholecystokinin with an 8 to 16 times higher potency than that of CCK (ERSPAMER et al., 1967). It has also been found in the skin of the South American leptodactylid frog *Leptodactylus pentadactylus labyrinthicus* and in that of the South African amphibian *Xenopus laevis* (ANASTASI et al., 1970; ERSPAMER and ANASTASI, 1968).

A similar peptide, the nonapeptide phyllocaerulein, Pyr-Glu-Tyr(SO_3H)-Thr-Gly-Trp-Met-Asp-Phe-NH_2, was extracted from the skin of the South-American hylid frog *Phyllomedusa sauvagei* by ANASTASI et al. (1969).

3. Cholecystokinin – Thyrocalcitonin

The sequence 16—23 of CCK · *Leu* · Asp · Pro·Ser · *His* · *Arg* · Ile · *Ser* · shows a similarity to the corresponding section · *Leu* · Asn · Asn · Phe · *His* · *Arg* · Phe · *Ser* · (POTT et al., 1968) of the molecule of porcine thyrocalcitonin.

4. Amidation of the C-Terminal Carboxyl Group

The amidation of the C-terminal carboxyl group is common, although not obligatory, in the low molecular weight, biologically active peptides. Amidated are: secretin, CCK, gastrin, calcitonin, the melanotropic hormones with 13 amino acids (LEE, LERNER and BUETTNER-JANUSCH, 1963), the 9 nonapeptides of the vasopressin-oxytocin group and the active peptides from the skin of amphibians, the decapeptide caerulein (ANASTASI, ERSPAMER and ENDEAN, 1967), the nonapeptide phyllocaerulein (ANASTASI et al., 1969) and the endecapeptides eledoisin (ERSPAMER and ANASTASI, 1962) and physalaemin (ERSPAMER et al., 1964). A C-terminal OH-carboxyl occurs in glucagon with 29 amino acids (BROMER, SINN and BEHRENS, 1957) and in ovine, bovine and porcine corticotropin with 39 amino acids (LEE et al., 1961).

The kinins, bradykinin, kallidin (FREY, KRAUT and WERLE, 1968, pp. 76—80) and phyllokinin (ANASTASI, BERTACCINI and ERSPAMER, 1966) and hypertensin (ELLIOTT and PEART, 1957) are proteolytic split products with the C-terminal nonamidated.

II. Biologically Active Breakdown and Synthetic Products

1. Secretin and Glucagon

For full secretin activity the intact whole chain of the heptacosapeptide is obligatory. Even the last member in the synthetic chain, the N-terminal histidine, is needed (ONDETTI, SHEEHAN and BODANSZKY, 1968). None of the C-terminal sequences assayed up to the tricosapeptide stage showed any significant degree of pancreatic stimulation. The hexacosapeptide amide, i.e. secretin minus the N-terminal histidine, showed a very weak biological activity. On replacing the α-aspartyl in position 3 with the β-aspartyl the potency drops to 0.6% of that of the ordinary secretin (ONDETTI, SHEEHAN and PLUŠČEC, 1970).

Synthetic porcine secretin and its synthetic N-terminal peptide 1—14 have a *lipolytic activity* as assayed *in vitro* on free fat cells or adipose tissue of rat and mouse but not of hamster, guinea pig, rabbit or pigeon (RUDMAN and DEL RIO, 1969). The C-terminal peptides 5—27, 9—27, 14—27 and 23—27 and the peptide 5—14 were inactive. Maximal response was attained by secretin at 1 μg/ml dose and ranged between 5.7 and 7.1 μEq FFA/g triglyceride/2 h.

BUTCHER and CARLSON (1970) found in their experiments with rat adipose tissue *in vitro* the secretin peptide 1—14 like the peptides 1—6, 1—23 and 15—27 to be inactive in amounts roughly equimolar to 0.025 μg/ml of secretin. Synthetic secretin stimulated lipolysis in a concentration of 0.0025 μg/ml.

Crystalline glucagon, 0.05 mg/kg subcutaneously inhibits both the histamine and pentagastrin stimulated HCl secretion in vagally innervated or denervated gastric pouch dogs. The inhibitor effect requires the integrity of all the 29 amino acids in the molecule (LIN and SPRAY, 1968). It is unrelated to hyperglycemia, because the N-terminal fragment containing 21—22 amino acids causes hyperglycemia without having any effect on the electrolytes, including gastric acid. The C-terminal fragment containing 11—12 amino acids and the synthetic C-terminal octapeptide of glucagon lack according to the authors, both the hyperglycemic and the electrolyte activities,

2. Cholecystokinin

The full activity of CCK both on the gallbladder and on the enzyme secretion from the pancreas could be recovered in the C-terminal tryptic octapeptide and in the fragments incorporating this octapeptide, namely in the C-terminal dodecapeptide and in the C-terminal heptacosapeptide obtained after splitting off the N-terminal hexapeptide of CCK with thrombin (MUTT and JORPES, 1968b).

Table 9. *Gallbladder contractile activities of synthetic C-terminal peptides of CCK-PZ* (RUBIN and ENGEL, 1972)

Peptide No.	L-Amino Acid Sequence	Guinea Pig Gallbladder Potency (i.v.) In Vitro	In Vivo
1	**Z-Trp-Met-Asp-Phe-NH_2	<1/1000	<1/1000
2	Met-Gly-Trp-Met-Asp-Phe-NH_2	<1/1000	<1/1000
3	Tyr(SO_3H)-Met-Gly-Trp-Met-Asp-Phe-NH_2*	1/10-1/5	7/10
4	Asp-Tyr(SO_3H)-Met-Gly-Trp-Met-Asp-Phe-NH_2	[1]	[1]
5	Asp-Arg-Asp-Tyr(SO_3H)-Met-Gly-Trp-Met-Asp-Phe-NH_2	1—2	2
6	Ile-Ser-Asp-Arg-Asp-Tyr(SO_3H)-Met-Gly-Trp-Met-Asp-Phe-NH_2	1—2	2/5

* Trifluoroacetate ** Benzyloxycarbonyl

RUBIN et al. (1969a, b) and RUBIN and ENGEL (1972) analyzed the biological characteristics of the synthetic C-terminal octapeptide of CCK, Asp-Tyr(SO_3H)-Met-Gly-Trp-Met-Asp-Phe-HN_2, identified as SQ 19,844, as to the effects on gallbladder contractility, intestinal motility, pancreatic protein (enzyme) secretion, gastric secretion, and on systemic blood pressure in guinea pigs, rats, dogs or cats. The contractile activities *in vitro* and *in vivo* of synthetic shorter or longer C-terminal portions of CCK (Table 9), as well as those of synthetic octapeptide analogs of SQ 19,844 (Table 10), all prepared by ONDETTI and associates (ONDETTI et al., 1970a, b, c; PLUŠČEC et al., 1970), were also determined on the guinea pig gallbladder.

Both the synthetic (ONDETTI, SHEEHAN and PLUŠČEC, 1970) and the natural C-terminal octapeptide were, on a weight basis, 10 times more potent than the pure natural CCK. The corresponding figure for the dodecapeptide was 4. The durations of the contractile effects were about one-half those of 10% pure CCK.

The same ratio between the action on the gallbladder and the "pancreozymin" activity was found in the synthetic octa- and dodecapeptides as had been found in the CCK preparations at different stages of the purification procedure (JORPES and MUTT, 1970b).

The synthetic protected C-terminal tetrapeptide was, given intravenously, less than 1/200 as potent as CCK on a weight basis in contracting the gallbladder of the guinea pig. VAGNE and GROSSMAN (1968b) found that C-terminal tetrapeptide trifluoroacetate, given i.v. in unanesthetized dogs, was 1/24 as potent as

Table 10. *Gallbladder contractile activities of synthetic octapeptide analogs of the C-terminal octapeptide, SQ 19, 844* (RUBIN and ENGEL, 1972)

Peptide No.	L-Amino acid sequence 1 2 3 4 5 6 7 8	Guinea pig gallbladder potency In vitro	(i.v.) In vivo
1	SO$_3$H | Asp-Tyr-Met-Gly-Trp-Met-Asp-Phe-NH$_2$	[1]	[1]
2	3′-SO$_3$H | Asp-Tyr-Met-Gly-Trp-Met-Asp-Phe-NH$_2$	1/72—1/36	1/32
3	Asp-Tyr-Met-Gly-Trp-Met-Asp-Phe-NH$_2$	1/300—1/150	1/125
4	SO$_3$H | Tyr-Asp-Met-Gly-Trp-Met-Asp-Phe-NH$_2$	1/660—1/330	1/450
5	SO$_3$H | Asp-Met-Tyr-Gly-Trp-Met-Asp-Phe-NH$_2$	1/300—1/150	1/140
6	SO$_3$H O O | ↑ ↑ Asp-Tyr-Met-Gly-Trp-Met-Asp-Phe-NH$_2$	—	1/80
7	SO$_3$H | Asp-Tyr-Leu-Gly-Trp-Leu-Asp-Phe-NH$_2$	1/12—1/6	1/14
8	SO$_3$H | Asp-Tyr-Met-Gly-Trp-Leu-Asp-Phe-NH$_2$	1/4—1/2	1/10
9	SO$_3$H | Ssp-Tyr-Leu-Gly-Trp-Met-Asp-Phe-NH$_2$	1/2—9/10	1
10	SO$_3$H | Asp-Tyr-Met-Gly-Trp-Met-Ala-Phe-NH$_2$	1/60—1/30	1/125
11	SO$_3$H | Ala-Tyr-Met-Gly-Trp-Met-Asp-Phe-NH$_2$	1/8—1/4	1/3
12	SO$_3$H | α-Abu-Tyr-Met-Gly-Trp-Met-Asp-Phe-NH$_2$	1/16—1/8	1/2
13	SO$_3$H | BOC-Asp-Tyr-Met-Gly-Trp-Met-Asp-Phe-NH$_2$	3/8—3/4	1/5
14	SO$_3$H | β-Asp-Tyr-Met-Gly-Trp-Met-Asp-Phe-NH$_2$	1.8—3.7	1/3

CCK on a weight basis. The C-terminal tetrapeptide had an activity about 1/143 of CCK on a molar basis. Gastrin I and gastrin II had equal activity, about 1/22 of that of CCK on a molar basis. Caerulein was 47 times as potent as CCK on a weight basis and 16 times on a molar basis.

3. Gastrin and Caerulein

TRACY and GREGORY (1964) demonstrated that the entire range of biological activities of gastrin was displayed by the C-terminal tetrapeptide sequence Trp-Met-Asp-Phe-NH_2. In studying the biological activity of about 500 synthetic compounds related to the tetrapeptide amide MORLEY (1970) found that within this tetrapeptide changes can be made in the positions occupied by the Trp, Met and Phe residues without resulting in loss of activity. Even the smallest changes at the Asp residue resulted in loss of activity, except when the aspartyl carboxymethyl side chain was replaced by a 5-tetrazolylmethyl side chain. The action of a number of gastrin analogues, including ICI 50,123 the pentagastrin, on the gastric and pancreatic secretion of the cat was reported by MORRIS, BESWICK, HOWAT and MORLEY (1970).

According to YALOW and BERSON (1970) plasma gastrin is heterogeneous, composed of two major components of immunoreactive gastrin; one component, H-LG, resembles the heptadecapeptide gastrin, the other is a larger molecule, BG (big gastrin), that appears to be composed of heptadecapeptide gastrin linked to a more basic peptide of about 5000 molecular weight. The two components exhibit qualitatively and quantitatively identical immunoreactivities and possibly equal biologic activities as well. The relation BG/H-LG is different in antral and duodenal extracts in normal and in disseased plasma. During short-term treatment with trypsin at 37°C, BG is converted to a component migrating with the mobility of the more acidic H-LG (YALOW and BERSON, 1970, 1972).

A number of analogues and split products of the decapeptide *caerulein*, Pyr-Gln-Asp-Tyr(SO_3H)-Thr-Gly-Trp-Met-Asp-Phe-NH_2, have been studied by ANASTASI et al. (1968) and by ANASTASI and ERSPAMER (1970) as to their action on the gastric and pancreatic secretion in the dog, on the gallbladder of the guinea pig and of the dog and on other parameters. The removal of the N-terminal tripeptide, Pyr-Gln-Asp-, did not cause any significant change in the activity. The position 7 of the tyrosine sulfate, counting from the C-terminal, seemed to be essential for the caerulein activity, since shortening or prolongation of the adjacent C-terminal hexapeptide chain gives only slightly active products.

In an extensive review article ERSPAMER (1972) deals with the pharmacological actions of caerulein on different organs in a number of species.

The question about active centers and the relations between structure and activity in the GI hormones were discussed by MORLEY (1972).

4. The Importance of the Tyrosine Ester Sulfate for the Biological Activity

In their original communications on the isolation and properties of the two gastrins, G I and G II, GREGORY and TRACY (1964), TRACY and GREGORY (1964) found them equally potent as stimulants of the gastric secretion. Likewise VAGNE and GROSSMAN (1968b) found them equally active on the gallbladder of the conscious dog, about 1/22 as potent as CCK on a molar basis. MORLEY (1970) reported that the sulfate-free synthetic human gastrin I and the natural hog gastrin II are equipotent as stimulants of gastric acid secretion in both Heidenhain and gastric fistula dogs. They found synthetic desulfated caerulein to be just as active in this respect or even more potent than the natural caerulein, containing the ester sulfate group (MORLEY, 1970).

ANASTASI and ERSPAMER (1970), however, found the desulfated peptides invariably to possess only a small percentage of the activity of the corresponding sulfate esters on secretory cells and to be almost free of any action on smooth muscle, including the gallbladder. Similar findings as to the action on the gallbladder of sulfated and desulfated CCK and caerulein respectively were made by AMER (1969), STENING and GROSSMAN (1969a), and JOHNSON, STENING and GROSSMAN (1970). AMER found gastrin I to be 10—30 times weaker than gastrin II in its action on isolated gallbladder strips, the isolated guinea pig gallbladder and the guinea pig gallbladder *in situ*. The desulfated caerulein was 40 to 60 times weaker than caerulein itself.

Similar findings were made by ONDETTI, SHEEHAN and PLUŠČEC (1970) with the C-terminal octapeptide of CCK. Whereas the O-sulfated tyrosyl octapeptide of CCK showed a potency of 30,000 Ivy dog units per mg in the *in vitro* and *in vivo* guinea pig gallbladder test, the corresponding sulfate free octapeptide had a potency of about 50 Ivy dog units per mg.

III. The Occurrence and Distribution of the Hormones in the Gastrointestinal Tract

1. Secretin

a) Occurrence

As stated by BAYLISS and STARLING (1903), *secretin occurs along the whole vertebrate series*. It has, according to DAVIDSON and DAVIES (1964), been found in all vertebrates in which it has been sought. They mention 17 different species including salmon and dogfish.

Secretin was extracted by BAGGENSTOSS et al. (1948) with the technique of IVY et al. (1929, 1930b) from *human material*, 35 adults and 20 children. It could be extracted up to fifteen hours post mortem and, by freezing the specimens, stored for up to 39 days without loss of activity. Even in the neonatal period secretin was present. No active fractions were obtained from a child, 16 months of age, suffering from mucoviscidosis. GIBBS and GERSHBEIN (1950), however, found a normal content of secretin in the intestinal mucosa in four cases with cystic fibrosis of the pancreas. The response of the pancreas to secretin, 1 U/kg in the ordinary secretin test, is known to be extremely poor or absent in this disease (HADORN, JOHANSEN and ANDERSON, 1968; HERMIER et al., 1969). The latter authors reported on a series of 51 cases.

As early as 1906 HALLION and LEQUEUX had extracted secretin from the intestine of two newborn infants and from a five months' foetus.

Secretin has been prepared from the spiral intestine of the skate (BABKIN, 1929). A sample from the species *Raia clavata* was found to be active in the dog (LEDRUT and ALECHINSKY, 1933) and hog secretin was active in the skate. The intestine of the holocephalian fish *Chimaera monstrosa* contains per weight 10% of the amount of secretin present in the first meter of the hog duodeno-jejunum (NILSSON, 1970). Extracts of the *lamprey* intestine show some secretin and pancreozymin activity (BARRINGTON and DOCKRAY, 1970), although the pancreatic gland is not yet fully developed in the agnathans (BARRINGTON, 1945).

The secretin mechanism does not seem to be restricted to vertebrates. LEDRUT and UNGAR (1937) found an extract of the spiral caecum of the *Octopus vulgaris* to be active in stimulating secretion from the hepatopancreas of the octopus and from the dog pancreas as well. Porcine secretin was active in the octopus.

The secretin content of the intestinal mucosa of hypophysectomized rats is about half of that of normal animals (DORCHESTER and HAIST, 1952b). Likewise vagotomy reduces the content of secretin and CCK in the rat intestine (DORCHESTER, 1959).

Secretin in birds. In birds the BRUNNER glands are absent and are replaced by duodenal Lieberkuhn's glands, secreting an opaque orangeyellow juice with amylase, sucrase and proteinase activities, having the osmolality of the blood and a reaction around neutrality. Secretin and extract of chicken intestinal mucosa increased the secretion into the duodenum by 3—4-fold (KOKAS, PHILLIPS and BRUNSON, 1967).

The histamine or gastrin stimulated secretion from the proventriculusgizzard of the chicken, assumed to be analogous to the mammalian stomach is strongly depressed by secretin and by duodenal distension, the latter mechanism being partly neural, partly hormonal (KOKAS and BRUNSON, 1969). CCK depresses the basal gastric secretion.

b) Distribution of Secretin in the Intestine

After DOLINSKI's demonstration in 1894 that pancreatic secretion can be provoked by acidification of the gastric juice, preferably with hydrochloric acid, and POPIELSKI's (1896, 1901) finding that the stimulation of the pancreas occurred first when the chyme or the acidified gastric contents entered the duodenum, the reflex was considered to be elicited from this part of the intestine, adjacent to the pancreas (PAVLOV, 1901). By filling ligated pieces of the upper third or fourth of the jejuno-ileum of the dog with acid *in vivo* WERTHEIMER and LEPAGE (1901c) extended the area to the latter parts of the intestine. No reaction followed the introduction of acid into the lower jejuno-ileum. BAYLISS and STARLING (1902b) found the secretin extracts of duodenum of the dog more active than those of the jejunum, whereas those of the ileum were inactive. The dog duodenal extracts of LALOU (1912) were 10 times as active as extracts of the ileum.

Only small amounts of secretin were claimed by DREWYER and IVY (1929) to occur in the pyloric mucosa of the dog. Our own experience is that the yield of secretin from this part of the stomach is practically nil.

In applying the extraction procedure of BAYLISS and STARLING, MELLANBY and HUGGETT (1926) found the relative distribution of secretin in the intestine of the goat to be as follows: In the fundic and pyloric parts of the stomach no secretin, in the upper and middle third of the small intestine 2.75 and 2.6 ml of pancreatic juice, respectively, in the lowest third of the small intestine 0.5 ml and in the ascending colon 0.2 ml. Using his alcohol extraction method, MELLANBY (1926) found that the secretin content of the hog intestine dropped from 100 units in the first foot below the pyloric sphincter to 76, 56, 48, 24, and 16 units in the subsequent 5 feet. In the goat the distribution of secretin extends to the large intestine with 100 units in the upper third of the small intestine, 90 units in the middle third and 18 units in the lower third. In the cat almost all the activity was found in the duodenum.

In 1927 WEAVER applied the technique of LUCKHARDT, BARLOW and WEAVER (1926) to different parts of the dog intestine, including the colon. The acid washings of the intestinal lumen were precipitated with sodium chloride, whereby practically histamine-free preparations were obtained. The small intestine was divided into five pieces of equal length. The yield from the duodenum was 2—3 times that from the uppermost fourth of the jejuno-ileum. In the third piece of the jejuno-ileum there was only a trace of secretin and in the fourth piece and in the colon, none (Table 11). The statements of WEAVER (1927) and of WERT-

Table 11. *Relative distribution of secretin on different parts of the dog intestine.* (Mean of 14 experiments) (WEAVER, 1927)

	Maximum	Minimum
	drops	drops
Duodenal extract	207	31
Intestine[2] extract	87	9
Intestine[3] extract	30	7
Intestine[4] extract	18	1
Intestine[5] extract	0	0
Colon-rectum	0	0

HEIMER and LEPAGE (1901c) that no secretin is eluted on introducing acid into the ileum of the dog but that a slight amount is obtained from the jejunum, successively diminishing with the distance from the pyloric sphincter, were recently confirmed by KONTUREK, TASLER and OBTULOWICZ (1971).

FRIEDMAN and THOMAS (1950b) found secretin to be present throughout the whole length of the small intestine in the dog, with the greatest concentration within the first 25 cm from the pylorus. The secretin content of the terminal 10 cm of the ileum was found to be only 2% of that found in the first 10 cm of the duodenum. The assay was performed under sodium pentobarbital anesthesia in dogs with the main pancreatic duct cannulated.

Acidification of the duodenum also results in pancreatic secretion in rats (HEATLEY, 1968a). The peak flow rate of pancreatic secretion decreases as more caudal segments of the rat intestine are perfused with acid, and there is no effect on perfusing segments more than 10 cm below the ligament of Treitz (RAMIREZ et al., 1966).

2. Cholecystokinin

The presence of CCK activity has been demonstrated even in the intestine of the holocephalian fish, *Chimaera monstrosa*, phylogenetically related to the elasmobranchs (NILSSON, 1970).

Since cholecystic agenesis is a fairly common phenomenon in the animal kingdom, the occurrence of CCK is not dependent upon the presence of a gallbladder. In reviewing the literature on the congenital absence of the gallbladder, VANDERPOOL et al. (1964) went back to ARISTOTLE, who had observed the phenomenon in the mule, ass, deer, camel dolphin and sea calf. MENTZNER (1929) mentioned 17 species of fish without a gallbladder, 9 species of birds and 26 mammalian species including the horse and the goat, animals that are primarily herbivores. Cholecystic agenesis in man is found in from 0.03 to 0.09% of necropsies (SMITH, 1964).

Little attention has been paid to the quantitative distribution of CCK in the different parts of the intestine. There are observations that indicate that the more distal parts of the intestine, known to be poor in secretin, contain considerable amounts of CCK, Thus Go, HOFFMANN and SUMMERSKILL (1968, 1969), applying their technique of perfusing the intestine with isotonic solutions of essential amino acids to different regions of the small intestine in man, found, on stimulating the duodenum and the areas 30 and 80 cm beyond the ligament of Treitz, for all three regions about the same pancreatic trypsin, lipase and amylase values as during stimulation with 0.25 Crick, Harper and Raper U/kg/min of "pancreozymin" intravenously, or values 3—4 times higher than those for basal pancreatic secretion during perfusion with saline. Combining intravenous administration of CCK and intraduodenal perfusion of essential amino acids doubled the enzyme secretion. Intravenous administration of the amino acids was without effect. Nor did perfusing the ileum 130 cm beyond the ligament of Treitz have any effect on the pancreatic secretion. The well-known release of CCK by fats in the duodenum and during the digestion of a fat meal is also in favour of such a view, particularly since the effect is elicited first when part of the neutral fat has been split by enzymes (SIRCUS, 1958).

In another series comprising 15 normal volunteers ERTAN et al. (1971) showed that jejunal perfusion with the solution of essential amino acids 40 cm beyond the ligament of Treitz releases endogenous CCK which is as effective a stimulus of pancreatic enzyme secretion as continuous i.v. CCK infusion.

3. The Distribution of Gastrin

The earlier literature on the occurrence and distribution of gastrin in the gastrointestinal tract was reviewed by GREGORY (1967a) and by ELWIN and UVNÄS (1966). By means of the radioimmunoassay technique the distribution of gastrin has recently been thoroughly mapped (BERSON, WALSH and YALOW, 1972; NILSSON, YALOW and BERSON, 1972; McGUIGAN, 1972; THOMPSON et al., 1972). Due attention has therewith been paid to earlier findings as to the occurrence of gastrin-like activity in the cardiac area of the stomach and in the duodenum (EDKINS, 1906; GREGORY and TRACY, 1961; EMÅS and FYRÖ, 1968).

GREIDER and McGUIGAN (1970) were able to identify cells binding fluorescein-labelled antibodies to gastrin in the human pancreas. They corresponded to the delta cells of the islets of Langerhans, staining positively with the argyrophilic HELLERSTRÖM-HELLMAN silver stain. Since the gastrin containing cells of the antral mucosa do not take up this stain, the difference may indicate that the two "gastrins" are not fully identical (McGUIGAN, 1972).

An attempt to determine by means of radioimmunoassay the amount of a hormone present in an intact organ has so far been made only with gastrin.(Table 12 and Table 13). The highest concentrations in the *antral mucosa* of the hog found by NILSSON et al. (1972) averaged 22 μg gastrin/g. The corresponding figures for human, dog and cat antral mucosa were 2, 0.6 and 2 μg/g respectively. The *duodenal mucosa* of man, hog, cat and dog contained gastrin, in man the quantities were nearly equal to those found in the antrum. Even the mucosa of the jejuno-ileum of the four species contained gastrin-like material in detectable amounts, distinguishable on electrophoresis from cholecystokinin by its negative electric charge.

As determined with the radioimmunoassay technique, the gastrin content of the plasma of fasting human subjects is about 30 ± 5 pg/ml (BERSON, WALSH and YALOW, 1972) or 63.3 ± 3 pg/ml (THOMPSON et al., 1972). Following feeding of a meal containing 240 gm of lean steak, serum gastrin levels were observed to rise from less than 30 pg/ml to from 100—345 pg/ml, with peak gastrin levels attained from 20—45 minutes following the start of the meal (McGUIGAN, 1972).

Table 12. *Mean tissue concentrations of gastrin as determined by radioimmunoassay of specimens from five dogs* (THOMPSON et al., 1972)

Tissue	Average gastrin concentration (pg/g)	Percent of antral mucosal concentration
Antral mucosa	5553	100
Gallbladder	653	12
Thyroid	199	4
Fundic mucosa	182	3
Pancreas	172	3
Jejunal mucosa	146	3
Duodenal mucosa	115	2
Uterus	111	2
Colonic mucosa	106	2
Fallopian tube	106	2
Ovary	100	2
Esophagus	97	2
Tongue	96	2

Table 13. *Tissue concentrations, ng/g, of gastrin in various tissues of different species. Results are expressed as the means of specimens from five animals* (THOMPSON et al., 1972)

	Antrum	Fundus	Duodenum	Pancreas	Plasma (pg/ml)
Frog (hibernating)	500	100	400	4500	24
Guinea pig	7160	300	4360	—	92
Rat	475	240	267	2020	125
Rabbit	11100	1200	5900	—	—
Hog	19400	400	—	—	—
Cat	5640	480	300	2800	31
Dog	5553	182	115	172	60

Extremely high basal concentrations are observed in patients with Zollinger-Ellison tumors of the pancreas (MCGUIGAN and TRUDEAU, 1968), with pernicious anemia, or with achlorhydria or hypochlorhydria (BERSON et al., 1972).

On analyzing, whole pancreatic tissue from skate and snake, containing A_1 cells, and isolated islet tissue from sculpin and hagfish, containing agranular cells, BLAIR et al. (1969) found no gastrin activity. The extraction procedure used gave a full yield of gastrin from the antral mucosa in mammals.

4. The Cell Layer of the Mucosa Carrying Secretin and Gastrin

In their communication BAYLISS and STARLING (1902b) reported that they could extract secretin from the desquamated epithelial layer of the duodeno-jejunal mucosa. In the same year WERTHEIMER (1902a, b) found that secretin goes into the acid washings of the lumen of the intestine, and in 1925 VOLBORTH in PAVLOV's laboratory at Leningrad found that all the secretin activity of the juice from the intestines of dogs with permanent Thiry-Vella fistulas was located in the sedimented desquamated epithelial cells and none in the supernatant. The secretin preparations obtained from this material through boiling with 0.4% hydrochloric acid and cautious neutralization were remarkably free of depressor substances, including Popielsky's "vasodilatin", as were the preparations of LUCKHARDT, BARLOW and WEAVER (1926), likewise obtained from acid washings of the intestinal lumen. In this respect these preparations differed markedly from those obtained by extracting the whole mucosa.

As to the location of secretin to different layers of the duodenal mucosa, clear-cut evidence was presented by KRAWITT, ZIMMERMAN and CLIFTON (1966). They sectioned pieces of frozen dog duodenal mucosa into four histologically clearly differentiated layers containing — a) villi only; b) villi with superficial portions of the crypt layer; c) crypt layer with basilar portions of villi; d) crypt layer only. Assay of the extracted material in rats showed that there was definitely no secretin activity in the crypt layer. The other three layers all contained secretin.

Since the Paneth cells are located only in the crypt area and the argentaffine cells are predominantly there, these cells are not involved in secretin production. The same applies to the goblet cells, which are abundant in both villous and crypt areas of the intestinal mucosa. The authors conclude that secretin originates either in cells located in the stroma of the villi or in the villous epithelial cells.

An opposite view was held by BUSSOLATI et al. (1971) who concluded from ultrastructural and immunofluorescence studies that secretin originates from the S cells lying mainly on the basal membrane of the crypts.

On the other hand, maximal *gastrin activity* is localized to the basal $^2/_3$ of the antral gland crypt region in the cat, the dog and man (BROOME, FYRÖ and OLBE, 1968). The superficial $^1/_3$ of the antral mucosa of the cat contained no gastrin activity, whereas in the dog traces of activity were found in this part of the mucosa. Extracts from the submucosa of the cat antrum contained no gastrin activity, but in the submucosa of one dog out of three, low activity was found. The gastrin-producing cells seem to be located predominantly in the region of the middle and basal parts of the gland crypts.

By means of immunofluorescence technique MCGUIGAN (1968) found cells binding fluoresceinated antibodies to human gastrin I in porcine and human antral mucosa extending from a region just above the gland neck area to the lower third of the glands, with an accumulation in the middle third. He described them as irregular in shape, in some instances globular, in others triangular, with their bases placed against the basement membrane and their apices extending towards the lumenal surface.

5. Subcellular Distribution

The only study of the subcellular distribution of gastrin and secretin up till 1967 was that of BLAIR, SHERRATT and WOOD (1967). No activity was found in the particle-free supernatant of the homogenate of the mucosa from the upper small intestine of the chicken. The particles were extracted with 0.01 N HCl at 100°C for 1 min. Assays were performed in cats. The distribution of both the gastrin (cholecystokinin ?) and the secretin activity followed very closely the distribution of succinodehydrogenase and protein, with 22% and 15% respectively in the nuclei, 66% and 67% in the mitochondria and 12% and 18% in the microsomes. A similar distribution was found in the mucosa of the guinea pig small intestine.

Similarly BROWN and GINSBURG (1969) found 20—33% of the total gastrin in the mitochondrial plus microsomal fraction on differential centrifugation in sucrose of homogenates of guinea pig antral mucosa. Centrifugation of the "nuclei-free" supernatant at 20,000 g for 20 min, however, yielded gastrin particles distinct from mitochondria but not clearly separated from lysosomes.

IV. The Release of the Gastrointestinal Hormones

1. Neural Influences on the Release of the Gastrointestinal Hormones

a) Gastrin

It was early observed (ZELIONY and SAVICH, 1911—1912; SAVICH and ZELIONY, 1913; SAVICH, 1922), that after cocainization of the pyloric mucosa, application of meat extract into the pyloric pouch of the dog does not stimulate any acid secretion from the stomach.

Since a moderate dose of atropine (1 mg subcutaneously) abolishes the gastric response to secretagogues or distension of the stomach (LIM, IVY and MCCARTHY, 1925) without interfering with the secretory response to injected gastrin extracts, the suggestion was made (GRAY, 1937; IVY, 1941a) that atropine prevents the release of gastrin. The discussion about the role played by vagel stimuli in the liberation of gastrin was followed up by GROSSMAN (1950, p. 40) with particular attention to the evidence brought forward by UVNÄS (1942) and KAHLSON (1948). Further evidence was presented by LIM and MOZER (1951), who worked with dogs equipped with an antral pouch and two isolated gastric pouches, one of them denervated. After cocainization of the antral pouch, sham feeding did not result in any secretion from the innervated fundic pouch. Likewise, WOODWARD et al. (1954) found that application of a cocaine or atropine solution to the mucosa of the isolated dog antrum prevents the secretion of gastric juice in response to application of foods to the antrum.

The inhibition of gastrin release by means of anesthetics is thus observed whether the stimulus is of vagal origin, is distension, is blood-borne or operates from the mucosal surface. Both completely ionized anesthetics, like lignocaine benzyl chloride, the quaternary ammonium derivative of lignocaine, and those which are ionized only at an acid pH, like cocaine and lignocaine, are equally active (REDFORD and SCHOFIELD, 1965). Acid secretion stimulated by acetylcholine in the antrum is, however, not inhibited.

After vagotomy the pancreatic secretion after a meal is highly reduced (PINCUS, THOMAS and LACHMANN, 1948; HENRIKSEN, 1969b). HENRIKSEN found that the gastric acid secretion of the dog in the period 0—30 min after feeding was reduced, on an average, by 84% after vagotomy. As a result of the reduced HCl secretion, the volume and bicarbonate output from the pancreas during the 0—60 min period were reduced by 84% and 89% respectively. The protein output was reduced, on an average, by 57%. Stimulation with Urecholine, 1 mg/h in continuous i.v. infusion, elevated the secretion level above the normal.

b) Cholecystokinin

In conscious dogs with a Thiry-Vella duodenal loop, irrigation of the loop with 0.1 N or 0.2 N HCl, milk, corn oil, 5% peptone solution, protein hydrolysate or 5% solution of essential amino acids increased the biliary pressure, but irrigation with 10% glucose or sucrose or 2% $NaHCO_3$ did not (HONG, MAGEE and CREWDSON, 1956; HONG, 1960). With the common duct occluded, the pressure was much greater and more prolonged. The intensity of the response was much less in pentobarbital narcotized animals. The local administration of 2% procaine into the loop prevented the biliary response to irrigation with HCl but failed to prevent the increase in biliary pressure following intravenous administration of cholecystokinin. Hexamethonium chloride, given systemically, itself produced a drop in the biliary pressure and prevented the pressure response to either irrigation with HCl or feeding. It had no effect on the results of cholecystokinin injection. The author concluded (HONG, 1960) that substances causing release of cholecystokinin from the duodenum do so by stimulating procaine sensitive receptors which are connected to the cells producing cholecystokinin by a pathway that can be blocked by hexamethonium chloride.

In pigs provided with an external pancreatic fistula, a duodenal fistula, antrectomy and low gastroenterostomy, the application of the local anesthetic oxethazine hydrochloride intraduodenally, 20 ml 2 mg/ml, reduced the usual increase in volume and enzymes following intraduodenal applictaions of peptone and oleic acid (HONG and MAGEE, 1970). Atropine and pentolinium tartrate significantly reduced the enzyme response to all intraduodenal stimuli. After HCl intraduodenally the volume response was reduced. Pentolinium blocked the increase in volume, amylase and protein output after 10 units of secretin. In consequence the authors concluded that the release of CCK depends on a cholinergic mechanism with at least one synapse and a local anesthetic susceptible mucosal receptor.

The importance of this mechanism for the release of CCK in man was demonstrated by GAMBLE (1970) in 9 patients who had undergone vagotomy and pyloroplasty at least one year previously and showed steatorrhea. The lipase output from their pancreas during intraduodenal perfusion with a solution of essential amino acids, 53.9 KU/h, was reduced to almost half of that occurring under similar conditions in 16 control subjects, which was 85.2 KU/h. The pancreatic enzyme output after i.v. CCK was the same in both groups.

The release of secretin requires a similar mucosal receptor. It may be facilitated by a cholinergic mechanism, but it seems unlikely that it requires one.

c) Secretin

The above discussion also applies to secretin. Five percent cocaine, 2% oxethazaine, 1—2% xylocaine or panthocaine solutions perfused through a Thiry-Vella loop in the dog depress the pancreatic secretion by 30—80% (SCHAPIRO and WOODWARD, 1965; THOMAS and SWENA, 1963). SLAYBACK, SWENA, THOMAS and SMITH (1966, 1967) perfused a Thiry-Vella loop in anesthetized dogs with 0.075 N HCl or 5% Bactoprotone solution, 1.5 ml/min during 30 min, before and after perfusion with a 0.4% oxethazaine-HCl solution. The topical anesthesia caused an 86% decrease in pancreatic secretory volume and a 94% drop in the lipase and amylase excretion in the subsequent perfusion experiment.

2. Chemical Stimuli for the Release of Secretin and CCK

a) The Release of Secretin

Besides food like meat, meat extract and sugar, and digestion products like peptones, glycine and fatty acids, a number of compounds and products such as alcohol, chloral hydrate, chloroform, urea and mustard oil were listened as stimulants for the release of secretin, when introduced into the duodenum (DELEZENNE and POZERSKI, 1912a, b; GLEY, 1912; IVY, 1930 pp. 306—311).

The action of acid in the duodenum was first observed and correctly interpreted by LEURET and LASSAIGNE (1828), who introduced acetic acid into the intestine. The specific stimulation mechanism for the release of secretin, that by means of HCl, was discovered by DOLINSKI (1894) and POPIELSKI (1896) prior to the discovery of secretin.

The acid threshold for causing a significant amount of secretion from the pancreas in the dog digesting raw meat was estimated by THOMAS and CRIDER (1940) to be near pH 4.0, an acidity which, according to the authors, is commonly found in the dog's duodenum during meat digestion. Of 210 samples taken from the uppermost part of the dog's duodenum during meat digestion, only 11 fell outside the pH range of 3.0 to 4.8, and of 166 samples collected from a point between 15 and 20 cm from the pylorus, only 13 had a pH above 4.8 (THOMAS, 1940).

The distribution of secretin in the intestine with an accumulation to the uppermost part of the duodenum is in harmony with the prevailing acidity of the duodenal contents. Following a meat meal in the dog, the bulbar pH is 3.4 to 3.7 and the midduodenal pH 5.5 to 5.5, as measured with miniature glass electrodes in the duodenum by BROOKS and GROSSMAN (1970b). 55% of the titratable acidity of the acid chyme was neutralized during passage through the first 15 cm of the duodenum.

The amount of secretin set free on duodenal acidification is fairly independent of vagal stimulation. The pancreatic secretion in response to infusion of hydrochloric acid in the duodenum of conscious dogs with duodenal and gastric fistulas is not changed after vagotomy (HENRIKSEN and RUNE, 1969b). Stimulation with Urecholine, however, considerably enhanced the pancreatic response to acid in the duodenum, an effect considered by the authors to be due to an enhanced liberation of endogenous secretin.

The relation between the maximal pancreatic secretion of bicarbonate during constant intravenous secretin infusion in man and the highest obtainable endogenous release of secretin was determined by RUNE and WORNING (1970). The ratio was in the series of 20 persons 100:60 and the maximal endogenous release amounted on an average to 0.5 U/kg/h.

The volume of pancreatic secretion and the total output of bicarbonate obtained by means of duodenal perfusion with hydrochloric acid in the cat was in the experiments of KONTUREK, DUBIEL and GABRYS (1969) 90% of that obtainable by means of exogenous secretin.

b) The Release of CCK

Both LYON's (1919) test, 20 ml 33% $MgSO_4$ solution introduced into the duodenum by means of a rubber cannula, and BOYDEN's (1925, 1926) test, the raw yolks of five eggs and half a pint of cream taken by mouth, were developed to stimulate bile flow to the intestine prior to the advent of CCK into the discussion. BOYDEN based his test on the finding that in cats the gallbladder is almost completely empty a few hours after a meal of egg yolk and cream, whereas the ingestion of lean meat gives an incomplete emptying and carbohydrates an insignificant one (BOYDEN, 1923). It was fully confirmed that the fatty meal invariably causes evacuation of a normal gallbladder (WHITAKER, 1926; HIGGINS and MANN, 1926). No definite opinion was held at that time, as to the mechanism of action of the fatty meal.

Sorbitol, 15 g dissolved in 30 ml water at 37°C and administered by duodenal intubation, has been used for the same purpose (PLESSIER, 1960; CAROLI, PLESSIER and PLESSIER, 1960; SVATOS, BARTOS and BRZEK, 1964).

An extensive literature, not cited here, deals with the role of fats and split products of neutral fats in the release of CCK. *The lipolytic split products formed during digestion are the active stimulants for the release of CCK as shown by* SIRCUS *(1958).* In consequence there is a latent period of 15—30 min before fats in the small intestine inhibit gastric secretion in the dog.

Besides acids and fats, *peptones and some of the amino acids* are effective stimulants for the *release of CCK* from the intestinal mucosa.

Instillation into the intestine of the dog of 5% mixtures of amino acids or polypeptides causes a secretion rich in enzymes from the transplanted pancreas (WANG and GROSSMAN, 1951).

An amino acid mixture, simulating beef hydrolysate, gives in healthy normal subjects the highest sustained output of lipase, trypsin and amylase from the pancreas, equalling the maximal effect after CCK administration (GO, HOFMANN and SUMMERSKILL, 1970a). A mixture of the eight essential amino acids gave the same maximal response, whereas a mixture of the non-essential amino acids behaved like the saline in the control periods. Most active were L-phenylalanine, L-valine and L-methionine. In the same concentration, a mixture of the essential amino acids is significantly more potent than any one given individually. In experiments on dogs with gastric and pancreatic fistulas, D-phenylalanine was found to be inactive in this respect (MEYER and GROSSMAN, 1970a). The same authors (MEYER and GROSSMAN, 1970b) found L-methionine to be ineffective in this respect and phenylalanine and tryptophan to be about equally effective on a molar basis.

In the anesthetized rabbit, protein secretion from the pancreas was stimulated by perfusing the upper duodenum with 0.1 mM methionine, serine, glycine, glutamic acid, threonine and lysine (ROTHMAN, 1972). Phenylalanine was effective first in a concentration of 10 mM.

c) Influence of Bile Salts on the Release of Secretin and Cholecystokinin

The question of the participation of the bile salts in the release of secretin and CCK has been almost completely neglected until recently, although it was taken up at an early date by MELLANBY. He found (MELLANBY, 1926b) that introduction into the duodenum of a urethanized cat of an emulsion of bile, 2 ml ox bile + 8 ml physiological saline solution, causes within 5 min a secretion of pancreatic juice lasting for 2 h and an augmentation of the flow of bile. A similar injection of bile into the ileum (MELLANBY, 1927) augmented the secretion of bile but had no effect on pancreatic secretion.

The author (MELLANBY, 1926b, p. 434) considered the effect of the bile salts on the pancreatic secretion to be a result of an increased release of secretin, "carried into the portal blood associated with the bile salts contained in the intestinal fluid". The hypothesis has, of course, its weak points, particularly since the bile salts are absorbed to the greatest extent in the distal part of the ileum.

The question was actualized through the recent work of FORELL and coworkers. Introduction of human or ox bile into the duodenum by means of a duodenal tube or emptying of the gallbladder by means of hypophysin was found to stimulate pancreatic secretion, mainly the enzyme secretion (FORELL, STAHLHEBER and SCHOLZ, 1965). This detail strongly influenced the outcome of the secretin test or the combined secretin-CCK pancreatic function test in man (FORELL and STAHLHEBER, 1966). After cholecystectomy or in case of a non-functioning gallbladder the values for both volume and enzyme output were reduced to about half of those in persons with a normally functioning gallbladder (Fig. 12). The effect exerted by the bile in the duodenum was significantly reduced by means of atropine. Probantheline, 15 mg i.v., had little effect on the water and bicarbonate secretion but almost blocked the ecbolic effect of the bile salts (FORELL, 1972). The author thought it most likely that the stimulation of the pancreatic secretion was an indirect one due to release of hormones, the possibility of a local nervous reflex not being excluded. FORELL et al. (1971) found the sodium salt of 3α-12α-dihydroxy-5β-cholanic acid on intraduodenal application to be the most active stimulant of the pancreatic secretion in man. Pure glycocholic acid evoked no secretion. When the dose of bile introduced into the duodenum is sufficiently large the increase in pancreatic secretion is as large as after the simultaneous i.v. administration of 1 U/kg of secretin and 1 U/kg of CCK.

The effect of bile salts on the antral gastrin release was studied by BEDI et al. (1971).

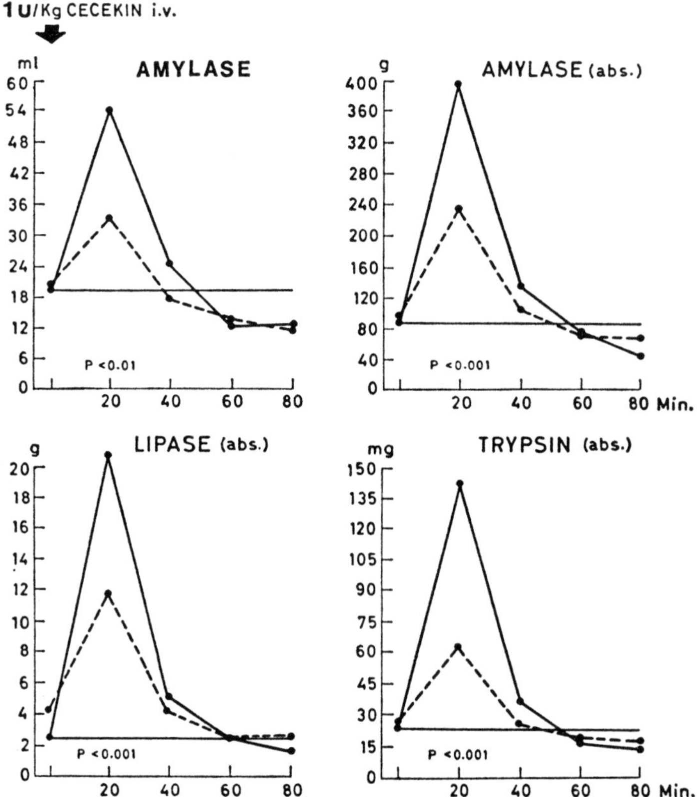

Fig. 12. Pancreatic secretion after CCK stimulation, 1 U/kg i.v., in normal, ○—○, and cholecystectomized, ○----○, subjects. Number of tests 37 and 18 respectively (FORELL and STAHLHEBER, 1966)

3. Ionic Mechanisms for the Accumulation and Release of Secretin, Gastrin and CCK

a) The Prosecretin of Bayliss and Starling

Although weak acids like acetic acid introduced into the duodenum stimulate pancreatic secretion, as do solutions containing ethanol, ether, neutral fat, chloral hydrate, Witte peptone, cane sugar, glycine or urea, it has been recognized since PAVLOV's days that mineral acid alone, usually 0.2—0.4% hydrochloric acid, is an efficient stimulant in this respect. BAYLISS and STARLING (1902a, b,

1904) and STARLING (1913) therefore expressed the view that secretin could be stored in the cells as a prosecretin, which was activated by hydrochloric acid through some kind of hydrolysis. Their view was not generally accepted. French authors, DELEZENNE and POZERSKI (1904), as well as MELLANBY and HUGGETT (1926) for different reasons claimed that it must be preformed in the mucosal cells (See STILL, 1931, p. 334).

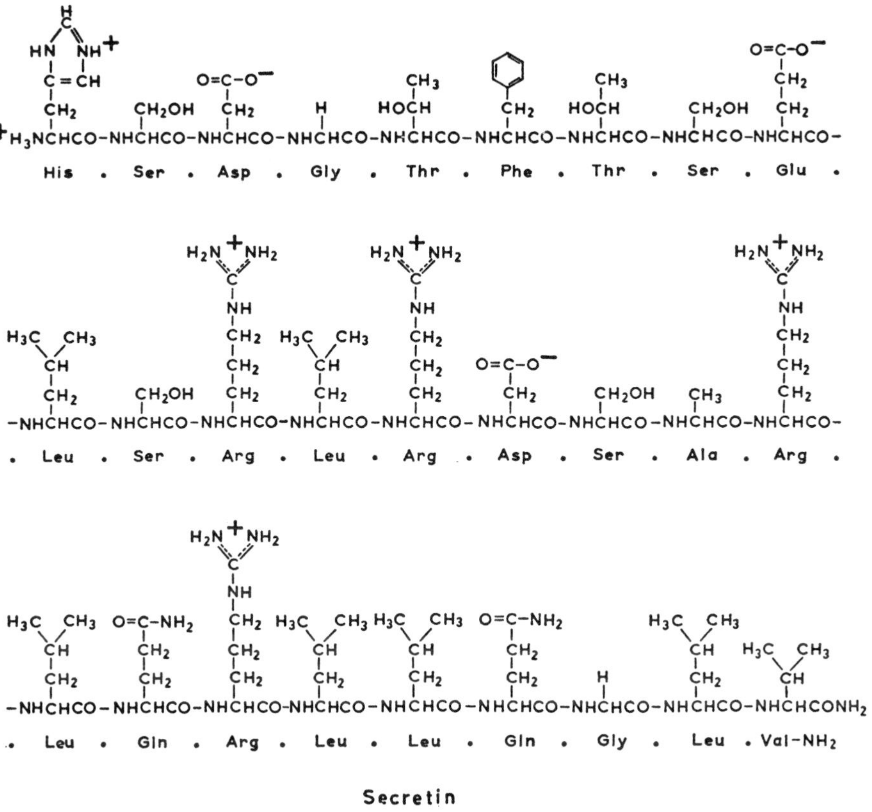

His . Ser . Asp . Gly . Thr . Phe . Thr . Ser . Glu .

. Leu . Ser . Arg . Leu . Arg . Asp . Ser . Ala . Arg .

. Leu . Gln . Arg . Leu . Leu . Gln . Gly . Leu . Val-NH_2

Secretin

Fig. 13. The primary structure of secretin

Our present knowledge permits us to accept the view of BAYLISS and STARLING in a certain sense (MUTT and JORPES, 1968a; JORPES, 1968, 1972a). Being a strongly basic peptide of low molecular weight, secretin is at neutral reaction electrostatically bound to ionized carboxyl groups of the tissue proteins. In fact the basicity of secretin is its most outstanding physico-chemical property. The C-terminal valine and the γ-carboxyl group of two of the three glutamic acid units are amidated. In addition to the N-terminal histidine, four arginines project their positive charges into the surrounding space (Fig. 13) thereby practically covering the surface of the molecule with an ionic shell. At neutral reaction, that is, at a pH above the isoelectric point of the tissue proteins, there are plenty of negatively charged carboxyl groups capable of holding the basically charged, low molecular weight secretin. As a consequence, secretin is not easily extracted with water unless the negative charge of the proteins is reduced or they acquire a positive charge. This is what happens when hydrochloric acid enters the duodenum. Secretin is set free from its electrostatic binding to the cellular or tissue proteins and appears as a hydrochloride in a highly ionized state, allowing its free diffusion.

The importance of strong acidity for the release of secretin from the mucosa was early demonstrated by GROGAN and LUCKHARDT (1924). All the secretin was eluted *in vivo* from the duodenal mucosa of anesthetized dogs only after repeated washings with 0.4% HCl.

PRESHAW, COOKE and GROSSMAN (1966) found the flow rate of pancreatic secretion and the bicarbonate output in conscious fistula dogs to be related to the amount of titratable acid introduced into the duodenum per unit time.

In an extensive study in dogs with permanent gastric and pancreatic fistulas, MEYER, WAY and GROSSMAN (1970a) convincingly demonstrated that secretin release involves an ionic mechanism as well as neural influences. By perfusing the uppermost 100 cm of the intestine with acids they found that the magnitude of the pancreatic response was proportional to the rate of entry of acid titratable at pH 4.5. Sulfuric, hydrochloric and phosphoric acids were nearly equipotent as releasers, when measured as acid titratable at pH 4.5. The organic acids, lactic and citric acid, were considerably less potent, due to their lower degree of dissociation.

The authors concluded that the relation of response to amount of titratable acid entering the intestinal segment per unit time depends on the pH at the mucosal site where receptors for release of secretin are located. The pH in its turn determines the nature and magnitude of the electric charge carried by the proteins, in this case a loss of negative charges with acquisition of positive ones. Likewise, HONG, NAKAMURA and MAGEE (1967) observed in dogs as well as in pigs a release of secretin in progressively increasing amounts as the duodenal pH fell.

The same mechanism can function for *the accumulation and release of CCK*, which shares with secretin the site of formation, the uppermost part of duodenojejunum. Among the 33 amino acid units there are, in addition to the N-terminal lysine, one lysine, one histidine and three arginine units in the molecule (MUTT and JORPES, 1968b). The C-terminal phenylalanine is amidated as are two of the six dicarboxylic acid units; thus there is a total excess of 2 basic charges. The location of both lysine and arginine in the N-terminal hexapeptide without any acidic units makes the N-terminal end of the molecule strongly basic.

b) The Linkage of Histamine to Proteins

The binding and release of secretin is analogous to that of other low molecular weight basic compounds like histamine and serotonin, as shown by UVNÄS, ÅBORG and BERGENDORFF (1970).

Histamine-rich granules isolated from mast cells, lysed with distilled water, thus in a salt-free medium, lose their histamine in proportion to the amount of Na^+ or H^+ added, when NaCl or acid are added to the surrounding medium. At 0.1 M NaCl (Fig. 14) or pH 3.5—4.0 (Fig. 15) release is 95 or 80—90% complete, respectively. The almost complete release of histamine even at pH 4.0 indicates that it is not linked to the sulfate groups of heparin in the mast cells but to poorly ionizable carboxyl groups in a heparin-protamine complex. By means of ^{14}C-histamine and $^{22}NaCl$ the authors demonstrated that there is a stoichiometric exchange of histamine and Na^+ between the mast cell granules and the surrounding medium.

During the digestion of a meal, the release of secretin therefore does not need to depend solely upon the acidity in the duodenum. Once pancreatic secretion has started, the Na^+ ions from the pancreatic juice can participate in the ion exchange along with the H^+ ions and release secretin from the mucosa even at pH values above 4.5. The French authors who refused to accept the prosecretin theory of BAYLISS and STARLING extracted secretin from the duodenal mucosa with physiological saline solutions.

The flocculation of secretin together with bile acids on acidification is due to the same mechanism. Most authors, however, found it dififcult to repeat MELLANBY's (1926) procedure of precipitating secretin with bile acids, an obstacle which is to be expected, since crude secretin extracts never are salt-free.

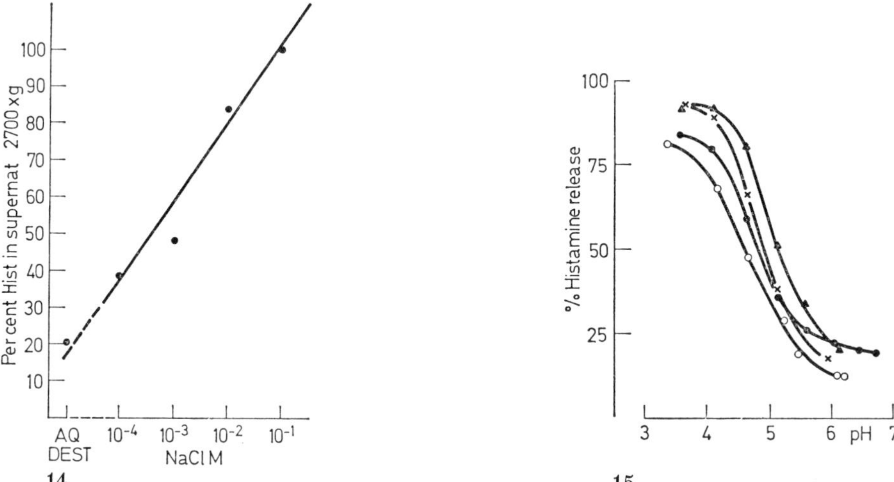

Fig. 14. Liberation of histamine from isolated rat peritoneal mast cell granules suspended in NaCl solutions of different concentrations (UVNÄS, ÅBORG, BERGENDORFF, 1970)

Fig. 15. The influence of acidification upon the liberation of histamine from isolated rat peritoneal mast cell granules suspended in distilled water (UVNÄS et al., 1970)

c) The Inhibition by Acid of the Release of Gastrin from the Antral Mucosa

The observation that acid inhibits gastric acid secretion dates back to the finding by SOKOLOV (1904) in PAVLOV's laboratory that injection of 0.5% HCl into the dog's stomach depresses its secretory response to a meat meal. As a result of a series of investigations in dogs, WILHELMJ et al. (1936, 1937a, b, c) outlined a theory for the regulation of acid secretion in the stomach. They found that during acid secretion, evoked by partially digested fresh, finely ground beef liver, an inhibitory regulatory process sets in when the acidity reaches 0.06 N and that inhibition is very marked or complete at 0.1 N. The response to histamine was not affected by the acid reaction in the stomach.

Two new concepts were introduced into the discussion with KOMAROV's (1938, 1942a, b) demonstration that the gastric antrum in fact contains gastrin and UVNÄS' (1942) finding that gastrin is liberated from the antral mucosa during the cephalic phase of stimulation. In order to eliminate the cephalic phase mediated by the vagus, DRAGSTEDT et al. (1951) performed experiments with an isolated antral pouch transplanted to the colon of the dog. Gastric hypersecretion in the Heidenhain pouch followed. If the transplanted antrum contained a collar of acid-secreting mucosa, the effect was modified. Removal of the acid-producing rim of the transplant restored the excess acid secretion in the Heidenhain pouch. Rinsing the isolated antral pouch with acid likewise abolished the basal secretion from the vagally innervated stomach (OBERHELMAN et al., 1952). WOODWARD, LYON, LANDOR and DRAGSTEDT (1954) found that suspensions of food substances which are effective in stimulating an isolated antrum to release gastrin at neutral or faintly acid pH, are ineffective or block gastrin release when they are more strongly acid. The blocking is complete at pH 1.5 (WOODWARD and DRAGSTEDT, 1960) and at pH 3 it is fully developed (UVNÄS, 1962).

The topic was reviewed by STATE (1962) and by ANDERSSON (1967). The findings of OBERHELMAN et al. (1952) eliminated the possibility of an inhibitory reflex elicited by the acid. Furthermore, REDFORD, SAVAGE and SCHOFIELD (1962) and REDFORD and SCHOFIELD (1965) demonstrated that release of gastrin took place after rinsing an isolated antral pouch with a neutral 0.1% acetylcholine solution in spite of prior anesthesia. Acidification of the pouch, however, blocked the effect of acetylcholine.

The possibility that an antral chalone functions as an inhibitor of gastric secretion has been tested by a number of authors as reviewed by THOMPSON (1966) and DRITSAS and KOWALEVSKY (1968). In reviewing the literature pertaining to this question, STATE (1962) found no evidence for the existence of an inhibitory hormonal mechanism, nor did DRITSAS and KOWALEVSKY (1968). Referring to his own experiments, STATE stated, that inhibition begins in both dog and man as soon as the digestion products reaching the pyloric antrum have a pH of 3.0 or lower. Likewise, DRAGSTEDT (1967) stated that his group after much experimental effort has abandoned the idea of an inhibitor in favour of the idea that an acid environment in the antrum per se inhibits the release of gastrin. The main evidence against the inhibitor hypothesis was obtained in Heidenhain pouch dogs, supplied with two separate antral pouches (LONGHI et al., 1957; DRAGSTEDT et al., 1959). When one pouch was stimulated, either by contact with food or by distention, the application of acid solution to the other pouch failed to block the stimulating response in the Heidenhain pouch. According to DRAGSTEDT, SCHOFIELD has supplemented this experiment by demonstrating that acidification of the stimulating food in the first pouch in fact caused prompt cessation of the acid secretion.

SCHOFIELD (1962) discussed the possible existence of a final common pathway for the local and vagal mechanisms for gastrin release. In this case antral acidity would influence gastrin release via a surface pH-sensitive receptor and a local nervous link to the effector cell. Preliminary experiments with local anesthetics, however, did not produce positive evidence for such a nervous connection. Since acid inhibits release of gastrin by acetylcholine even after local anesthetization of the mucosa, acid must act at the gastrin-releasing cell without nervous intermediation. This being the case, the acidification of the milieu of the antral mucosa per se seemed to be the most reasonable explanation of the reduced release of gastrin during the nervous phase of gastric secretion, as suggested by ANDERSSON and OLBE (1964).

In analogy the gastrin release by ethanol, introduced into the duodenum, is inhibited by acidification of the pyloric contents. The passage of ethanol through the mucosa proceeds without interference even at pH 1, thus allowing the alcohol to reach the gastrin producing cells (ELWIN, 1971). Nevertheless gastrin is not delivered to the blood.

Evidently the same principle is operating here as in the case of secretin, although in the opposite direction. Gastrin is strongly acidic due to its 5 glutamic acid units and one aspartic acid and its lack of basic amino acids (GREGORY, H. et al., 1964). Gastrin II is even more acidic due to an additional ester sulfate group.

The antral phase of gastric secretion, as measured in conscious dogs with denervated gastric pouches, is most active when the pH of the antral contents is 5.5—6.5, irrespective of whether the stimulation is exerted by 5% peptone, gastrin, acetylcholine or metacholine (ANTINONE, BLUVAS and MAGEE, 1967).

During meat digestion in the dog, the content of the pyloric antrum shows pH values between 1.6 and 3.0 (THOMAS, 1940). Of 199 samples, only 3 had a higher, and one a lower, pH value.

When the pH of the antral contents is 4.0 or below, the non-diffusible proteins at the surface of the superficial cells and in the intercellular space have acquired a positive charge capable of keeping the negatively charged low molecular weight gastrin peptide electrostatically anchored to them, preventing its uptake by the blood capillaries.

In discussing the inhibitory action of acid in the antrum on the release of gastrin, GREGORY (1962) called attention to the similarity between this situation and that when secretin is liberated under the action of duodenal acidity, a pH around 2.5 (1.4—3.2) being necessary in both situations. In fact, one and the same reaction takes place. Proteins of the tissue fluid acquire, in proportion to the degree of acidity, positive charges, which bind the negatively charged gastrin in the former case and repel the positively charged secretin molecules in the latter case, in both cases in a phase in which the liberation of the hormone is no longer dependent upon neural influences.

4. Absorption from the Intestine

Because of the lability of secretin towards digestive enzymes an enteral administration has been found unsuitable (MATSUO, 1912—1913). Early experiments of WERTHEIMER and DUVILLIER (1910) showed, however, that an absorption of secretin from the intestine is possible. On introducing an acid secretin extract into a loop of the distal ileum of the dog, where introduction of hydrochloric acid produces no effect, the authors obtained a marked pancreatic secretion. If the extract had been neutralized before administration no effect followed. In the latter case the secretin had been either enzymatically destroyed or electrostatically bound to the epithelial cell proteins in the same way as in BAYLISS and STARLING's "prosecretin".

V. The Disappearance of the Gastrointestinal Hormones from the Circulating Blood

1. Half-life Times

The gastrointestinal hormones, like the active hypophyseal peptide hormones, disappear from the circulating blood very quickly.

The half-life of exogenous secretin was calculated by LAGERLÖF, EK and NYBERG (1962) to be 17.9 min in man; LEHNERT et al. (1969) found the corresponding value in the dog to be much lower, 3.2 min. The corresponding figure for CCK is 1.8 min in the anesthetized dog (LEHNERT et al., 1970). In discussing the disappearance of gastrin and pentagastrin from the circulating blood, BLAIR et al. (1970) reviewed the pertinent literature giving half-life times for arginine-vasopressin between 3½ and 7 min in dogs and rats, for glucagon 5—10 min in rabbits and man (UNGER et al., 1961) and for vasopressin less than 1 min in the intact male rat and 3 min in the rabbit. The authors found the half-life of pentagastrin in the circulating arterial plasma of the anesthetized cat to be 1.50 min and of synthetic human gastrin I to be 2.65 min. The corresponding figure found by THOMPSON et al. (1972) for human synthetic gastrin I infused into dogs was 3.1 min. FABIAN et al. (1968) found the half-times for the disappearance of oxytocin and lysine-vasopressin from the plasma after i.v. injection in man to be 3.2 min and 4.6 min respectively.

In the early literature attention was mainly paid to *the destruction of secretin and CCK ("pancreozymin") in the blood and during passage through the liver.* In contrast to the vasodilating agent in the extracts used, the secretin activity soon disappeared, particularly under the influence of the digestive enzymes.

In demonstrating an inactivation of secretin by whole blood, plasma and urine, GREENGARD, STEIN, Jr. and IVY (1941a) found some evidence indicating the presence of a specific "secretinase". Likewise, GREENGARD, STEIN, Jr. and IVY (1941b) and GREENGARD, GROSSMAN, WOOLLEY and IVY (1944) found CCK and "pancreozymin" preparations to lose activity during 6 h incubation with dog serum. ROGERS (1951) also found the chloroform-activated purified serum protease highly active in this respect. The destruction of secretin was completely inhibited by the soybean trypsin inhibitor. Secretin is also inactivated by plasmin at pH 7.0—7.4, and by a catheptic enzyme preparation from the liver at pH 3—5 (BRIDGEWATER et al., 1962). In perfusing isolated dog pancreas with the dog's own blood, HERMON-TAYLOR (1968) found that 10—20 clinical units of secretin are used up in the circulating blood during the course of 40 minutes. Consequently it seems logical to assume that a certain amount of secretin will be inactivated by enzymes of the blood.

2. Loss of Secretin during Passage through the Liver

The question as to the destruction of secretin in the blood during its passage through the liver is of particular interest. The pancreatic function test with secretin, usually lasting for one hour, shows considerably higher figures for the volume of the duodenal aspirate in patients with liver cirrhosis, which could indicate less extensive destruction of the secretin.

Both secretin and glucagon can be assumed to be partially degraded during the passage through the liver because of the presence in the liver as well as in the spleen of a dipeptidyl aminopeptidase, cathepsin C, which stepwise eliminates pairs of amino acids from the N-terminal end of both secretin and glucagon (McDONALD, CALLAHAN, ZEITMAN and ELLIS, 1969). Thus successively 8 pairs of amino acids could be split off from glucagon and 10 pairs from secretin. The enzyme was by the authors considered to be identical with the glucagon degrading enzyme of the liver, described by previous authors. Furthermore more or less specific peptide-splitting enzymes, including cystine aminopeptidases (SJÖHOLM, 1964) that split oxytocin, vasopressin and angiotensin, are normal constituents of the blood plasma (SJÖHOLM and YMAN, 1966, 1967). The pertinent literature has been reviewed by TUPPY (1968) and by YMAN (1970).

According to WERTHEIMER (1902a, b), secretin is taken up by the portal venous system and not by the lymph vessels. On introducing mustard oil as irritant into a jejunal loop, secretin activity was demonstrated in the portal blood in two dogs but was absent in the thoracic duct of a third dog. MELLANBY (1926) came to the same conclusion. After introducing dilute bile (2 ml ox bile, 8 ml physiological saline solution and 0.05 ml N HCl) into the duodenum of a cat, the flow of pancreatic juice was not affected by ligation of the thoracic duct, nor was there any secretin in the chyle. Likewise, CCK and gastrin enter the bloodstream through the portal circulation. BOYDEN (1926) showed that the expulsion of bile from the gallbladder after a fat meal takes place freely in cats with the thoracic duct ligated, but not if the portal vein is ligated. McGUIGAN (1972) concluded from his measurements of the gastrin concentrations in the thoracic duct lymph and in the portal venous blood and the flow rates of the two fluids, that substantially more than 99% of the gastrin reaching the peripheral circulation is transported via the portal vein. A similar view was held by THOMPSON et al. (1972). Since secretin and CCK thus enter the portal circulation, the question of their stability during passage through the liver is essential.

Early workers, cited by BABKIN (1928, p. 589) and by MELLANBY (1926), found a weaker pancreatic secretory response following the injection of crude secretin extracts into the portal vein than after injection into a systemic vein. MELLANBY (1926b) made the same observation when using crude alcoholic extracts of hog duodenal mucosa, but not when he used a purified material. Nor did HART and CLARKE (1959) find such a difference. The latter authors injected 1–10 clinical units of secretin alternately into a femoral and a splenic vein in six anesthetized dogs. The mean average volume of the pancreatic juice secreted was 4.06 ml in 30 min in response to 17 injections into the femoral vein versus 4.20 ml after the same number of injections into the splenic vein.

In recent work, however, both NECHELES, OGAWA, CHILES and LEVINSON (1959) and SKILLMAN, SILEN and HARPER (1962) found 30 per cent smaller volumes of pancreatic juice after intraportal injection than after systemic injection of secretin.

The former group injected 2–10 units of secretin alternately into the portal vein and a peripheral vein in 13 experiments on 11 anesthetized dogs and registered the numbers of drops of fluid secreted from a pancreatic fistula. After the intraportal injections the mean number of drops was 69.5 per cent of that after the ordinary i. v. injections. In contrast, the response to an injection directly into a major pancreatic artery was very large, 62 and 46 drops respectively, in 30 minutes after 2 units of secretin, a dose which when given intravenously did not stimulate the pancreas to secrete above the control value, 4 to 5 drops in 30 minutes.

The latter authors infused secretin into adult anesthetized dogs, 5.3 U/min (2.80 U/ml) for periods of 15 minutes alternately via the portal and systemic route, 3 pairs of infusions in each of five dogs, and measured the volume of pancreatic juice collected from the cannulated major pancreatic duct. In each pair of infusions, portal and systemic, the volume of pancreatic juice was always greater when secretin was given by the systemic route, the mean of all the values after portal infusion being 30 per cent lower than that after systemic infusion; exactly the same relationship was found by NECHELES et al. (1959).

Conclusive evidence was presented by WAY, JOHNSON and GROSSMAN (1969), working with unanesthetized dogs with chronic gastric and pancreatic fistulas and with a plastic catheter in the portal vein. Portal administration of 0.06 µg/kg/h of synthetic secretin gave volume and bicarbonate responses 75% as great as when it was given systemically. There was no difference in response to a dose of 0.24 µg/kg/h when given by the two routes.

Similarly, CHEY, LEE and LORBER (1970) found that secretin infused in a dose of 2 U/kg/30 min in dogs with a gastric fistula and a portal vein cannula was in large measure inactivated during passage through the liver, the inhibitory effect on the pentagastrin stimulated gastric acid secretion and the gastric motility being used as indicators. Intraportally administered ^{3}H-labelled secretin was destroyed to the extent of 68.6% during passage through the liver.

There are clinical findings *in patients with cirrhosis of the liver* which could be interpreted as a result of *a reduced destruction of secretin.* FRIEDMAN and CHENG (1961) and van GOIDSENHOVEN et al. (1963) found in series of 25 patients each, that the duodenal volume response to 1 clin. u. of secretin per kg was markedly or excessively increased in 75 and 48% of the patients respectively (Fig. 16). Similar earlier findings were summarized by von GOIDSENHOVEN et al.

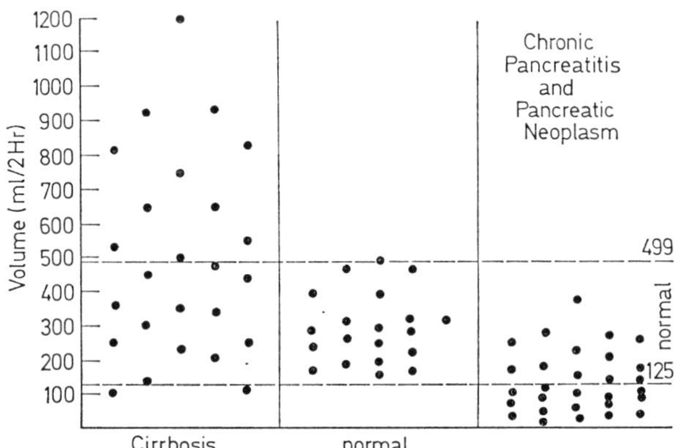

Fig. 16. Volumes of postsecretin duodenal aspirate in normal subjects and patients with cirrhosis of the liver, chronic pancreatitis, and pancreatic neoplasma (Van GOIDSENHOVEN et al., 1963)

On analyzing five cases of hemochromatosis with liver cirrhosis, PERMAN and BONERA (1964) found that the secretin test gave excessively high values for volume (550–1,026 ml) and bicarbonate (30–36 mEq) instead of the normal values 125–250 ml and 8–25 mEq respectively. They considered deficient destruction of secretin in the cirrhotic liver to be the cause of the abnormal outcome of the test. In a series of 29 patients with portal cirrhosis and 5 patients with fatty liver, ZIEVE and MULFORD (1967) observed in two-thirds of the cases volumes of the 30 min duodenal aspirates after 90 U of secretin and 100 U of "pancreozymin" which exceeded the highest recorded in 18 normal men. The values for the volumes of the duodenal aspirates were in some cases up to 5–9 times higher than the upper limit in the normal subjects. The increase in volume was frequently followed by a decrease in bicarbonate concentration. There was usually no increase in the amount of bile pigment which could indicate an admixture of bile.

3. The Fate of CCK, Gastrin, Pentagastrin and Glucagon during Passage through the Liver

GREENGARD (1941) and GREENGARD et al. (1941 b) reported a certain slow inactivation of CCK in blood serum. BRIDGEWATER et al. (1963), however, found that neither the route (portal *versus* systemic) nor the mode of injection (single dose *versus* constant infusion) changed the amylase or trypsin concentration of the pancreatic secretion. Nor was there any difference in response in the series of WAY et al. (1969) when 0.25 U/kg/h of CCK or 0.15 μg/kg/h of caerulein were administered intraportally or systemically in the chronic pancreatic fistula dogs.

Gastrin behaves similarly (GILLESPIE and GROSSMAN, 1962). When injected into the portal vein in three dogs with Heidenhain pouches, it gave as great a secretory response as when injected into a systemic vein. By contrast, the response to histamine injected into the portal vein was only 24 per cent of that obtained by systemic venous injection.

Similarly, LICK et al. (1967) found no reduction in the action of gastrin, a 90% reduction of the histamine response and a 75% reduction in the response to the synthetic C-terminal tetrapeptide amide of gastrin after passage through the liver.

Quite opposite results were obtained by THOMPSON et al. (1969, 1970, 1972) on infusing the portal vein and the inferior vena cava of conscious fistula dogs with solutions of gastrin, ^{14}C-pentagastrin and histamine and analyzing both the effect on the acid production in the Heidenhain pouch and the content of gastrin, pentagastrin and histamine, respectively, in the blood obtained from the catheterized hepatic vein. There were losses of 48%, 91% and 75% of the three agents, respectively, as measured by the acid secretion and of 45%, 93% and 95% as measured across the liver. Digestion of human synthetic gastrin I at 37° for 2 hours with slices of liver, kidney, lung, fundus ventriculi and muscle, respectively, resulted in a heavy loss of activity, almost total, 99%, in the batches with kidney tissue (Table 14).

Table 14. *Loss of activity of human gastrin I during 2 h digestion at 37° with slices of liver, kidney, lung, fundus ventriculi and muscle as measured in the living animal and with radioimmunoassay technique* (THOMPSON et al., 1972).

Tissue	Gastrin inactivation	
	Bioassay %	RIA %
Liver	82*	86*
Kidney	99*	99*
Lung	75	86*
Fundus	42	58*
Muscle	21	77*

According to Le VEEN and BOREK (1969), twice as much human gastrin is needed to evoke an identical secretory response in man when it is injected into the portal vein system rather than into a systemic vein. Portacaval shunt causes gastric hypersecretion.

As to the mechanism for the rapid disappearance of gastrin from the circulating blood, BLAIR et al. (1970) considered diffusion into the extracellular fluids to be an important factor, although not sufficient to explain the rapid drop in the concentration in plasma. The drop is too sudden and the extravascular water volume too small for it to be due to equilibration through free diffusion. Elimination and some kind of destruction must be assumed. In fresh cat plasma, however, there is no destruction of added pentagastrin or synthetic human gastrin I either at +4°C during 27 h or during storage for 30 min at 37°C.

Since the C-terminal carboxyl of both secretin and CCK is amidated, it is of particular interest that an amidase, capable of splitting off the C-terminal NH_2-group in the N-acylated C-terminal tetrapeptide amide of gastrin, occurs in the liver and intestinal mucosa of the rat (LASTER and WALSH, 1968). Thereafter the molecule is accessible for further destruction by decarboxylases and aminopeptidases.

As to *glucagon*, the experiments of von HEIMBURG and HALLENBECK (1964) and of KOCK, DARLE and DOTEVALL (1967) showed that no appreciable destruction of glucagon takes place during its passage through the liver. The former authors measured the inhibition of HCl secretion by vagally innervated and vagally denervated gastric pouches of dogs, the latter authors recorded in man the inhibition of motility in the jejunum and colon, appearing after 30 to 60 sec and lasting 4–8 min after injection of 0.05–0.1 mg of glucagon. In both series of experiments the effect was the same irrespective of whether glucagon was administered via the portal vein or a systemic vein.

In another series DOTEVALL, KOCK and VALAN (1970) found that there was consistently a pronounced decrease of the volume of gastric secretion and acid output following intraportal injection of 2 mg of glucagon in 7 patients with a fine plastic tube introduced into a peripheral omental vein in connection with a previous operation.

C. Biological Actions of the Gastrointestinal Hormones*

I. Actions of the Gastrointestinal Hormones on the Pancreas

1. Oxygen Consumption of the Pancreas under the Influence of Secretin and Cholecystokinin

In applying the then newly developed techniques of determining blood gases quantitatively BARCROFT and STARLING (1904) demonstrated that the oxygen uptake of the pancreas from the blood is in the dog much greater during secretin stimulation than in the resting gland.

In 1933 STILL and his co-workers measured the oxygen consumption of tissue slices of *rat pancreas* in Warburg vessels with and without secretin (GERARD and STILL, 1933). The secretin prepared by them had no effect on the vasomotor system even in amounts equivalent to 200 maximal secretory doses. There was a consistent increase of about 30% in the respiration in the tissue slices in each of the six experiments performed. Of other tissues examined, brain, diaphragm, kidney and liver, only the latter showed an increase in one single experiment.

A similar conclusion was drawn by STILL, BENNETT and SCOTT (1933) who measured the flow of blood through the dog pancreas *in situ* with a stromuhr of their own construction and the gaseous exchange in the gland. Within 10 min after the administration of secretin there was a rise in the O_2 consumption from 0.58 ml/min to 1.45 ml/min with no change in the blood flow. In some cases there could be a 50% drop in the blood flow in spite of increased secretion and O_2 consumption.

Using Warburg vessels, KIYOHARA (1934) also found that secretin, added to a suspension of slices of *rabbit pancreas* in concentrations of 10^{-6}–10^{-4}, regularly increased the oxygen uptake by 6–11%. No change whatsoever took place when slices of pancreas atrophied after duct ligation, or slices of the rabbit liver or the adrenal cortex were used. In connection with their study of the influence of acetyl choline + eserine on the oxygen uptake and secretion of the parotid gland,

* The biological actions of secretin were dealt with in a number of early review articles among which only those of LA BARRE (1936) and GROSSMAN (1950, 1958) will be mentioned here.

DEUTSCH and RAPER (1936) included a series of Warburg experiments using slices of *cat pancreas*. The oxygen uptake increased fivefold after the addition of secretin as well as after adding acetylcholine + eserine. The very crude extract of hog intestinal mucosa used as secretin was fully active after boiling for half an hour at pH 6.4 or 7.5, but totally inactive if boiling took place at pH 8.7.

Using a similar technique and pieces of *cat pancreas*, DAVIES, HARPER and MACKAY (1949) confirmed the results of the previous authors. Following the admixture of 0.2–2 mg % of a pancreozymin-free secretin preparation, the O_2 consumption and CO_2 production of the pieces were consistently elevated by 20 to 40% of the control values. About the same increase followed the admixture of 3–30 mg % of pancreozymin, or 0.1–10 mg % of acetyl choline + the same amount of eserine. The effect of the latter drugs, but not that of pancreozymin, was inhibited by atropine. Histamine in a concentration of 0.1 mg % had no effect. Pancreozymin and acetyl choline + eserine caused marked changes in the histologic picture during the course of the 60 min the experiment lasted, resulting in an extrusion of zymogen granules from the acinar cells. Secretin promoted no reduction of the zymogen granule content. In anaerobic experiments, the rate of glycolysis and the histological appearance of the cells were unaffected by the addition of acetyl choline with eserine, either alone or with ATP.

A similar effect, with a reduction of zymogen granules of the acinar cells, had been demonstrated by HARPER and MACKAY (1948) in the *living cat* by stimulating the dorsal vagus trunk electrically or administering pancreozymin. No change took place during secretin stimulation. DICKMAN and MORRILL (1957) incubated excised whole *mouse pancreas in vitro* with the parasympathomimetic drugs pilocarpine and Carbachol, and with the hormones pancreozymin and secretin. The first three substances stimulated both the rate of respiration and the rate of enzyme secretion, whereas secretin stimulated only the respiratory rate. The secretory and respiratory effects of pancreozymin were not decreased by atropine. In confirmation of the results of DAVIES et al. (1949), secretin was found to stimulate the respiratory rate in the gland by approximately 15%. The authors observed a potentiation of the action of a suboptimal dose of Carbachol by secretin, causing a 16% rise in the excretion of ribonuclease to the medium. Histamine in concentrations from 5×10^{-8} to 5×10^{-5} had no significant stimulatory effect on the enzyme secretion. DAVIES et al. (1949), using cat pancreas, and HOKIN (1956) using mouse pancreas found that enzyme secretion was blocked when the Warburg vessels were filled with nitrogen, even in the presence of pilocarpine or pancreozymin.

Both the synthesis and the secretion of the pancreatic enzymes are dependent upon oxygenation (SCHUCHER and HOKIN, 1954). The authors followed the synthesis of lipase and ribonuclease in slices of *pigeon* pancreas incubated in oxygenated physiological saline solution. The formation of the enzymes was abolished by 10^{-4} M 2,4-dinitrophenol or by anaerobic incubation. In slices depleted of their stores of free amino acids by preincubation, addition of amino acids stimulated enzyme synthesis. Carbamylcholine stimulated the secretion of amylase, lipase and ribonucelase, to the same extent for all three enzymes. The stimulation of enzyme secretion was not accompanied by increased enzyme synthesis.

In their further studies of enzyme production in slices of pigeon pancreas suspended in a bicarbonate saline medium, sometimes supplemented with a casein hydrolysate or with a suitable mixture of amino acids, HOKIN and HOKIN (1956, 1962) found that "*pancreozymin*", like the cholinergic agents acetylcholine (+ eserine), carbamylcholine and pilocarpine, stimulates the excretion of amylase ribonuclease and lipase into the medium. Simultaneously there was an increase in the incorporation of phosphates into the phospholipids, mainly into the phosphoinositide fraction. The phospholipids formed were assumed to participate as carriers in the transport of zymogens across lipid membranes.

There is, with one single exception, full agreement that secretin, impure or pure, increases the respiratory rate of the pancreatic tissue *in vitro* and that CCK, like the cholinergic drugs, does the same, and furthermore provokes extrusion of enzymes from the acinar cells.

Applying the usual technique with Warburg vessels and pieces of rat pancreas suspended in a Krebs-Ringer phosphate buffer, pH 7.4, BAUDUIN of Brussels found acetyl choline $1 \cdot 10^{-3}$ M—$1 \cdot 10^{-4}$ M + eserine to be without effect on the respiratory rate of the tissue (BAUDUIN et al., 1964). The same was true of a secretin preparation, active on the human pancreas in a dose of 1 clin. U/kg, irrespective of whether or not soybean trypsin inhibitor was present in the medium (BAUDUIN and REUSE, 1965a). On the other hand, pancreozymin, 0.06 U/ml, increased the respiratory rate of the rat pancreas by 15%. A reduction of the respiratory quotient, like that caused by acetyl choline, $5 \cdot 10^{-7}$ M, was masked by a production of CO_2 due to the liberation of carbonic anhydrase (BAUDUIN and REUSE, 1965b). The experiments were repeated using the pure natural porcine secretin in various media, but the results were the same (BAUDUIN, 1967).

There can, however, be no doubt that the secretory activity of the pancreatic gland is dependent upon oxygen consumption. In addition to all the previous evidence, this was most clearly demonstrated by NARDI et al. (1963) and by ROTHMAN and BROOKS (1965a, b). NARDI et al. perfused a dog pancreas *in situ*, after ligation of the normal vascular connections, with freshly collected heparinized dog blood, with pH, p CO_2, p O_2 and the temperature equilibrated within physiological ranges. The perfusion pressure was 100 mm Hg, the flow rate 50—80 ml/min. The gross appearance of the gland, the integrity of the cellular structures as observed under the microscope and the electron microscope on biopsy samples, the production of pancreatic juice of normal composition, oxygen consumption in the range of that of the *in vivo* gland and the ability of the preparation to incorporate labeled amino acids into protein, all indicated the viability of the gland. In a control experiment the oxygen uptake of the pancreas of intact anesthetized dogs averaged 1.57 ml/min. The average oxygen uptake of six perfused glands was 1.29 ml/min. The addition of secretin to the perfusion medium caused a slight increase in the oxygen consumption. The addition of both secretin and cholecystokinin (pancreozymin), 25 units of each, was followed by a two-fold increase in the mean oxygen uptake.

In similar experiments of HERMON-TAYLOR (1968), the oxygen pressure of the effluent venous blood was greatly reduced under the action of CCK infusion, an expression of the increased oxygen consumption of the gland.

ROTHMAN and BROOKS (1965a, b) studied the secretion from the isolated rabbit pancreas mounted together with the duodenal loop and the mesoomentum on a polyvinyl-chloride frame and incubated in a bath with a suitable salt solution according to ROTHMAN (1964b). Since the rabbit pancreas is nearly as thin as the omentum, arterial perfusion becomes superfluous. In such a preparation secretion ceased when inhibitors of glycolysis and aerobic metabolism were added to the bath.

2. Action of Secretin on the Pancreatic Blood Flow

KUZNETSOVA (1963a) reviewed the older literature concerning the blood supply to the pancreas during digestion. The story begins with CLAUDE BERNARD's (1856b) famous remarks about the gross appearance of the pancreas of the dog during fasting and after a meal. It was a topic of great interest for the PAVLOV school. When secretin preparations free of vasodilating properties became available, it seemed reasonable to assume that the hormonal activity was independent of the gland's blood supply (BAYLISS and STARLING, 1902a, b; LUCKHARDT, BARLOW and WEAVER, 1926; WEAVER, LUCKHARDT and KOCH, 1926; WEAVER, 1928). As late as 1957, TANKEL and HOLLANDER concluded in a review article that "the evidence presently available does not warrant the conclusion that pancreatic secretion is dependent on the blood supply to the organ."

Through the communication of MALTESOS and WATSON (1939) about a fourfold increase in flow of blood through the pancreas of the dog after injection of a secretin preparation free of vasodilating activity, the question about the connection between blood flow and secretin stimulated pancreatic secretion became highly actualized. Referring to recent Russian modifications of the REIN thermoelectric technique for determining the rate of flow of blood, KUZNETSOVA (1963a) reported on a series of results of her own obtained with a similar technique. There was in the dog, in sham feeding experiments, a definite correlation between the rate of flow of blood through the pancreatic artery and the secretion of pancreatic juice, the increased blood flow occurring 1.5 to 3.0 min sooner than the secretion and often ending somewhat later. When dilute HCl was introduced into a duodenal loop, the pancreatic blood flow began to increase after 1 to 2 min and reached a maximum after 5 to 7 min. Secretion from the pancreas started 2—3 min after introduction of the acid and lasted 15 to 20 min. The volume ranged from 3 to 12 ml. A secretory vascular reaction of this kind was observed in 75 out of 81 experiments.

With the crude preparations available in the past, it was impossible to decide whether the increased blood flow through the gland was due to impurities in the preparations. In 1960, HOLTON and JONES, using a photocell, amplifier and recorder equipment, measured the blood content of a portion of the cat's pancreas under transillumination. The fairly impure secretin and "pancreozymin" preparations used caused an immediate vasodilation lasting 2—5 minutes, which was not affected by atropine and mepyramine. When using pure secretin, however, HILTON and JONES (1963) found that there was no change whatsoever in the blood pressure or the venous outflow from the pancreas in the cat even during strong secretin stimulation. Nor did UNGER et al. (1966) find any significant change in the blood flow through the dog pancreas after the injection of 25 units of a sample of crude secretin. The vasodilation observed in the past could, of course, be explained as being due to a plasma kinin produced by pancreatic kallikrein activated by the "pancreozymin" stimulation.

In spite of these observations, there is a unanimous opinion that the hormonally elicited pancreatic secretion is accompanied by an increased blood flow through the gland (JACOBSON, 1967; BARLOW, GREENWELL, HARPER and SCRATCHERD, 1968; ROSS, 1969).

NARDI et al. (1963) reported on perfusion experiments with the isolated dog pancreas *in situ*, a technique first elaborated by BABKIN and STARLING (1926). Although the introduction of secretin or pancreozymin caused a rapid fall in perfusion pressure which preceded secretion, the stimulated gland was able to maintain secretion of pancreatic juice at a constant rate. Increasing the flow rate to restore perfusion pressure to 100 mm Hg did not alter the rate of pancreatic juice production. Acetylcholine also caused marked alteration in perfusion hemodynamics, but did not evoke a secretory response from the pancreas at any time. Their preliminary experiments indicated that the vasodilatory effects of the hormones stimulating the pancreas may be independent of their effect on the exocrine activity. Alterations in pancreatic blood flow did not influence pancreatic secretion within the limits studied.

The same correlation between the hemodynamic state and secretory activity of the pancreas as found by KUZNETSOVA during sham-feeding of the dogs, was also observed by MACKOWIAK, FRIEDMAN and HORN (1967) in anesthetized dogs in which the rate of arterial inflow of blood to the pancreas was measured with a gated sine-wave electromagnetic flow meter and perivascular probe. Pure secretin, in doses adequate to elicit submaximal rates of pancreatic secretion, produced concomitantly a 20—30% increase in mean pancreatic blood flow, and the onset of pancreatic secretion due to secretin was almost always *preceded* by augmentation of the blood flow. The duration of pancreatic secretion in response to secretin could be correlated with the duration of augmented arterial flow rates.

According to the authors, the effect of the "sapocrinine" stimulation of the pancreas could be distinctly differentiated from the secretin effect. The onset of pancreatic secretion due to soap extracts of intestinal mucosa, "sapocrinine", was not accompanied by changes in the local blood flow.

That *vasodilation in the pancreas precedes the onset of secretion in response to secretin and gastrin* was convincingly demonstrated by HERMON-TAYLOR (1968) working with the isolated canine pancreas. The sample, wet weight 100—115 g, was perfused with the dog's own blood, 20—25 ml/min or 0.2 ml/g/min, and kept at 37° C, intermittently irrigated with warmed Ringer solution. The resting volume of pancreatic secretion was 0.1 ml per 5 min with a mean bicarbonate concentration of 35 mEq per litre. Arterial blood pressure was 75 to 90 mm Hg. After infusing Boots secretin in the arterial line in doses of 0.4 to 1.6 U/min, the volume flow of secretion increased with each rise in secretin dosage, reaching a maximum of 4.5 ml per 5 min between 0.8 and 1.6 units per min, with a mean bicarbonate concentration of 110 mEq per litre. With a mean pancreatic weight of 50 g, maximum bicarbonate output per unit weight of pancreas was 0.032 mEq per g per 15 min. The blood pressure dropped to 30 mm Hg as an expression of a decrease in the pancreatic vascular resistance, and the venous oxygen saturation dropped from 60—70% to 50—55%, indicating increased metabolic activity.

A similar effect was obtained after injecting 1 U, 0.25 μg, of *pure secretin* in a single dose. Even the *pure CCK*, added to the perfusion fluid in amounts of 0.08—0.16 μg/min caused a similar reaction (HERMON-TAYLOR and BEAUGIE, 1972).

The sequence of events following infusion of *pure gastrin II* was similar to that found with secretin. The maximal effect of an infusion of gastrin II was obtained with the dose 0.08 μg/min. The volume of pancreatic secretion rose from 0.1 to 0.6 ml/5 min, the bicarbonate concentration from 22 to 60 mEq/litre. There was a sharp fall in arterial pressure immediately preceding the onset of the pancreatic exocrine secretory response, and an increase in the metabolic activity of the preparation.

As determined by the radiopotassium clearance technique (DELANEY and GRIM, 1964, 1966), blood flow through the pancreas of the anesthetized dog increased from 0.63 ml/min/g of pancreas, the mean for 9 control animals, to 0.97 ml/min/g, after intravenous injection of 1 U/kg of secretin (Boots), whereas epinephrine infusion, 1 μg/kg/min reduced the value to 0.41 ml/min/g. The most profound reduction was elicited by pitressin. Administration of histamine or norepinephrine did not cause statistically significant changes.

In anesthetized dogs with the pancreatic duct, the pancreatico-duodenal vein, the superior mesenteric vein and the portal vein cannulated, GERBER et al.

(1967) measured the pancreatic blood flow in the pancreatico-duodenal artery using an electromagnetic flowmeter. Simultaneously cardiac output, hepatic, gastric, carotid and periferal blood flow was measured. The O_2 consumption was derived from blood flow and O_2 saturation. The effect of 1 U/kg of pure secretin on the three parameters pancreatic secretion, pancreatic blood flow and O_2 consumption were as given in Fig. 17.

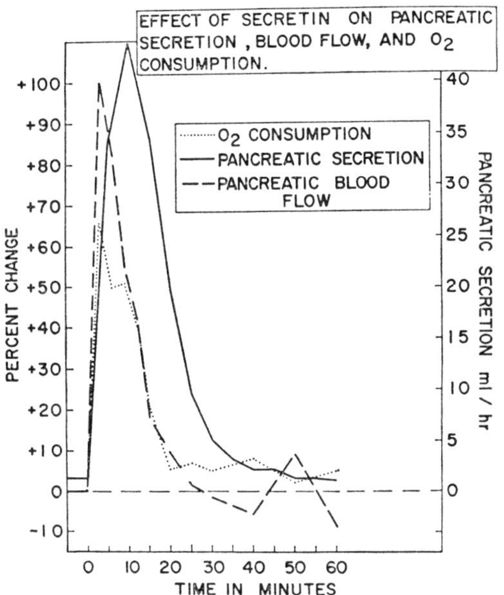

Fig. 17. Following injection of secretin, 1 U/kg, there is in the anesthetized dog, a prompt increase in pancreatic secretion reaching a peak within 10 to 15 min. There is also a marked increase in pancreatic blood flow corresponding to the increase in pancreatic secretion. Pancreatic O_2 consumption parallels the increase in secretion and blood flow although not of the same magnitude. Results are shown as a mean of 15 experiments (GERBER et al., 1967)

Similar findings were made by ROSS (1969). Rapid injection of glucagon (1—10μg) or of secretin (1—10 μg) in anesthetized cats produced dilation of the mesenteric vasculature and constriction of the hepatic arterial vascular bed but had no effect on the renal vessels. Since the pattern of vascular responses differed from those after isoprenaline, the vasomotor changes induced by these hormones were, according to the author, probably not mediated by β-receptors.

According to DORIGOTTI and GLÄSSER (1968) all the agents, secretin, "pancreozymin", caerulein and ICI 50.123, known to stimulate the external pancreatic secretion, are able to increase arterial blood flow to the gland by locally reducing vascular resistances. In the anesthetized dog, caerulein in doses 2—30 ng/kg i.v. causes a dose related increase in the blood flow through the pancreatico-duodenal artery, reaching its peak in 40—60 sec and lasting no more than 6 min. Similarly "pancreozymin" in doses of 0.1—1.5 IDU/kg causes a dose related increase in the pancreatic blood flow with a similar peak effect and duration without signs of tachaphylaxis. The gastrinlike pentapeptide ICI 50.123 was about 25 times less active. Secretin stimulated pancreatic secretion at doses far lower than those active on blood flow. None of the substances had any influence on the blood pressure, heart rate or total femoral flow.

GOODHEAD, HIMAL and ZANBILOWICZ (1970) confirmed the results of DORIGOTTI and GLÄSSER (1968) that not only secretin but also CCK, Urecholine and pentagastrin augment the pancreatic blood flow as well as the pancreatic perfusion rate. The blood flow to the pancreas and other abdominal organs was measured by the radioactive rubidium, ^{86}Rb, fractionation technique. In their experiments, secretin (BOOTS) had a marked stimulatory effect on the cardiac output, and the perfusion rate and blood flow to the stomach, gallbladder, jejunoileum and colon were increased under the action of the above-mentioned stimulants. The action on the pancreas and duodenum was more pronounced. The relationship between an increased secretion rate and increase in pancreatic blood flow was clearly demonstrated.

Glucagon likewise exerts a strong hemodynamic effect, causing an increase in flow by 36% in the ascending aorta and by almost 200% in the superior mesenteric artery (SHOEMAKER et al., 1959). The hemodynamic response to glucagon is not influenced by variations in the blood sugar concentration, or by the presence or absence of the liver. It counteracts the vasoconstriction induced by catecholamines in the mesenteric region but not the vasoconstriction in the skin and the muscle regions (TIBBLIN, KOCK and SCHENK, 1970).

The views presented concerning hormonal influence on the hemodynamic state of the pancreas during secretion have been fully substantiated through recent microcirculation studies (HEISIG 1966, 1968). The author developed a chamber technique for microscopy of the rabbit pancreas *in situ* under physiological conditions and without any displacement of the organs except for the O_2 and N_2O anesthesia and the opening of the abdomen. During intravenous infusion of 10 Ivy dog units/kg/hr of *a 10% pure CCK preparation* there was, in a large series of experiments in the capillaries of the pancreas with a diameter of 10 μ or less, a constant increase in the corpuscular velocity from the mean 848 μ/sec to a mean of 1195 μ/sec. The difference was statistically highly significant. The increase was apparent 3 min after beginning the CCK injection, and there was a return to the initial speed after cessation of the stimulation. There was no change in the diameter of the capillaries, but there was a marked increase, up to 20%, in the diameter of the main arteries and veins of the lobules and their larger branches. There were no changes in the arterial and venous blood pressure or heart rhythm of the animal, and no change in the rhythmically intermittent flow through the capillaries of the gland, or in the lymph vessels. As was to be excepted, zymogen granules were emptied from the acinar cells. *The increased perfusion during increased glandular activity was confined to the pancreatic circulation.* The corpuscular velocity in the capillaries of mesenteric fatty tissue remained the same before, during and after the CCK injection.

Secretin in Pancreatic Angiography

Anticipating an increased flow of blood through the pancreas during the secretory phase, KISSELER, LEISTNER and BARTH (1964a, b; 1965) tried to opacify the pancreas in the roentgenogram after Urografin by combining the ordinary endo- and perigastric gas technique with an intravenous injection of 1 U/kg of secretin. A clearly discernible opacification of the pancreas occurred forty min after injection in each of the 26 subjects studied. In a subsequent communication, KISSELER et al. (1965) reported on 34 cases. The normal tissue filled with blood was distinctly discernible from the surroundings. In 7 cases the technique settled the diagnosis. The technique was modified by TAYLOR, MACKEN and FIORE (1966), who passed a catheter, by means of a percutaneous transfemoral approach, selectively into the celiac and/or superior mesenteric arteries, and injected 150 U of secretin directly into the vascular system of the gland, immediately followed by the contrast medium. In three normal patients studied, an excellent delineation of the pancreatic vasculature was obtained in the arteriographic picture.

Plessier et al. (1967) combined in 25 cases the simultaneous administration of 75 U of secretin and 30—50 ml of the iodinated contrast medium into the coeliac artery with duodenal intubation. In all normal cases the whole gland was visible in the pancreatographic picture with the vasculature clearly discernible.

Rosenbusch and Cen (1969) reviewed the pertaining literature and reported on a series of experiments of their own.

Udén (1969) performed combined celiac and superior mesenteric angiography in 22 patients with and without prior intraarterial secretin injection, 1—2 U/kg. After secretin stimulation the rate of blood flow through the pancreas increased. The mean time for the appearance of opacity in the portal vein was, without secretin, 9.3 sec and with secretin 7.0 sec. The maximal venous phase was reached in the portal vein after an average of 16.7 sec without, and 13.1 sec with secretin. The mean increase in the diameter of the gastroduodenal artery was from 3.8 mm to 4.8 mm, without any widening of the hepatic artery proper. There was a more intense opacification of the pancreas during the capillary phase. The venous phase in the portal vein and its branches was more clearly depicted allowing the two vascular systems of the liver to be studied. The opacification due to a higher degree of contrast filling in neoplastic small vessels and capillaries and around tumors and cysts, as a consequence of the increased number of capillaries opened, was considered by the author to be a valuable diagnostic parameter. He did not, however, share the view of Bennet et al. (1967) that absence of opacification after secretin *per se* would imply carcinoma or pancreatitis.

3. The Action of Secretin, CCK, Gastrin and Glucagon on the Pancreatic Secretion

a) Secretin

The findings of the Pavlov school had clearly indicated that the stimulus exerted by hydrochloric acid in the duodenum influenced the *volume* and the *alkalinity* of the pancreatic juice. The two mechanisms, the humoral and the neural, acting on the pancreatic secretion were also clearly distinguished by Mellanby (1925). "Secretin stimulates the cells of the pancreas to produce a copious flow of a dilute solution of sodium bicarbonate, which carries the pancreatic enzymes with it. The mechanism of the enzymes of the pancreas, however, appears to be under the control of the vagus nerves, and in this respect the results confirm the previous conclusions of Babkin and Savich". The importance of the vagus nerves for the enzyme secretion was demonstrated by Mellanby in an anesthetized cat in which both vagi were cut in the neck; after secretion of two portions of pancreatic juice, 3 ml each, under the influence of secretin, three additional 3 ml quantities were collected. The alkalinity of the juice remained practically unchanged but the enzyme concentration dropped heavily, an effect comparable with that after the intravenous injection of atropine (Table 15).

The function of secretin is, according to Mellanby, to "ensure the presence in the intestine of an adequate supply of sodium bicarbonate to preserve the neutrality of the intestinal contents and thus to secure an optimal medium for the activity of the enzymes."

Table 15. *The bicarbonate and enzyme secretion from the pancreas of an anesthetized cat before and after cutting both vagal nerves* (MELLANBY, 1925)

	Before vagal section		After vagal section		
$NaHCO_3$ N	.134	.138	.138	.132	.128
Trypsinogen	1250	800	330	180	100
Amylase	520	200	75	75	50
Lipase	30	19	9	2	5

The correctness of MELLANBY's view has later on been fully confirmed. HARPER and VASS (1941), THOMAS (1952a, b) and others came to the same conclusion. It could be demonstrated that secretin preparations of different degrees of purity did not affect the basal output of enzymes from the pancreas of dogs (WANG, GROSSMAN and IVY, 1948; PRESHAW and GROSSMAN, 1965a) or of man (LAGERLÖF and WELIN, 1937; LAGERLÖF, 1942; BANWELL, NORTHAM and COOKE, 1967). In their first experiment with highly purified secretin, WERNER and MUTT (1954) likewise found no stimulatory effect on the enzyme secretion, nor did SUN and SHAY (1960), CHEY (1962) and FORELL et al. (1965) working with pure secretin.

After the first injection of secretin a moderate secretion of enzymes is generally observed, usually interpreted as being due to a "wash-out" phenomenon, a flushing out of enzymes already present in the ducts (WANG, GROSSMAN and IVY, 1948). Under prolonged action of the hormone the concentration of proteins in the pancreatic juice falls.

A dissociation of the two components of the pancreatic secretion is observed in the "pancreozymin"-secretin test on children with cystic fibrosis (HADORN et al., 1968). The test, administration of 2 U/kg of each of the hormones with a 20 min interval, was performed on a group of 10 cases with no clinical symptoms of exocrine pancreatic insufficiency. The volume response was small, and the secretion had a very low bicarbonate content but an abnormally high enzyme concentration.

All the different schools are unanimously of the opinion that secretin stimulation results only in a secretion of water with a concomitant exchange of HCO_3^- and Cl^- ions from a state in which their concentration is isosmolar with that of the plasma to a preponderance of HCO_3^- ions at the expense of the Cl^- ions, the sum of their concentrations remaining constant (BALL, 1930b). The sodium and potassium concentrations are equal to those in plasma at any secretory rate (BALL, 1930a, b; BALL et al., 1941; JANOWITZ and DREILING, 1962).

The characteristics of the pattern of external pancreatic secretion were clearly demonstrated by NARDI et al. (1963) in their perfusion experiment with the isolated dog pancreas in situ. The addition every 20 minutes of from 1 to 18 units of secretin to the dog blood used as perfusion fluid was followed by a steady increase in the flow of pancreatic juice with a steep drop in the secretion of enzymes (Fig. 18), whereas the combination of secretin and "pancreozymin", up to 25 units of each, resulted in a constant high volume output, but after 100 min in a sharply reduced output of enzymes. The authors attributed this to enzymatic destruction of the "pancreozymin" during the time of perfusion. It is also possible and more likely that the enzyme—producing capacity of the pancreas was slowly exhausted. It is a common observation that the amount of protein secreted under the action of "pancreozymin" gradually diminishes on repeated stimulation. On the other hand, the gland seems to be able to go on secreting water and bicarbonate under secretin stimulation almost indefinitely as long as the general condition of the animal permits. Thus LALOU (1912), by injecting secretin every 20 min during the course of 8 hours, obtained no less than 1300 ml of pancreatic juice from a 42 kg dog. CARLSON et al. (1916) concluded from their experience that "pancreas is not readily fatigued by secretin".

Following heavy intoxication, however, as after X-ray irradiation of dogs with 500 r, there develops, concomitant with other symptoms of illness, an almost complete inability of the pancreatic gland to react to hydrochloric acid in the duodenum and to exogenous secretin. Secretin formation in the intestinal mucosa is evidently also impaired (KUZNETSOVA, 1963b). After three months, normal conditions were restored.

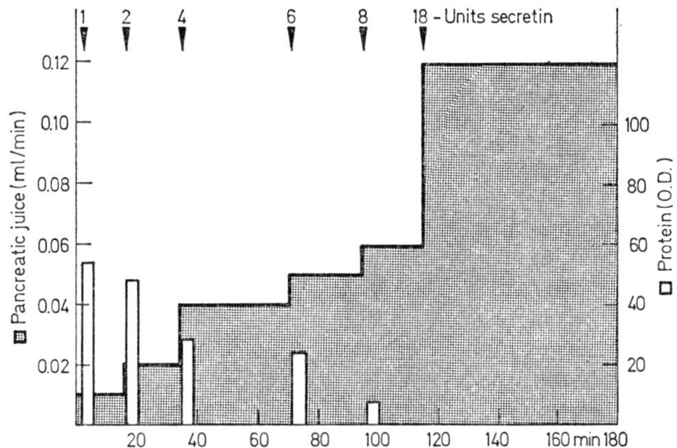

Fig. 18. Effect of secretin on the volume and protein content of secretion from the perfused canine pancreas (NARDI et al., 1963)

After injecting synthetic secretin in dogs, HENRIKSEN (1968) found an increase in the rate of protein excretion from the pancreas lasting for 2 min. A more pronounced effect followed after larger doses, 4—6 U/kg. There was, however, no relation between the secretion rate of protein and the dose of secretin used. When single injections of smaller doses of secretin were superimposed on a background stimulation with the hormone, no increase in the protein secretion rate was observed. The brief increase in the protein secretion was interpreted as a "wash-out" phenomenon.

WORMSLEY (1968a) did not accept the concept of "wash-out" as an explanation for the initial 10 min rise in enzyme output, which then decreases to a plateau level during continued stimulation. According to him, there is a biphasic response to secretin in man; at low levels of stimulation up to 1 U/kg/h there is an increase in the output of trypsin. Higher doses reduce the trypsin secretion.

In studying the relationship of dose and response to pure secretin in chronic gastric and pancreatic fistula dogs, STENING, JOHNSON and GROSSMAN (1969a) found that all doses of secretin were associated with a "wash-out" phenomenon in the first 15 min infusion period and in all periods the output of protein was significantly above the basal level, indicating a weak stimulation of enzyme secretion from the dog pancreas as well.

According to CASE, HARPER and SCRATCHERD (1968, 1970) there is in the cat, in which there is no basal secretion from the pancreas during starvation, a continuous basal secretion, which in the absence of secretin stimulation causes a build-up of enzymes within the duct system and results in the "wash-out" phenomenon.

According to DREILING (1969) experimental findings provide evidence, albeit inconclusive, for a continuous pancreatic secretion in man like that in the dog and unlike the situation in the cat, in which no continuous secretion occurs.

The basal flow is augmented by hormonal, neural and vascular factors. The 24 hour volume is estimated to be 1200—3000 ml; pH 7.5—8.8; Na^+ 138 mEq/litre; K^+ 4.4—5.6; HCO_3^- 60—150 and Cl^- 60—80.

Under the action of secretin the concentration of bicarbonate in the pancreatic juice bears a curvilinear relationship to the rate of flow (BALL, 1930a; HART and THOMAS, 1945; DREILING and JANOWITZ, 1956). At high rates of flow the curve becomes asymptotic at a level of approximately 154 mEq/l, in man and in experimental animals. There is an inverse relationship between the concentrations of HCO_3^- and Cl^- at all rates of flow (BALL, 1930a), their sum equalling approximately 154 mEq/l (WASTELL, RUDICK and DREILING, 1969). The corresponding figure given by MELLANBY (1925) was 140 mEq/l and by BERNIER and LAMBLING (1962) 143 mEq/l. In contrast to the findings in man, the dog and the cat, COMLINE et al. (1969) found the chloride concentration of the pancreatic juice of the horse to exceed that of the bicarbonate concentration at all rates of flow. The bicarbonate concentration did not exceed 60—70 mEq/l. The basal secretion from the pancreas was high.

The question of the pancreatic secretion of fluid and electrolytes with and without hormonal stimulation has been reviewed by JANOWITZ and DREILING (1962), HARPER (1967), JANOWITZ (1967), CASE, HARPER and SCRATCHERD (1968, 1969b, 1970) and WAGNE (1969).

Under all conditions the Na^+ and K^+ ion concentrations in the pancreatic juice correspond to those of the blood plasma, except for the transient increase in the K^+ concentration of the juice from the perfused isolated cat pancreas observed by CASE et al. (1969b, 1970) following a rapid secretin injection. The calcium concentration, 1.3 mEq/l (GOEBELL, HORN, GOSSMAN and BODE, 1970) or 1.7 mEq/l (JANOWITZ and DREILING, 1962), is much lower than that of the plasma, 4—5 mEq/l. It is further reduced under the action of secretin as a result of the water secretion. Following administration of CCK, the calcium concentration of the duodenal contents increases, mainly due to the admixture of bile with its high concentration of Ca, 10—20 mEq/l (GOEBELL, STEFFEN and BODE, 1970; GOEBELL, BODE and HORN, 1970). The latter authors also considered the possibility that calcium is secreted from the acinar cells under the influence of CCK. They found the secretin-stimulated pancreatic juice of conscious and barbital anesthetized dogs to contain 0.6 and 0.8 mEq/l of Ca, concentration being independent of the rate of flow. I.v. injection of 2.5 U/kg of CCK induced a sharp rise in the Ca concentration parallel to the increase in protein content and reaching in the first five minutes of CCK stimulation the same concentration as the ionized plasma calcium, 3—4 mEq/l, the Na^+ and K^+ ion concentrations not being significantly altered.

Working with dogs anesthetized with Pernocton® or Nembutal® intravenously and with the pylorus ligated, LEHNERT et al. (1969) found a straight log dose: volume relationship with an exponential fall of the secretion curve after doses of from 0.5 to 4 CRICK, HARPER and RAPER secretin units/kg.

A linear relationship between the output of pancreatic juice and log dose of secretin was observed on infusing 2—16 U/kg/h to unanesthetized cats with a chronic pancreatic fistula (WAY and GROSSMAN, 1970). The maximal response was for volume 4.8 ml/15 min and for bicarbonate 509 $\pm$ 30 μEq/15 min. The maximal response was not reached with 16 U/kg/h but could be calculated from the dose response curve. Cholecystokinin alone did not elicit a volume response from the pancreas. *In combination with a background of 2.0 U/kg/h of secretin, however, it potentiated the effect of secretin*, varying doses of cholecystokinin, from 2 to 16 U/kg/h, giving a graded increase in volume, bicarbonate, and protein output. The threshold dose of cholecystokinin was lower for volume response than for protein output.

KONTUREK (1969) found 3.2 U/kg/h of the present Swedish secretin to be the dose giving maximal volume and bicarbonate output in the conscious cat.

The three parameters, volume, bicarbonate output and bicarbonate concentration following administration of 0.1, 0.3, 0.9 and 2.7 U/kg of the new standard secretin to 6 healthy subjects were as shown in Fig. 19 (KONTUREK, 1970). The

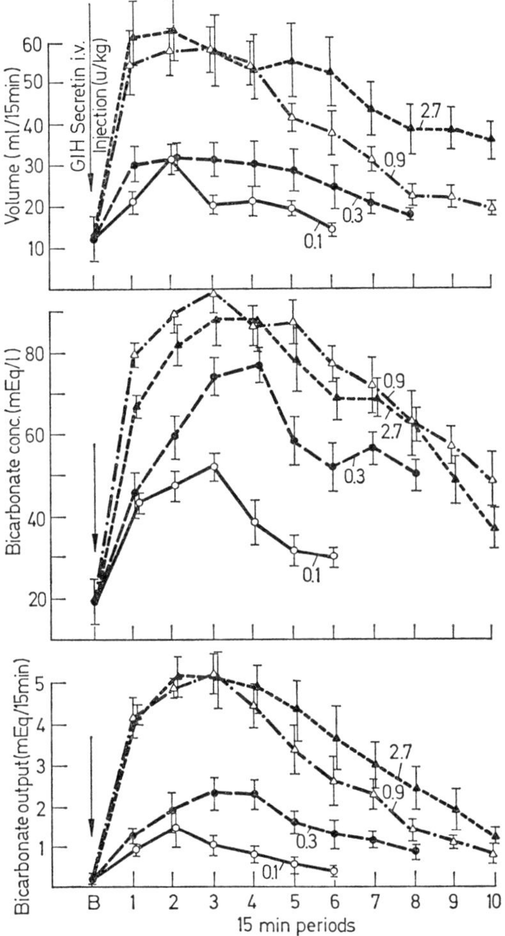

Fig. 19. Pancreatic volume flow, bicarbonate concentration, and bicarbonate output per 15-min period in response to single rapid intravenous injections of different doses of secretin. In this and subsequent figures each line represents the mean of tests performed on the same 6 subjects. The vertical bars indicate the standard error of the mean. In all figures the doses are plotted on a logarithmic scale (KONTUREK, 1970)

author found no difference in the effect whether the secretin was given i.v. in a rapid single injection or as a constant rate infusion.

Maximal flow rates (1.7 $\pm$ 0.1 ml/15 min) in the anesthetized cat were attained by WAY and DIAMOND (1970) with 0.5, 1.0 or 2.0 U/kg of the Swedish secretin. The flow remained maximal for 15 min and subsided within 30—40 min. During the maximal secretion rate the concentration of HCO_3^- was 137 + 7 mM, the Cl^- concentration was 40 mM (Table 16).

Table 16. *Ionic composition of cat serum and pancreatic juice*

	$[Na^+]$	$[K^+]$	$[Cl^-]$	$[HCO_3^-]$
Serum	149 ± 1 (27)	3.6 ± 0.1 (27)	113 ± 3 (17)	24 ± 3 (7)
Secretin-stimulated juice	158 ± 2 (7)	3.3 ± 0.1 (7)	40 ± 3 (7)	137 ± 7 (7)
Resting juice	158	3.3	148	29 ± 3 (25)

The table gives average values (in mM) ± S. E., with the number of determinations in parentheses. The values for $[Na^+]$, $[K^+]$, and $[Cl^-]$ in resting juice are assumed, not measured, values: $[Na^+]$ and $[K^+]$ were taken as equal to the values in secretin-stimulated juice, and $[Cl^-]$ was taken as ($[Cl^-]$ + $[HCO_3^-]$) in secretin-stimulated juice *minus* $[HCO_3^-]$ in resting juice, since the values of $[Na^+]$, $[K^+]$, and ($[Cl^-]$ + $[HCO_3^-]$) in pancreatic juice are independent of flow rate. Way and Diamond (1970).

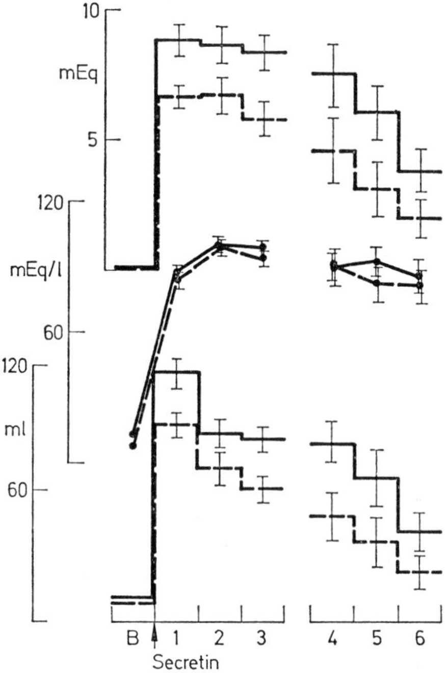

Fig. 20. The mean values with standard errors of the bicarbonate outputs, bicarbonate concentrations, and volumes of duodenal juice collected in 20-minute periods before (B) and after (1—6) an intravenous injection of one clinical unit of pure natural secretin per kg body weight. In 11 females (broken line) and 15 males (unbroken line) the examinations included three post-secretin 20-minute periods. In 6 females and 8 males the examinations were prolonged to include three further 20-minute periods (Petersen, 1970)

Route of Administration of Secretin

Experiments performed with the old secretin preparations showed a poor or no effect when the secretin was administered subcutaneously in cats and dogs (Matsuo, 1912—1913; Mellanby, 1928; Ågren, 1934). Similar findings were made in dogs also with the highly purified secretin (Preshaw and Grossman, 1965b). Later on, however, the pure secretin, the natural as well as the synthetic one, was found to be fully active irrespective of the way of administration, intravenously or subcutaneously both in dogs (VAGNE and GROSSMAN, 1968a) and in man (ISENBERG and GROSSMAN, 1969a) (Fig. 21). There is in the dog a difference in the response. Higher doses were required subcutaneously as compared with intravenously for the same 15 min peak response. But instead after a subcutaneous injection the total response to a definite dose lasted much longer and exceeded that after an intravenous injection. There was in each case a complete parallelism between the volume of pancreatic secretion, the concentration of bicarbonates and the output of bicarbonate with the pancreatic juice. When administered subcutaneously CCK stimulated the enzyme secretion and gastrin both the water, bicarbonate and enzyme secretion.

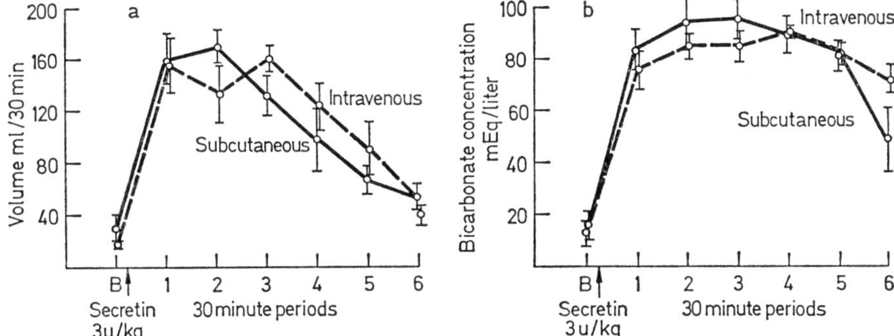

Fig. 21. Pancreatic volume response and bicarbonate concentration per 30 min period. The solid line represents the response following subcutaneous secretin, the broken line represents the response following intravenous secretin, and b represents the basal period. Each point represents the mean of five studies. The vertical lines indicate the standard error of the mean (ISENBERG and GROSSMAN, 1969a)

b) The Function of the Ductular System under the Action of Secretin

CCK and stimulation of the vagus nerve, either alone or in combination, produce morphological changes within the acinar cells, as an expression of their secretory activity (HARPER and MACKAY, 1948; DICKMAN and MORRILL, 1957; NARDI et al., 1963; HEISIG, 1966). Nothing similar is known about the site of action of secretin.

In a preliminary note, JOHANSEN, HADORN and ANDERSON (1968) reported histological changes in the epithelium of the rectal mucosa of children, obtained by rectal suction biopsies 15 min after administering 2 U/kg of secretin. The nuclei of the epithelial cells seemed to be displaced towards the luminal surface and the basilar region of the cells was swollen; the picture was clearly distinguishable from the normal.

GROSSMAN and IVY (1946) *found a markedly decreased responsiveness to secretin in alloxan diabetic dogs.* In four dogs rendered diabetic for 18—30 days by the i.v. injection of 75 mg/kg of alloxan, the threshold dose of secretin was increased tenfold. Their findings were confirmed by TISCORNIA, JANOWITZ and DREILING (1968). Degenerative changes in the intralobular cells and the ductule cells as well as the disappearance of the β-cells from the islets had been observed in alloxan diabetic animals (GOLDNER and GOMORI, 1943). Since *alkaline phosphatase*, secreted with the pancreatic juice, was believed to occur only in the cells lining the ductules and not in the acinar cells (GOMORI, 1941; JACOBY, 1946a, b), it was assumed that it is produced by the ductule cells. The phosphatase could be demonstrated both histologically in the intralobular ducts and in the centroacinar cells of the dog, rabbit and man as well as chemically in the pancreatic juice of the same species (GROSSMAN, WANG and WANG, 1951). In other species, the rat, the guinea pig and the cat, however, the enzyme was not demonstrable in either the tissue or the juice. An attempt to follow the secretion of amylase and alkaline phosphatase during the stimulation of the pancreas with secretin and pancreozymin (WANG, GROSSMAN and IVY, 1970) gave little information as to the site of action of secretin.

Recent findings (WARNES, HINE and KAY, 1970) that alkaline phosphatase occurs in both islets and acini of human pancreas may explain the negative outcome of these experiments.

The study of *the distribution of carbonic anhydrase* in the different types of cells in the pancreas proved to be more informative. The enzyme is concentrated in the ductal epithelium, whereas the acinar epithelium contains very little or none (MANZKE, 1959, quoted by BECKER, 1962). Blocking the enzyme by means of acetazolamide, 2-acetylamino-1,3,4-thiadiazole-5-sulfonamide, Diamox, depresses both the histamine-stimulated gastric secretion of acid in dogs (JANOWITZ, COLCHER and HOLLANDER, 1952) and the fluid outflow and bicarbonate secretion from the pancreas in response to secretin in dogs (HOLLANDER and BIRNBAUM, 1952; BIRNBAUM and HOLLANDER, 1953; JANOWITZ, COLCHER and HOLLANDER, 1952) and in man (DREILING, JANOWITZ and HALPERN, 1955). Acetazolamide, 10 mg/kg, reduced the flow of pancreatic juice and HCO_3^- output to half normal (RAWLS et al., 1963). Severe hyperventilation has a similar effect. About half of the HCO_3^- output normally depends on an uncatalyzed reaction and half on the reaction catalyzed by carbonic anhydrase.

Likewise, acetazolamide reduces the secretin-stimulated bile secretion in man (WAITMAN, DYCK and JANOWITZ, 1969). Working with cholecystectomized patients with a T-tube in the common duct, the authors found that under the action of secretin, 1 U/kg, the bile volume increases by an average of 119%, the bicarbonate output by 283%, the Na^+ and K^+ output by 115% and 104% respectively, the Cl^- by 100%, but, as expected, the taurocholate output by only 16%. There was a 20—40% reduction in these parameters and in the basal bile flow when acetazolamide, 50 mg/kg/h, had been infused during the hour preceding a repeated i.v. injection of the same dose of secretin. The authors accepted the view of WHEELER (1965) that the site of elaboration of the bicarbonate-containing fluid is the bile ductules or ducts distal to the canaliculi.

WHEELER (1965), in discussing the secretion of water and bicarbonate superimposed upon the bile secretion from the liver under the action of secretin, considered it very likely that this secretion takes place in the bile ductules and ducts. He called attention to the observation of ROUS and MCMASTER (1921) that isolated canine bile ducts under some circumstances elaborate an alkaline fluid. His own perfusion experiments could be interpreted to favour this view. Secretin, 2 U/min, injected into the cannulated hepatic artery of 2 unanesthetized dogs consistently gave a larger volume of bile than if the same dose was injected into the splenic vein or a peripheral vein. Other experiments supported the idea that peripheral parts of the ductular system participate in the secretin-stimulated bile secretion.

Likewise, a modification of the primary secretion during its passage down the duct system has been assumed for the pancreatic secretion (HART and THOMAS, 1945; DICKSTEIN and BIRNBAUM, 1960; JANOWITZ and DREILING, 1962; CASE, HARPER and SCRATCHERD, 1969a, b, 1970). The most expressive change is the reciprocal exchange of the HCO_3^- and Cl^- ions, more closely studied by HART and THOMAS (1945) in the dog, by DREILING and JANOWITZ (1959),

JANOWITZ and DREILING (1962) and by BERNIER (1962) in man and by CASE, HARPER and SCRATCHERD (1966, 1968, 1969a, b, 1970) in the cat. The pertinent literature has recently been reviewed by HARPER (1967), by JANOWITZ (1967) and by CASE, HARPER and SCRATCHERD (1968, 1969b).

The latter authors (CASE et al., 1966, 1969a) perfused the main pancreatic duct of the anesthetized cat either with pancreatic juice collected at maximal secretory rates or with fluid having a similar concentration of the essential ionic components. By regulating the rate of flow through the duct, the different secretion rates produced by continuous infusion of secretin at various concentrations could be simulated. When the changes in the bicarbonate and chloride concentrations were plotted against the rate of flow during the perfusion of the duct, curves identical with those for secretin-stimulated pancreatic juice were obtained (Fig. 22).

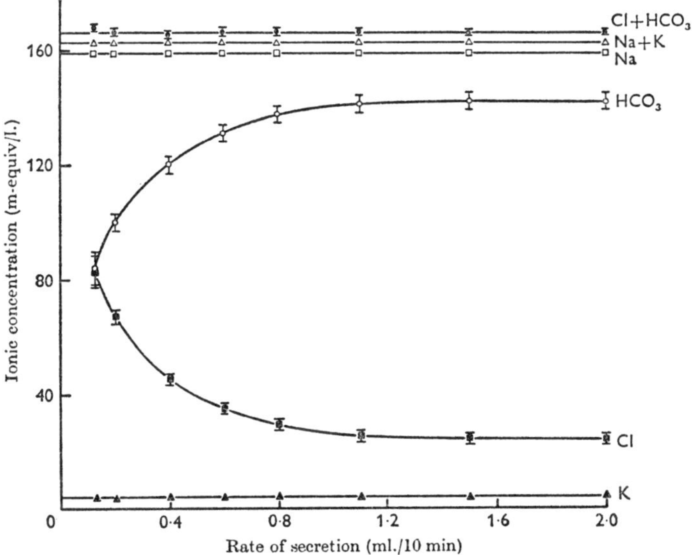

Fig. 22. The electrolyte composition of pancreatic juice at different rates of secretion. In each of six experiments, concentrations of Na^+, K^+, HCO_3^- and Cl^- were plotted against secretory rate, and the best curve fitted by inspection. The concentration at each of eight selected flow rates was combined for all six experiments and the results expressed as mean ±S.E. of mean (CASE, HARPER and SCRATCHERD, 1969b)

WASTELL, RUDICK and DREILING (1969) perfused in a similar manner the duct of the dog pancreas *in situ* from the tail to the head of the gland. Their results were identical with those of CASE et al. (1969a, b). Both groups of authors accepted the view expressed by HART and THOMAS (1945) that the primary secretion consists mainly of a solution of sodium bicarbonate, isosmolar with the extracellular fluid, which is then modified during its passage along the duct system, bicarbonate being exchanged for chloride from the extracellular fluid. At a slow flow rate there is greater opportunity for an exchange, under strong secretin stimulation a juice with the assumed initial high bicarbonate and low chloride concentration is delivered.

REBER, WOLF and LEE (1969) applied the technique of CASE et al. (1969b) in perfusing the main duct of the rabbit pancreas both *in vivo* and *in vitro* in the pancreas chamber described by ROTHMAN (1964b). During perfusion of the main duct, there was, as in the experiments of CASE et al. (1969b), HCO_3^- reabsorption from, and Cl^- secretion into the perfusate, with no net flux of water, Na^+ or K^+. The quantity of ion flux was directly related to perfusion rate. At low rates, the composition of the collected perfusate approached that of the blood or the solution in the bath. The results were similar even when 10^{-5} M DNP was added.

Recent applications of the micropuncture technique have helped in demonstrating the function of the ductular system. In their early micropuncture experiments, REBER and WOLF (1968) could not find any evidence indicating that the ducts of the extralobular collecting system play an active role in the secretion of bicarbonate and chloride. They found the chloride and bicarbonate concentrations in the extralobular collecting system in the anesthetized rabbit, including ductules 58 μ to over 400 μ in diameter, to be the same as in the main pancreatic duct. Samples for analysis were taken with the renal micropuncture technique. The intralobular and the intercalated ducts were not accessible for study.

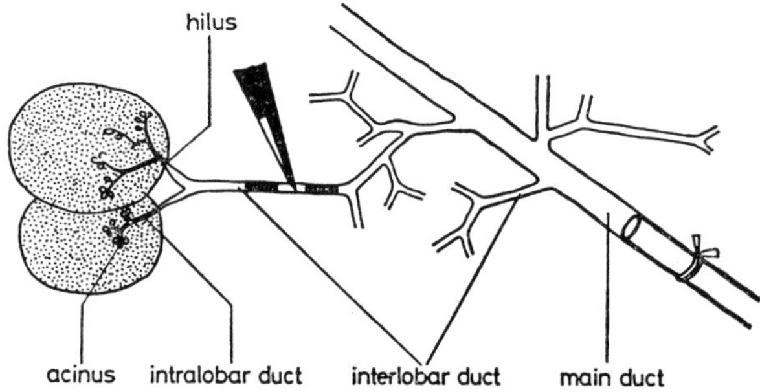

Fig. 23. Scheme of rabbit pancreas and the "stopped flow microperfusion method". An interlobar duct is punctured with a double-barreled pipette, one barrel containing colored ricinus oil, the other one a sample of plasma from the same animal. An oil droplet is injected and split by the plasma sample (SCHULZ et al., 1969)

SCHULZ (1969) used stepwise micropunctures to follow the changes in the composition of the pancreatic juice, arising under the action of secretin, along the ductular system. Microsamples for Cl^- analysis, 1—2 nl, were collected under *free flow conditions from different sites in the duct system* with the technique of ULLRICH and THURAU (1962), and water and bicarbonate ion secretion were studied with the *stopped flow microperfusion* method (SHIPP et al., 1958). In the latter technique, as applied to the rabbit pancreas by SCHULZ, YAMAGATA and WESKE (1969), the pancreatic duct is punctured at different sites with double-barreled pipettes, one barrel containing colored ricinus oil, the other a sample of plasma obtained from the same animal. A small amount of ^3H- or ^{14}C-labelled inulin is added to the plasma sample. After the pancreatic duct is punctured, an oil droplet is injected and split by injecting the plasma sample (Fig. 23). After 3—6 min this sample is withdrawn and analyzed for chloride and for labelled inulin.

The Cl^- concentrations of *free-flow micropuncture samples* after secretin stimulation, 34 U/h in intravenous infusion, were plasmalike in the intralobular ducts and decreased towards the main duct: the mean concentration was 92 mEq/l in the intralobar duct, 90.5 mEq/l at the hilar region, 74.2 mEq/l in the interlobar duct and 62.3 mEq/l at the end of the main duct. The mean chloride concentration of the plasma was 99 mEq/l (Fig. 24). With no secretin stimulation the Cl^- concentration increases towards the main duct. Secretin did not significantly change the Cl^- concentration *in acinar fluid*, mean: 87.4 mEq/l, and after stimulation, 87.6 mEq/l, or the Cl^- concentration in the duct segment near the aciin. With increasing flow rate the Cl^- concentration in the fluid secreted decreases and the HCO_3^- concentration incraeses.

In the *stopped flow microperfusion experiments* the mean Cl^- concentration of the plasma probes injected into the interlobular ducts was, after 3–6 min, 92.4 mEq/l without stimulation and 69.4 mEq/l after subsequent secretin stimulation. The labelled inulin was correspondingly diluted, an expression of the water secretion into the lumen of the interlobar duct diluting the plasma probe.

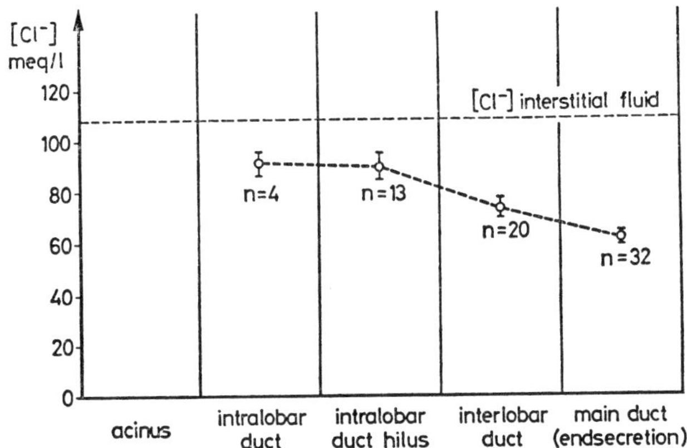

Fig. 24. Free-flow chloride concentrations in micropuncture samples of pancreas fluid. The samples are obtained at different sites of the duct system after secretin stimulation. The chloride concentration of the interstitial fluid is marked by a horizontal dotted line (Schulz et al., 1969)

Very early, attention was drawn to the ductular cell system of the pancreas (Bensley, 1912). The cytological structure of the centroacinar cells that line the alveoli was found to be identical to that of the intralobular duct cell and quite different from that of the acinar cells with their zymogen granules and long mitochondrial filaments. Recent electron microscopic findings likewise support the view that the centroacinar cells, the intercalary duct cells and the intralobular duct cells form a homologous cell system, different from the acinar cells and having a secretory function of their own (Ekholm, Zelander and Edlund, 1962). There are marked similarities in their ultrastructure, with a sparse endoplasmic reticulum and relatively few small mitochondria, details which make it unlikely that they participate in any protein production or high energy requiring process such as osmotic work. The apical surface of all of them has micro-villi, with blebs progressively increasing in number and size towards the intralobular duct cells. The presence of these blebs and intraluminal bleblike formations, according to the authors, could be taken as an indication of secretory activity of the cells.

Having accepted this view of the specific function of the ductular system as producer of the final bicarbonate solution secreted it follows, as pointed out by Thomas (1952b), that the intracellular mechanism for secretion of HCl by the stomach and of bicarbonate by the pancreas may be identical. "If by some trick", he said, "we could turn the cells around so that their luminal border faced the blood stream and the base of the cell the lumen we should be secreting bicarbonate into the lumen and HCl into the blood. The centroacinous cells would have the position that the parietal cells would have if the gastric glands were turned inside out." This is possibly more than an amusing coincidence, the author concluded.

As to the source of energy for the secretion process, CASE et al. (1969b) found in their perfusion experiments with the isolated cat pancreas *in situ* that glucose, lactate or pyruvate are essential components of the perfusion fluid for an undisturbed secretion.

c) The Mechanism of the Water and Electrolyte Secretion from the Pancreas

As to the nature of the action mechanism of secretin, no general concept seems to have been accepted. According to JANOWITZ and DREILING (1962) the participation of carbonic anhydrase in the HCO_3^- production speaks in favour of an active cellular process. CASE et al. (1969b, 1970) pointed out that the carbonic anhydrase inhibitor acetazolamide only reduces the maximal rate of secretion after secretin stimulation but does not alter the pattern of exchange of bicarbonate and chloride as found in their experiments in perfusing the main pancreatic duct of the cat. Referring to their observation that a transient increase in the K^+ concentration of the pancreatic juice occurs following a rapid secretin injection, CASE et al. (1970) stated that "there arises under the action of secretin a disturbance of the intracellular ionic balance which may trigger the active secretory processes, dependent upon a membrane-bound ATP-ase".

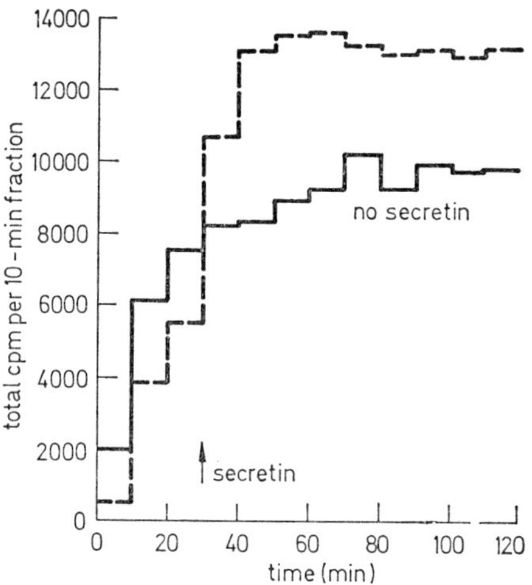

Fig. 25. Effect of secretin (480 U/l bathing fluid) on excretion of ^{22}Na by the isolated rabbit pancreas *in vitro* after addition of 20 μC $^{22}NaCl$ to the bathing fluid. Average increase for four secretin experiments and four control experiments: 39 (S.E.: 2.1)% (RIDDERSTAP, 1969)

An Na^+-K^+-activated ATP-ase, inhibited by ouabain, does occur in the dog pancreas (RIDDERSTAP and BONTING, 1969a, b). The water secretion from the pancreas under the action of secretin, 0.5 U/min by i.v. infusion, was in their experiments on the anesthetized dog reduced by 15, 55 and 86% after cumulative doses of ouabain, 13, 26 and 39 μg/kg respectively, consistent with the assumption that an ATP-ase is an intermediate in the secretion process. There was no change in the bicarbonate concentration. Following secretin administration there is, however, a sudden remarkable increase in the Na^+ excretion with the pancreatic juice as demonstrated by RIDDERSTAP (1969). The addition of secretin, 480 CHR units/l, to the bath resulted in a sudden increase of the sodium excretion, mean 39%, which closely corresponded to the increase in volume, 35% (Fig. 25).

According to the authors, secretin stimulates pancreatic secretion by increasing active sodium extrusion rather than by increasing bicarbonate secretion. The active transport of sodium by means of the Na^+-K^+-activated ATP-ase is assumed to be the primary and rate-limiting step in the fluid and electrolyte secretion by the pancreas, as it is for the secretion of aqueous humor in the rabbit and the cerebrospinal fluid in the cat, as found by other authors. According to this theory, the water follows passively through osmotic equilibration, as has been shown to be the case for the movement of water through the mucosa of the gallbladder and the intestine, and in the ciliary body and the choroid plexus. The enzyme secretion of the pancreas is not coupled to the sodium pump, responsible for fluid and electrolyte secretion (RIDDERSTAP and BONTING, 1969a, c).

Working with an isolated rabbit pancreas mounted together with the duodenal loop and meso-omentum on a polyvinyl-chloride frame and incubated in a plexiglas chamber containing a 95% O_2 and 5% CO_2 aerated Krebs-Henseleit salt solution at 30°C, according to ROTHMAN (1964a, b), ROTHMAN and BROOKS (1965b) followed the secretion when the gland was submitted to Cl^- or HCO_3^--free environments or to a low concentration of Na^+. They presented evidence for the view that the major electrolyte constituents of pancreatic secretion are primarily moved transcellularly and not intercellularly, by filtration and/or diffusion, and may even be the product of a single cell. The "unicellular" model for the gastric secretion of HCl, suggested by DAVIES (1948, 1951), functions for pancreas as a "stomach working in reverse". H^+ ions inside the cell are exchanged for extracellular Na^+ on the membrane facing the blood. The OH^- ions in the cell combine with CO_2 to form HCO_3^-. SOLOMON (1952) interpreted the variation of the ratio $[HCO_3^-]/[Cl^-]$ with the rate of the pancreatic secretion as an expression of active HCO_3^- secretion. The cation transport could, according to him, be either active or passive. ROTHMAN and BROOKS pointed out that Na^+ and K^+ are present in essentially similar concentrations in extracellular fluid and pancreatic secretion. Nevertheless, pancreatic cells separating them exhibit high intracellular K^+ and low Na^+ concentrations. Consequently, two additional concentration gradients are of significance: movement of K^+ from low bath concentrations (approximately 6.0 mM) to relatively high intracellular K^+ concentrations (over 100 mM), and movement of Na^+ from low intracellular concentrations (about 45 mM) to high Na^+ concentrations in the secretion (approximately 150 mM). They consequently assumed that there is active transport of the cations.

WAY and DIAMOND (1970), however, considered an active HCO_3^- transport to be the primary effect of secretin stimulation. The active Na^+ transport, proposed to be a driving force for pancreatic secretion of water and electrolytes by ROTHMAN and BROOKS (1965a, b) und by RIDDERSTAP and BONTING (1969b), seemed to the authors to be less well documented, because almost all mammalian cells possess an ouabain-inhibited, Li-rejecting Na^+-K^+-pump to regulate cell volume and intracellular ion concentrations. Disruption of this pump might well cause failure of other cell functions.

Applying the values for the potential difference between the duct lumen and the blood, and the concentrations of Na^+, K^+, Cl^- and HCO^- in the serum and in the juice during maximal secretin-stimulated secretion in the NERNST equation, the authors came to the conclusion that the effect of secretin must depend upon an active HCO_3^- transport and that the Na^+, K^+ and Cl^- ions diffuse passively into the pancreatic juice. In principle their views were accepted by MAKHLOUF and BLUM (1970). WAY and DIAMOND found the PD between the duct lumen of the resting pancreas and the blood in the anesthetized cat to be $+2.0 \pm 0.3$ mV, the duct lumen being positive to the blood. A dose of secretin, 0.5, 1.0 or 2.0 U/kg, causing maximal secretion, shifted the duct potential in a negative direction by 7 mV to -4.9 ± 0.2 mV, with return to the resting value parallel with the decline in flow of juice.

Earlier measurements of the electric potential difference across the wall of the pancreatic duct made by SCHULZ (1969), SCHULZ et al. (1969) and by REBER et al. (1969) gave similar results except that these authors found the lumen of the duct to be negative to the interstitium even in the unstimulated rabbit pancreas.

d) Cyclic AMP and Pancreatic Secretion

Adenosine 3′,5′-monophosphate, cyclic AMP, has been found to be a mediator in the action mechanism of a number of hormones (SUTHERLAND, ØYE and BUTCHER, 1965; ROBISON, BUTCHER and SUTHERLAND, 1968). The hormone is thought to influence a tissue-specific adenyl cyclase, located in the cell membrane, promoting the formation of cyclic AMP from adenosine triphosphate (ATP). The compound is inactivated by hydrolysis to adenosine -5′-monophosphate by an enzyme, cyclic 3′,5′-nucleotide phosphodiesterase (Fig. 26), which can be blocked in the presence of methyl xanthines.

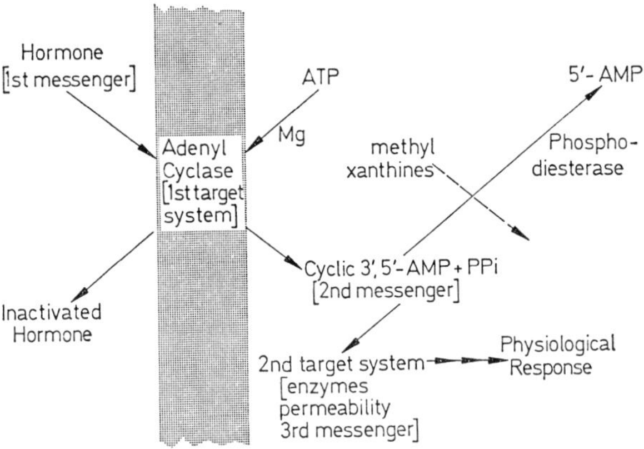

Fig. 26. The role of cyclic AMP as the intracellular mediator of hormone action as envisaged by SUTHERLAND, ØYE and BUTCHER (1965). The shaded area represents the cell membrane

The findings so far indicate that cyclic AMP is also an intermediate in the series of reactions following stimulation of the pancreas cell with secretin or CCK or both. The first communication on this line by KULKA and STERNLICHT (1968) showed that cyclic AMP and its monoburyl and dibuturyl derivatives and theophylline like "pancreozymin" and carbamylcholine in suitable concentrations stimulated amylase secretion from the isolated mouse pancreas. Protein synthesis was not stimulated. Similar findings were made by RIDDERSTAP and BONTING (1969a) and by KNODELL, TOSKES, REBER and BROOKS (1970) using isolated rabbit pancreas, mounted according to ROTHMAN and BROOKS (1965a) in a Krebs-Henseleit bath, pH 7.2, with glucose. Theophylline (10^{-2} M) stimulated protein secretion from the gland maximally by 155%, and α-amylase secretion by 80%. Cyclic AMP (10^{-3} M) increased protein secretion by an average of 64%, while α-amylase secretion was maximally stimulated by 31%. Theophylline (10^{-2} M) potentiated the stimulatory effect of "pancreozymin" (RIDDERSTAP and BONTING, 1969a).

A different view is held by British authors. In a preliminary communication, CASE, LAUNDY and SCRATCHERD (1969) suggested that secretin may act on the pancreatic cell via an intracellular cyclic AMP. On perfusing the isolated cat pancreas *in situ* with saline according to CASE, HARPER and SCRATCHERD (1968), CASE, LAUNDY and SCRATCHERD (1969) found that addition of N^6-2-0-dibuturyl 3′,5′-cyclic AMP (dibuturyl cyclic AMP) at a concentration of 1 mM, to the perfusate stimulates, in the absence of secretin stimulation, a small but sustained flow of pancreatic juice. Theophylline at a concentration of 0.5 mM potentiates this response (Fig. 27).

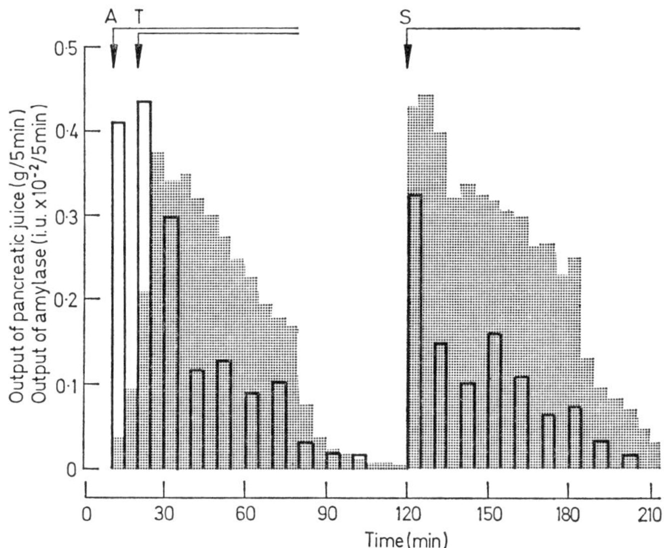

Fig. 27. The output of pancreatic juice (shaded) and enzyme (columns) from a rested, perfused cat pancreas. At A, dibutyryl cyclic AMP (10^{-3}M) was added to 40 ml perfusion fluid, followed, at T, by theophylline (4×10^{-4}M), and this fluid was recirculated through the gland for the length of the bars. At S, 80 μg secretin was added to a further 40 ml fluid, recirculated for the length of the bar. The large output of enzyme associated with the first response, and the smaller output with the second, is probably a "wash-out" phenomenon (CASE, LAUNDY and SCRATCHERD, 1969)

The electrolyte concentration of the pancreatic juice secreted in response to cyclic AMP and theophylline, either alone or in combination, was, according to SCRATCHERD and CASE (1972), the same as that obtained with secretin stimulation at similar rates of flow, but the rate never approached that which is achieved with secretin. A small increase in the output of enzymes in the pancreatic juice following addition of dibuturyl cyclic AMP to the perfusate was interpreted as a wash-out phenomenon.

After the intravenous injection of secretin, either as a single injection or as a continuous infusion, the concentration of cyclic AMP in the pancreatic tissue rises markedly and within 30 sec has trebled the basal level before any visible secretion occurs, and remains elevated as long as secretion is in progress (JOHNSON, SHERRATT, CASE and SCRATCHERD, 1970). If either pancreozymin or acetylcholine is injected during a plateau of secretin stimulation, a further rapid elevation of cyclic AMP occurs within 30 sec, returning to pre-stimulation levels in about one minute, and is accompanied by enzyme secretion. SCRATCHERD and CASE (1972) reviewed the present findings.

In *in vitro* experiments with rat adipose tissue cells and homogenates of isolated fat cells BUTCHER and CARLSON (1970) observed an increase in the concentration of the cyclic AMP in the presence of secretin, 2 U/ml. Coffein acted synergistically with secretin, whereas nicotinic acid and prostaglandin, PGE, were strong antagonists.

In view of the similarities in structure and a number of biological actions between secretin and glucagon RODBELL, BIRNBAUMER and POHL (1970) studied the effect of secretin upon the adenyl cyclase system or systems, known to be potentially stimulated by glucagon in the liver cells, heart muscle and fat cells. The authors selected purified plasma membranes from rat liver and ghosts of isolated rat fat cells for study. The latter contain an adenyl cyclase system which is activated by glucagon, catecholamines and a number of hormones. It is also activated by secretin in half or one third of the concentration valid for glucagon. The two hormones act on one and the same enzyme system. Secretin was also more active than glucagon in stimulating lipolysis in isolated fat cells. Since pretreatment of the adipose tissue with trypsin decreased by 44% the lipolytic response of isolated fat cells to glucagon but had no effect on their response to secretin the authors concluded that the two hormones activate adenyl cyclase via different receptors.

e) Cholinergic Stimulation over the Vagus Nerve of the Pancreatic Secretion.

In a review article THOMAS (1967) discussed the neural regulations of the pancreatic secretion.

Distension of the stomach in the dog, producing an amount of acid in the stomach corresponding to 40% of the maximal response to histamine or gastrin, results in only a small pancreatic response, the increase in volume being only 6% of the maximal response to endogenous secretin (VAGNE and GROSSMAN, 1969). The increase in protein output was 20% of the response to a large dose of exogenous CCK, as could be expected from a neural reflex stimulation.

PINCUS, THOMAS and LACHMAN (1948) found that the pancreatic secretion after a meal was reduced to ½ to ⅓ of normal in dogs submitted to transthoracic vagotomy.

Vagotomy in the dog, leading to an 85% reduction of the acid secretion in the stomach in response to a meal, secondarily causes a similar reduction in the pancreatic secretion of fluid and bicarbonate and a 57% reduction in the enzyme secretion (HENRIKSEN and RUNE, 1969b). On the other hand, vagotomy had no effect upon *the basal pancreatic secretion* in the dog nor did it change the response to exogenous hormonal stimulation (HENRIKSEN, 1969b).

MORELAND and JOHNSON (1970) found transthoracic vagotomy in dogs to significantly reduce the protein secretion in response to secretin and the volume, bicarbonate and protein output after duodenal acidification with 10 and 40 mEq HCl/h.

Electrical stimulation of the vagus nerve just above the diaphragm causes in the conscious dog a significant increase in water secretion from the pancreas with a still greater increase in the enzyme secretion and no change in the bicarbonate concentration (BOURDE, ROBINSON, SUDA and WHITE, 1970b). The authors (BOURDE et al., 1970a) developed a special technique of placing electrodes around the anterior and posterior vagal trunk above the diaphragm in order to reduce the effects of vagal stimulation on circulation, respiration and the sympathetic nervous system. The electrodes stayed in place for 1 to 3 months. The anode was preferably proximal and the stimuli varied between 10 and 30 volts, 10—50 pulses per second with a duration of 1 to 2.5 milliseconds. The three major enzyme groups responded to the vagal stimulation in a strictly paralleled fashion.

In the pig, stimulation of the pancreas through the vagus nerve is extraordinarily strong (HICKSON, 1963). This is consistent with a more prolific parasympathetic innervation of the gland in the pig than in other species. Cholinergic nerves and ganglia do occur more abundantly in the pancreas of the pig than of the dog and cat (COMLINE, HICKSON and MESSAGE, 1964). In the pig, stimulation of the vagus nerves causes a profuse flow of pancreatic juice with a high content of bicarbonate in addition to enzymes. Atropine suppresses the secretion of enzymes but fails to diminish the flow of a bicarbonate-rich juice. Stimulation of the vagus nerve and injection of acetylcholine are effective even after resection of the stomach and the intestine, which excludes a hormonal stimulation (HICKSON, 1970a, b).

f) The Action of CCK on the Pancreas

In their original communication on "pancreozymin", HARPER and RAPER (1943) reported that in the anesthetized cat "pancreozymin" must be given with secretin to elicit a measurable response. They found the secretagogue effect on the pancreas *in vivo* to be unaffected by doses of atropine sufficient to abolish enzyme secretion brought about by cholinergic stimulation.

In a series of papers, HARPER (1946, 1959) and HARPER, BLAIR and SCRATCHERD (1962) reported on the effects of "pancreozymin" and of the vagus nerve on the pancreas. Attention was also paid to the effect on the histological appearance of the pancreas as compared with its appearance during vagal nerve stimulation. It had been shown by BABKIN, RUBASHKIN and SAVITCH (1909) that stimulation of the vagus nerve in the neck elicited histological changes with loss of granulation in the acinar cells of the cat pancreas. Similar observations were made by HARPER and VASS (1941). In a series of investigations, HARPER and MACKAY (1945/46, 1948) and DAVIES, HARPER and MACKAY (1949) demonstrated in cats that stimulation of the dorsal vagus trunk or the administration of "pancreozymin" resulted in a marked decrease in the enzyme granules of the acinar cells. Secretin, even in large doses, caused no histological changes.

CCK has no effect on the volume rate of pancreatic secretion in the cat (CASE et al., 1970). The secretion of water and bicarbonate is due to the action of secretin and therefore the secretory effect of CCK can only be studied during the simultaneous administration of secretin. Under adequate secretin stimulation, 3 clinical units every 30 minutes, we found that 12—48 "pancreozymin" units, as defined by CRICK, HARPER and RAPER (1949), produce an optimal secretion of pancreatic juice, 1.5—2 ml in 15 min, in a cat. Without secretin, however, a dose of 250 units of "pancreozymin" gives not more than 0.1—0.2 ml of juice.

Nor did LIN and IVY (1957) find that administration of "pancreozymin" or parasympathomimetic agents increased the volume of pancreatic secretion sustained in anesthetized pancreatic fistula dogs with 20 U of secretin every 20 min. Only when small doses of secretin are administered can an increase in volume result.

The specific action of CCK on the enzyme secretion from the pancreas has been treated in a review article by HARPER (1967). The total output of protein into the duodenum after CCK is in normal patients linearly related to the log dose of CCK (JORPES and MUTT, 1954; LIN and GROSSMAN, 1956; HANSCOM and LITTMANN, 1963; HANSCOM, JACOBSON and LITTMAN, 1967). In the experiments of the latter authors, the output of enzyme protein after 0.37 to 3 U/kg of CCK was during the first 15 min after the i.v. injection three times that during each of the two following 15 min periods. Secretion was kept up with 1.5 U/kg/h of secretin in infusion. In pathological cases the protein output after the different doses of CCK was about half of the normal output.

Besides proteolytic enzymes, nucleases and alkaline phosphatase are secreted into the duodenum under the action of secretin and CCK (WARNES, HINE and KAY, 1970). The authors found the output of alkaline phosphatase into the duodenum under the action of the hormones to be greatly reduced in complete biliary obstruction as compared with the output in normal persons. The authors made no statements about the purity of the hormone preparations used.

The picture of the pancreatic secretion as outlined by the previous authors may have to be slightly modified in view of the recent findings as to the effect of CCK upon the water and bicarbonate secretion. Pure secretin has been shown to activate the enzyme mechanism of the pancreas in man (WORMSLEY, 1968a, c). Pure CCK, added in an amount of 0.08—0.16 μg/min to the perfusion fluid during perfusion of the isolated canine pancreas in the experiments of HERMON-TAYLOR and BEAUGIE (1972), caused not only an enzyme secretion but also a rise both in the volume flow of pancreatic juice and in the bicarbonate concentration. The latter increased from 41 mEq/l to 71 mEq/l during the course of 30 min stimulation. Like secretin pure CCK causes an immediate vasodilation in the perfused gland accompanied by an increase in metabolic activity.

Events on the subcellular level in the enzyme-secreting cells of the pancreas under the influence of "pancreozymin" are dealt with in a separate chapter of this volume (Chapter III, p. 195). Previous review articles dealing with this topic were published by SCHRAMM (1967) and by ROTHMAN (1969).

Recent electron microscopic studies of the subcellular elements of the acinar cells during the different phases of hormone stimulation have given a fairly clear picture of the intracellular transport of the secretory proteins from their site of synthesis, the rough endoplasmic reticulum, to the zymogen granules. All the subcellular organelles involved in the protein transport can be isolated and accounted for by labelling with ^{3}H-leucine. The transport is an enzymatic process, inhibited by low temperature but highly dependent upon mitochondrial energy production. JAMIESON (see Chapter III) considers the transport to be independent of stimulation by CCK. The cholinergic stimulation exerted by CCK acts primarily on the mechanism leading to the discharge of the content of the zymogen granule into the ductular lumen. This process involves movement of the granule to the cell apex followed by fusion of the granule membrane with that of the cell surface (PALADE, 1959).

Not only the transport, but also the synthesis of the enzyme proteins can be uncoupled from the discharge process (HOKIN and HOKIN, 1962). The refilling of the load of enzyme proteins after CCK stimulation follows at a later moment than the maximum of secretion (WEBSTER, 1969b). Even the intracellular transport can be uncoupled from protein synthesis. In the presence of a dose of cycloheximide which blocks the protein synthesis by $>95\%$, the transport goes on with 75—80% efficiency.

The literature dealing with the early attempts to follow the incorporation of labelled amino acids into proteins and ^{15}N-glycine or ^{14}C-orotic acid or ^{3}H-uridine into nuclear fractions under cholinergic stimulation of the pancreas cell has been reviewed by WEBSTER (1969b) and MORISSET and WEBSTER (1971). In summarizing the findings of the previous authors and his own results, WEBSTER stated that when secretion is stimulated *in vivo* by cholinergic agents, protein synthesis is also initiated. Using *in vitro* systems, a dissociation of the secretory and the synthetic processes is observed. Cholinergic drugs and "pancreozymin" have a secretory effect but no effect on either RNA or protein synthesis (SCHUCHER and HOKIN, 1954; HOKIN and HOKIN, 1962; DICKMAN, HOLTZER and GAZZINELLI, 1962; YANG and DICKMAN, 1966).

Besides the synthesis and turnover of zymogen proteins *a synthesis of certain phospholipid fractions takes place in the acinar cells under the action of acetylcholine or "pancreozymin"* as convincingly demonstrated by HOKIN and HOKIN and their coworkers (HOKIN and HOKIN, 1956; HOKIN, L.E., 1967; HOKIN, M. R., 1968). A synthesis of membrane phospholipid can be observed both in the GOLGI and the rough surfaced endoplasmic reticulum (HOKIN and HUEBNER, 1967). The cholinergic stimulation accelerates the turnover of phosphatidylinositol and phosphatidylethanolamine but not that of phosphatidylcholine (see RUBIN, 1967).

g) The Trophic Effects of the Gastrointestinal Hormones

A trophic effect resulting in an increased synthesis of proteins, including enzymes, in the secretory glands has been demonstrated for the cholinergic drug, carbamylcholine, and for CCK, gastrin and pentagastrin.

"Pancreozymin", 20 U/kg, when injected subcutaneously 3 times a day for 4 days in rats, caused in the experiments of ROTHMAN and WELLS (1967) a significant increase in the weight of the pancreas, from 800 to 1350 mg, attributable to hypertrophy of pancreatic acinar cells. In the enlarged pancreas, tissue concentrations of trypsinogen, chymotrypsinogen and amylase were significantly increased. Secretin, 20 U/kg, or metacholine, 5 mg/kg, administered in the same way had no such effect.

The incorporation of ^{14}C-leucine into homogenates of gastric and duodenal mucosa of rats *in vitro* increases by at least 100% if the animals have been pretreated with pentagastrin 60 min before killing (JOHNSON, AURES and YUEN, 1969). Likewise, the intraperitoneal introduction in rats of ^{14}C-leucine together with doses of human synthetic gastrin (20 µg/kg) or pentagastrin (250 µg/kg), known to give 80–90% of the maximal acid secretory response, resulted within 2 hours, after which time the animals were killed, in an 11 to 32% stimulation of protein synthesis in tissues from the duodenum and stomach but had no effect on liver or skeletal muscle (JOHNSON, AURES and HÅKANSON, 1969).

A marked effect on the *growth of the parietal cell system*, with no effect whatsoever on the peptic cells, was exerted by pentagastrin (ICI 50,123) in rats equipped with chronic gastric fistulas (CREAN, MARSHALL and RUMSEY, 1969). Pentagastrin, 2×2 mg/day for 21 days was administered in depot form. During the third week of the period there was a 4-fold increase in the acid output, an increase in the height and weight of the fundic mucosa, in the number of parietal cells per unit area of the mucosa and in the total number of these cells. Histamine, 2×6 mg/day administered in the same way in a second group, caused no morphological changes but doubled the acid output. In spite of the high rates of acid secretion, there was no evidence of peptic ulceration.

The course of reactions following administration of labelled L-^{14}C-valine during carbamylcholine (CCh) stimulation of the rat pancreas *in vivo* was demonstrated by MARCHIS-MOUREN and REGGIO (1970). During the first 180 min of the intraperitoneal infusion of CCh there was a reduction of the amylase, lipase and protein content of the pancreas due to enzyme secretion. The incorporation of L-^{14}C-valine into amylase and total protein was slow during the first 100 min of stimulation and very intense during the period 100 to 200 min after starting the infusion. "Pancreozymin", 3 U/kg/h when perfused alone or with secretin, 3 U/kg/h, increased the amylase and protein synthesis tenfold as compared with the controls. Perfusion of secretin alone had no effect. Nor did „pancreozymin" modify the rate of valine incorporation into liver proteins. As to the action mechanism of "pancreozymin", the authors left it an open question whether the effect on enzyme synthesis is direct or indirect, stimulated by a feed-back mechanism when the enzyme content of the gland is lowered.

WEBSTER and TYOR (1966) studied the incorporation of labelled L-^{14}C-phenylalanine into slices of pigeon pancreatic tissue incubated for 60 min in a bath containing a suitable amino acid mixture and glucose. If the bird had been sacrificed 60, 90 or 120 min after administering 50 units of "pancreozymin", incorporation was constently twice or more than twice that when saline had been injected in similar experiments. As an expression of the secretory effect of "pancreozymin" there was, besides the protein synthesis, a decrease in the pancreatic tissue amylase.

As a result of subsequent studies along this line (SAHBA, MORISSET and WEBSTER, 1970) a modification of this view seems to be desirable. CCK in doses from 10 to 100 IVY dog units/kg invariably caused a strong amylase secretion from the pancreas of the birds. After treatment the amylase content of the gland tissue was reduced. In slices of the pancreas from birds pretreated with CCK, 40 U/kg, 30 to 120 min prior to sacrifice, no increase of incorporation of ^{14}C-L-phenylalanine over the controls was observed. At first a dose of 100 U/kg caused in slices from fasted birds the same increase of incorporation as produced by feeding. The conclusions to be drawn are consistent with the view expressed by HOKIN and HOKIN 1962) that *secretion and synthesis in the pancreatic tissue are independenly controlled processes and that secretion may proceed without synthesis.* Likewise MELDOLESI (1970) concluded from experiments, performed with caerulein, 2.5 ng/ml, in vitro with slices of guinea pig pancreas, that stimulation of the pancreas secretion does not affect *per se* the rate of synthesis of digestive enzymes. Only a prolonged treatment of fasted animals with caerulein resulted in an increased incorporation of labelled L-leucine.

LEROY, MORISSET and WEBSTER (1971), however, found a close correlation between the synthetic and the secretory responses of the rat pancreas in vivo after administration of CCK. There was furthermore an almost linear increase in L-phenylalanine-^{14}C incorporation into protein after intraperitoneal single injections of CCK in doses ranging from 1 to 4 U/kg. Maximum incorporation occurred with 8—16 U/kg.

In similar experiments with pancreatic slices from pigeons treated 45 min before killing with 50 units of "pancreozymin" i.v. or 1.25 mg methacholine i.m., WEBSTER, GUNN and TYOR (1966) found an increased rate of oxidation and incorporation of ^{14}C-labelled palmitate into triglyceride and phospholipid as compared with experiments with slices from starved animals. The changes in the lipid metabolism corresponded to those found in slices from birds fed ad libitum. *The authors concluded that "pancreozymin" and methacholine not only are associated with extrusion of zymogen granules from the pancreatic acinar cell but in addition cause an increase of the rate of pancreatic lipid metabolism.*

„Pancreozymin" influences like Urecholine upon the metabolism of the transfer RNA inhibiting the incorporation of labelled orotic acid into the heavy nuclear fraction of RNA. It did not inhibit the incorporation into the ribosomal precursor type of nuclear RNA (DICKMAN and YANG, 1966; YANG and DICKMAN, 1966).

h) The Action of Gastrin on the Pancreas

According to BLAIR, HARPER, LAKE, REED and SCRATCHERD (1961a), a crude extract of minced and boiled *hog antral mucosa*, precipitated with 20 volumes of acetone, yield 11 mg/g mucosa, gives in a dose of 5.5 mg in the vagotomized, anesthetized cat 0.67—2.0 m.eq. HCl, depending upon the rate of infusion, and a small output of pepsin. The same dose greatly increased the *output of pancreatic enzymes* without having any effect on the volume of pancreatic secretion. The preparation was claimed to be free of any cholecystokinin-like activity. As an expression of endogenous hormone stimulation, the same effect was observed after introduction of meat extract in the antrum or distension of the stomach or the antrum of the cat (BLAIR, CLARK, HARPER, LAKE and SCRATCHERD, 1961b). The active principle was considered to be an *antral pancreozymin* (HARPER et al., 1962; HARPER, 1963). These findings were confirmed by PASSARO and GROSSMAN (1963) who found that irrigation of a separated pouch of the pyloric gland area of the stomach with acetylcholine or liver extract stimulated secretion from a transplant of the pancreas to the mammary gland of the dog.

The pancreozymin-like activity of the antral extracts paralleled their ability to cause acid secretion by the stomach (BLAIR, HARPER, LAKE and REED, 1963), a clear indication that the active component of the extracts was gastrin. In their first communication on *pure gastrin*, GREGORY ynd TRACY (1964) also reported that a dose of 50 μg of both gastrins I and II caused an increase in pancreatic secretion in conscious and anesthetized dogs. Because of the similarity in the chemical structures of gastrin and CCK, with the C-terminal pentapeptide and a nearby sulfated tyrosine unit in common (Fig. 11), it is to be expected that gastrin, like CCK, should preferentially stimulate the enzyme secretion from the pancreas, which has also been found to be the case.

Working with crude extracts of hog pyloric mucosa, PRESHAW and GROSSMAN (1965a) first excluded any interfering action of histamine. An intravenous infusion of 4 mg/hr of histamine dihydrochloride, which caused a strong acid secretion from the stomach of a conscious fistula dog, had only a slight initial stimulatory effect on volume flow and bicarbonate output by the pancreas. The values quickly returned to the control levels, provided that the gastric secretion had been effectively drained through a gastric fistula. In contrast, the gastrin preparation exerted a long-lasting stimulus on the pancreas. A crude gastrin preparation, given in infusion in a dose equivalent to 2.5—10 g wet pyloric mucosa, which produced 6.07 m.eq/15 min of gastric acid, caused a pancreatic secretion of 8.2 ml with 270 mg of protein per 15 min as compared with the volume 12.5 ml/15 min containing 373 mg of protein obtained after administering 75—150 IDU of CCK. Similar extracts made from the fundic mucosa did not stimulate pancreatic secretion.

Further evidence for hormonal stimulation of the pancreatic secretion by antral products was presented by PRESHAW, COOKE and GROSSMAN (1965a, b). In dogs with a transplanted pancreas, stimulation of the antral pouch with acetylcholine chloride caused a gastric secretory response and an increase in protein output by the pancreas. In other dogs with a total pancreatic fistula and a transplanted antral pouch, a pancreatic and a gastric secretory response were observed on perfusion of the antral pouch with acetylcholine chloride or liver extract. Both gastric and pancreatic responses were abolished by acidification of the antral pouch.

The effect of *pentagastrin* on pancreatic secretion in the dog was found by EMÅS, BILLINGS and GROSSMAN (1968) to be similar to that of gastrin. The dose of gastrin or pentagastrin that produced maximal bicarbonate and protein responses from the pancreas also produced maximal or close to maximal acid responses from the stomach. In man, pentagastrin produces no demonstrable bicarbonate or protein response from the resting pancreas (WORMSLEY, MAHONEY and NG, 1966). Against a low background stimulation with secretin, however, a rapid intravenous injection of the pentapeptide increased both bicarbonate and protein output, but the dose required was higher than that producing maximal gastric acid response.

Likewise VAGNE (1970a) found that pentagastrin causes only an insignificant increase in the volume and bicarbonate secreted by the pancreas of a patient carrying a pancreatic fistula.

PETERSEN, BERSTAD and MYREN (1971) failed to show in 3 healthy subjects any significant effect of i.v. infusion of pentagastrin (0.15, 0.9 and 5.4 μg/kg/h) on resting and secretin (0.1, 0.5 and 2.5 U/kg/h) induced pancreatic secretion of bicarbonate and enzymes.

The same applies to the *decapeptide caerulein*, which with the exception of a single amino acid, threonine in caerulein and methionine in CCK, shares the C-terminal octapeptide with CCK. In comparing the two gastrins and caerulein with CCK with respect to their action on the pancreatic flow, protein output and bicarbonate output in dogs with gastric and pancreatic fistulas, STENING and GROSSMAN (1969a) found that on a molar basis caerulein was on intravenous infusion about 3 times as potent as CCK, and gastrins I and II one-third as

Table 17. *Pancreatic flow, protein output, and bicarbonate output in response to various stimulants* (STENING and GROSSMAN, 1969a)

Parameter	Test Substance	Basal	Dose, μg/kg-hr		
			Gastrin I and II		
			1.0	2.0	4.0
			Caerulein		
			0.03	0.15	0.75
			Cholecystokinin		
			0.67	1.33	2.67
Flow, ml/15 min	Gastrin I	0.6 ± 0.2	2.1 ± 0.6	2.9 ± 0.5	4.3 ± 0.5
	Gastrin II	0.4 ± 0.1	2.3 ± 0.6	3.1 ± 0.7	3.8 ± 0.5
	Caerulein	0.6 ± 0.1	1.2 ± 0.4	2.9 ± 0.7	4.2 ± 0.6
	Cholecystokinin	0.6 ± 0.1	1.7 ± 0.3	2.9 ± 0.7	3.9 ± 0.4
Protein output, mg/15 min	Gastrin I	31.5 ± 3.9	179.9 ± 20.1	273.2 ± 29.6	356.3 ± 25.6
	Gastrin II	29.7 ± 4.7	173.7 ± 16.0	267.1 ± 15.5	366.8 ± 10.7
	Caerulein	40.8 ± 4.6	84.8 ± 8.3	283.4 ± 31.2	442.6 ± 27.2
	Cholecystokinin	30.6 ± 4.2	169.9 ± 22.4	292.3 ± 17.2	393.1 ± 47.4
Bicarbonate output, mEq/15 min	Gastrin I	26.6 ± 6.9	105.9 ± 19.5	169.5 ± 31.2	290.7 ± 46.9
	Gastrin II	29.1 ± 7.6	117.7 ± 27.1	157.9 ± 27.5	285.4 ± 19.9
	Caerulein	23.2 ± 8.2	62.7 ± 8.5	223.3 ± 25.1	282.5 ± 36.7
	Cholecystokinin	21.9 ± 5.2	78.1 ± 21.9	198.9 ± 22.3	362.5 ± 57.5

Values are means ± SEM. N = 6.

potent as CCK for enzyme secretion, and caerulein about 3 times as potent as CCK and the gastrins one-half as potent as CCK for pancreatic flow (Table 17). ANASTASI and coworkers (1968) had found that on a weight basis caerulein was 15 times as potent as CCK and 50 times as potent as human gastrin I as a stimulant of pancreatic volume flow in the dog. The corresponding figures found by STENING and GROSSMAN (1969a) were, expressed on a weight basis, 9 times and 11 times, respectively.

The threshold dose for stimulant action on the pancreatic secretion in the dog is, according to BERTACCINI et al. (1969), 1—5 ng/kg by rapid i.v. injection, 0.25—1 ng/kg/min by i.v. infusion and 50—100 ng/kg by subcutaneous injection.

i) Effect of Glucagon on the Pancreatic Secretion

According to NECHELES (1957) glucagon depresses the external pancreatic secretion in *anesthetized dogs*. At first there is a transient stimulation of secretion in 30 to 70% of the animals after an intravenous dose of 6—40 µg/kg or 40—570 µg/kg, respectively. A depression followed in practically all the tests and lasted for 15—120 minutes. In some tests, pancreatic secretion ceased entirely for up to 100 min. Injection of glucose, 0.5 g/kg, produced no change or a slight decrease in pancreatic secretion.

Glucagon, 2 mg, given intravenously *in man* induces hyperglycemia but does not, according to DREILING et al. (1958), affect the rate of flow, bicarbonate concentration or the rate of enzyme secretion by the pancreas in patients with or without pancreatic inflammation. Likewise KAESS, BRECH and SCHLIERF (1968) found after intravenous administration of 7 µg/kg of glucagon in healthy normal subjects no change from baseline levels in the secretion of bicarbonate and amylase from the pancreas, whereas blood glucose and plasma insulin rose rapidly. The reaction after secretin BOOTS, 1 U/kg, was as expected.

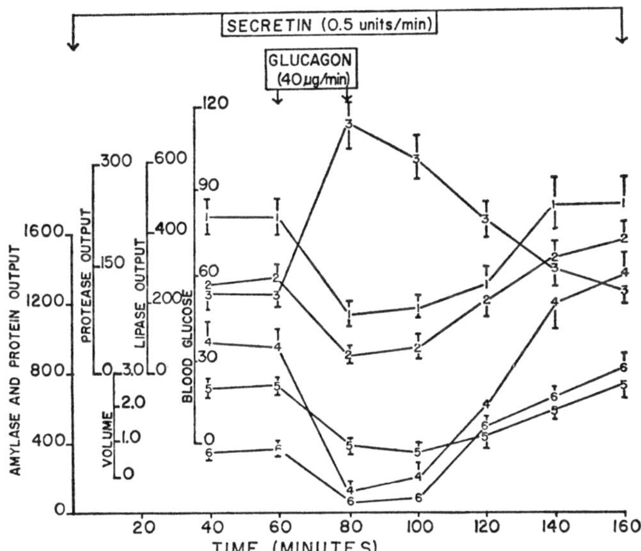

Fig. 28. Effect of glucagon (40 µg/min i.v.) on blood glucose, and volume and contents of pancreatic secretion. Each point represents the mean of 12 experiments in 12 dogs; the vertical bars indicate S.E. of the mean. (1) Lipase, $\times 10^{-4}$ mEq NaOH/5 min. (2) Protease, mg tyrosine/5 min. (3) Blood glucose, mg/100 ml. (4) Amylase, mg maltose/5 min. (5) Pancreatic juice, ml/5 min. (6) Protein, $\times 10^{-3}$ mg bovine albumin equivalent/5 min (NAKAJIMA and MAGEE, 1970c)

ZAJTCHUCK et al. (1967), however, found in 2 patients with an external pancreatic fistula following trauma, that infusion of glucagon, 40 µg/kg, decreased the volume and amylase output of pancreatic juice by 90%. The blood sugar level during the infusion was 200 mg/100 ml, a level which causes only a 10—15% reduction. First on increasing the level to 400 mg/100 ml did the volume and amylase concentration drop by 60% to 70%.

In dogs supplied with Thomas cannulas opposite to the bile duct and the major pancreatic duct and under constant endogenous secretin stimulation, induced by HCl perfusion of the duodenum, 1 mg i.v. of glucagon caused within 15—30 min a doubling of the control bile flow with a porportional increase in Na^+, Cl^- and HCO_3^- output (SWEETING, 1968). From the pancreas, however, there was a reduction in flow volume by 30—60% of the control level, with corresponding reduction in Na^+ and HCO_3^- outputs. There was a return to normal after 1—1½ h.

DYCK et al. (1969, 1970) administered glucagon by single intravenous injection in doses of 1.0, 5.0, and 10.0 µg per kg to 7 subjects after a steady state of pancreatic secretion had been reached during continuous intravenous infusion of secretin (3 U/kg/h) and CCK (1 U/kg/h). 1 µg/kg reduced both volume and protein concentration and 5 µg/kg caused near maximal suppression of both parameters.

Nor did glucagon produce any significant stimulation of the secretion from the resting pancreatic gland in the dog (DYCK et al., 1969).

NAKAJIMA and MAGEE (1970c) found that an i.v. infusion of 1.9 ml/min of 40% glucose produced in unanesthetized fistula dogs a reduction of secretin-stimulated (0.5 U/min) pancreatic secretion, with respect to volume, protein, amylase, lipase and protease output, almost identical to that produced by an infusion of 40 µg/min of glucagon (Fig. 28).

j) Other Hormonal Influences on Pancreatic Secretion

In analogy with the reduction in rate of salivary flow under the influence of the antidiuretic hormone *vasopressin* (KRAINTZ, 1960), ADH depresses secretin-stimulated or histamine-stimulated pancreatic secretion (PERKS, SCHAPIRO and WOODWARDS, 1964). It is active in a threshold dose of 4.2 mU/kg in conscious dogs carrying a Thomas duodenal cannula allowing cannulation of the pancreatic duct. There is a straight line log dose-response relationship up to 33 mU/kg and 75% inhibition of the secretion stimulated by 1 U/kg of secretin. The blood flow through the pancreas is not affected. Simultaneous with the resorption of water there is an isosmotic reabsorption of electrolytes from the lumen of the tubules, the sodium, potassium and bicarbonate concentrations of the pancreatic juice remaining constant. Oxytocin, even in large doses, had no such effect.

In similar experiments with conscious dogs carrying pancreatic and gastric cannulas BANKS et al. (1967, 1968) found during the first 5 min after injection of 2—32 mU/kg of ADH an 18—44% reduction in volume of the response to 1 U/kg of secretin and a 4—19% reduction in bicarbonate concentration after 8—32 mU/kg. With secretin given in intermittent doses there was an 18—30% rise in potassium concentration and a rise of 45% in 10 min samples after 32 mU/kg of ADH.

In a patient carrying an external pancreatic fistula for 5 months after drainage of a pancreatic pseudocyst, somewhat resembling Mr. MARTIN, Doctor BEAUMONT's Canadian trapper, SCHAPIRO et al. (1967) were able to study the influence on the pancreatic secretion of oral alcohol, exogenous and endogenous secretin, pitressin and anticholinergic drugs. In 2 studies the authors found that 35 mU/kg of pitressin caused a 37% decrease and 50 mU/kg a 56% decrease in volume of the basal pancreatic secretion, which had been 6—53 ml/30 min. Atropine and cholinergic drugs likewise reduced the volume of the basal secretion.

ADH is assumed to increase the permeability of cell walls and membranes by enlarging pore size, possibly by stimulating production of cyclic adenosine 3′,5′-monophosphate, which increases the permeability of membranes to water (WAKIM, 1967).

k) Influences on Iron Absorption

A number of authors (vide PLESSIER et al., 1967; DAVIS and BIGGS, 1967) have studied the effect of the pancreatic secretion, whether stimulated by a meal or by means of secretin and cholecystokinin, on iron absorption. Most authors found a reduction of iron uptake. Thus BENJAMIN, CORTELL and CONRAD (1967) found that 25 CRICK units of a crude secretin, given intraperitoneally to guinea pigs 15 min prior to, and then 30 and 75 min following an oral dose of labelled ferrous sulfate, reduced the iron absorption by 50%. The bicarbonate ions of the pancreatic juice are said to chelate with the ferrous ions. Of course there are many pitfalls involved in studying the absorption and metabolism of iron and these complicate our understanding the events in this situation.

A very unclear picture was obtained by KAVIN et al. (1967) in experiments with double isotope radio-iron in 83 rats, 16 dogs and 40 adult patients. Only in rats did "pancreozymin" (10 U) alone or with secretin (20 U) diminish iron absorption. No depression was observed with secretin alone or with smaller doses of the hormones or when the iron dosage was increased from 10 to 100 μg.

l) Secretin and the Flux of Ions through the Intestinal Epithelium

In contrast to the effect of secretin upon the pancreatic and bile secretion, an i.v. submaximal dose of secretin, as determined by its action on the pancreatic exocrine activity, fails to influence the net fluxes of bicarbonate, chloride, sodium or potassium in fluid perfusing the ileum of the rat (HUBEL and COLBERT, 1967).

II. Secretin, Glucagon, CCK and the Brunner's Glands

In their extensive studies on the physiology of Brunner's glands, FLOREY and HARDING (1935a, b) presented convincing evidence that their secretory activity is controlled by a humoral mechanism, in which secretin seemed to be the active agent. They found that impure intestinal extracts and crude secretin preparations stimulated the flow of liquid from these glands. FOGELSON and BACHRACH (1939) in confirming their results suggested that the secretion could be secondary to an increase in motility. The field was covered in two early review articles by GROSSMAN (1958a) and by GREGORY (1962).

Using dogs with innervated pouches of the Brunner's gland area, COOKE and GROSSMAN (1966) found that fundic extracts, jejunal extracts, crude gastrin, crude secretin preparations of the kind used by the above-mentioned workers and a CCK-PZ preparation containing 250 IVY dog units per mg were potent stimulants of both motility and secretion in the Brunner's gland area. Pure samples of gastrin I and of secretin, however, were inactive. Rapid intravenous injection of crude secretin evoked a dose-related secretory response. The juice contained pepsin in low concentration and a lower bicarbonate concentration than blood plasma. Urecholine stimulated motility without any secretory response. The contemporary state of the question about the hormonal regulation of the secretion from Brunner's glands was reviewed by COOKE (1967).

In 1968 LOVE, WALDER and BINGHAM, however, found pure and synthetic porcine secretin to be fully active as stimulants of the secretion from a transplanted denervated duodenal pouch of the dog (Fig. 29). In a subsequent study, STENING and GROSSMAN (1968, 1969b) demonstrated that synthetic secretin, pure gastrin, pure cholecystokinin and caerulein stimulated secretion from Brunner's gland pouches in both cats and dogs. Maximal responses to secretin, 2 μg/kg/h, were 0.8 ml/15 min in dogs and 0.7 ml/h in cats, compared with the highest rate of secretion, 1.0 ml/15 min and 0.7 ml/h respectively attained by ad libitum feeding. CCK, 4 U/kg/h, and caerulein 0.15 μg/kg/h evoked a somewhat smaller volume response.

In continuation of these experiments, LOVE et al. (1970) confirmed that secretin in adequate doses is an effective stimulant of Brunner's gland secretion in dogs and cats. The response to secretin is sustained for the duration of the intravenous infusion of the hormone. A high initial secretion in response to a CCK infusion, not sustained on continuation of the infusion, could be a result of the stimulation of duodenal motility exerted by CCK.

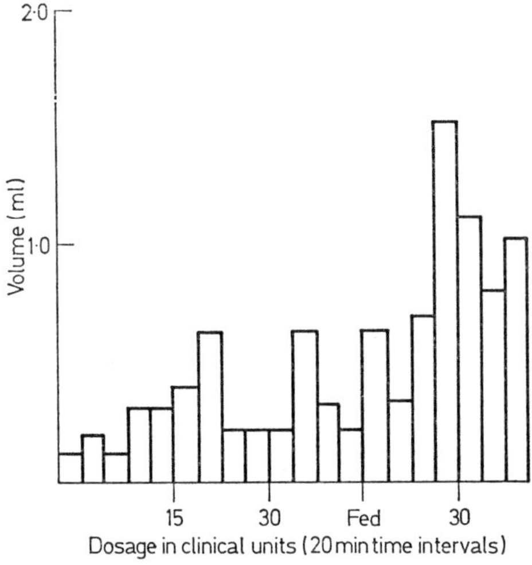

Fig. 29. Duodenal secretion in response to synthetic secretin and to feeding in the same dog (LOVE et al., 1968)

Glucagon infused into conscious dogs with a proximal duodenal pouch caused in doses of 8 to 64 μg/kg/h a dose related increase in the volume of secretion from the duodenal pouch (STENING and GROSSMAN, 1969b). The maximal response 1.4 ml/min was produced by 64 μg/kg/h of glucagon. Glucose infusion did not stimulate the pouch secretion nur did oral glucose administration (JONES and HALL (1969).

III. Action of the Gastrointestinal Hormones on the Liver and the Gallbladder

1. The Influence of the Hormones on the Bile Flow

a) The Ågren–Lagerlöf Effect

In working with the secretin test, ÅGREN (1934) and ÅGREN and LAGERLÖF (1937) found that a few minutes after injecting secretin intravenously in normal subjects, the bile-stained duodenal juice became colourless and remained so for 10—20 minutes. Evidently the gallbladder takes up all the bile and concentrates it for storage temporarily. The continuous presence of bile in the duodenal juice during the course of the secretin test would therefore indicate either the absence of the gallbladder or an abnormally functioning one. The authors suggested that this detail be used for the study of the functional state of the gallbladder.

LAKE (1947) considered this test of gallbladder function to be comparable to LYON's method and to GRAHAM's test (GRAHAM and COLE, 1924). SNAPE, FRIEDMAN and SWENSON (1948) found a high degree of correlation between the findings in the cholecystogram and those in the secretin test with an indwelling duodenal tube. In 55 of 65 patients the conclusions drawn from cholecystography and the secretin test were the same and fitted well with the clinical diagnosis. DUNCAN et al. (1953) confirmed the findings of ÅGREN and LAGERLÖF. MARKS (1959) found the variations in the icteric index of the different 10 min. portions of the duodenal aspirates during the 60 minutes following a secretin injection and the 20 minutes following a subsequent "pancreozymin" (cholecystokinin) injection to conform to a characteristic pattern in patients in whom the biliary tract and the pancreas were normal, with a filling of the gallbladder during the post-secretin hour and gallbladder emptying following the subsequent administration of "pancreozymin". If the gallbladder is absent or nonfunctioning, the bilirubin content of the different portions of the duodenal fluid is constant.

b) The Choleretic Effect of Secretin

At the time of the discovery of secretin, French authors described the choleretic effect in bile fistula dogs of perfusing the duodenum with dilute hydrocholric acid, and interpreted it as being partly due to a nervous reflex stimulation in the old Pavlovian sense and partly to a humoral transmission (WERTHEIMER, 1903; FALLOISE, 1903; FLEIG, 1903).

In their very first communication on secretin, BAYLISS and STARLING reported stimulation of bile secretion from the liver by secretin. Later on a number of authors reported similar findings (LA BARRE and GOFFIN, 1937 and GROSSMAN, 1950, ref. no. 1, 2, 135, 186, 286, 287, 296, 328, 383, 427, 431). MELLANBY (1927) believed that metabolic products of pancreatic activity pass into the portal blood, stimulating the liver cells to secrete bile. That this cannot be the case was demonstrated by STILL, MCBEAN and RIES (1931) and by TANTURI, IVY and GREENGARD (1937). They observed the same effect even after removal of the pancreas in the cat and the dog or after anastomosing the portal vein with the inferior vena cava by means of a Crile cannula.

STILL and coworkers found that the effect on the liver was parallel to that on the pancreas as the strength of the secretin preparations was increased; the increase in bile volume, however, was only $^1/_7$ of the increase in the pancreatic secretion. Likewise LUETH and KLOSTER had found in 1928 that a vasodilatin-free secretin in doses of 1 mg gave in the dog, after a latent period of 7—9 minutes, an increase in the bile flow approximately 10 per cent of the increase in the flow of pancreatic juice.

Unwilling to engage in a discussion as to the possible effect of CCK, shown three years earlier by IVY and OLDBERG to be present in the crude secretin preparations, STILL et al. (1931) of the Physiology Department, University of Chicago, claimed that their own experiments "express valid evidence that secretin *per se* is the agent stimulating the flow of bile". Under the influence of their purest secretin preparations the total amount of the bile acid secreted in chronic bile fistula dogs was increased, but not in proportion to the increase in bile volume. The effect of secretin was considered to be due to a direct stimulation of the hepatic cells and not to local or general circulatory changes.

In cholecystectomized dogs with the cystic duct and the accessory pancreatic duct ligated (see THOMAS, 1950), FRIEDMAN demonstrated that secretin injections regularly doubled the output of bile in fasting animals but caused no additional secretion of bile once the animal was in a digestive phase. FRIEDMAN and SNAPE (1945) considered the possibility that there are two substances affecting the liver, one affecting the liver only, *hepatocrinin*, and secretin, acting on both the liver and the pancreas.

MELLANBY and SUFFOLK (1938) found in the *anesthetized cat* a 50% increase in the volume of the bile under secretin stimulation without any increase in the excretion of bile salts, that is, a purely hydrogogue action of secretin.

GROSSMAN, JANOWITZ, RALSTON and KIM (1949) found a similar increase in the bile secretion *in man* after intravenous injection of 15 mg of a purified Eli Lilly secretin in five female cholecystectomized patients with choledochus fistulas. The preparation had a 20 times higher potency than that of the S_I secretin of IVY et al. (1930b), 0.7 mg of which corresponded to one dog dose or one clinical unit. The amount of secretin injected should thus correspond to 428 clin. u., a dose about 6 times larger than that used in the ordinary secretin test in man. The authors consistently found an increase in the volume of bile excreted, lasting for 80 minutes, the largest increase for each patient within any twenty-minute period ranging from 60 to 325% of the average basal secretion. The increase in the volume of bile was accompanied by a parallel decrease in viscosity and in the cholic acid and bilirubin concentrations.

Extending the studies of WHEELER and RAMOS (1960) on the influence of bile salts on the formation and excretion of bile, PREISIG, COOPER and WHEELER (1962) studied the effects of intravenous secretin in *unanesthetized fistula dogs*. During a constant infusion of 1.3% sodium taurocholate solution in 5% dextrose, 2.5 units of the Eli Lilly secretin were administered per min intravenously with or without simultaneous infusion of the cholinergic blocking agent, pipenzolate methylbromide, 0.1 mg/kg/5—10 min. The excretion rate of the taurocholate itself was approximately equal to the rate of infusion and it was unaltered by either secretin or pipenzolate methylbromide administration. Irrespective of whether the blocking agent was given, secretin elicited at all levels of taurocholate excretion nearly constant increments in chloride, bicarbonate and water output, about 0.3 μEq/min, 0.25 μEq/min and 0.3 ml/min respectively. The chloride and bicarbonate concentrations of the bile were increased.

The old secretin preparations, however, with the possible exception of a few of STILL's, HAMMARSTEN's and HARPER and MACKAY's (1948) preparations, were highly impure, containing less than one pro mille of secretin. The secretin preparations of ÅGREN (1934) and of GROSSMAN et al. (1949) probably all contained CCK as well, irrespective of the authors' claims to the contrary. Since CCK preparations stimulate bile secretion to the same extent as does a meal (PLESSIER, 1960; EDHOLM, JONSON and THULIN, 1962), a prerequisite for the interpretation of the earlier findings was that pure secretin should become available.

As soon as secretin preparations free of CCK were obtained, WERNER and MUTT (1954) administered the highly purified secretin intravenously to an anesthetized dog and found a 50 per cent increase in the basal rate of bile flow. Using a similar preparation of ours, THOMAS found an approximately 100 per cent increase over the basal flow in cholecystectomized dogs with bile fistulas (personal communication). EDHOLM, JONSON and THULIN (1962) and JONSON, SUNDMAN and THULIN (1964) performed a series of experiments with *the pure porcine secretin* in unanesthetized cholecystectomized dogs provided with a new type of permanent common duct fistula (JONSON, 1963) allowing the 24 hour bile volume under standard conditions to be measured with a standard deviation of about 5%.

After a 23 to 27 hours' fast the bile flow was determined during 6 to 10 hours, during which period secretin, cholecystokinin or a normal meal supplemented with bile was given. Secretin and CCK were given by continuous intravenous infusion. The volume of the basal bile flow during ½ hour, amounting to about 2—4 ml, was designated by n. A definite increase over the basal flow was obtained in two dogs after giving in intravenous infusion about 2½ U/kg/h of secretin. By increasing the dose of secretin up to 10 U/kg/h the n value was slightly more than doubled. A further increase had only an insignificant effect.

Taking into account that a fairly large dose of secretin is necessary to double the volume of bile over the basal flow in the unanesthetized dog, as compared with the 3—6 times the basal volume obtainable in connection with a meal supplemented with bile, JORPES et al. (1963, 1965) concluded that secretin can hardly play an important role as a stimulant for normal bile secretion.

The experiments of GROSSMAN et al. (1949) and of PREISIG et al. (1962) left the question open as to what extent secretin participates in the stimulation of bile secretion in man. This uncertainty could be eliminated when similar experiments were performed using the pure natural porcine secretin (SCRATCHERD, 1965; JONES and GROSSMAN, 1969). SCRATCHERD (1965) found a tenfold increase in the bile secretion of *the cat* after injection of 0.5 μg, 2 U, of the pure natural porcine secretin. As a result of stimulation with secretin the bicarbonate concentration of the bile increased linearly with the rate of flow. JONES and GROSSMAN used fistula dogs. The bile was collected through a polyethylene tube inserted 5—6 cm into the common bile duct through a Thomas cannula in the duodenal wall. The gastric secretion was collected through another Thomas cannula inserted into the stomach. Throughout each experiment a continuous intravenous infusion of 0.15 M NaCl containing 0.5% sodium taurocholate was given. The lowest dose of secretin, 0.0625 U/kg/h, was doubled for each successive experiment until 8 U/kg/h had been given, and two experiments were performed in each of three dogs for each of the 8 doses. The test substance, secretin or histamine dihydrochloride, 40, 80 and 160 μg/kg/h, was infused during 8 15-min periods and the means taken of the values for volume, bicarbonate, chloride, bile acid, sodium and potassium concentration of the bile, obtained during the last six 15-min periods. The rate of bile flow increased with increasing doses of secretin. It reached twice the basal level of secretion after a dose of 1 U/kg/h of secretin and was three times the basal value after 8 U/kg/h. The mean bicarbonate concentration of the bile rose from 27 mEq/l to between 45 and 58 mEq/l for all the doses above 0.0625 U/kg/h. The bicarbonate output rose proportionally with increasing secretin doses, from 60 to 403 μEq/15 min. There was a similar increase in the chloride concentration of the bile, which rose from 80 to 110 mEq/l. The increase in the ionic concentration of bicarbonate and chloride was counterbalanced by a corresponding fall in the concentration of bile acids, from 60 to 20 mEq/l. Histamine exerted similar although not identical effects. At low rates of flow the electrolyte composition of bile stimulated by histamine is different from that of bile stimulated by secretin. As a choleretic, secretin was on a molar basis 29,000 times more potent than histamine.

In general the figures given for the increase in volume of the bile secretion in dogs correspond to those found by EDHOLM et al. (1962) and by JONSON et al. (1964). The discrepancy in the dose necessary to double the secretion volume, 10 U/kg/h as given by JONSON et al. instead of 1—2 U/kg/h as found in the experiments of JONES and GROSSMAN (1969), can be explained as being due to the use in the earlier series of a secretin assayed against a standard which had only 25% of the potency of the standard preparation used in our laboratory from the beginning of 1966.

Fully identical results with regard to the bile flow and bicarbonate output were obtained when synthetic secretin was administered in similar experiments to unanesthetized fistula dogs (VAGNE, STENING, BROOKS and GROSSMAN, 1968) and to sheep (HEATH, 1970).

In a series of 10 patients with low level T-tube drainage after cholecystectomy, KONTUREK, DABROWSKI, ADAMCZYK and KULPA (1969) studied the effect of the pure GIH-secretin, 1 U/kg/h in intravenous infusion, upon the flow of bile and the concentration and output of bicarbonate. The volume was elevated to threefold the basal level during 1½ h and the bicarbonate output with the bile was increased fivefold during the same period. The concentration of bile salts slightly decreased and the output of bile salts was significantly increased. The gastrin-pentapeptide, 8 μg/kg/h, and histamine. 2 HCl, 40 μg/kg/h, administered in the same way did not influence the bile flow or the bicarbonate output.

In analyzing bile from 10 patients with a T tube in the common bile duct after cholecystectomy, WAITMAN et al. (1969) found the electrolyte composition to resemble that of the plasma. Secretin augmented the flow and stimulated the secretion of a bicarbonate rich fluid. The effect was partially inhibited by prior infusions of the carbonic anhydrase inhibitor acetazolamide.

Contrary to the findings in man, the dog, the hog, the cat and the sheep no choleretic effect could be observed after administering secretin or CCK to rabbits (AFFOLTER, PILLER and GUBLER, 1964; SCRATCHERD, 1965) or to rats (CLODI and SCHNACK, 1967). AFFOLTER et al. worked with series of unanesthetized rabbits with indwelling cannulas for the collection of the bile and the gastric secretion. After a 20 min control period, 2.5, 5, 10 or 20 units of secretin or CCK were given intravenously in addition to the continuous infusion through the gastric fistula of 0.2 ml/min of rabbit bile. The samples of secretin and CCK in doses of 1—10 U/kg exerted the expected effects on the pancreatic secretion, but *neither secretin nor CCK produced a constant choleresis* or any definite electrolyte changes, whereas Decholin, 100 mg/kg, induced, as expected, a 200% increase in bile secretion with depression of the chloride and bicarbonate concentrations of the bile.

Similar experiments were performed by SCRATCHERD (1965). The infusion into *rabbits* of active secretin preparations in no instance resulted in choleresis. Secretin prepared from rabbit intestine was active in this respect in the cat but not in the rabbit.

According to ERLINGER, DHUMEAUX, BENHAMON and FAUVERT (1969), however, the bile secretion, which is independent of the secretion of bile acids, is in the rabbit and probably also in the rat and the guinea pig even larger than the corresponding fraction of the dog bile, making up about 60% of the spontaneous bile flow of the rabbit.

Likewise, CLODI and SCHNACK (1967) were unable to demonstrate any choleretic effect of secretin or CCK in *bile fistula rats*.

Working with bile fistula rats ROZÉ and FELDMANN (1971) found no choleresis whatsoever after secretin. Intravenous infusion of 0.8 Harper units/min of pancreozymin during 25 min, however, caused a 30% increase in the flow of bile and an excess secretion of bile salts. According to the authors a hormone stimulated secretion from the ductular system seems to be lacking in this animal species.

In one respect the composition of secretin-stimulated bile differs from that of the pancreatic juice. In the former there is ordinarily an increased chloride concentration leading to an increased excretion of chloride, whereas the secretin-stimulated pancreatic secretion shows a drop in chlorides with an inverse relationship between the bicarbonate and the chloride concentrations. However, a bile secretion of the latter type with no change in the cation concentration was observed by HARDISON and NORMAN (1967) on perfusing the isolated hog liver with blood (Fig. 30). There was an adequate response to 1 CRICK unit of secretin/kg liver and a straight line relationship between the log dose of secretin and the volume of bile secreted up to a dose of 100 units of secretin. This type of secretion differs markedly from the bile secretion stimulated by bile acids.

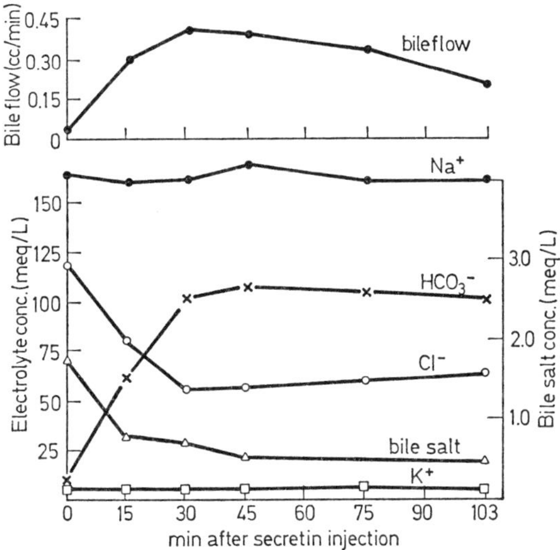

Fig. 30. Sequential changes in bile flow and electrolyte concentrations after injection of 100 units of secretin. As bile flow increases, bicarbonate concentration rises and chloride concentration falls. Bile salt concentration, low before injection, declines further after injection (HARDISON and NORMAN, 1967)

In similar liver perfusion experiments performed with hog livers, DOUGLAS et al. (1969) found that neither gastrin, gastrin pentapeptide, nor cholecystokinin (pancreozymin) influenced hepatic bile production, whereas secretin in doses even less than 0.1 U was found to be a potent hydrocholeretic. The smallest concentration of secretin in the portal vein which produced an increase in bile flow was only half of the concentration necessary in the hepatic artery.

In perfusion experiments with isolated calf liver, PISSIDIS et al. (1969) found secretin to have a significant hydrocholeretic and a direct hepatocyte stimulating effect. In contrast to the findings of NAHRWOLD, COOKE and GROSSMAN (1967) that stimulation of the gastric antrum induces choleresis in the dog and of MORRIS, SARDI and BRADLEY (1967) that glucagon does the same, the authors unexpectedly found that other proposed biliary secretagogues, Urecholine, gastrin and glucagon have no effect on the bile flow in the isolated calf liver preparation.

Secretin has so far been shown to have a choleretic effect on the liver in man, the dog, the cat and on the perfused isolated hog liver. No effect was seen in the rabbit or in the rat. In dogs, man and cats secretin causes a constant increment in the water, bicarbonate and chloride output regardless of the basal bile flow. *The increment is approximately constant at all levels of bile salt secretion, indicating the addition of an alkaline solution to the bile by a process altogether independent of the main bile production associated with bile acid secretion* (Wheeler, 1965; Brooks, 1969).

In sheep secretin, both exogenous infused into the portal vein and endogenous after duodenal acidification, stimulates the volume and bicarbonate output of bile to a greater extent than that of the pancreatic juice, the reaction thus being reversed to that in the dog, where the effect of secretin on the bile flow is only 10—20% of the effect on the flow of pancreatic juice (Caple and Heath, 1971). Nor was there any considerable difference between the responses to portal and jugular injections.

c) The Site of Action of Secretin on the Liver Tissue

As evidenced by the experiments of Preisig, Cooper and Wheeler (1962), Scratcherd (1965) and Jones and Grossman (1969), the bile secretion superimposed under the influence of secretin upon the cholate-induced basal secretion is of a different nature. In their extensive study of the stasis bile in man, Rous and McMaster (1921) came to the conclusion "that the duct walls, though intimately related to the tissue forming the bile, themselves secrete a fluid that is colorless even when the animal is jaundiced. The ducts fail to concentrate and thicken the bile with mucus, as the gallbladder does, but dilute it slightly with a thin secretion of their own that is colorless and devoid of cholates. It is slightly alkaline to litmus, clear, almost watery, practically devoid of cholesterol and of low specific gravity", all details that fit the properties of the liquid secreted under the influence of secretin both from the pancreas and the liver.

Likewise Sperber (1959) in his monograph on the secretion of organic anions in the formation of urine and bile stated that "it would seem that the bile duct system, including the finest branches, may be expected to have some modifying influence, especially with regard to biliary bicarbonate and chloride concentration, which are known to vary considerably both within and between different vertebrate groups".

Further evidence indicating that secretin acts upon the duct system was brought forward by Wheeler (1965), Wheeler and Mancusi-Ungaro (1966). Trained, unanesthetized, cholecystectomized dogs were infused with secretin via indwelling catheters in a hepatic artery, the splenic vein and a peripheral vein. The increments in bile flow were 1.5 times greater during hepatic arterial than during splenic venous infusion and 1.2 times greater during splenic venous than during peripheral venous infusion. Since the bile ducts are supplied mainly by the hepatic artery this suggests, according to the authors, that secretin acts mainly on the duct system. Furthermore the speed with which the indicator substance sulfobromophthalein was washed out during secretin or taurocholate choleresis suggested that the process responsible for secretin-induced choleresis occurs in some part of the biliary tract distal to the canaliculi.

Clinical observations of various kinds can also be taken as further evidence for the ductular origin of the non cholate-induced bile secretion. According to Erlinger and Preisig (1969), Erlinger et al. (1969) hydrocholeresis has been observed in cases of congenital malformations with dilation of the intrahepatic bile ducts. Likewise patients with preoperative bile duct obstruction show, besides the cholate-induced bile secretion, an additional large biliary output of a fluid rich in bicarbonate and chloride supposed to originate in the distended biliary tree (Preisig, Bucher, Stirnemann and Tauber, 1969; Stirnemann, Bucher and Preisig, 1969).

Thus all evidence so far available indicates that the processes leading to an increase in volume and bicarbonate concentration of the bile under the action of secretin take place in the duct system of the liver.

d) Stimulation of the Bile Secretion by Cholecystokinin

The experiments of HARDISON and NORMAN (1967, 1968) in using isolated hog liver and of PISSIDIS et al. (1969), who used calf liver, showed that secretin has a fairly strong choleretic effect on the isolated liver.

Recent perfusion experiments, using isolated canine pancreas and liver, indicate that CCK, as compared to secretin, is a rather weak stimulant of the bile secretion (HERMON-TAYLOR and BEAUGIE, 1972). A dose of 0.08 μg/min of pure CCK, perfused into the hepatic artery, which is maximal for the stimulation of secretion from the perfused pancreas, causes an increase in gallbladder pressure but has only a slight choleretic effect. A 60 times larger dose, 5 μg/min, was necessary to increase the basal secretion of bile within 10—15 min from 0.9 to 1.3 ml/5 min. Simultaneously there was a rise in the concentration of bicarbonate and chloride in the bile. Hepatic arterial vasodilation only occurred when the hormone was injected directly into the artery, not when released into the portal vein. Nor did the dose influence upon the metabolic state of the perfused canine liver.

A more pronounced effect in this respect was observed in earlier experiments in cholecystectomized bile fistula dogs (JORPES et al., 1965). In these series the presence of secretin in the CCK-preparations could have contributed to the outcome of the experiments. The elimination of the interplay between neural and hormonal stimulations in the isolated liver may also be of some significance.

e) Action of Gastrin on Bile Secretion

In discussing the question about the supposed "antral pancreozymin", BLAIR et al. (1961a), HARPER et al. (1962) reported that their antral preparations had little or no effect on the gallbladder tone or the hepatic bile flow. Furthermore, GREGORY and TRACY (1964) found that pure G I and G II given in a dose of 50 μg intravenously to lightly anesthetized cats and dogs caused only a slight rise in gallbladder tone (1—2 cm water) subsiding in a few minutes, and only a slight increase in the flow of hepatic bile, thus a reaction of a quite different order of magnitude than that after CCK.

In a subsequent communication, TRACY and GREGORY (1964) pointed out the difference between gastrin and CCK by stating that neither of the gastrins causes contraction of the gallbladder, nor does either significantly influence the rate of flow of hepatic bile. ZATERKA and GROSSMAN (1966), however, found that a dose of 4 μg/kg/h of G II given in intravenous infusion produces a choleresis like that after secretin in unanesthetized cholecystectomized dogs with a total gastrectomy. The concentration and output of bicarbonate in the bile were increased although not to the same degree as after secretin. Histamine-stimulated bile secretion behaved differently, the bicarbonate concentration being lowered and the chloride concentration increased.

That the pyloric antrum is the source of a choleretic agent released by vagal stimulation was demonstrated by JONES and BROOKS (1965, 1967), who showed that antrectomy in the dog abolished the choleretic response to insulin hypoglycemia.

Likewise, NAHRWOLD, COOKE and GROSSMAN (1967) found that perfusion of a separated antral pouch in the dog with acetylcholine at pH 7.0 caused a choleresis with increased bicarbonate concentration and output as well as a gastric acid secretion. If the perfusion fluid containing acetylcholine had a pH of 1.0, no response followed.

The choleretic effects of CCK, caerulein and gastrin II were determined in conscious fistula dogs by Vagne and Grossman (1968b) and by Jones and Grossman (1970). Each of the peptides produced increased bile flow and bicarbonate concentration with the relative choleretic potency decreasing in the order caerulein, CCK and gastrin II. The commonly used dose ranges were for caerulein 0.006—0.75 μg/kg/h, for CCK 1—8 unit/kg/h and for gastrin II 0.5—2.0 μg/kg/h.

f) Glucagon and Bile Secretion

In accordance with the similarity in structure between secretin and glucagon, the latter also induces bile secretion (Morris, Sardi and Bradley, 1967). Within 15 min after injection of 1 mg of crystalline glucagon into conscious, cholecystectomized dogs with a Thomas duodenal cannula, the bile flow increased two- to three-fold. The biliary output of taurocholate was increased by 50%. The Na^+, Cl^- and HCO_3^- output with the bile rose two- to three-fold. In all there was an increased secretion of taurocholate and an addition of fluid similar to that produced by secretin.

Jones et al. (1971) found secretin 5—6 times more potent as a choleretic than glucagon.

The i.v. dose of *caerulein* causing an increase in bile flow with increased HCO_3^- and Cl^- excretion is 0.1—0.5 ng/kg/min (Erspamer, 1972).

2. Action of CCK, Gastrin, Glucagon and Secretin on the Gallbladder

a) The Action of CCK on the Gallbladder

The action of CCK on the gallbladder has been dealt with in a series of review articles (Ivy, 1930, 1934; Grossman, 1950, 1968; Plessier, 1960). Although the active material usually made up only 0.1‰ of the old preparations, access to 1%, 10% and 100% pure preparations did not essentially change the picture as to the action of the hormone on the gallbladder. During the course of 15 min there is after 1 Ivy dog unit/kg i.v., as found in a series of 15 normal persons (Edholm, 1960), a progressive evacuation of up to 35% of the content of the gallbladder (Fig. 31). The average of the total amount of bile expelled was 45% of the initial volume, which varied between 60 and 14 ml, average 33 ml. Lescut (1963) found on an average a 50% reduction of the shaded area of the gallbladder in normal cholecystographies. According to Cozzolino et al. (1963), 50—80% of the content of the normal human gallbladder is evacuated in 15 min. Refilling of the gallbladder begins after another 15 min.

In studying a material of 96 Koreans, Park, Pae and Hong (1970) found that the gallbladder of healthy individuals contracts to 55% of its initial volume in 15 min and to 20.8% in 60 min after a fat meal and to 23.4% in 15 min and to 21.4% in 30 min after 1 IDU/kg of CCK.

Young healthy people seem to always react to 1 IDU/kg of CCK i.v. with a contraction of the gallbladder. In larger cholecystography series, however, about 15% of the patients have a non-reacting gallbladder (Tomenius et al., 1958; Tomenius and Backlund, 1959; Lescut, 1963). Cholelithiasis without infection does not in general affect the reactivity of the gallbladder to CCK.

The C-terminal octapeptide of CCK shares the pharmacological properties of the original molecule, acting directly on the smooth muscle cell of the gallbladder, but indirectly via a nervous pathway on the ileum. Its molar activity on the gallbladder and the ileum *in vitro* is comparable to that of caerulein, about 3 times that of CCK and 1000 that of pentagastrin (HEDNER, 1970).

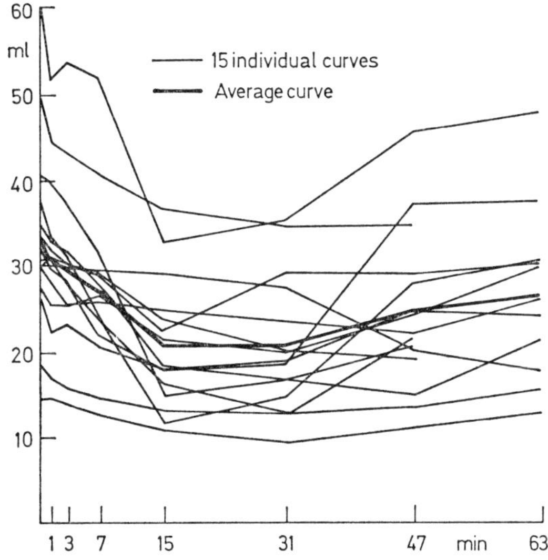

Fig. 31. Changes in gallbladder volume after injection of 75 U of CCK intravenously during the course of 30 sec in healthy young persons (EDHOLM, 1960)

The activity on a molar basis of *porcine gastrin II* on the gallbladder is, according to AMER (1969), only 3—5% of that of CCK. The synthetic gastrin pentapeptide was found to be only weakly cholecystokinetic. Caerulein possessed about half the molar activity of CCK in the 3 assay systems applied by the author (Table 18).

Table 18. *Relative molar potency* of the different cholecystokinetic peptides on three systems as determined by parallel line assays* (AMER, 1969)

Peptide	Relative molar potency*		
	Isolated rabbit gallbladder strips	Isolated guinea pig gallbladder	Exposed guinea pig gallbladder *in situ*
Cholecystokinin	1	1	1
Caerulein	1:2.0 ± 0.24 (8)	1:1.37 ± 0.20 (4)	1:2.1 ± 0.10 (3)
Porcine gastrin II	1:20.3 ± 2.1 (3)	1:33.6 ± 4.8 (3)	1:27.3 ± 5.0 (3)
Desulfated caerulein	1:80 ± 9.9 (10)	1:68.3 ± 9.5 (4)	1:122 ± 37.4 (3)
Porcine gastrin I	1:420 ± 50 (3)	1:987† ± 38.1 (3)	1:366† ± 82.8 (3)
Pentapeptide	1:4400 ± 560 (12)	1:3433 ± 378 (3)	1:1592 ± 135 (4)

* The molar activity of cholecystokinin was taken as unity. Its specific activity was taken as 3000 Ivy Dog Units/mg (9). The estimates are given ±SE. The number in parentheses is the number of determinations.

† Based on the initial contraction.

b) Caerulein

Caerulein closely mimics the effects of CCK. On a weight basis it is 10 times more potent than CCK on the gallbladder of the anesthetized guinea pig, 13—20 times more potent on the jejunal loop of the dog, 47 times more potent on the gallbladder of the conscious dog (VAGNE and GROSSMAN, 1968b) and at least 50 times more potent as a relaxant of the sphincter of ODDI contracted by morphine.

In large doses, 0.4—0.5 μg/kg i.v. or 3—4 μg/kg subcutaneously, caerulein causes emesis and evacuation of the bowel in the dog. Contraction of the dog's gallbladder in situ is elicited by 1 ng/kg/min in intravenous infusion.

A pertinent examination of the action of caerulein on the smooth muscle of the gastrointestinal tract and on the gallbladder in 9 species of mammals was performed by BERTACCINI, DE CARO, ENDEAN, ERSPAMER and IMPICCIATORE (1968). Doses of 1—5 ng/kg i.v. have a spasmogenic action on jejunal loops of the dog and slightly larger doses contract the small intestine of the cat. The threshold dose for the action on the isolated gallbladder *in vitro* was for the guinea pig 0.5—2 ng/ml, the rabbit 0.1—0.25 ng/ml, the cat 1—2 ng/ml, the sheep 0.1—0.2 ng/ml and for the cow 0.03—0.1 ng/ml. (ERSPAMER et al., 1967).

The i.v. dose of caerulein causing a contraction of the gallbladder in man and the dog is, according to ERSPAMER (1972), 0.1—0.5 ng/kg/min.

CAMERON, PHILLIPS and SUMMERSKILL (1969) studied the effect of the hormones on muscle strips of the human gallbladder suspended in a prewarmed, moistened atmosphere of 95% oxygen and 5% carbon dioxide. Krebs solution with or without added hormone dripped down the surface of the strips. An admixture to the solution of 4 U/100 ml of *CCK* (10% purity) or more resulted in a progressive shortening of the strip and an increase in the frequency but not in the amplitude of superimposed contraction waves. The mean duration of the action was 18 min. The initial latent period was dependent upon the dose, being 6 min with 4 U, 1.3 μg,/100 ml, 3 min with 10 U, 3.3 μg,/100 ml and 0.83 min with 25—30 U/100 ml. The concentration of CCK in the *in vitro* experiments was calculated to be 25 times greater than that necessary to produce an effect *in vivo*. Under similar experimental conditions, *synthetic human gastrin I*, 10 μg/100 ml or 47.3×10^{-9} M, had no effect on the muscle strips, nor had *crystalline natural glucagon*, 10 μ/100 ml or 28.8×10^{-9} M. *Synthetic secretin*, however, in a concentration of 10 U, 2.5 μg/100 ml had about one sixth of the activity of a similar concentration of CCK.

c) The Action of Secretin on the Gallbladder

Exogenous secretin, 2 U/kg, as well as endogenous secretin released by HCl in the duodenum consistently causes a higher pressure response from the gallbladder after 1—8 U/kg of CCK than when CCK is given alone to chronic gallbladder and gastric fistula dogs (STENING and GROSSMAN, 1969c). Secretin alone, 4 U/kg, did not alter the basal gallbladder motility. *Pentagastrin*, 1—4 μg/kg/h given alone, behaved similarly.

d) Neural Components in the Action Mechanism

Working with a CCK preparation with a strength of 22 Ivy dog units of cholecystokinin per mg, NAITO, IWATA and SAITO (1963) studied the influence of neural components on the action mechanism. They found that CCK in a concentration of 1—2.5 Ivy dog units per liter, corresponding to 0.3—0.75 ng of the pure hormone per ml, caused contraction of a circular segment of the dog's gallbladder aerated with oxygen at 38°C in a Ringer solution. On administering CCK intravenously to nembutalized dogs, rabbits and guinea pigs they found that bilateral vagotomy did not suppress the contraction of the gallbladder and the acceleration of intestinal peristalsis caused by CCK. *Atropinization of the animals suppressed the effect of CCK on the intestine but not that on the gallbladder.* CCK exerts a specific action on this organ, different from that on the intestine, an action which is independent of the state of the autonomic nervous system.

Prior to the work of NAITO et al. (1963), HARPER (1959), HARPER et al. (1959), and BROWN et al. (1963) demonstrated that right vagal stimulation in the cat facilitates the effect of CCK on the gallbladder tone. According to PALLIN and SKOGLUND (1964), the response after stimulation of the peripheral end of the right vagal trunk combined with i.v. CCK was stronger than the sum of the pressures obtained with vagal and humoral stimulation alone. Electrical stimulation of the right splanchnic nerve had an inhibitory effect on the response to i.v. administered CCK. LIEDBERG (1969), working with the anesthetized cat, confirmed the findings of NAITO et al. (1963) that vagal section has no influence on the changes in pressure in response to CCK. Vagotomy, however, caused a decrease in the resting gallbladder pressure and in the resting activity of the duodenum and its response to CCK.

After vagotomy in man, TINKER and COX (1969) found a hypersensitivity to cholinergic and hormonal stimulation. A dose of CCK, 0.06 IDU/kg, which was a subthreshold dose in 10 persons with intact vagi, caused within 30 min a 26.6% reduction in gallbladder area in 10 patients submitted to truncal vagotomy. Still more efficient was a subthreshold dose of Carbachol (75 μg).

DANHOF (1966) measured the motility of four portions of duodenum and upper jejunum of the dog with balloons in situ. CCK, given intravenously in doses of 0.35—1.0 U/kg elicited within 50—60 sec a 6—8 min sustained motility in the first part, but had no action on the fourth portion of duodenum and upper jejunum. Removal of the second portion of the duodenum abrogated the motor response of the gallbladder to CCK almost entirely. CCK injection after infiltration of the common duct with a 1% or 2% procaine solution or transection of the duct resulted in duodenal motility, but the gallbladder showed only a minimal, transient, and incomplete emptying response. *The author concluded that the gallbladder motor response to CCK is mediated by stimulation of the duodenal pacemaker and requires intact ductal innervation to effectively empty the bile.*

e) The Sensitivity of the Gallbladder to CCK as Influenced by the Sexual Hormones

Clinical observations indicate that gallbladder distress in women is more frequent at the time of menstruation. In consequence the French clinicians have created the terms "la sympathie cholécysto-ovarienne" and "le syndrome hépato-endocrinien" (BINET and JAHIEL, 1934). Referring to earlier clinical observations on the connection between biliary dyskinesia and the menstrual cycle, ADLERCREUTZ (1953, 1966) reported on a series of cases of his own in which progesterone therapy caused a remarkable improvement or complete relief of symptoms especially in cases of postcholecystectomy syndrome.

In his monographs CHABROL (1950, 1954) claimed that certain biliary dyskinesias are due to "hyperfolliculism" which in some of his cases could be successfully treated with corpus luteum hormone.

LASZLO and GÖRGEY (1960) treated a group of patients consisting of 143 posthepatitic dyskinesia cases and 56 cholecystectomy cases with a corpus luteum preparation every second day for 2—3 weeks. In 67% of the cases the symptoms disappeared and in 20% no improvement took place.

Referring to a material of 1930 cases of cholecystectomy, BODVALL (1964) selected for progesterone treatment, GESTANYN® (PHARMACIA, AB), 5 mg daily, a group of 54 patients, 47 women and 7 men, suffering from continuous severe postoperative biliary distress. The test lasted for 5 to 18 months. 76% of the patients were completely relieved of their symptoms and only 5% were unimproved.

The reduced sensitivity of the gallbladder toward CCK during a period of the menstrual cycle and during gravidity means that female guinea pigs are less suitable for the assay of CCK activity (Caroli et al., 1960; Plessier et al., 1961). Recent cholecystographic findings also indicate that gallbladder atony with impaired emptying and reduced sensitivity to cholecystokinin can occur in the middle of the menstrual cycle. In analyzing 10 healthy young women by means of oral cholecystography on the 14th and 21st day of the menstrual cycle, *i.e.* the time for the oestrogen and the progesterone peaks in the blood respectively, Nilsson and Stattin (1967) found in 8 cases out of 10 a reduced emptying during the latter phase (Fig. 32). The difference was in two cases 31 and 32% and in one case 15.8%. The hormonally induced gallbladder hypotony is in harmony with the fact that progesterone relaxes smooth muscles in many organs, the alimentary tract, the uterus and the blood vessels.

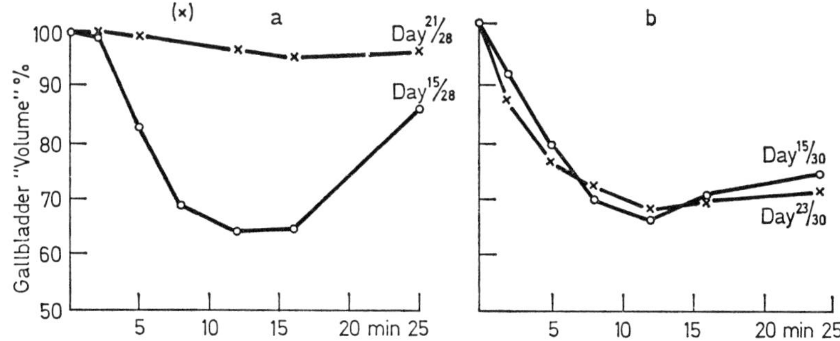

Fig. 32a. Gallbladder emptying in case 2, a 20-year-old woman. During the estrogen peak (day 15/28) the emptying is substantial while the gallbladder is essentially atonic during the progesterone peak (21/28). (Nilsson and Stettin (1967)

Fig. 32b. Gallbladder emptying in case 8, a 20-year-old woman. In this case no difference can be seen between emptying during the estrogen peak (day 15/30) and the progesterone peak (day 23/30). (Nilsson and Stettin, 1967)

IV. Influence of Secretin, CCK and Glucagon on Gastric Secretion

1. The Acid Secretion from the Stomach

a) The Duodenum and the Inhibition of Gastric Acid Secretion

In their review article of 1959, Jones and Harkins pointed out that Sokolov (1904), while working in Pavlov's laboratory, observed that gastric juice, when placed into the duodenum of a dog, markedly decreased the gastric acid secretion from a Pavlov pouch.

Since that time, a considerable volume of conflicting experimental data concerning this subject has been accumulated. Ivy and McIlvain (1923) claimed that acid in the duodenum stimulated gastric secretion. Similar observations were made by Sircus (1953).

The predominant effect of a duodenal infusion *in situ* with dilute hydrochloric acid is, however, an inhibition of gastric secretion. CODE and WATKINSON (1955) found acid in the duodenum to inhibit the secretory response to a meal in the vagally innervated but not in the vagally denervated gastric mucosa of the dog. Referring to a series of experiments of their own in humans, SHAY, GERSHON-COHEN and FELS (1942) confirmed the findings of the Pavlov school that a mechanism which depresses gastric secretion is elicited when acid from the stomach reaches the duodenum.

In both Pavlov and Heidenhain pouch dogs, with the proximal duodenum transected at the pylorus and cannulated, and a gastrojejunostomy performed, JONES and HARKINS (1959) demonstrated that infusion into the duodenum of 0.1 N HCl depressed the acidity of the secretion from the denervated Heidenhain pouch by 73.6%. The secretion was stimulated by an alcohol test meal. The infusion of normal saline or 0.1 N $NaHCO_3$ slightly increased the gastric acidity. The depression lasted for 3—4 hours, as long as the pH of the duodenal content was 2.5 or lower. However, the pouch secretion was inhibited by only 15%.

In similarly operated dogs with the antrum and the duodenum excluded, ANDERSSON (1960a) found that instillation of hydrochloric acid or gastric juice into the excluded antral-duodenal regions effectively inhibited the fasting secretion in Pavlov as well as Heidenhain pouch dogs. Only a slight inhibitory effect was observed during the perfusion of the isolated antrum. When acid secretion was stimulated in these animals by a test meal of 50 g or 250 g meat, the inhibitory effect of acid in the duodenum was more pronounced than that produced by acid in the antrum. The secretion from both the Pavlov and Heidenhain pouch dogs was equally inhibited (ANDERSSON, 1960b). Perfusion of the antrum alone with 0.1 N HCl for 60 min caused no depression of the acid secretion in two series and a 22% reduction in a third, whereas perfusion of the duodenum in 5 series produced during the first hour 87, 92, 88, 89 and 75% reduction of the control values. This clearly indicates that the inhibitory agent is not to be found in the antrum of the stomach but in the duodenum. In a subsequent series ANDERSSON (1960c) showed that perfusion of the duodenum with acid inhibited the action of a gastrin preparation administered by intravenous infusion. The inhibitory mechanism thus acts in the area of the parietal cells. This applies to the physiological stimulation of gastric secretion in connection with a meal.

It does not, however, apply to gastric secretion stimulated by histamine. ANDERSSON (1960d) found that the gastric secretion induced by histamine (0.17—0.34 μg/kg/min) was only slightly inhibited by the perfusion of the duodenum with 0.1 N HCl. There was no difference between the responses of the Pavlov pouch and the Heidenhain pouch dogs. In summarizing, ANDERSSON concluded that the inhibition of gastric secretion is exerted by one or several humoral factors liberated from the duodenal mucosa by dilute hydrochloric acid and that the physiological stimulation in connection with a meal is much more sensitive to these inhibitors than the stimulation produced by histamine.

b) The Role of Secretin

The same inhibitory effect on gastric acid secretion as elicited by dilute hydrochloric acid in the duodenum can also be produced by intravenous secretin.

In 1957 GREENLEE, LONGHI, GUERRERO, NELSEN, EL-BEDRI and DRAGSTEDT showed in dogs that *crude secretin preparations* (Lilly) exert a pronounced inhibitory effect on the secretory response of the vagally denervated Heidenhain pouches to food and to perfusion of antral pouches with liver extract, that is, an inhibition of the gastrin phase of the gastric secretion. The preparations did not inhibit secretion of hydrochloric acid by Heidenhain pouches in response to histamine or the responses of innervated total gastric pouches or Pavlov pouches to hypoglycemia induced by insulin. Their findings were confirmed by JORDAN and PETERSON (1962), WORMSLEY and GROSSMAN (1964) and by JORDAN and DE LA ROSA (1965), who all used *pure secretin*. KAMIONKOWSKI, GROSSMAN and FLESHLER (1964) found the same effect from intravenous pure secretin *in humans* whose gastric secretion was stimulated by broth as an antral stimulant. MCILRATH and HALLENBECK (1964) found that the amount of pure secretin, 20 clin. units, necessary to cause a 40% depression of the gastric secretion was 10 times larger than that which produced a maximal secretion of pancreatic juice. Secretin in large doses inhibited the gastric secretory response to exogenous gastrin in the absence of the antrum, suggesting that the site of action is at or near the parietal cell. KENNEDY and HALLENBECK (1963) and GRYBOSKI and MENGUY (1964) demonstrated that the inhibitory action of secretin, both of impure samples and the pure polypeptide, on gastric secretion persisted even after pancreatectomy or ligation of the pancreatic ducts, causing complete acinar atrophy, eliminating the possibility that the secretin effect was secondary to the passage of pancreatic secretion into the duodenum.

GILLESPIE and GROSSMAN (1964b) found that rapid intravenous injection of 75 clinical units of pure secretin depressed the acid response of Heidenhain pouch dogs to continuous intravenous gastrin infusion by about 60% of the control value. The effect lasted for ½ h.

In their analysis of the inhibition of gastrin and histamine induced acid secretion in the Heidenhain pouch and the innervated stomach of dogs with a gastric fistula, WORMSLEY and GROSSMAN (1964) found that acidification of the duodenum, following closure of the gastric fistula, reduced the acid output in the pouch in response to both gastrin and histamine by about 50 per cent. The reduction in acid secretion could be mimicked by injection of secretin, but not if the secretion had been induced by ordinary doses of histamine. Since acidification of the duodenum was capable of depressing the histamine induced secretion as well, the authors concluded that the release of secretin could not be the sole inhibitory mechanism elicited by endogenous acid in the duodenum.

The difference in the behaviour of secretin towards histamine stimulation and gastrin stimulation of the gastric secretion was further demonstrated by GRYBOSKI and MENGUY (1964). Secretin, even in large doses, did not alter the pouch response to subcutaneous histamine, which gave 50% of the maximal acid response. NAKAJIMA, NAKAMURA and MAGEE (1969) observed that with dose levels at or below 0.5 mg histamine/h the acid outputs from the Heidenhain pouch were significantly less with secretin than without it. With high doses of histamine (1.2 mg/h), producing near maximal or maximal rates of acid secretion, no significant difference was noted between the responses to histamine plus secretin and the responses to histamine alone.

JOHNSON and GROSSMAN (1968, 1969a) found the histamine stimulated Heidenhain pouch secretion in the dog to be unaffected by secretin, irrespective of the dose of histamine used.

Pure natural secretin, 1 U/kg/h, in i.v. infusion reduces by 64—80% the acid output from the Heidenhain pouch of the dog stimulated by porcine gastrin II, 1 μg/kg/h, caerulein, 0.15 μg/kg/h or desulfated caerulein 0.6 μg/kg/h (BROOKS, JOHNSON and GROSSMAN, 1969).

JOHNSON and GROSSMAN (1969b) (Fig. 33) considered secretin to be a stronger inhibitor of gastrin stimulated acid secretion in the stomach of the dog than it is a stimulator of pancreatic secretion. The dose required for 50% inhibition of gastric secretion was 0.4 U/kg/h, whereas the dose required for 50% maximal pancreatic stimulation was 1.2 U/kg/h. PRESHAW (1969), however, found the water and bicarbonate secretion from the pancreas to be a more sensitive mechanism in response to acidification of the duodenum in Heidenhain pouch dogs than is the inhibition of gastric acid secretion. As to the action mechanism of secretin as an inhibitor of gastrin activity, JOHNSON and GROSSMAN (1969b) found the Michaelis-Menton analysis of the dose-response curves to gastrin alone and gastrin plus 0.5 U/kg of secretin to be typical for a noncompetitive inhibition. On the

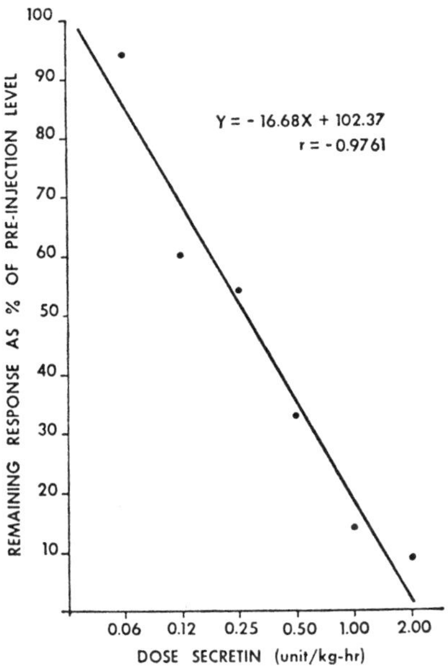

Fig. 33. Percent response remaining to stimulation by 0.8 g/kg/h gastrin during inhiibtion by secretin in doses doubling from 0.06 to 2.0 U/kg/h. Percentages are derived from responses during last 30 min of secretin infusion and 30 min before secretin infusion began. Means of two observations in each of 4 dogs. Correlation coefficient and equation of line are given (JOHNSON and GROSSMAN, 1969b)

other hand, the action of CCK on the gastrin induced gastric secretion was found to be typical for a competitive inhibition (JOHNSON and GROSSMAN, 1970a). The kinetics of the inhibition of secretion produced by duodenal acidification are non-competitive and identical to those of secretin.

Secretin, 2 U/kg/h, has in the antrectomized dog no effect on the acid response to 0.5 U/kg of insulin or 0.15 g/kg of 2-deoxyglucose (WAY, 1970). Thus it does not inhibit direct cholinergic stimulation of the parietal cell. In this study, however, the secretion elicited by Bethanechol, β-methylcholine carbamate (Urecholine), was in fact inhibited by secretin. Before antrectomy, secretin strongly inhibited the response to insulin, 2-DG and to Bethanechol, an effect probably mediated through endogenous gastrin released by vagal stimulation (JOHNSON and GROSSMAN, 1970b).

In man

As to the action of secretin on the gastric secretion in man, CHEY, HITANANT, HENDRICKS and LORBER (1968) found like KAMIONKOWSKI et al. (1964) that pure secretin (1 U/kg) administered intravenously caused a decrease in the mean acid output of histamine stimulated secretion in 7 subjects from 14.52 mEq/30 min to 9.52 mEq (34.4%). Similarly in 5 subjects the mean acid output of pentapeptide stimulated secretion decreased from 10.39 to 4.74 mEq (54.3%). In 3 subjects in whom both preparations produced a similar secretory response, secretin had a greater inhibitory effect on pentapeptide stimulated acid secretion (45.1%) than on the response to histamine (20.5%). "Cecekin" (1 U/kg) caused a similar degree of inhibition of pentapeptide stimulated acid secretion in 4 subjects (38.6%).

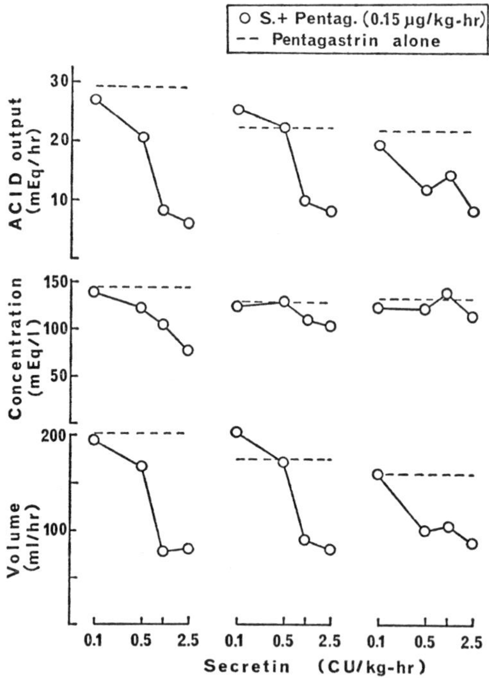

Fig. 34. The inhibitory effect of secretin, 0.1—2.5 U/kg/h, on the action of pentagastrin, 0.15 µg/kg/h, in man (BERSTAD and PETERSEN, 1970)

The basal gastric secretion of man is depressed by 50% both in volume and acid output by 1 or 2 U/kg of secretin, pure or impure (DINOSO, CHEY and LORBER, 1966).

The inhibitory action on acid secretion in man was limited to small doses of pentagastrin and histamine acid phosphate, 0.12 µg/kg/h and 0.02 mg/kg/h respectively. The response to 6 µg/kg/h of pentagastrin and 0.04 mg/kg/h of histamine acid phosphate was not influenced by 1 U/kg of secretin (CHEY et al., 1972). 1 U/kg of CCK in man inhibits acid secretion after 0.12 µg/kg/h of pentagastrin to the same extent as 1 U/kg of secretin. Similar results as to the action of secretin were reported by BERSTAD and PETERSEN (1970) (Fig. 34).

Using Secretin Boots, WOODS (1965) found that 1 to 1.5 U/kg injected intravenously in man reduced the gastric HCl production by 43% of basal levels and that approximately one third of the patients became temporarily achlorhydric.

Likewise PETERSEN (1969) fond a significant decrease in the basal gastric acid secretion (on an average 43%) in the first post-secretin 20 min period after

1 U/kg of pure natural porcine secretin in a group of 26 healthy young persons. In the third 20 min period there was a significant rebound effect.

Brooks and Grossman (1970a) characterized the inhibitory action of secretin in man as something between the extremes of canine sensitivity and feline resistance. Applying a technique with a balloon placed in the duodenum which prevented reflux of duodenal contents into the stomach, the authors found a 21% inhibition of the response to a maximal dose of pentagastrin by 2 U/kg of pure natural secretin.

In the cat

Contrary to the findings in the dog, the rat and in man, pure *secretin* in doses which produce maximal inhibition of gastric secretion in the dog and maximal pancreatic secretion in the cat *has no inhibitory effect on the gastrin and the CCK stimulated gastric secretion in the cat.* In dogs, supramaximal doses of gastrin or histamine inhibit histamine or gastrin stimulated acid secretion from the vagally innervated stomach. In cats, the corresponding doses cause no inhibition of the histamine stimulated acid secretion (Emås and Grossman, 1967b). In both species, however, rapid gastrin injection against background stimulation with histamine results in an increased pepsin secretion. In analogy, the inhibitory effect of endogenous secretin after acidification of the duodenum is much smaller in the cat than in the dog (Stening, Johnson and Grossman, 1969a; Johnson and Grossman, 1969b; Konturek, Gabrys and Dubiel, 1969). Identical doses, however, produce strong stimulation of pepsin secretion both in the cat and the dog.

Even in other respects the cat behaves differently from the dog. The gastric stimulant property of CCK is in cats not markedly sensitive to inhibition by secretin (Way and Grossman, 1970). Working with animals with gastric fistulas, Way, Johnson and Grossman (1970) found that dogs are more sensitive than cats for acid stimulation by gastrin. With synthetic human gastrin the D_{50} for dogs was 0.84 ± 0.4 µg/kg/h and for cats 2.6 ± 0.5 µg/kg/h.

The species specificity thus observed for the action of secretin also applies to another inhibitor of the gastrin effect, namely the synthetic "Antigastrin" [2-phenyl-2-(2 pyridyl) thioacetamide], SC-15, 396, found by Bedi, Gillespie and Gillespie (1967) and by Cook and Bianchi (1967) to inhibit the action of endogenous and exogenous gastrin and of pentagastrin in rats and dogs. Given in doses adequate for conscious dogs and anesthetized rats, no inhibition of the gastrin effect was observed in anesthetized gastric fistula cats (Sewing, Gorinsky and Lembeck, 1968).

In view of the behaviour of the cat and man in this respect, a generalization cannot be made. In the cat, secretin has no inhibitory effect on the gastrin and the CCK stimulated gastric secretion (Emås and Grossman, 1967b). Referring to his own findings in a human material, Wormsley (1968b) concluded that, in contrast to the impression gained from the studies in dogs, the overall effect of the duodenal hormones on the human stomach is stimulatory rather than inhibitory, particularly in doses likely to be encountered under physiological circumstances.

In rats

Nor does secretin, 75 U/kg, according to Johnson and Tumpson (1970) depress the acid secretion after doses of 5—40 mg/kg of histamine dihydrochloride, both drugs being administered subcutaneously in conscious gastric fistula rats.

Chey et al. (1970b), however, found that synthetic secretin infused in a dose of 2 U/kg/h in rats causes a 79% inhibition of the maximum acid response to histamine, an even larger inhibition than that of the gastrin stimulated secretion (50%).

In rats secretin acts as in dogs, preventing in adequate doses the response to maximal and supramaximal doses of pentagastrin (TUMPSON and JOHNSON, 1969).

c) CCK and the Gastric Acid Secretion

The Heidenhain pouch secretion stimulated by even small doses of histamine, not influenced by secretin, is markedly reduced by CCK (GILLESPIE and GROSSMAN, 1964b). 75 Ivy dog units of an impure preparation of CCK caused an inhibition lasting for an hour with a maximal reduction of the control value by 78%. Even responses to small doses of histamine, 0.125 mg histamine dihydrochloride per hour, upon which secretin had no influence, were depressed by CCK. No depression took place after infusion of 0.25 mg histamine dihydrochloride per hour, indicating that histamine stimulation is more resistant than that by gastrin to the inhibitory influence of CCK. The sample of CCK had a potency of only 250 Ivy dog units per mg, thus was only 10% pure. An infusion of about the same amount of CCK, 0.5 IDU/kg/min or more of a 50% pure preparation was found by MURAT and WHITE (1966) and by MAGEE and NAKAMURA (1966) to cause an inhibition of the gastric secretion.

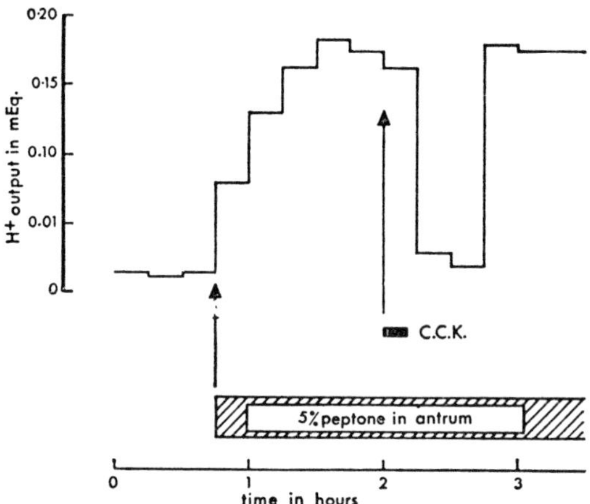

Fig. 35. Acid output from the Heidenhain pouch was stimulated by perfusing the denervated antrum with 5% peptone solution in water. CCK represents a 10-minute intravenous infusion of 1.0 unit/kg cholecystokinin. There is marked depression of acid secretion, lasting for 30 minutes, then a return to control levels (BROWN and MAGEE, 1967)

In 1967 BROWN and MAGEE (Fig. 35) presented evidence for an almost complete blocking of the endogenous gastrin effect in Heidenhein pouch dogs through intravenous infusion of 1 IDU/kg of CCK during 10 min. The gastrin effect was elicited by perfusing the antral pouch with 0.1% acetylcholine in 0.9% saline or with a 5% peptone solution in water. BEDI, GOVAERTS, MASTER and GILLESPIE (1967) showed that the same inhibitory effect on the histamine or gastrin stimulated secretion in the Heidenhain pouch is elicited by *pure CCK*. According to the authors, the degree of inhibition from a rapid single intravenous injection of 75 Ivy dog units of CCK in the dog was approximately the same, irrespective of whether the stimulation had been exerted by gastrin, histamine dihydrochloride,

0.125—0.5 mg/h i.v., the gastrinlike pentapeptide, 20 μg/h i.v., choline esters or by feeding a meat meal. They made the observation that in dogs with both a Heidenhain pouch and a simple fistula into the normally vagally innervated gastric remnant, and in whom antrectomy had been performed, a single rapid intravenous injection of "Cecekin", a CCK preparation of 10% purity, had no effect on the Heidenhain pouch responses to histamine and that the acid output from the main gastric remnant was increased. The authors discussed the possibility that the results might be accounted for by the absence of the pyloric antrum in the second group of dogs.

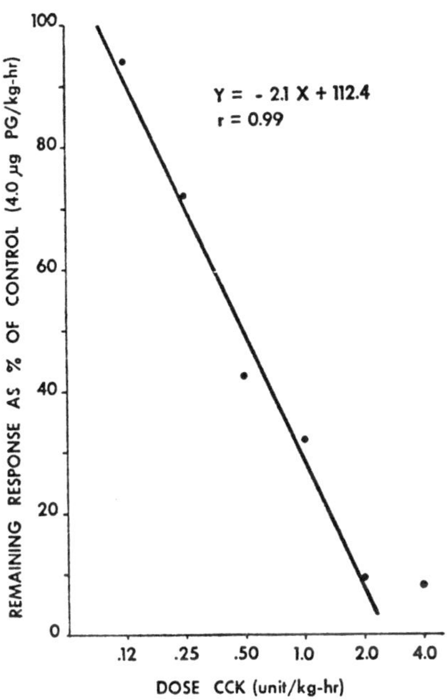

Fig. 36. Percent response remaining to stimulation by 4.0 μg/kg/h pentagastrin during inhibition by CCK in doses doubling from 0.12—4.0 U/kg/h. Percentages were derived from responses during last 30 min of CCK infusion and 30 min before CCK infusion began. Means of two observations in each of four dogs. Correlation coefficient and equation of line are given (JOHNSON and GROSSMAN, 1970a)

The inhibition of pentagastrin stimulated gastric secretion was studied by JOHNSON and GROSSMAN (1970a) *in dogs* with Heidenhain pouches and open gastric fistulas, using CCK preparations with 250 or 3000 IDU/mg, the latter sample consisting of pure CCK (Fig. 36). An infusion of about 0.5 IDU/kg/h was required for 50% inhibition and 2.0 IDU/kg/h for maximal (95%) inhibition. The experimental data fitted in with a competitive inhibition of the gastrin effect, as could be expected from the similarity in structure between CCK and gastrin. Since the dose of CCK needed for half maximal pancreatic enzyme response was about 3 U/kg/h, CCK, like secretin, is *in the dog* a more powerful gastrin antagonist than it is a stimulant of the pancreatic secretion.

On the other hands, 1 U/kg of CCK administered to *conscious gastric fistula cats* against a background stimulation with histamine. 2 HCl, 40 μg/kg/h, or pentagastrin, 4 μg/kg/h, increased the acid output from the stomach by 30% and 20 U/kg by 60% within 30 min (SVENSSON and EMÅS, 1970).

d) CCK as a Stimulant of Gastric Acid Secretion

A quite different picture is obtained when small doses of CCK are administered. PRESHAW and GROSSMAN (1965a), PRESHAW, COOKE and GROSSMAN (1965a) found that small doses of secretin or CCK sometimes stimulated the gastric secretion in conscious *pancreatic fistula dogs*. Then, in two concomitant publications, MURAT and WHITE (1966) and MAGEE and NAKAMURA (1966) showed in a large series of dogs with a denervated Heidenhain pouch that *CCK behaves like gastrin, acting in small doses as a stimulant and in large doses as an inhibitor of gastric secretion*, the ratio between the dose required to inhibit and that to stimulate gastric secretion being about hundred to one. Irrespective of whether the dogs were fasting, pretreated with acetylcholine, 0.2 μg/min, or fed with a proprietary food to a high secretory plateau, a continuous infusion of 0.003—0.005 Ivy dog units of CCK/kg/min caused an immediate significant rise both in volume and in acid. After the CCK was discontinued, the volume and the acid returned to their previous levels. If the dose of CCK was 1—5 IDU/kg in a single injection or 0.5 IDU/kg/min in infusion or higher, it inhibited gastric secretion. In these series the strength of the CCK preparation used was 1,500 Ivy dog units per mg as compared with 3,000 units in the pure hormone. The action was no doubt due to the hormone itself.

In sham feeding experiments in Pavlov pouch dogs, which more closely correspond to the physiological conditions. CCK enhances the effect of vagal stimulation of the gastric secretion, when given in doses of 0.75—3 U/kg/h in i.v. infusion (SJÖDIN, 1971).

In man

CELESTIN (1967) found that 0.5 U of CCK, or 0.17 μg/kg/h, in intravenous infusion increased both the volume and the concentration of acid in the stomach, leading to a steady level of secretion (12 mEq/h). About the same effect (14 mEq/h) was produced by an infusion of 0.5 μg/kg/h of the C-terminal gastrin tetrapeptide (Leo), 10 μg/kg of which induced a maximal response when given subcutaneously. On the other hand, 4 U/kg/h of both the 10% pure and the pure CCK inhibited the acid secretion in man stimulated by pentagastrin, 4 μg/kg/h, by 33% (BROOKS and GROSSMAN, 1970a).

In the rat

Both CCK and its synthetic C-terminal octapeptide in doses of 2—16 U/kg/h cause only hypersecretion. The maximal acid output stimulated by 1 μg/kg/h of pentagastrin or 80—160 μg/kg/h of histamine was increased by 378 and 180% respectively (CHEY et al., 1970b).

In birds

Inhibition of the basal, histamine and gastrin stimulated acid secretion, by intravenous secretin or CCK or 0.4% HCl in the duodenum likewise takes place in birds (KOKAS and BRUNSON, 1969).

Isolated Gastric Frog Mucosa

The stimulating effect of small doses of CCK on the gastric secretion in the dog (MURAT and WHITE, 1966; MAGEE and NAKAMURA, 1966), in the cat (EMÅS and FYRÖ, 1968; WAY and GROSSMAN, 1970), the rat (CHEY et al., 1970b) and in man (CELESTIN, 1967) has also been demonstrated in the *isolated gastric mucosa of the bullfrog*, suspended in a bath duly aerated with oxygen at room temperature (Davidson, Urushibara and Thompson, 1969a; Charters et al., 1969). In these series a 50% pure CCK preparation was used, in which there were no active contaminants. The maximal secretory response of the bullfrog mucosa to porcine gastrin, pentagastrin and CCK was achieved at 2.5×10^{-8}, 2.5×10^{-6} and 2.5×10^{-6} M, respectively. On a molar basis, porcine gastrin was 25—35 times as potent as CCK and the latter was 2—3 times as potent as pentagastrin. Synthetic human gastrin showed a potency equal to that of pentagastrin (Davidson et al., 1969b).

e) Gastrin and Caerulein

Murat and White (1966) found it remarkable that gastrin and CCK are almost equally potent with respect to their stimulating, as well as to their inhibitory effect on gastric secretion. The similarity in action caused Magee and Nakamura (1966) to suggest that the 50% pure CCK preparations may contain duodenal gastrin. This assumption later proved superfluous, when it was found that the active centre of both gastrin and CCK is located in the C-terminal end of the molecule and that the C-terminal pentapeptide is the same in both of the two hormones.

The effect of the subcutaneous administration of 1 μg per kg of *gastrin II* or 6 μg per kg of the *synthetic gastrin-like pentapeptide (ICI 50,123)* in man is, with respect to acid and pepsin secretion and to the behaviour of the electrolytes with the inverse relationship between sodium and hydrogen ions, similar to that following the subcutaneous injection of 40 μg of histamine acid phosphate per kg (Abernethy et al., 1967; Makhlouf et al., 1966, 1967). 6 μg per kg of the gastrin-like pentapeptide (t-butyloxycarbonyl-β-Ala-Trp-Met-Asp-Phe-NH_2) and 1.5 mg per kg of the cholinergic drug betazole (3-β-aminoethyl-pyrazole dihydrochloride) give, when injected subcutaneously in man, similar 15 and 30 min peak responses of acid secretion (Wormsley, Mahoney and Kay, 1967; Isenberg, Brooks and Grossman, 1968). Histamine and gastrin extracts given intravenously in appropriate doses produce the same *maximal rate of acid excretion* from the vagally innervated stomachs of unanesthetized dogs (Passaro and Grossman, 1964) and cats (Emås and Grossman, 1967a, b). *The latter authors observed pronounced differences between the dose-response curves for dogs and those for cats when supramaximal doses of histamine or gastrin were given.* The supramaximal doses depressed both acid and pepsin secretion in the dogs but not in the cats. In cats as in man (Barabas et al., 1966), supramaximal doses of histamine and gastrin were as effective as the maximal dose in stimulating acid secretion.

In view of the similarity in structure between CCK and gastrin, Venables, Rudick, Kark and Dreiling (1969) compared the stimulating effects of CCK and gastrin on the gastric secretion in gastric fistula dogs. In doses of 0.5—4 "pancreozymin" units/kg/h, CCK stimulated the gastric acid secretion but not to the same extent as gastrin. Against a background stimulation with 125 μg/kg/h of metacholine chloride (Mecholyl) there was an overall 80% increase in acid output after CCK. On the other hand, the effect of gastrin was increased through metacholine by only 14%. As a stimulant of the pepsin secretion CCK was as active as gastrin. The cholinergic background enhanced the pepsin output for both secretagogues equally.

In a review article Chey et al. (1972) summarized their observations on the effects of secretin and cholecystokinin on gastric emptying and basal gastric secretion of acid as well as on secretion of acid stimulated by pentagastrin and histamine in man.

The effect of *caerulein on gastric secretion* of the dog, the rat and the frog was studied by BERTACCINI, ENDEAN, ERSPAMER and IMPICCIATORE (1968). The threshold subcutaneous dose in the denervated fundic pouch dog was 0.15—0.5 μg/kg and on i.v. infusion 0.25—0.5 μg/kg/h. On a molar basis, caerulein was approximately twice as active as human gastrin I on volume and acid output and 4 times as active on pepsin output. Acid secretion elicited by caerulein is inhibited by atropine. The isolated mucosa of the frog stomach was extremely sensitive.

In analogy with the similarity in action between CCK and caerulein, STENING, JOHNSON and GROSSMAN (1969b) pointed out that both CCK and caerulein react in a similar way to histamine stimulated gastric acid secretion. CCK, 4 U/kg/h in infusion, consistently produced a 90% inhibition of gastric secretion stimulated by a dose of gastrin producing maximal acid secretion from the Heidenhain pouch of the dog. A dose of 0.2 μg/kg/h of caerulein caused a 65% depression. The same dose of CCK and 0.1 μg/kg/h of caerulein acted in a similar way on histamine stimulated secretion. Both slightly reduced the response to 0.01—0.02 mg/kg/h of histamine-dihydrochloride and both strongly increased the response to 0.04 to 0.08 mg/kg/h of histamine-dihydrochloride.

The C-terminal heptapeptide amide of CCK and caerulein, each in a dose of 0.1 μg/kg/h added to the i.v. perfusion fluid, produced about 70% inhibition of the pentagastrin, 1 μg/kg/h, stimulated gastric acid output in man (BROOKS et al., 1970).

Here again the species difference between the dog and the cat is very pronounced. In the cat, both CCK and caerulein behave as full agonists for gastric secretion. The maximal acid output to a high dose of CCK was about the same as that produced by a near maximal dose of histamine (WAY, 1971). The slope of the regression lines and the maximal rates of secretion were the same for CCK and gastrin although on a molar basis gastrin is about 6 times as potent as CCK.

f) The Influence of Glucagon on Gastric Secretion

As could be expected because of the similarity in structure between secretin and glucagon, both peptides having not less than 14 amino acid units in common in the same positions, glucagon also inhibits gastric secretion. Given intravenously, it inhibits the basal acid secretion in animals as well as in man (ROBINSON, HARRIS, HLAD and EISEMAN, 1957; DREILING and JANOWITZ, 1959; SOLOMON and SPIRO, 1959; DOTEVALL and WESTLING, 1960) and the food induced secretion in animals (CLARKE, NEILL and WELBOURN, 1960). It inhibits the secretion of HCl by vagally innervated and vagally denervated pouches in dogs in response to exogenous gastrin (von HEIMBURG and HALLENBECK, 1964). Histamine induced gastric acid secretion is, however, not inhibited (DOTEVALL and WESTLING, 1960; CHARBON, SEBUS, KOAL and HOEKSTRA, 1963; CUMMING and PERCIVAL, 1967).

The secretion taking place in response to both vagal nerve stimulation and pentagastrin infusion in dogs is moderately depressed (CUMMING and PERCIVAL, 1967). Likewise the gastric acid secretion after a submaximal pentagastrin infusion, 0.06 μg/kg/min, in man is reduced by about 50% by 2 mg glucagon given intravenously in a single dose (DOTEVALL, KOCK and WALAN, 1969).

In analogy with the action of small doses of CCK on the basal gastric acid and pepsin secretion, DOTEVALL, GILLBERG, KOCH and VALAN (1970a, b) observed in man *a significant increase in acid and pepsin output* during the second half hour of infusion of 0.001 μg/kg/min of glucagon. When 0.01 μg/kg/min of glucagon was infused there was a significant decrease during the second half hour period. A marked inhibition took place on infusion of 0.1 μg/kg/min.

2. Hormonal Influences on the Secretion of Pepsin

a) Action of Gastrin and Cholecystokinin

In his review article Ivy (1930 pp. 286—299) told of "a thirty year attempt to understand the mechanism of the chemical excitation of the gastric glands on the ingestion of food. Although", he said, "the attempts have resulted in establishing by means of transplantation and vivo-dialysis a humoral mechanism for gastric secretion, they do not prove whether the humoral agent is secretagogic or hormonal (gastrin)." The "gastric secretin" discovered by Edkins (1905, 1906) was considered by most authors to be histamine (Sacks, Ivy, Burgess and Vandolah, 1932; Bucher, Ivy and Gray, 1941) until Komarov (1938, 1942a, b) convincingly demonstrated that histamine-free antral extracts had gastrin activity. In referring to the findings of the Russian school that mechanical or chemical irritation of the pyloric mucosa stimulates pepsin secretion (Zeljony and Savich, 1914; Savich, 1922), to Grossman's findings (1947) that distension of the main stomach by a balloon results in pepsin secretion from a subcutaneously transplanted pouch stomach, and to his own experiments, showing that distension of the pyloric part of the stomach in dogs caused an increased pepsin output from a gastric fistula, Uvnäs (1948) concluded that there is sufficient evidence for the existence of a pepsigogue principle in the pyloric mucosa.

Once isolated (Gregory and Tracy, 1964), gastrin, both GI and GII, was found to be a powerful stimulant of the secretion of both acid and pepsin. In unanesthetized dogs with denervated fundic pouches, single subcutaneous injections of GI or GII within the range 0.25 to 2.5 μg per kg body weight stimulated acid and volume flow of gastric juice in proportion to the dose administered. Single subcutaneous injections of *larger doses of GI or GII*, 4 to 5 μg per kg, caused a remarkable change in the nature of the response. The acid and volume secretion were depressed, but the juice contained large amounts of pepsin. Similar findings were made by Konturek and Grossman (1965b) in vagally denervated, histamine stimulated Heidenhain pouch dogs.

The pepsigogue effect of supramaximal doses of gastrin was not observed in secretions obtained from gastric fistulas in the innervated stomachs.

Not only gastrin but also other *inhibitors of histamine stimulation such as acetazolamide and cholecystokinin in sufficient intravenous doses*, 7.5 mg and 10 unit per kg respectively, *strongly stimulate pepsin secretion from denervated Heidenhain pouches*; simultaneously there is a depression of the histamine stimulated water and acid secretion (Heitmann, Jungreis and Janowitz, 1967). The output of pepsin rose to levels 8 and 5 times higher, respectively, than that found during the control period.

Similarly active are the C-terminal tetra- and pentapeptides of gastrin (Gregory and Tracy, 1964) and their synthetic analogues and derivatives (Morley, Tracy and Gregory, 1965; Wormsley, Mahoney and Ng, 1966; Makhlouf, McManus and Card, 1966, 1967; Abernethy et al., 1967; Kay, 1967; Køster, Rødbro and Petersen, 1968). The hormonal action of these preparations on the stomach was usually expressed in relation to that of histamine so extensively studied in the past.

The stimulating action of gastrin on the fundic mucosa also extends, at least in the rat, to the enzyme activity which regulates *histamine formation* (Aures, Johnson and Way, 1970). In comparing the histidine decarboxylase activity of the oxyntic gland area of antrectomized rats to that in sham-operated control animals, Johnson, Jones, Aures and Håkanson (1969) found that pentagastrin caused an approximately 10-fold increase in enzyme activity in both groups of animals and that feeding increased the histidine decarboxylase activity 15-fold in sham-operated animals, but only 5-fold in antrectomized ones.

Similarly HÅKANSSON and LIEDBERG (1970) concluded that the activation of gastric histidine decarboxylase in the rat is a specific and physiological effect of gastrin.

b) Action of Secretin on the Output of Pepsin

After injection of a crude secretin preparation with an activity of 10 clinical units per mg, PRATT (1940) observed a pepsin concentration equivalent to that elicited by 5 mg of acetylcholine + eserine in a fasting cat under chloralose anesthesia.

FRIEDMAN et al. (1944) observed that instillation of HCl into the small intestine of Pavlov pouch dogs, secreting in response to insulin or food, increased the pepsin content of the gastric juice.

Initially, there was a search for a gastric equivalent to "pancreozymin" stimulating pepsin secretion.

In 1953 BLAIR, HARPER and LAKE reported that extracts of the mucosa of the upper part of the dog intestine and of the antrum stimulated pepsin secretion in anesthetized cats, atropinized and non-atropinized, with their vagus and splanchnic nerves cut, but had only a slight effect on gastric acid secretion. Since the extracts did not affect the volume or enzyme content of the pancreatic juice and thus could be considered to be free of "pancreozymin", the authors suggested the name "gastrozymin" for the pepsin stimulant.

BLAIR, HARPER, PEARSON and REED (1964) found that extracts of hog upper small intestine, when injected intravenously in cats, produced a well-marked increase in pepsin output from the stomach with *no* increase in the rate of acid output. The stimulation of pepsin secretion was effective in doses which had no "pancreozymin" effect but which showed secretin activity. The authors then found *pure secretin, when injected intravenously in anesthetized and atropinized cats, to be a strong stimulant for pepsin secretion.*

Working with Heidenhain pouch dogs and using pure secretin, MAGEE and NAKAJIMA (1968) and NAKAJIMA et al. (1969) found that administration of 3 units of secretin/min during continuous histamine stimulation caused *a sharp rise in pepsin output to a level eight times that obtained during the control period.* The output of pepsin in response to graded doses of i.v. secretin increased progressively as the dose of secretin was increased. The pepsin responses to combinations of histamine with secretin were significantly greater at doses of histamine above 0.5 mg/h than those to histamine alone (Fig. 37). A given dose of secretin was a more potent pepsin stimulant at high histamine doses than at low ones.

Both natural and synthetic hog secretin, on intravenous infusion in doses submaximal for the stimulation of pancreatic secretion, cause strong stimulation of pepsin secretion in both dogs and cats (STENING, JOHNSON and GROSSMAN, 1969a).

Pure secretin of standard potency was used in 1969 by BROOKS, ISENBERG and GROSSMAN in studying the effect of secretin on pepsin secretion in 7 human subjects. Since the dose administered, 1 or 4 clinical units per kg, depressed both the acid secretion and the volume of the gastric secretion, the gastric contents were emptied by means of continuous gastric perfusion with 100 mM HCl. The mean peak 30 min pepsin output was three times larger than during the pretest period. Perfusion of the duodenum with dilute hydrochloric acid caused a more prolonged increase in the pepsin output. Secretin was consequently claimed by the authors to be a pepsigogue.

Brooks and Grossman (1970a) found that in man 2 U/kg of secretin caused a 21% inhibition of acid output and 35% increase in the pepsin output whereas 4 U/kg of CCK inhibited acid output by 33% without any significant effect on pepsin output.

A prolonged dissociation between the pepsin and acid secretion, lasting for two hours, was observed by Berstad (1969), Berstad and Petersen (1969)' Berstad et al. (1970) and Petersen et al. (1970) after a single intravenous injection of 1 U/kg of pure secretin in a series of fasting healthy subjects. The highest mean output *of pepsin* after histamine administration was found in the first 15-minute period, whereas the highest mean output after secretin was found in the third 20-minute period. The total one-hour output after histamine injection was 336 per cent and the one-hour output after secretin injection was 242 per cent

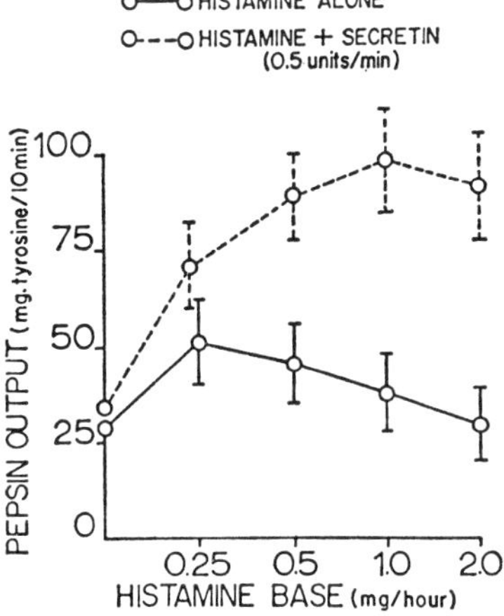

Fig. 37. Dose-response curves for pepsin output in response to histamine alone and histamine plus a fixed dose of secretin. Each point is the mean of 10 experiments in five dogs, the vertical bars represent SEM (Nakajima et al., 1969)

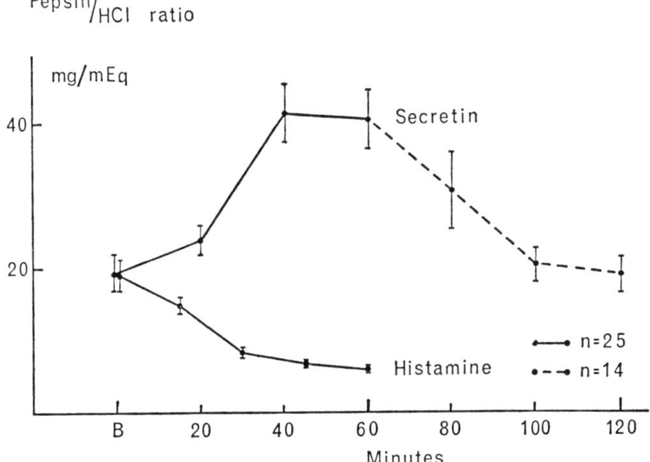

Fig. 38. Pepsin/HCl ratio calculated as the ratio between pepsin and HCl concentration in the samples of gastric juice before (B) and after injection of secretin and histamine respectively. Vertical bars = standard error of the means (Berstad and Petersen, 1962)

of the output during the hour before injection of the stimulants. The *pepsin/HCl ratio* increased to more than twice the unstimulated value in the second and third 20-minute samples after administration of secretin. After injection of histamine, the pepsin/HCl ratio decreased continuously to below one-third of the unstimulated value in the fourth 15-minute sample (Fig. 38).

According to the authors, the findings show that histamine stimulates the parietal cell acid secretion more strongly than the chief cell pepsin secretion. Secretin, on the other hand, preferentially stimulates pepsin secretion, resulting in a high pepsin concentration in the gastric juice.

The hormone stimulated secretion of pepsin is accompanied by a secretion of *the intrinsic factor* (KØSTER, FABER and RØDBRO, 1968).

c) Action of Glucagon

In spite of the many similarities between secretin and glucagon with respect to their chemical structure and their effects on bile flow (MORRIS, SARDI and BRADLEY, 1967), insulin liberation (SAMOLS, MARRI and MARKS, 1965) and inhibition of gastric secretion (LIN and SPRAY, 1968), glucagon in the dose 0.025 mg per kg intravenously has no effect on pepsin secretion (BROOKS, ISENBERG and GROSSMAN, 1969). Other authors (DREILING and JANOWITZ, 1959; COHEN, MAZURE, DREILING and JANOWITZ, 1960) observed a reduction by about 60% or more in both volume and pepsin output after 2 mg of glucagon intravenously in man.

3. "Enterogastrone"

In a review article on "The intestinal hormones as inhibitors of gastric secretion", JOHNSON and GROSSMAN (1970b) summarized the views as to the existence of a specific inhibitory hormone besides secretin and CCK put forward by different authors over the years. They pointed out that such a concept was developed prior to the discovery of the action of secretin in this respect, deriving from the findings of FARRELL and IVY (1926a) that feeding fat inhibited by a humoral mechanism the motility of a transplanted gastric pouch in the dog. KOSAKA et al. (1932), FENG, HOU and LIM (1929) and QUIGLEY, ZETTLEMAN and IVY (1934) extended the experiments of FARRELL and IVY. The active principle supposed to inhibit the gastric secretion and motility in the Heidenhain pouch of the dog in response to a meal and to histamine, without having any effect on the pancreatic secretion, was named "*enterogastrone*" by KOSAKA and LIM (1930a, b). GREENGARD et al. (1946) discussed the possibility of its use in the prophylaxis of recurrences of experimental and clinical peptic ulcer.

The idea of an "enterogastrone" has now been kept alive for four decades without any materialization as a specific hormone. Because of the interest of the medical profession in disturbances in gastric acid secretion, strenuous efforts have been made over the years to isolate the supposed hormone.

In the meantime it was found that secretin (GREENLEE et al., 1957) and CCK (GILLESPIE and GROSSMAN, 1964b) have "enterogastrone"-like properties. The literature dealing with the topic has been reviewed by IVY (1941a, b), GREENGARD (1948), GROSSMAN (1950), GREGORY (1962, 1967b, pp. 469—477) and by JOHNSON and GROSSMAN (1970b).

a) The "Enterogastrone"-Like Activity of Secretin

When secretin and CCK recently became available in pure form, the question of their inhibitory action on gastric acid secretion was actualized.

The inhibition of the gastrin stimulated acid secretion emanates from the uppermost part of the duodenum (KONTUREK and GROSSMAN, 1965a). Excision of the pyloric sphincter in Heidenhain pouch dogs with a gastric fistula did not change the rate of secretion of HCl from the main stomach in response to gastrin. After transplanting the middle portion of the duodenum to the jejunum, the mean rate of acid secretion rose by 62% over the control level. A further increase in acid secretion to about 100% above the control level followed after excision of the duodenal bulb. No further change was seen when the remainder of the duodenum was resected.

In their attempts to localize the site of release of the factor inhibiting gastrin stimulated gastric acid secretion, ANDERSSON, NILSSON and UVNÄS (1967) perfused, in both Pavlov dogs and Heidenhain dogs, duodenal pouches, one proximal and one distal to the entrance of the main pancreatic duct, with 0.1 N HCl. The secretory response to gastrin was not significantly inhibited on perfusing the distal pouch, nor was the response to histamine inhibited by bulbar acidification. A strong effect was observed on perfusing the bulbar pouch.

By performing cross-transfusion tests in four patients against three control cross-transfusions, JOHNSTON and DUTHIE (1966) demonstrated that the secretion depressing factor is humoral, circulating in the blood. The duodenum of the donor was perfused with an adequate amount of 0.1 N HCl. In the recipient, gastric secretion, stimulated by i.v. infusion of small doses, 0.05—0.1 μg/kg/min, of histamine acid phosphate, was depressed during the infusion of blood and 5—15 min thereafter by about 50%.

In view of the capacity of secretin to inhibit gastric acid secretion and gastric motility and to stimulate bicarbonate secretion from the pancreas and the liver, GROSSMAN (1966) describes secretin as "nature's antacid", which might one day be employed in the treatment of peptic ulcer, an idea put forward already in 1946 by GREENGARD et al. According to JOHNSON and GROSSMAN (1969b), the threshold dose of secretin for inhibition of gastrin stimulated acid secretion in the dog is approximately 0.05 U/kg/h, whereas five times this dose is needed to stimulate pancreatic secretion (MEYER, WAY and GROSSMAN, 1970b). In fact an infusion of 2 U/kg/h of secretin prevents the formation of erosions and peptic ulcers in the jejunum during pentagastrin stimulation, 16 μg/kg/h, for 24 hours, in cats with intact or resected duodenum (KONTUREK, 1968).

JOHNSON and GROSSMAN (1968) found that perfusion of the duodenum with 40 ml 160 mM HCl or intravenous injection of 4 U/kg/h of pure secretin gave in four dogs with fistulas in the Heidenhain pouch, the innervated stomach and the duodenum almost identical effects both upon the gastrin stimulated and upon the histamine stimulated gastric secretion. In these experiments, secretin, given in what was considered physiological doses, 4 U/kg/h intravenously, could account for all the inhibition of the gastric secretion produced by acid in the duodenum, which could indicate that secretin is the only "enterogastrone" released by acid in the duodenum.

JOHNSON and GROSSMAN (1970b) pointed out that *in the cat* diverting the gastric acid into the duodenum causes a 400% increase in pepsin secretion from a Heidenhain pouch (KONTUREK, GABRYS and DUBIEL, 1969). Irrigating the intact duodenum of *the dog* with 160 ml/h of 0.16 N HCl also results in a 3—6 fold stimulation of the pepsin output (HARRISON and JOHNSON, 1970), an effect which could be ascribed to a release of secretin, which strongly stimulates pepsin secretion. In the cat and in the rat, however, CCK also stimulates gastric acid secretion (WAY and GROSSMAN, 1970) and in no way behaves as an "enterogastrone" (WAY, 1971).

Unlike CCK, i.v. secretin (JOHNSON and GROSSMAN, 1969b) and acid in the duodenum (HARRISON and JOHNSON, 1970) both inhibit in the dog gastrin stimulated acid secretion via a non-competitive reaction mechanism. The authors (JOHNSON and GROSSMAN, 1970a, b) were therefore inclined to doubt that endogenous CCK plays a significant role in the inhibition of gastric secretion. According to their original view (JOHNSON and GROSSMAN, 1968), as supported by PRESHAW (1969) *secretin is the only enterogastrone of physiological significance, so far known, released by acid from the dog duodenal mucosa.* PRESHAW found a relationship between the rate of pancreatic secretion and the degree of inhibition of gastric secretion in response to duodenal acidification in chronic pancreatic and gastric fistula dogs.

b) "Enterogastrone"-Like Activity of CCK

Other authors (JOHNSON and MAGEE, 1965a, b; NAKAMURA, NAKAJIMA and MAGEE, 1968) called attention to the similarities in action between CCK and "enterogastrone". Whereas secretin inhibits only the gastrin stimulated acid secretion and strongly stimulates the pepsin secretion, CCK in adequate doses inhibits the total gastric secretory activity and the gastric motility as well, as it is supposed that "enterogastrone" should do. An inhibition by CCK of the Mechylol stimulated pepsin secretion was observed by NAKAJIMA and MAGEE (1970b) in conscious Heidenhain dogs with the duodenum separated from the stomach. The pepsin secretion sustained by 2 μg/min in i.v. infusion of acetyl-β-methylcholine (Mechylol) dropped after adding 1 IDU/min of CCK to the infusion fluid by 41% within 10 min and by 85% later. Unlike secretin, which stimulates the pepsin secretion, the 10% pure CCK preparation showed "enterogastrone"-like activity both with respect to acid and to pepsin secretion.

Furthermore, MAGEE and NAKAJIMA (1969) and NAKAJIMA and MAGEE (1970a) made an observation that could indicate that a factor other than secretin inhibiting gastric secretion is released from the duodenal mucosa of the dog on acidification. On lowering the pH in the duodenum from pH 7 to pH 3, the gastric acid secretion from the Heidenhain pouch, stimulated by the pentapeptide, histamine or metacholine, was reduced and the pepsin secretion augmented, an effect ascribed to secretin, but on further acidification down to pH 1, both acid and pepsin secretions were depressed. Since CCK inhibits pepsin outputs whether unstimulated or stimulated by secretin, and secretin stimulates pepsin secretion, the authors concluded that duodenal acidification releases secretin over the pH range 5.0—3.0 and CCK at a lower pH. ODORI and MAGEE (1970) extended the study using 10 dogs carrying a Heidenhain pouch and a Thiry-Vella loop, extending from 1 cm below the pancreatic duct to 10 cm below the ligament of Treitz. For each parameter, 20—30 experiments were performed. It was found that acidification of the Thiry-Vella loop depressed the pentagastrin stimulated acid output, whereas when metacholine was used as stimulator the acid output was almost invariably increased. Fat in the Thiry-Vella loop depressed acid secretion after pentagastrin significantly, but augmented the metacholine stimulated secretion. Peptone had a similar effect. A 20% glucose solution in the loop did not influence the secretion.

In view of the fact that CCK in adequate doses inhibits gastric acid secretion in response to histamine, gastrin and pentagastrin and potentiates the effect of metacholine stimulated acid secretion, as shown by NAKAMURA et al. (1968), the authors felt that under the conditions of the experiments CCK is the predominant inhibitory hormone released by acid or fat in the duodenum.

The findings of CHEY et al. (1968), DINOSO et al. (1969) and of VAGNE et al. (1968) as to *the inhibitory action of both secretin and CCK on the gastric motility* were confirmed by SUGAWARA, ISAZA, CURT and WOODWARD (1969) (Fig. 39). The authors concluded that secretin and CCK constitute a significant portion of the "enterogastrone complex", by which the small intestine inhibits gastric motor function. Like other authors, they considered the concept of a single substance, "enterogastrone", to be an oversimplification.

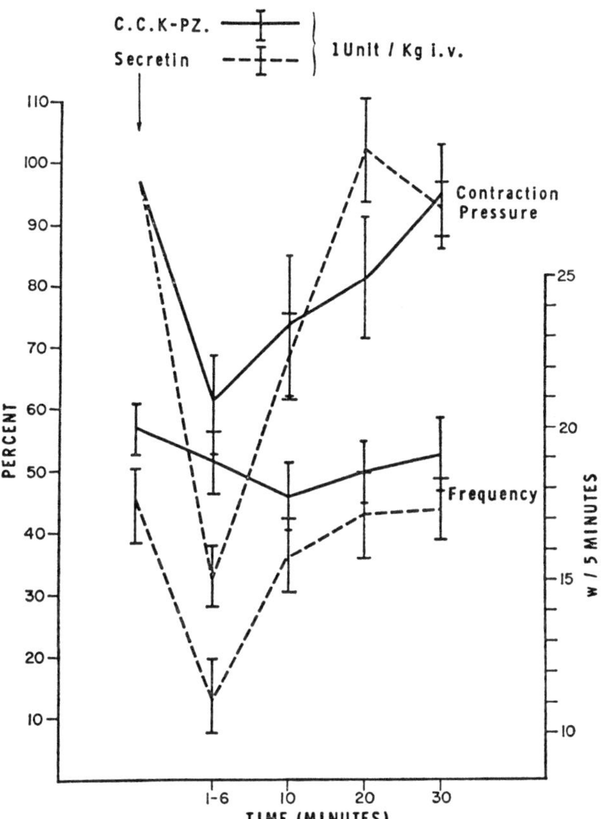

Fig. 39. Influence of a continuous infusion of cholecystokinin or secretin, in a dose of 1 U/kg/h on the frequency and contraction pressure of innervated antral pouches. Mean of 24 experiments in 4 dogs (SUGAWARA et al., 1969)

Some authors, however, left the field open for the existence of still more substances with "enterogastrone"-like activity. After having demonstrated that pure CCK is capable of inhibiting the acid response of Heidenhain pouch dogs to both gastrin and histamine, BEDI et al. (1967 b) thought it quite likely that endogenous duodenal acidification may release another, as yet unidentified, humoral inhibitory agent, or that secretin and/or cholecystokinin may act in collaboration with each other or with another inhibitor.

Evidence for the existence of one or several "enterogastrones" other than secretin and CCK in the duodenal mucosa was also obtained (JOHNSON and GROSSMAN, 1969 a) when an emulsion of 10 g corn oil/15 ml, (Lipomul, Upjohn) was instilled every 5 min during 30 min into the duodenum of dogs during optimal histamine stimulation, 0.04 mg/kg/h in i.v. infusion. The gastric secretion was reduced by more than 50%. The inhibition could not be mimicked by doses of either pure secretin or 10% pure cholecystokinin, 2 U/kg/h, which were near maximal for pancreatic secretion, and which, when given alone, each produced a stronger pancreatic response than the fat. The combination of 2 U/kg/h of secretin and CCK failed to produce any diminution of the gastric secretory response to histamine.

An early observation by WORMSLEY and GROSSMAN (1964) that acidification of the duodenal contents depresses the histamine induced secretion, against which secretin is poorly active, could be interpreted in the same direction. This is also true of the findings of LUCAS et al. (1968) that acidification of the duodenum in conscious dogs with a Heidenhain pouch and a duodenal fistula or a Thiry-Vella loop causes a heavy increase in the acid secretion stimulated by metacholine, 4 μg/min, whereas the secretion after the gastrin pentapeptide, 2 μg/min, is inhibited. Secretin reduces the response to both stimuli to ½ and ⅓ respectively.

BERSTAD, PETERSEN and MYREN (1971) likewise concluded that the inhibitory effect of duodenal acidification in man cannot be due to endogenous secretin alone. In 17 healthy young persons the duodenal acidification with 400 ml 0.1 N HCl and 0.05 N NaCl per hour caused a depression by 45% of the pentagastrin, 0.15 μg/kg/h, stimulated acid secretion with no effect on the pepsin secretory response to 6.0 μg/kg/h of pentagastrin. In a previous series BERSTAD and PETERSEN (1970) found 54% inhibition of acid secretion and 69% increase in the pepsin secretion in response to the corresponding doses of pentagastrin.

Lately different workers have analyzed the biological activity of a number of peptide fractions deriving from hog intestinal mucosa as obtained from the extracts used for the isolation of secretin and CCK. BROWN (1967) and BROWN and PARKES (1967) discussed the possibility of the occurrence in the duodenum of *a factor stimulating gastric motility*, an antagonist to secretin in this respect.

Particular attention has been paid to the inhibitory effect of CCK preparations (JOHNSON and MAGEE, 1965a, b; CHEY et al., 1967, 1968, 1969, 1970b; LORBER et al., 1972).

c) The Gastric Inhibitory Polypeptide (GIP) of J.C. Brown and Coworkers

BROWN and PEDERSON (1970) presented physiological evidence for the existence of a gastric inhibitor, other than cholecystokinin-pancreozymin. In experiments in dogs in which they monitored gall-bladder pressure, H^+ and pepsin secretion, and motor activity in fundic and antral pouches they were able to demonstrate that a "40%" pure CCK was a better stimulator of H^+ secretion than a "10%" pure material. They concluded that in purifying CCK an inhibitory material for gastric acid secretion was removed. This conclusion supported the earlier observations of BROWN et al. (1969) who demonstrated that a side fraction from the purification of CCK possessed potent inhibitory activity for gastrin stimulated H^+ and pepsin secretion, antral and fundic motor activity. In those experiments antral pouches were being perfused with 0.1% acetylcholine in 0.9% saline, to release endogenous gastrin. On the other hand, SJÖDIN (1971) in performing sham feeding experiment in Pavlov pouch dogs, found that both the 10% pure CCK and the pure hormone tended to enhance the vagal stimulation of the parietal cells. There was no indication that the 10% pure material, from which the polypeptide of BROWN derives, should in the doses applied, 0.75 to 3.0 U/kg/h, exert an enterogastrone like activity. BROWN et al. (1970) described the further purification of this inhibitory material and demonstrated that it was a polypeptide. They demonstrated inhibitory activity for pentapeptide stimulated H^+

secretion and that the polypeptide contained < 2.0 U/mg CCK activity. They were unable to show changes in blood pressure in the aneasthetized rabbit. The gastric inhibitory activity was destroyed by digestion of the polypeptide with trypsin. Amino acid analyses revealed the absence of proline, a high content of glutamine and a preponderance of lysine over arginine. The authors, however, had reservations about the physiological status of the polypeptide until further physiological criteria had been satisfied. BROWN (1971) revealed the probable amino acid composition of the polypeptide to be:

Ala_3 Arg_1 Asx_6 $Glx_{(5-6)}$ Gly_2 His_1 Ile_4 Leu_2
Lys_5 Met_1 Phe_2 Ser_3 Thr_2 Trp_2 Tyr_2 Val_1

making a total of 42—43 amino acid residues and the N-terminal amino acid was tyrosine, distinguishing the polypeptide from other gastrointestinal hormones. The partial sequence of the polypeptide, based on work on the tryptic peptides has been shown by BROWN (1970) to be as follows:

Tyr-(Ala(2),Asx,Glx,Gly,Ile(2),Phe,Ser(2),Thr,Tyr)-Met-Asp-Lys-Ile-Arg-
Gln-(Ala,Asx(2),Glx(2—3),Leu(2),Phe,Trp,Val)-Lys-Gly-Lys-Lys-Ser-Asp-
Trp-Lys-His-(Asn,Gln,Ile,Thr).

Recently the complete amino acid sequence has been reported by BROWN and DRYBURGH (1971) to be:

Tyr-Ala-Glu-Gly-Thr-Phe-Ile-Ser-Asp-Tyr-Ser-Ile-Ala-Met-Asp-Lys-Ile-Arg-
Gln-Gln-Asp-Phe-Val-Asn-Trp-Leu-Leu-Ala-Gln-Gln-Lys-Gly-Lys-Lys-Ser-
Asp-Trp-Lys-His-Asn-Ile-Thr-Gln

making a total of 43 amino acid residues and a molecular weight of 5105. The authors also reported similarities in the structure of GIP, glucagon and secretin (Table 19a).

In the table, it can be seen that fifteen of the first 26 amino acids occur in the same position as they do in porcine glucagon, and 9 of the first 26 in the same position as in porcine secretin.

Table 19a. *Similarities in structure of "gastric inhibitory polypeptide" with porcine glucagon and porcine secretin*

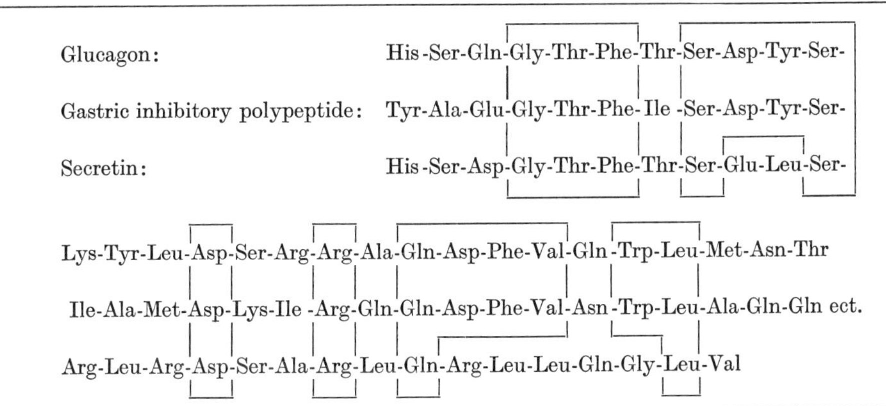
Glucagon: His-Ser-Gln-Gly-Thr-Phe-Thr-Ser-Asp-Tyr-Ser-
Gastric inhibitory polypeptide: Tyr-Ala-Glu-Gly-Thr-Phe-Ile-Ser-Asp-Tyr-Ser-
Secretin: His-Ser-Asp-Gly-Thr-Phe-Thr-Ser-Glu-Leu-Ser-

Lys-Tyr-Leu-Asp-Ser-Arg-Arg-Ala-Gln-Asp-Phe-Val-Gln-Trp-Leu-Met-Asn-Thr
Ile-Ala-Met-Asp-Lys-Ile-Arg-Gln-Gln-Asp-Phe-Val-Asn-Trp-Leu-Ala-Gln-Gln ect.
Arg-Leu-Arg-Asp-Ser-Ala-Arg-Leu-Gln-Arg-Leu-Leu-Gln-Gly-Leu-Val

d) The "Enterogastrone" of Lucien and Coworkers

By applying the extraction and purification technique elaborated by MUTT (1959b, d) and JORPES and MUTT (1961a) for the purification of CCK up to the

10% pure preparation with 250—300 IDU/mg, Lucien et al. (1969) obtained chromatographic fractions containing "enterogastrone" which in a dose of one mg inhibited histamine stimulated secretion (40—80 μg/kg/h) by 40% in the Heidenhain pouch dog. The preparations were free of secretin and CCK (Itoh, Lucien and Schally, 1970).

In view of the assumed inhibitory effects of "enterogastrone" on the gastric motility, Schally, Redding, Lucien and Meyer (1967) studied the effect of a purified "enterogastrone" preparation on hunger in mice. After 17 hours of fasting, the mouse was injected with 0.1—1 mg of the preparation. The reduced appetite observed is not unexpected after administration of an amount of substance1000—10,000 times as large per kg b.w. as the ordinary dose of 10% pure CCK administered in man.

e) "Urogastrone"

Considerable attention was paid to the occurrence of an antisecretory factor in the urine (Necheles, Hanke and Fantl, 1939). As to its origin, Culmer, Gray, Adkison and Ivy (1940) demonstrated, that it disappeared from dog urine after excision of the small intestine. A pyrogen-free active product, named "urogastrone", was prepared from human urine by Gray, Culmer, Wieczorowski and Adkison (1940) and its action on the histamine stimulated gastric secretion in man was studied by Gray, Wieczorowski and Ivy (1940).

Highly purified "urogastrone" from human urine is, according to Gerring (1969, 1970) and Gerring and Haworth (1970), a potent inhibitor of the acid secretion from the Heidenhain pouch of the dog, producing in a dose of 1 to 2 μg/kg a 70% inhibition. 5 μg/kg is equally active on innervated stomach preparations. After histamine stimulation of the innervated stomach, not only the volume but also the acid concentration were reduced by the preparation. It was without effect on the pancreatic exocrine secretion, the salivary secretion or on gastric motility in animals.

f) "Bulbogastrone"

Particular attention has been paid to the role of the bulbar region of the duodenum in the inhibitory mechanism. From their findings in dogs that perfusion of bulbar pouches with acid produced an inhibition of the secretory response to a meal, Andersson and Uvnäs (1961) concluded that the duodenal inhibitory mechanism may be located mainly in the duodenal bulb. The finding of Andersson, Nilsson and Uvnäs (1965, 1967) that no inhibition was achieved on acidification of the considerably larger segment of the distal duodenum strongly supported this concept.

In contradistinction to this the stimulation of the pancreatic secretion by acid in the duodenum was seven times more efficient when 45 cm of the proximal small bowel of the dog was perfused with 0.16 N HCl at 25 ml/15 min than when the upper 11.5 cm segment was perfused (Meyer, Way and Grossman, 1970b).

The bulbar inhibitory mechanism acted as effectively in the Heidenhain as in the Pavlov pouch group of dogs. The secretory responses to histamine, in contrast to gastrin, were not significantly inhibited by acidification of the duodenal bulb (Andersson, Nilsson and Uvnäs, 1967). The degree of inhibition of gastrin stimulated secretion was dependent upon both the dose of gastrin given and the pH in the bulbar pouch. At low secretory rates the reduction of pH to 3.1—4.1 produced significant inhibition. At high secretory rates the pH-level within the duodenal bulb had to be reduced to 2.0—2.5 before inhibition of the acid secretion occured (Andersson and Nilsson, 1969). It has been demonstrated in humans (ANDERSSON and GROSSMAN, 1966) and in dogs (BROOKS and GROSSMAN, 1970b) that there exists a steep pH-gradient between the duodenal bulb and the postbulbar duodenum. Even values below 2.0 were not uncommon in the duodenal bulb, which indicated that the pH normally might fall to the critical pH necessary for eliciting inhibition of gastric secretion. NILSSON (1969) was also able to demonstrate that vagally activated secretion, evoked by sham feeding, was highly susceptible to the inhibitory influence of bulbar acidification. Reduction of the pH to 4 resulted in decreased secretory responses to sham feeding.

It has further been reported that an inhibitory material, not containing significant amounts of either cholecystokinin or secretin, could be extracted from duodenal bulbs of hogs. The material, which was not wholly homogeneous, was able upon intravenous injection, to totally block pentagastrin induced secretion in Heidenhain pouch dogs in as low doses as 1.0 μg per kg b.w. It has been suggested that the extracted bulbar material contained a specific gastric secretory inhibitor, for which the name "bulbogastrone" has been proposed (ANDERSSON, NILSSON, SJÖDIN and UVNÄS, 1972; UVNÄS, 1971).

V. Potentiation of the Effect of the Gastrointestinal Hormones

A lively discussion has been going on concerning the interpretation of an enhanced response to stimuli acting together, i.e. whether the effect is purely additive or a result of potentiation.

A number of authors (GROSSMAN, 1963, 1969b; GILLESPIE and GROSSMAN, 1964a; MAGEE, NAKAJIMA and ODORI, 1968; HENRIKSEN, 1969a; WAY, 1969) have given their views on the criteria for potentiation. MAGEE et al. (1968) differentiated between pharmacological and true potentiation. In the latter, the mixture of the drugs acts on a common receptor, whose maximal response, *i.e.* the response in which all the receptor sites are activated, cannot be exceeded. Since the size of the response on doubling the dose depends upon where on the dose-response curve the dose falls, separate dose-response curves are needed for each of the single components and for the mixture. GROSSMAN (1969b) demanded that one must find doses of the two agents that give an equal response when given separately. If the response to half-doses of the two agents given together is equal to the response to the whole doses of the individual drugs, the action is additive. If the response is greater than the response to the whole doses, potentiation has occurred. SPINGOLA, MEYER and GROSSMAN (1970) concluded that there is potentiation between exogenous secretin and endogenous CCK because maximal volume, becarbonate, and protein response to the combination was greater than to either agent alone. In general, more attention has been paid to experimental findings than to terminology, particularly when the potentiating effect has been fairly evident.

a) The Mutual Potentiating Effect of Neural and Hormonal Stimuli

In his monograph, *The Secretory Mechanisms of the Gastrointestinal Tract*, GREGORY (1962, p. 21, 53—55) stated that vagal excitation of the oxyntic cell is an important factor conditioning its response to the antral hormone gastrin. Acetylcholine and the stable cholinesters, Urecholine and Carbachol sensitize the oxyntic cells. Given in subthreshold doses to dogs they greatly increase the otherwise small response of a denervated fundic pouch to a meal or to gastrin (GROSSMAN, 1961). In the special issue of *The American Journal of Digestive Diseases* of February 1966, dedicated to the memory of S. A. KOMAROV, UVNÄS and associates

(UVNÄS et al., 1966) discuss the question of the interaction of vagal impulses and *gastrin* in the control of gastric acid secretion. There is an interplay between them resulting in the normal response to a meal. After curtailment of antral function, the HCl-secreting glands respond poorly or not at all to vagal impulses, and the vagus-denervated fundic mucosa shows a very low sensitivity to endogenous or exogenous gastrin. The nervous and humoral mechanisms are unable to operate effectively independently of each other (UVNÄS, 1968). Exogenous gastrin can substitute for the antral function (UVNÄS, 1942) even in subthreshold doses (OLBE, 1964a, b, c; OLBE et al., 1968) and cholinergic drugs for the vagal impulses (ANDERSSON and GROSSMAN, 1965). Apparently the neural impulses are not strong enough to break through the resistance around or within the secreting cell without the support of a catalyzer, a kind of grease that gets things going. Accordingly, antrectomy diminishes the responsiveness of the fundic glands to humoral stimulation both in man (GILLESPIE et al., 1960), and in the dog (ANDERSSON and GROSSMAN, 1965).

A similar interplay also takes place in the pancreas between *secretin* and vagal stimulation.

As demonstrated by GAYET and GUILLAUMIE (1930), a dose of secretin which is too small to evoke any secretion or produces only a small amount will cause copious secretion if given while the vagi are being stimulated. In experiments intending to show that an elevated blood glucose level does not over the central nervous system stimulate pancreatic secretion, the authors cross-circulated the head of a dog, connected to the body only through the intact vagus nerves, with blood from another dog. Glucose injection in the donor dog did not stimulate pancreatic secretion in the recipient dog. In each experiment electrical stimulation of the vagus nerve was followed by a profuse secretion in excess of the basal secretion, 1—2 ml/10 min, sustained by a small dose of secretin (Fig. 40).

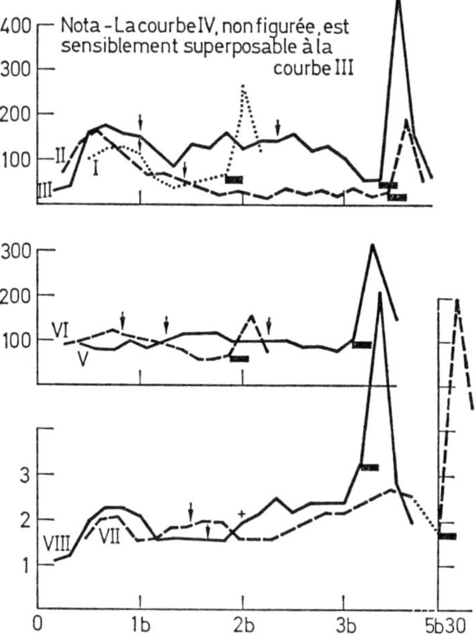

Fig. 40. The experimental series of GAYET and GUILLAUMIE (1930). At ↓ glucose injection in the donor dog; at + vagotomy in experiment VIII; at — electrical stimulation of the thoracal vagus. Ordinate: ml pancreatic juice secreted

Referring to the findings of GAYET et GUILLAUMIE (1930) that vagal stimulation greatly increases the volume of pancreatic secretion after secretin, and of THOMAS (1950) that previous injection of secretin potentiates the secretory response to subsequent vagal stimulation, BROWN, HARPER and SCRATCHERD (1967) showed that stimulation of the dorsal vagus trunk, or the administration of "pancreozymin" or antral extracts, which *per se* have little or no effect on the resting pancreas of the anesthetized cat, increase the rate of secretion, the concentration of bicarbonate and the output of enzymes in animals under secretin stimulation kept on a steady slow rate of secretion, 0.5—1.0 ml/15 min. The mean volume in 70 observations in 40 experiments before *stimulation of the vagus* was 0.80 ml/15 min. During stimulation there followed a mean increase of 0.66 ml, a strong potentiation of the secretin effect through nervous influences. Atropine caused only an insignificant reduction of the volume and bicarbonate response but abolished the increase in enzyme secretion. Hexamethonium abolished all the effects of vagal stimulation.

The type of close interdependence that exists between vagal stimulation and gastrin, both with respect to the release of the hormone and their mutual interactions, does not seem to be necessary for the action of secretin. In the rat the division of both vagi at the level of the oesophagus did not influence the effect of secretin on the pancreas in the doses used in the experiments of LIN and ALPHIN (1958) and of HEATLEY (1968a). Likewise in the dog, vagotomy did not change the pancreatic response to exogenous secretin (HENRIKSEN, 1969b), nor did Urecholine potentiate the secretin response in the experiments of PRESHAW, ADASHEK et al. (1965).

The integration of nervous and hormonal mechanisms for external pancreatic secretion has been discussed by GROSSMAN (1962, 1963, 1972b) and by PRESHAW (1967).

d) Interactions with Histamine

The potentiation of the gastrin effect by histamine and the combined effect of *gastrin* or *histamine* and *cholinergic drugs* have been extensively studied in Heidenhain pouch dogs by PASSARO, GILLESPIE and GROSSMAN (1963), GILLESPIE and GROSSMAN (1964a), MARKS, KOMAROV and SHAY (1966) and COOKE (1969).

A potentiation of the effects in man between the pentapeptide (ICI 50,123) and histamine was reported by KONTUREK and OLEEKSY (1967).

Gastrin or Urecholine, 0.04 mg/kg/h, causes an essential potentiation of the histamine effect on the gastric acid output in the conscious gastric fistula dog (JOHNSON and GROSSMAN, 1969c; BROOKS, JOHNSON and GROSSMAN, 1970) but not in man (MAKHLOUF, McMANUS and CARD, 1966; BROOKS, JOHNSON and GROSSMAN, 1970). Combining 0.04 mg/kg/h of histamine dihydrochloride with 0.2 g/kg/h of a crude gastrin preparation or 0.04 mg/kg/h of Urecholine in the intravenous infusion more than doubled the maximal response as compared with that to the dose of histamine alone. The observed peak response was considerably higher than the calculated maximal response to histamine or gastrin alone (JOHNSON and GROSSMAN, 1969c). It is, according to the authors, unlikely that the small dose of gastrin can double the gastric response to maximal stimulation by merely increasing mucosal blood flow, particularly since HARPER, REED and SMY (1968) found that the increase in blood flow did not itself produce increased gastric secretion in the cat.

The ulcerogenic effect of pentagastrin causing duodenal ulcers in the rat is strongly potentiated by the simultaneous subcutaneous infusion of histamine or Carbachol (ROBERT, STOUT and DALE, 1970).

Cholecystokinin behaves similarly. In studying the combined effect of CCK and the cholinergic drug metacholine, MAGEE and NAKAMURA (1966) observed a potentiating effect of the cholinergic drug on the stimulating action of small doses of CCK on gastric acid secretion. In continuation, NAKAMURA, NAKAJIMA and MAGEE (1968) used dogs with double pouches made from the whole denervated stomach with the antrum separated from the fundic part by a mucosal septum. The mean acid response at 1 to 4 U/min of CCK with background metacholine, 2 μg/min in infusion, was in all the 9 animals significantly larger than the additive effects. The mean response to 1 μg metacholine/min with 2 units of CCK as background was likewise significantly more than additive. With 8 μg/min of metacholine as background, the inhibitory effect on the gastric acid secretion was observed already at the level of 3 U/min of CCK. There was a drop of 18.6% as compared with the response to 2 U/min of CCK. When CCK was given with background metacholine, a dose response relationship for pepsin was evident. Without metacholine, the pepsin response was unrelated to dose.

The findings of MURAT and WHITE (1966) and MAGEE and NAKAMURA (1966) were confirmed by VENABLES, RUDICK, KARK and DREILING (1969) using 4 gastric fistula dogs, on one of which a pyloroplasty had been performed earlier. 0.5—4 units of "pancreozymin" per hour infused intravenously stimulated the secretion of acid and enzymes. The acid secretion was 3—5 times the basal secretion. The peak output of acid increased over 100% if potentiated by Mecholyl (metacholine chloride), 125 μg/kg/h. The peak pepsin output after "pancreozymin" equalled that stimulated by the gastrin pentapeptide. A cholinergic background enhanced the pepsin output as well for both "pancreozymin" and gastrin, thus demonstrating the similarity in action between CCK and gastrin with respect to the gastric secretion.

c) Mutual Potentiation of Action of Secretin and CCK

In the experiments of BROWN et al. (1967), "*pancreozymin*" and *antral extracts* in suitable doses caused potentiation of the secretin effect equal to that obtained by stimulation of the vagus nerve, the mean volume before "pancreozymin" being 0.81 ml/15 min and the mean increase in volume under the action of "pancreozymin" 0.49 ml/15 min. The effect of "pancreozymin" on the volume, bicarbonate concentration and enzyme output was uninfluenced by atropine or hexamethonium. Neither CCK nor gastrin stimulated the flow of pancreatic juice when given alone in the cat, but when combined with secretin they potentiated the effect of the latter. The authors discussed the likelihood that the effect of "pancreozymin" on the water and bicarbonate secretion is due to increased vascular perfusion in the gland.

In analogy with the findings of BROWN et al. (1967) in the cat that "pancreozymin" or stimulation of the dorsal vagus trunk potentiates the effect of secretin, WORMSLEY (1969a, b, c) found that "pancreozymin" combined with a barely superthreshold dose of secretin elicited a bicarbonate response in man which was greater than the maximal responses to the two components in a mixture. The secretion of pancreatic enzymes in response to the combined hormones was additive. According to the author, the combination of the two hormones results in a more efficient secretion of bicarbonate than after secretin alone.

Working like BARON et al. (1963) and HANSKY et al. (1964) with unanesthetized duodenal fistula dogs carrying a gastric fistula, HENRIKSEN and WORNING (1967) observed a potentiating effect when *secretin* and *CCK* stimulation were combined. The rates of secretion of fluid and bicarbonate after the combined stimulation were, over a wide dose-range, greater than the sum of the secretion rates after administering secretin and CCK separately. The maximal rates of secretion of fluid and bicarbonate after stimulation with secretin or CCK were obtained with 6—8 U/kg of secretin or with 12—16 U/kg of "pancreozymin". The secretion rates after combined secretin-CCK stimulation (1 U/kg of each) were on an average 93% (fluid) and 97% (bicarbonate) of the maximal secretion rates thus obtained.

A potentiation was also observed by SPINGOLA, MEYER and GROSSMAN (1970) between exogenous secretin, 0.25—2 U/kg/h, and endogenous CCK, released by perfusing the intestine of pancreatic and gastric fistula dogs with 0.13 M, pH 7, isosmotic phenylalanine (PA) solution. Maximal responses to secretin and PA were 34 ml/15 min and 4.0 mEq/15 min of bicarbonate versus 24.2 ml and 3 mEq respectively, which was the maximal responses to secretin (8 U/kg/h) alone. The protein output exceeded by 400% that after secretin alone.

On finding that the combination of threshold inhibitor doses of both secretin and CCK results in a greater degree of inhibition of the gastrin-stimulated acid secretion than was obtained with twice the dose of either agent alone, BEDI et al. (1969) concluded that a potentiation of the inhibitor effect had taken place. They were working with dogs with innervated or vagally denervated gastric pouches.

Exogenous secretin, 2 U/kg, as well as endogenous secretin released by HCl in the duodenum potentiates the effect of 1—8 U/kg of CCK on the gallbladder, causing a higher pressure response than when CCK is given alone to chronic gallbladder and gastric fistula dogs (STENING and GROSSMAN, 1969c). Secretin alone, 4 U/kg, did not alter the basal gallbladder motility.

The combined effect of *secretin* and *gastrin* on the pancreatic secretion in conscious gastric and pancreatic fistula dogs is, however, according to HENRIKSEN and WORNING (1969), purely additive. The doses used by the authors were 1 U/kg of secretin and 2 U/kg of gastrin. Nor was there any potentiation of the pancreatic response to gastrin when gastrin was given against a background stimulation with 1 mg/h of Urecholine intravenously (PRESHAW et al., 1965a).

To the contrary the experiments of BERSTAD and PETERSEN (1970) indicated that a potentiation may exist between secretin and pentagastrin in stimulation of pepsin secretion in man.

VI. The Action of Secretin, CCK, Gastrin and Glucagon on Gastric Motility

1. Secretin

JOHNSON and MAGEE (1965a, b) studied in a series of dogs with a totally denervated Heidenhain pouch the effect on gastric motility of the pure natural secretin and a 10% pure CCK preparation. Secretin infused intravenously during a period of 10 min in a dose of 1 U/kg exerted no influence on the gastric motility, nor did 10 μg of serotonine. In a subsequent series of 8 fasting healthy young human subjects, JOHNSON, BROWN and MAGEE (1966) infused one after the other pure secretin and 10% pure CCK, 0.05 U/kg/min of each intravenously, in total 0.5 U/kg during 10 minutes. After CCK, but not after secretin, there followed in each of the subjects a prompt, complete and fairly prolonged gastric motor inhibition. CUMMINS et al. (1966) likewise found in 19 studies on 12 human subjects and 16 experiments on 8 dogs with gastric cannulas that pure secretin, 1 U/kg, did not alter the motility or tone of the stomach.

The findings of the above authors as to the action of secretin on the spontaneous motor activity of the stomach in man and the dog have not been substantiated in more recent series of investigations.

Already in 1965, LORBER, CHEY and LEWI consistently found a reduction of the motility of both the main stomach and the Heidenhain pouch of conscious dogs after 1.5, 3 and 6 U/kg of secretin.

Both the pure secretin and Secretin Boots have been found to cause an inhibition of both spontaneous and Urecholine-stimulated gastric motor activity lasting for 15 min or longer. The duodenal motility is similarly affected. In dogs, both the natural and the synthetic forms of secretin produce inhibition of spontaneous motor activity of the stomach and duodenum (CHEY, LORBER, KUSAKCIOGLU and HENDRICKS, 1967; CHEY et al., 1969).

The mean basal rate of the 15 min emptying of the stomach, 85%, dropped after injection of one U/kg of secretin, synthetic or natural, in 5 dogs to 64% (CHEY, KOSAY, HENDRICKS and LORBER, 1968).

Intravenous injection of 1 U/kg of the pure natural or the synthetic secretin in 10 normal persons caused a retardation of the emptying rate of stomach. Instead of a normal emptying rate of 83% in 15 min, the rate was reduced to 42%, a retardation of the same order of magnitude as that caused by 0.5 U/kg of CCK intravenously (CHEY, HITANANT, HENDRICKS and LORBER, 1968, 1970).

DINOSO, CHEY, HENDRICKS and LORBER (1969) reported on a study of the gastric motor function in 19 healthy human subjects and 7 patients. One U/kg of the pure secretin consistently reduced the number and mean amplitude index of the spontaneous or Urecholine-induced contractions of the stomach to about one fifth for the next 10 min with a return to normal after 20—30 min. The poor response to secretin seen in the series of JOHNSON, BROWN and MAGEE (1966) was considered by the authors to be due to the lower dose of secretin used, 0.5 U/kg during a 10 min infusion. The more plausible explanation is that the unit of secretin available before 1966 had a several times lower potency than that manufactured by the GIH Research Unit at Karolinska institutet, Stockholm, beginning in January 1966.

These observations are in accordance with the findings made by VAGNE, STENING, BROOKS and GROSSMAN (1968) in comparing the potency and action spectrum of the pure natural and the synthetic porcine secretins in dogs. The motility of both the fundic part of the stomach and an innervated antral pouch was recorded. Three doses of natural and synthetic secretin were given alternately during each of 4 experiments performed on 2 dogs. In all instances there was a decreased motility after injection of secretin. After 0.63 U/kg of natural secretin the antral motility was abolished for 4 min and the decrease lasted for 10 min. The fundic motility was reduced to a lesser degree and was never abolished completely.

As a supplement to the experiments of CHEY et al. (1969), in which only one dose of secretin was given i.v., VAGNE and ANDRE (1971) administered 0.125, 0.395 and 1.250 U/kg of the pure porcine secretin i.v. infusion to 2 healthy persons. The volume of the test meal remaining in the stomach 20 min after ingestion increased with increasing doses of secretin. The doses of secretin were not maximal for pancreatic secretion.

Fully convincing evidence as to the action of pure secretin on the gastric motility was also presented by KELLY, WOODWARD and CODE (1969) by measuring the gastric myoelectrical activity in conscious dogs during a steady state of gastric contractions. A number of monopolar Ag-AgCl electrodes had been implanted on the antral serosal surface of the stomach 2 weeks before the experiment.

Water (10 ml/min) was instilled into the stomach via a gastric cannula by means of a constant-infusion pump, and the gastric antral action potentials excited by the constant infusion of water were recorded during 15 min. periods, during which a continuous intravenous infusion of physiological saline solution without or with secretin, 0.1 U/kg/min, was given.

The incidence of antral action potentials began to decrease within 2 min after the start of the secretin infusion in 11 of 12 tests. By 10 min the incidence of antral action potentials was reduced by 69—100% (Table 19b). The incidence of

Table 19b. *Effect of Secretin on Incidence of Antral Action Potentials during Constant Intragastric Infusion of Water.* (Kelly, Woodward, Code, 1969)

	Percentage of antral PP with action potentials*			
Period:	1	2	3	4
Dog	Control	Secretin	Control	Secretin
1	90	21	79	16
	48	7	76	8
	47	0	88	0
2	45	0	45	20
	78	10	90	20
	32	6	36	20
3	47	27	53	13
	33	10	60	19
	87	10	80	16
4	50	13	53	17
	80	24	73	10
	42	13	90	16

* During 6-min interval begun 7 min after start of each period; results of three tests on each dog on different days are given.

antral action potentials increased within 3 min after secretin infusion was stopped in three of the four dogs and within 5 min in the fourth; after 10 min it had returned to control levels. In contrast, cholecystokinin infusion, 0.1 U/kg/min, produced small and inconsistent changes in the incidence of antral action potentials. The frequency and velocity of conduction did not change significantly during infusions of secretin or cholecystokinin.

The action of secretin on the lower esophageal sphincter

In accordance with the inhibitory action of secretin on the gastrin stimulated gastric motility and gastric acid secretion secretin, both endogenous and exogenous, is in man a sensitive inhibitor of the gastrin stimulation of the lower esophageal sphincter (Cohen and Lipshutz, 1971). The ordinary rise in sphincter pressure from 15 to 75 mm Hg, caused within 3 min by 0.5 μg synthetic gastrin I intravenously, can be completely blocked by previous i.v. injection of 1 U/kg of secretin or by intraduodenal acidification.

2. Cholecystokinin

Even before the discovery of CCK, Ivy and Farrell (1925, 1926), Farrell and Ivy (1926a) observed that fat introduced into the duodenum inhibited the motility of a transplanted fundic pouch, an effect assumed to be elicited by a specific duodenal hormone, "enterogastrone", an "analogue" of secretin, inhibiting both gastric motility and secretion (vide Grossman, 1950). Kosaka and Lim (1930a, b) discussed the mechanism of inhibition.

JOHNSON and MAGEE (1965a, b) found that the 10% pure *CCK* in a dose of 0.3—1 Ivy dog unit per kg caused a total cessation of the spontaneous pressure contractions both in the denervated fundic pouch and in the innervated stomach. The effect on the stomach of 1 U/kg lasted for 12 minutes and on the denervated pouch for up to 2 hours, the duration of inhibition being, within the range 0.3 to 2 U/kg of CCK directly proportional to the dose administered. The activity was, like the activity on the gallbladder, destroyed by digestion with an enterokinase activated pancreatic juice. Both activities were resistant to boiling in water for 2 hours. Instillation of 20 ml of an olive oil emulsion into the duodenum of the dogs produced an inhibition of similar intensity, the instillation of a peptone solution a weaker inhibition. 0.1 N HCl had a variable effect. The authors pointed out that the CCK preparations exerted a physiological activity similar to that previously ascribed to "enterogastrone".

Likewise, JOHNSON. BROWN and MAGEE (1966) found a prompt, complete and fairly prolonged gastric motor inhibition in man after infusion of 0.05 U/kg/min during 10 min of the 10% pure CCK.

In the experiments of CHEY, HITANANT, HENDRICKS and LORBER (1968, 1970) CCK of the same purity given intravenously in a dose of 0.5 Ivy dog units/kg to 5 normal human subjects reduced the mean emptying rate of the stomach to 44% from the normal value 80%, as measured by the Hunt method employing phenol red as indicator. DINOSO et al. (1969) found in a series of 6 persons that the number and mean amplitude index of gastric contractions were reduced to about one fifth, remaining at that low level for 20 min after slow intravenous injection of 1 U/kg of the 10% pure CCK.

The findings of CHEY et al. (1967, 1968, 1969, 1970) and LORBER et al. (1965) as to the inhibitory action of secretin and a 10% pure preparation of CCK on the gastric motility were fully substantiated by SUGAWARA, ISAZA, CURT and WOODWARD (1969). Secretin, 1 U/kg injected rapidly or 4 U/kg/h in constant infusion, reduced the frequency of contractions in the isolated vagally innervated pyloric antrum of the dog to 74% and the amplitude to 42% of the control. The corresponding figures after similar doses of CCK were 75% and 63% respectively (Fig. 39).

CAMERON, PHILLIPS and SUMMERSKILL (1967) found an increase in amplitude of chymographically registered rhythmic contractions of gastric antral strips, cut from surgical specimens. The prewarmed KREBS solution, dripped down the surface of the strips, contained 1 U/100 ml of CCK. With fundic strips no effect was seen.

The recent results as to the action of secretin and CCK on the gastric motility in man and the dog were summarized by LORBER et al. (1972).

3. Gastrin

BLAIR et al. (1961b) found that crude gastrin causes an increase in the gastric tone in the anesthetized cat. The pure gastrins, both gastrin I and II, were found by GREGORY and TRACY (1964) to cause a rapid and powerful brief contraction of the Heidenhain pouch when administered i.v. in doses of 10 to 50 µg. 25—50 µg of gastrin II stimulated antral contractions in man when given as a single intravenous injection (SMITH and HOGG, 1966). Accordingly, gastrin or the synthetic pentagastrin (ICI 50,123) in a concentration of 0.4—0.6 µg/ml produces contractions in isolated strips of the human gastric muscle *in vitro*, the upper and lower small intestine being unresponsive (BENNETT, MISIEWICZ and WALLER, 1967; BENNETT and MISIEWICZ, 1967).

According to SUGAWARA, ISAZA and WOODWARD (1969), endogenous gastrin or i.v. administrated pentagastrin, 3 µg/kg/h, causes in dogs a sharp increase in frequency and simultaneously an equal fall in the amplitude of the contractions of the innervated isolated antral pouch without influencing the gastric tone.

ISENBERG and GROSSMAN (1969b) compared the action of crude gastrin, gastrin I and gastrin II in doses submaximal for gastric acid secretion by counting the number of contractions and measuring the amplitude of each wave both in the intact stomach and in the innervated antral pouch of dogs. The samples stimulated rhythmic antral contractions in both kinds of preparation. The synthetic antigastrin SC 15396 decreased the acid secretion stimulated by gastrin, but did not influence the gastrin stimulated antral motility.

A delayed emptying of the stomach was observed on infusing porcine gastrin II in two human subjects (HUNT and RAMSBOTTOM, 1967).

4. Glucagon

Intravenous administration of glucagon, 2 mg, either in a single injection or by infusion, abolishes the gastric hunger contractions and the sensation of hunger in man (STUNKARD, van ITALLIE and REIS, 1955). SCHULMAN et al. (1957) performed a similar experiment with 10 persons for a period of five weeks, 1 mg glucagon being given intramuscularly before each meal. A significant reduction in caloric intake and body weight was recorded.

In reviewing the earlier literature, NECHELES, SPORN and WALKER (1966) added some experiments of their own, performed in dogs. In the anesthetized dog glucagon depressed the motility of the stomach, duodenum and colon in about half of the tests. In unanesthetized animals, the motility and tone of the same organs were distinctly inhibited in most tests.

In summary it can be said that gastrin stimulates and secretin and glucagon inhibit both the spontaneous and the Urecholine stimulated contractions of the gastric muscle. To what extent the hormones contribute to the physiological motor function of the stomach in connection with meals remains to be seen, when information has been gathered about the concentration of the hormones in the circulating blood. The conclusive statements we can now make as to their activity on gastric motility could not have been made without access to the pure natural and synthetic preparations of gastrin and secretin. Since the CCK preparations of 10% purity still contain impurities which inhibit gastric motility (JOHNSON and MAGEE, 1965a, b; BROWN et al., 1969; BROWN, MUTT and PEDERSON, 1970) more studies are to be performed using pure CCK and its strongly active C-terminal octa- and dodecapeptides.

VII. Influence of CCK on the Sphincter of Oddi and on Intestinal Peristalsis

The early *CCK preparations* caused contraction of the guinea pig ileum *in vitro* (JUNG and GREENGARD, 1933). SANDBLOM, VOEGTLIN and IVY (1935) after injecting vasodilatorfree CCK in anesthetized dogs, noted an increase in the duodenal motility in 87% of the tests in which the gallbladder contracted. The increase was periodic followed by a decrease. A primary increase in the resistance to the flow of bile through the common bile duct into the duodenum was due to the increase in the tone of the duodenum. If the hormone had a specific action on the sphincter of ODDI, it was inhibitory rather than excitatory.

IVY (1955) reported unsuccessful attempts to separate the intestinal contracting factor from the gallbladder contracting activity. Both activities were destroyed at the same rate by treatment with heat and alkali and serum enzymes. "The evidence indicates", he said, "but does not categorically establish, that the CCK in extracts of the mucosa of the upper intestine is a motor excitant of the smooth muscle of the intestine, colon, stomach, uterus and urinary bladder, the gallbladder musculature being the most sensitive, the duodenal musculature ranking second."

I. The Sphincter of Oddi

Working with conscious dogs with a Thiry-Vella duodenal loop and the common bile duct cannulated, HONG, MAGEE and CREWDSON (1956) demonstrated that irrigation of the loop or injection of duodenal extract caused a contraction of the gallbladder accompanied by a relaxation of the sphincter of Oddi. Both procaine and hexamethonium prevent the release of CCK from the duodenum, the former when applied locally and the latter when given systemically.

The effect of cholecystokinin on the sphincter of Oddi and on the motility of the duodenum has been studied by a number of authors: ADLERCREUTZ, JORPES, MUTT and WEGELIUS (1957), ADLERCREUTZ, PETTERSSON, ADLERCREUTZ, GRIBBE and WEGELIUS (1960), ALESSANDRINI, PALAGI, RAMORINO and COLAGRANDE (1961), ALLEGRI, BALDRIGHI and MONTEMARTINI (1957), BIZARD and PARIS (1960a, b), BOSSI (1961), COLAGRANDE et al. (1960), PARIS, ROBELET, SALEMBIER and DU BOIS (1962), PLESSIER and MARSICO (1960), RAMORINO, COLAGRANDE, MONTI and SISTI (1960), TORSOLI, RAMORINO, COLAGRANDE and DEMAIO (1961a), GRILL et al. (1963).

According to TORSOLI et al. (1961a, b) the terminal part of the common bile duct is constricted during the first 30 seconds after injection of cholecystokinin. Then follows a relaxation of the musculature and a dilation of both the intramural and extramural parts of the common duct. Even when the intramural part is originally obstructed, relaxation is still evident in the extramural part. Cholecystokinin may at least temporarily reduce pure Oddi hypertonicity. It was considered by the authors to be the most powerful relaxing agent of the sphincter of ODDI we have today. BIZARD and PARIS (1960a, b) pointed out that it is the only agent simultaneously causing contraction of the gallbladder and dilation of the sphincter of Oddi. Other physiological and pharmacological agents act on both of them in only one direction. ADLERCREUTZ et al. (1960) made kymographic records of duodenal tone and motility prior to, during and after injection of cholecystokinin in 15 cases, 3 of which exhibited pathological conditions of the bile ducts. In the normal cases, 4 mg of CCK with 22 IDU/mg brought about initial dilation and decrease in duodenal tone, followed by increased tone and markedly accelerated peristalsis when the secretion of bile had commenced. This effect failed to occur in the absence of a gallbladder. The results were verified roentgenologically.

The choledocho-duodenal junction, interposed between the duodenum and the common bile duct is according to CRISPIN et al. (1970) characterized by a zone of elevated pressure distinguishing it from the adjacent structures. Administration of atropine to conscious dogs resulted in decrease in the pressure suggesting that a cholinergic mechanism is partly responsible for the maintenance of the resting pressure in the choledocho-duodenal junction. At the same time there was no change in the duodenal pressure and only a slight decrease in pressure in the common bile duct.

Immediately after an injection of CCK, an increase in pressure in the common bile duct and, after a while, increased peristaltic activity in the duodenum are recorded (DAHLGREN, 1966). Thereupon there occurs, within 5—10 minutes, a narrowing of the diameter of the common duct and a decrease in the density of the contrast medium, possibly due to contraction of the duct or to relaxation of the sphincter (BLASBERG, EDMUNDS and FINBY, 1964).

2. A Neural Component in the Action of CCK on the Intestine

Using a sample of the pure CCK with a potency of 3 Ivy dog units per μg, HEDNER et al. (1967), HEDNER and RORSMAN (1968) repeated the experiments of NAITO et al. (1963). On segments of guinea pig ileum CCK was active in a concentration of 40 ng/ml, the action of one μg being equal to or greater than the effect of 1 μg of acetylcholine hydrochloride. Atropine in doses of about 0.1 μg completely inhibited the action on the intestine of 1 μg of each of the two substances. Even large doses of ACTH and insulin had no effect on the preparation. *Nor had CCK under similar conditions any effect on the guinea pig colon or uterus.* Circular strips of the gallbladder responded to CCK in lower doses than those required for contraction of the ileum, the lowest effective dose being 3 ng/ml in the medium. Unlike the effect on the jejunum, atropine even in large doses did not affect the response of the gallbladder to CCK. Like NAITO et al. the authors concluded that the action of CCK on the jejunum and on the gallbladder is mediated through different mechanisms. It seemed, according to the authors, plausible to assume that the hormone may play a role in the regulation of intestinal motility.

Since the *choledochal junction* contains a sphincter of its own (BOYDEN, 1957; HAUGE and MARK, 1965), capable of operating independently of the duodenal wall and being under cholinergic nervous stimulation, the question arises about the relationship of its smooth muscle to that of the gallbladder and of the intestine. In fact, on atropinization and CCK stimulation it behaves like the gallbladder muscle (HEDNER and RORSMAN, 1969). Even after atropinization CCK antagonized a contraction of the sphincter caused by bradykinin.

RAMIREZ and FARRAR (1970) studied the intraluminal pressure in a *jejunal loop* of conscious dogs after i.v. injection of *CCK*, 0.1 U/kg and 0.4 U/kg. Both doses caused a prompt and moderate increase in amplitude and rate of pressure waves. *Secretin*, on the other hand, in analogy with glucagon in doses of 0.25 to 1 U/kg, elicited an almost complete inhibition of jejunal activity lasting for 10 min or longer. Intravenous injection of 0.26—1.0 mg of *glucagon* in man inhibits for a period of 10—15 min the motility in the jejunum and the sigmoid colon induced by means of neostigmine and morphine (DOTEVALL and KOCK, 1963; KOCK, DARLE and DOTEVALL, 1967). NECHELES et al. (1966) found the same to be the case in dogs.

In experiments similar to those performed by KELLY et al. (1969) for the demonstration of the inhibitory effect of secretin on gastric motility, HERMON-TAYLOR and CODE (1970) showed that pure secretin exerts in conscious dogs an analogous inhibition of the small bowel myoelectric activity. The action potentials after feeding were inhibited along the entire small bowel, more consistently and for longer periods in the duodenum and jejunum.

3. The Action of Gastrin, Caerulein and Glucagon on the Intestine

An effect on the intestine similar to that elicited by CCK is also exerted by *gastrin* and *caerulein*. Crude antral extracts given intravenously in *anesthetized cats* increase the tone and motility of the small intestine (BLAIR et al., 1961a, b). Both gastrins I and II are active in this respect in the fasting conscious dog (GREGORY and TRACY, 1964). According to BENNETT (1965) who worked with muscle strips of the guinea pig jejunum, gastrin seems to act either on acetylcholine receptors in the muscle or, more likely, on the postganglionic parasympathetic nerves at a site not blocked by hexamethonium to cause release of acetylcholine. Both gastrin and pentagastrin (ICI 50,123) in a concentration of 0.4—0.6 μg/ml cause contractions of isolated strips of human gastric muscle, but upper and lower small intestine are unresponsive (BENNETT and MISIEWICZ, 1967; BENNETT, MISIEWICZ and WALLER, 1967).

On comparing the action of CCK on the sphincter of Oddi in conscious dogs with that of pentagastrin, caerulein and glucagon, LIN and SPRAY (1969) found that 0.5—10 μg/kg of pentagastrin, 0.01—2 μ/kg of CCK and 5—100 ng/kg of caerulein lowered the choledochal resistance and increased the bile flow. The relaxation occured after 3—5 minutes and the effect lasted for ½—2 hours depending upon the dose. In their series even glucagon proved to relax the choledochus.

The i.v. dose of caerulein acting on the smooth muscle of the small intestine in man and the dog is 0.3—1 ng/kg/min (ERSPAMER, 1972) and that acting on the choledocho-duodenal junction of the dog < 0.1 ng/kg/min.

Threshold stimulant doses of caerulein in man are 1—2 ng/kg i.v. and 10 to 20 ng/kg i.m. Doses of 500—750 ng/kg markedly accelerate the transit of radio-opaque material through the ileum (BERTACCINI and AGOSTI, 1971).

4. Cholecystokinin for the X-Ray Analysis of the Jejuno-Ileum

An accelerated passage of X-ray contrast medium through the intestine under the influence of CCK was described in 1961 by FRANZEN of the University of Mainz, Germany. Three hours after administering the barium emulsion, gallbladder contraction was elicited by giving an egg-yolk meal or a cholecystokinin injection. In both cases peristalsis was markedly intensified, particularly after CCK, with a corresponding reduction of the passage time. After CCK the effect was almost immediate. In a normal subject, part of the emulsion had already passed the valvula Bauhini within 2 min after the slow injection, which lasted 8 min, and half of it within 10 min. After a carbohydrate meal with no increased peristalsis and no emptying of the gallbladder there was no acceleration of the passage.

This effect has been most extensively studied by DAHLGREN (1964, 1966, 1967) at Upsala. Using cholecystokinin preparations of three different strengths, 25, 250 and 3000 Ivy dog units per mg, the last a sample of pure cholecystokinin, he proved that *the peristalsis inducing effect is elicited by the hormone itself* and not by any contaminating peptides. The effect is elicited even after cholecystectomy or ligation of the common duct in the dog and is thus independent of the stimulus exerted by the bile salts. Likewise MONOD (1964) found the effect of CCK on the intestine to be normal in 4 cholecystectomized cases. After injecting 1 unit/kg of CCK intravenously, DAHLGREN found that duodenal peristalsis followed within one minute and continued for 2—5 min. After production of mechanical ileus in the dog or the rabbit, whether in the duodenum or the ileum, pronounced peristalsis was induced by CCK (DAHLGREN and THORÉN, 1967). Since CCK had a peristalsis-promoting effect even in the immediate postoperative period, DAHLGREN considered it possible that the effect could be useful in the treatment of paralytic ileus. The symptoms provoked by CCK in patients with the chronic afferent loop syndrome allow a diagnostic differentiation of this syndrome from the efferent loop dumping syndrome (DAHLGREN, 1964).

The French radiologists MONOD (1964), MORIN and coworkers (1965, 1966) and GRALL (1967) found CCK most useful in the radiological analysis of the jejuno-ileum. When the barium emulsion, 150 g barium sulfate in a volume of 150 ml after about 20 min reaches the upper jejunum, 75 Ivy dog units of CCK are administered intravenously. For four minutes the jejunum is immobilized. The accelerated peristalsis then carries the emulsion down to the coecum during the course of 10 min, sometimes even 3 min. During the last 4 minutes passage through the small intestine can be followed by radiocinematography, by means of which important details of anatomy and function can be distinguished. In 11 of 19 pathological cases the diagnosis was confirmed, in 8 of them processes in or around the small intestine were observed which had escaped detection in the ordinary X-ray analysis. As an accelerator of peristalsis CCK was superior to sorbitol, prostigmine and serotonin.

BACKLUND (1970) reported on a material of 186 patients in whom fluoroscopy of the intestine was performed in connection with an X-ray analysis of the stomach. The latter being completed, the patient was laid on his right side for 15 min until the contrast medium appeared in the duodenum. At that moment 40 IDU of CCK were injected intravenously. The medium was visible in the coecum after 5 min in 30% of the cases and within 15 min in 70%.

The mean small intestine transit time for the ordinary 40% (by weight) barium sulfate suspension was found by KIM (1968) to be 80 and 87 min respectively for younger and more elderly patients, 315 cases in all. The time varied between 15 min and 2 h.

VIII. Miscellaneous Biological Effects of Secretin and Cholecystokinin

1. The Diuretic Effect of Secretin and Glucagon

The antagonism between secretin and the antidiuretic hormone as to the pancreatic secretion discussed in Chapter I p. 84 does also apply to the renal activity (BARBEZAT, ISENBERG and GROSSMAN, 1972). Diuresis was sustained by i.v. infusion of 0.15 M NaCl, 0.4 ml/kg/min, in 3 female dogs. The addition of secretin, 0.5—1.0 μg/kg/min, or glucagon, 0.25 or 0.5μg/kg/min caused a significant increase in urinary volume, sodium and potassium output (Table 20).

Table 20. *Urinary volume and output of sodium and potassium (Mean ± SEM) during or within 30 min after hormone infusion, as per cent of preinfusion level* (BARBEZAT, ISENBERG and GROSSMAN, 1972)

	Volume	Na^+ output	K^+ output
NaCl control	93 ± 7%	101 ± 9%	102 ± 14%
Secretin 0.5	165 ± 31%	162 ± 24%	162 ± 25%
Secretin 1.0	173 ± 38%	160 ± 31%	167 ± 43%
Glucagon 0.25	152 ± 31%	149 ± 16%	114 ± 14%
Glucagon 0.5	161 ± 8%	188 ± 13%	133 ± 18%

2. The Release of Insulin

The early observations by DUPRE (1964a, b), MCINTYRE, HOLDSWORTH and TURNER (1964, 1965), PFEIFFER et al. (1965), DUPRE et al. (1966), UNGER et al. (1966, 1967) that secretin stimulates the insulin release from the islet cells of the pancreas opened up a new field in gastrointestinal physiology at the same time as new facts were added to the discussion about the disposal of an oral glucose load. The field is under intense investigation using newly developed immunoassay techniques (PFEIFFER et al., 1968, 1972; UNGER, 1972) and can be more adequately treated at a future date.

A factor or factors which enhance glucose-induced insulin release by rat islets and pieces of rat pancreas *in vitro* was extracted from pork ileum + jejunum by MOODY et al. (1970). The activity was not caused by secretin and probably not by CCK. It seemed to be associated with glucagon-like immunoreactive fractions of the gut extract. Synthetic secretin did not increase insulin release by the isolated islets. CCK was only slightly active.

3. Release of Free Fatty Acids

A release of glycerol and FFA from rat adipose tissue *in vitro* under the influence of secretin has been reported. With 0.1 U/ml of secretin the speed of

Table 21. *Effect of gastro-intestinal polypeptide hormones on the release of glycerol (μmol/g/hr.) from rat adipose tissue incubated in vitro. Mean value ± standard error of the mean is given* (CARLSON, 1969)

Addition per ml medium	0	Nor-adrenaline 0.05 μg	Secretin 0.01 U	Secretin 0.1 U	Chole-cystokinin 0.1 U	Secretin 0.1 U PGE$_1$ 1 μg	Secretin 0.1 U Nor-adrenaline 0.05 μg
Exp. 1	2.20 ± 0.20	4.62 ± 0.53	—	5.16 ± 0.28	2.13 ± 0.12	—	6.34 ± 0.43
Exp. 2	1.79 ± 0.10	—	3.03 ± 0.21	4.19 ± 0.44	—	—	—
Exp. 3	1.62 ± 0.16	—	—	3.41 ± 0.29	—	2.20 ± 0.11	—

Adipose tissue of fed rats (180 g) was incubated in Krebs-Ringer bicarbonate buffer with 2% albumin and 0.1% glucose. There were 6 incubation flasks in each group.

liberation of glycerol was doubled, whereas 0.1 U/ml of CCK had no influence (CARLSON, 1969) (Table 21). Likewise LAZARUS et al. (1968) found that "pancreozymin" (0.63 U/ml) and gastrin (0.15 μg/ml) had no effect and 0.1 U/ml of secretin markedly stimulated the release of free fatty acids from the rat fat pads *in vitro*. The activity of secretin was 30—600 times that of an equivalent dose of glucagon. None of the three hormones showed in rat liver perfusion experiments any glucagon-like hyperglycemic or glycogenolytic activity, not even in doses of 10—20 U/ml of "pancreozymin", 1—10 μg/ml of secretin and 10 μg/ml of gastrin. All three seemed, when injected in rats in doses of 0.3 U, 0.1 U and 0.5 μg resp., to increase the circulating insulin levels.

In the experiments of BUTCHER and CARLSON (1970) secretin raised the concentration of cyclic AMP in isolated fat cells and increased its formation from ATP in homogenates of isolated fat cells.

4. The Influence of Secretin and CCK on the Thoracic Lymph Flow

The literature concerning the influence of the enteric hormones on the formation of lymph in connection with meals has been reviewed by VEGA, APPERT and HOWARD (1967). After 100 U of Secretin Lilly i.v. RAZIN, FELDMAN and DREILING (1962) found in adult dogs an increase of 0.5 to 0.9 ml/min over the normal values of 0.61—0.60 ml/min. The return to normal values followed after 90 min. 100—200 U of "pancreozymin" gave a similar increase in the lymph flow. The increase was accompanied by increased peristaltic activity and villous motion. VEGA et al. (1967), however, found in dogs with a cannulated thoracic duct no change in the flow of lymph but consistently a manifold increase in the concentration of lipase and amylase, much higher in the lymph than in the serum, during infusion of 95 units of Secretin Boots over a 30 min period. The contradictory results may be due to impurities in the preparations used. The necessity to repeat the experiments with pure preparations of the hormones is evident, particularly since CCK also influences upon the intestinal motility.

LJUNGBERG (1969b) found a slight but statistically significant increase in the *flow of lymph*, from 1.01 ml/h to 1.23 ml/h, in anesthetized rats with the thoracic duct cannulated during administration of 1 IDU/kg of the 10% pure CCK intravenously every 30 min.

5. Toxic Effects of Secretin and Cholecystokinin Preparations

Toxic effects of different types are to be expected from the use of less pure extracts of the intestinal mucosa. Thus DENTON and GERSHBEIN (1966) reported on toxic effects on the isolated heart of crude CCK preparations. In one series (HANSCOM, PINTO and LITTMAN, 1963) not less than 7 of 10 patients developed nausea, backage and rigors after 1 or 2 h infusion of 1.5 U/kg/h of a less pure secretin preparation. Pure secretin has proved to be free from side reactions even when administered i.v. in large doses.

The 10% pure CCK with 250—300 IDU/mg has been extensively used intravenously in man without any drawbacks. HANSCOM and LITTMAN (1963) gave the 10% pure CCK-PZ in doses of 4.5 U/kg to 30 patients and 6 U/kg to 3 patients with no apparent side reactions.

No toxic effects were observed when even large doses of CCK, up to 2000 IDU/kg of the 10% pure preparation, were given intravenously to mice (LJUNGBERG, 1969b). Doses of 0.2 to 32.0 IDU/kg, given intravenously to urethane anesthetized rabbits, did not influence upon the *arterial blood pressure*. Nor could any *tachaphylaxis* be observed in series of 33 doses of 0.2 IDU/kg given during the course of 330 min to each of 9 male anesthetized guinea pigs as used in the ordinary assay technique. Doses up to 0.03 IDU/ml elicited no contraction of the surviving *guinea pig uterus* as employed in the aerated water bath for oxytocin standardization.

D. The Bioassay of Secretin and Cholecystokinin

I. The bioassay of secretin

1. In dogs

At an early date IVY and coworkers (IVY and OLDBERG, 1928; IVY et al., 1928; IVY, KLOSTER, DREWYER and LUETH, 1930) elaborated a technique for measuring the biological activity of secretin in *anesthetized dogs* with the duct of Santorini cannulated. They expressed the activity in a dog unit of secretin, based on the findings in a large number of animals. *The dog unit* was defined by IVY as that amount of dried material dissolved in normal saline solution which, when injected i.v. in an anesthetized dog weighing from 10 to 20 kg during 10 or 15 sec, will cause a 10 drop (0.4 ml) increase in the rate of flow of pancreatic juice from the cannulated duct during a period of 10 min, the control or basal flow being not more than one drop in 2 min. Because of the variations in sensitivity, both between different animals and in the same animal during the course of an experiment, comparison with a standard preparation proved necessary. The dog method was extensively applied (Luckhardt et al., 1926; Weaver et al., 1926; Still, 1930; Gershbein et al., 1949; Friedman and Thomas, 1950b). The technique of the Ivy group for assaying secretin in anesthetized dogs and cats was described in detail by Ivy and Janecek (1959). A cat unit of secretin was defined in similar terms, one dog unit corresponding to 2 cat units.

Later the influence of anesthesia was eliminated by cannulating the pancreatic duct in dogs carrying a permanent gastric fistula and a duodenal fistula according to Thomas (1941) or Stening (1969), a technique found to be extremely useful for the accurate assay of secretin samples in *the conscious animal* (Preshaw and Grossman, 1965a, b; Stening, Vagne and Grossman, 1968; Vagne, Stening, Brooks and Grossman, 1968; Stening, 1969). It has also been successfully applied in cats (Konturek, 1969; Konturek, Gabrys and Dubiel, 1969; Way and Grossman, 1970). The technique as applied in dogs was described by Spingola and Grossman (1972).

2. In cats

For economical reasons, anesthetized cats have been used by most authors. The Swedish group used this animal exclusively.

Instead of measuring the volume or counting the number of drops of pancreatic juice secreted, Hammarsten et. al. (1928) introduced the principle of titrating the alkali, the amount of alkali secreted with the pancreatic juice being within the straight line part of the dose-response curve, in cats (Wilander and Ågren, 1932) as well as in man (Hammarsten et al., 1937; Werner and Mutt, 1954) almost stoichiometrically proportional to the dose of secretin injected.

The Hammarsten cat unit (HCU) of secretin was defined as the amount of secretin which in the anesthetized cat induces secretin of 0.1 ml of 0.1 N bicarbonate in the 15 min period following injection.

The technique of performing the assay in cats was greatly improved by Mutt and Söderberg (1959), partly by cannulating the pancreatic duct instead of using filter paper to collect the juice around the papilla of Vater in the opened duodenum, and partly by keeping the cats in good condition under Placidyl anesthesia for up to 4—5 days. The long-acting anesthetic, Placidyl (Abbott), is administered into the jejunum through an indwelling plastic tube. The gastric juice is continuously evacuated through another tube, the bladder is emptied, and penicillin is given at regular intervals. Through this arrangement the necessity of time-consuming daily operations was eliminated. Furthermore, since the anesthesia lasts for at least 12 h, the animals can, with adequate temperature control, be safely left without supervision overnight.

The details of the technique for the secretin assay in cats according to Mutt and Söderberg were given by Jorpes and Mutt (1966b). Injections of the hormone are made every 30 min, or, if the secretin activity of the injected dose is low, after 20 min. The pancreatic juice flowing from the cannulated pancreatic duct is collected in small 25 ml Pyrex flasks of the Erlenmeyer type containing 0.2 or 0.3 ml of N HCl during the 20- or 30-min period following the injection, depending upon when the secretion ceases. It is brought to a boil, and the excess acid is titrated with 0.1 N NaOH, using methyl red-methylene blue 5:1 0.05%

alcoholic solutions as indicator. The number of ml of 0.1 N alkali secreted by the pancreas multiplied by 10 gives the number of Hammarsten cat units (HCU) in the amount of secretin injected. The amount of secretin injected should be such that it elicits a secretion of about 1.0 to 3.0 ml of 0.1 N alkali.

According to the requirements of most pharmacopoeias 2 doses of the standard in the strength ratio 1:2 are compared with 2 doses of the test solution, adjusted as closely as possible to the strength of the standard. A number of series of tests are then submitted to 4-point analysis.

For routine work, equally good or even better results are obtained if only one dose each of the sample and the standard are used, the test dose being adjusted so that it does not deviate more than 10—20% from the standard. There are weak points in the pharmacopoeia method, mainly the variability in the animal's reaction during the course of 2 hrs. Two consecutive injections are liable to give more reliable responses, allowing a 10 per cent differentiation in strength with fewer series.

3. In rats

Since rats are cheap and readily available in quantities, some laboratories have preferred to use this animal species. A technique for using rats was elaborated by LOVE (1957) of the Oxford group. In rats starved overnight and anesthetized with urethane, pancreatic juice was collected from a cannula in the terminal part of the bile duct which drains the pancreas, as suggested by COLWELL (1951), and the volume measured in a calibrated capillary. In some instances the bile was by-passed through another cannula from the upper part of the choledochus implanted into the first portion of duodenum. The basal secretion was maesured before the injection and after cessation of the secretin stimulation. The total volume of secretion under secretin stimulation minus the basal secretion was taken as the response. Over a certain range, 1.8—5.5 Hammarsten cat units (HCU) per animal i.v., the dose-response curve was linear with variations in the slope of the curve for different animals. At least 2 standard doses of secretin differing in strength by 1:3 were used for plotting the dose-response curve on which the doses of the unknown were read off.

In the same year SVATOS and JELINEK (1957) published a similar method. A fine glass cannula, attached directly to a horizontally placed calibrated capillary tube, was kept in position in the pancreatic duct (SVATOS and PADR, 1957; SVATOS, KOZLIK and VERISOVA, 1960).

An extensive study of the secretin assay in rats has been made by DEBRAY et al. (1961, 1962a, b). They counted the number of drops of pancreatic juice secreted under the influence of secretin during the course of 1 h, and subtracted the basal secretions. There was a linear relationship between the response and the logarithm of the dose administered. In these series the basal secretion from the pancreas, probably due to the operative technique with no ligation of the pylorus, was several times higher, than in the series of LOVE (1957), SVATOS and JELINEK (1957), SVATOS et al. (1960), LIN and ALPHIN (1962) and HEATLEY (1968a). The accuracy of the analysis was thereby reduced. In order to get satisfactory accuracy the authors found that the administration of two doses of the test and the standard in the ratio 2:3, each to four rats was not sufficient, twelve animals being necessary.

From their own experience with both dogs and rats, LIN and ALPHIN (1962) were very reluctant to use rats for the assay of secretin and "pancreozymin" (cholecystokinin). They found the average basal secretion from the pancreas to be 3.12 (2—6) μl/10 min in anesthetized rats and 57.2 (30—110) μl/10 min in unanesthetized rats. Likewise the response to secretin was greater in the conscious animals. There was a straight line relationship between the log dose and response in anesthetized rats. In their experiments anesthetized dogs were nearly 40 times as sensitive to secretin as the rat. They concluded that "in view of the sensitivity of the dog to these hormones and especially in view of the reproducibility (in a given dog) of rate of flow and volume output after identical doses of secretin (LIN and IVY, 1957) and of amylase output after identical doses of pancreozymin (LIN and GROSSMAN, 1956), the dog is still the animal of choice for the bio-assay of secretin and pancreozymin."

In refining the technique elaborated by LOVE (1957) to the utmost precision, HEATLEY (1968a) proved that the rat method properly applied offers a means for accurate assay of secretin preparations. Particular attention was paid to the cannulation technique. The alkalinity of the pancreatic juice was titrated. Contrary to the findings of LIN and ALPHIN (1962) that ether, chloroform and pentobarbital were unsuitable as anesthetics for rats, the author found a combination of ether and urethane anesthesia quite useful. The basal secretion was elevated by 50% under urethane but secretin response was only slightly higher. There is responsiveness within a 64-fold range (0.9—57 HCU), the log dose-response curve being roughly linear. A linear dose-response curve was obtained over a 3-fold range, 1.8—5.5 HCU, in accordance with SVATOS and JELINEK (1957), who found the relation to be linear over a 4-fold range. As found by other authors, there were frequent changes in the sensitivity of the rats causing fluctuations in the response to secretin during an assay. The operative technique took less than half an hour for one animal, 4—5 animals being used simultaneously. Mortality at operation was 4—5 per cent with no difference between male and female rats. Male rats gave a significantly larger response to a given dose of secretin than females. 3—6 h after preparation the basal secretion in a series of 68 urethanized rats was 2.60 ± 0.84 µl/min/kg and the mean pancreatic response (total volume minus basal secretion) 20.0 ± 5.39 µl after 5.5 HCU and 11.1 ± 3.4 µl after 1.8 HCU. The response to secretin in the rats was roughly three times that reported by SVATOS and JELINEK (1957) and seven times that reported by LIN and ALPHIN (1962). Hence the author did not share the view of the latter authors as to the superiority of the dog over the rat. When standard and unknown were compared in the same rat the method had a coefficient of variation of 15.6% for single determinations. By paying due attention to the details of the technique, the rat method can thus be safely used.

On comparing the strength of the rat unit suggested by LOVE with that of the Hammarsten cat unit, one rat unit was found to correspond to 4.48 HCU. The same figure 4.4 HCU = 1 rat unit, had been found by NEWTON et al. (1959). Since the strength of the Ivy dog unit of secretin is equal to the clinical unit suggested by ÅGREN and LAGERLÖF (1936), DEBRAY et al. (1962b, p. 574) were anxious to choose a rat unit of equal strength. One rat unit in their terminology is equal to the clinical unit. The rat unit of the Oxford group was $^1/_4$—$^1/_5$ of the clinical unit.

CRICK, HARPER and RAPER (1949) used the strength of 0.1 mg of an arbitrarily chosen standard preparation of their own as a secretin unit. The average amount of pancreatic juice found by them to be secreted in the 12 min period following the i.v. injection of 0.1 mg of this preparation in cats, anesthetized with chloralose, was 1.2 ml. According to this, the strength of the Crick, Harper and Raper unit of secretin would be about 12 HCU or about half of the clinical unit.

The potency of the Crick, Harper and Raper unit of secretin has been found to be $^1/_8$—$^1/_9$ (STENING et al., 1968, VAGNE et al., 1969) or $^1/_{10}$ (KONTUREK, 1969) of that of the new secretin standard.

Evidently any of the methods discussed above can be used for the assay of secretin. The dog method of IVY gives accurate values, particularly when applied to unanesthetized animals carrying a duodenal fistula, but it is suitable only for physiological laboratories with ample housing facilities and trained personnel.

The cat method as elaborated by MUTT and SÖDERBERG has many advantages. Once the pancreatic duct is cannulated, an approximate estimation of the strength of a sample can be made within 2 hours and an accurate assay, preferably with two cats, within a few hours. If the cat stays alive under Placidyl anesthesia for a second, third or fourth day, it functions somewhat like the chronic duodenal fistula cat. There is no basal secretion. There is a straight line relationship between the log dose of secretin injected and the amount of alkali secreted. A prerequisite for the successful performance of an assay of secretin activity is, however, that solutions are prepared with sterile physiological saline, containing about 0.001 N HCl, in meticulously cleaned sterile glassware (IVY and JANECEK, 1959). The dilutions should be frozen immediately or kept in ice water during the course of a test.

The rat method as elaborated by LOVE and HEATLEY, by DEBRAY et al. and by SVATOS and JELINEK can function as a substitute when cats or dogs are not available. There are two serious drawbacks to the use of rats, the very high basal secretion and the difficult technique of collecting the pancreatic secretion. Furthermore, the number of animals recommended by the authors would make the assay time-consuming.

In the rabbit the pancreatic tissue is dispersed in the duodenal mesentery and in the duodenal wall and there is a high level of spontaneous secretion. Therefore this animal species has been used for the assay of secretin preparations in only one laboratory (DORCHESTER and HAIST, 1952a). The isolated rabbit pancreas secretes at rates of up to 600 μl/h without external stimulation (RIDDERSTAP and BONTING, 1969a).

4. Secretin standards

Mucous membrane dried with acetone and ether and extracted by boiling with dilute acid was used as a standard secretin preparation by STEPP (1912) and by BURN and HOLTON (1948). To obtain a stable preparation, the acetone-dried dog duodenal mucosa was immediately ground in a mortar and passed through a No 100 sieve and then extracted with acetone in a Soxhlet apparatus for 4 hours. After being kept *in vacuo* over P_2O_5 for 24 hours, the powder was distributed in small tubes which were left *in vacuo* over P_2O_5 for 2 days. The desiccator was then filled with *dry air* and the tubes taken out and sealed immediately, the elimination of moisture being the most important step for the preservation of the activity. BURN and HOLTON considered their desiccated dog duodenojejunal mucosa to be stable for many years. The extract prepared by boiling for 1 min with 0.15 N HCl and neutralization, 1 ml of which was equal to 40 mg dry powder, was found to lose activity after 24 hours, the extraction procedure itself being a weak point in a quantitative technique.

LOVE (1957) used a dried ethanol extract of the salt precipitate from an acid extract of acetone-dried pig duodenal mucosa, designated, 'LHP 18'. It had an arbitrary potency of 2 Love units/mg, one Love unit corresponding to 4.4 and 4.48 HCU as compared with two Swedish standard preparations from 1957 and 1952 respectively. It was stored over $CaCl_2$ in the dark at room temperature and seemed to be stable for 5 to 10 years.

Since 1926 when CHIRAY and his coworkers (CHIRAY et al., 1926, 1930; CHIRAY and BOLGERT, 1936; BOLGERT, 1935, 1948) in France introduced secretin, as prepared by Penau and Simonnet (1925), as a diagnostic tool in medicine, numerous attempts have been made to obtain stable secretin preparations for use in the study of the secretory capacity of the pancreas. Most of the preparations obtained contained only a few clinical units of secretin activity per milligram and sometimes gave more or less severe side reactions. The pharmaceutical houses, Byla, Paris, Astra, Södertälje, Sweden, and Wyeth Co., Philadelphia, therefore soon dropped their manufacture of secretin, while the Eli Lilly Company, Indianapolis, continued to supply a well standardized secretin on a non-commercial basis for experimental purposes until 1961.

Purified preparations of the type "S I" (Gershbein et al., 1949; Ivy et al., 1930) with a potency of 1.5—4 dog units/mg were used as standards by the American authors.

In their attempts to make standard preparations of purified fractions, Jorpes and Mutt (1966b) met with considerable difficulty. Lyophilized preparations containing 420 or 3500 U/mg stored in ampoules with rubber caps at room temperature or even in the cold were highly unreliable after 3—4 years. The acetate of pure secretin was particularly unstable, both as dry powder and in sterile solution. After introducing the principle of adding cysteine hydrochloride as stabilizer to the distilled water before dissolving the secretin, 1 mg of the hydrochloride per ampoule containing 75 U, 19 μg, of pure secretin, sterile filtration and lyophilization in ampoules could be performed without any loss of activity. The exclusion of moisture from the lyophilized product proved to be of the utmost importance. If stored in the deep freeze or even in the cold room in sealed glass ampoules under nitrogen, secretin seems to keep its original potency for a couple of years, as evidenced by repeated comparisons with ampoules of newly prepared lots. In fact the new lots used to assay at 3,500 U/mg of pure porcine secretin during the summer months and at 4,000 U/mg during the winter.

5. The levels of strength of the different secretin units and standards

In human series the clinical unit of Ågren and Lagerlöf (1936) and the Ivy dog threshold unit are used almost exclusively. Fortunately they were found to be very similar in strength. One Ivy dog unit is equal to 16 (Wilander and Ågren, 1932; Greengard and Stein, 1941) or approximately 20 (Greengard and Ivy, 1938) Hammarsten cat units. For the sake of simplicity the figure 20 is usually used (Heatley, 1968a).

The great problem today is to reproduce the clinical unit of secretin.

An approximate level of strength can, of course, be reached by including a larger number of animals. Ivy and Janecek (1959) used 16 dogs and 10 cats for the assay of our first secretin standard. In 209 single tests on cats the following results were obtained (Fig. 41) (Jorpes and Mutt, 1966b). 1 μg of the standard produced 1.11 $\pm$0.17 ml of pancreatic juice in the anesthetized cat (46 injections), 1.5 μg 1.38 $\pm$0.32 ml (20 injections), 2 μg 1.68 $\pm$0.163 ml (118 injections) and 3 μg 2.40 $\pm$0.51 ml (25 injections). The potency was determined to be 8400 HCU/mg or 420 clinical units/mg. Another approach would be to compare the results obtained in man in the numerous series of secretin tests performed. This would seem to be a rather futile task because of the variations found among the different series as summarized by Lagerlöf (1967) and Petersen (1969, 1970). In spite of meticulous application of the experimental techniques, figures varying from one U/kg [Lagerlöf, 1942 (Astra); Dreiling and Janowitz, 1962 (Boots); Petersen, 1969 (Gih Res. Unit, Karolinska Institutet); Christensen, 1963 (Vitrum)] to 2—3 U/kg (Hartley et al., 1966) or to 8—16 U/kg [Lagerlöf,

SCHÜTZ and HOLMEN, 1967 (Vitrum); SARLES et al., 1966 (Vitrum)] have been given as the amount of secretin necessary for the production of a nearly maximal secretory response. Such large differences must be attributed mainly to the lability of the secretin and the manufacturers lack of experience in handling it.

LAGERLÖF et al. (1967), using 7.5 U/kg of the Vitrum secretin, obtained during the first hour a volume of 316 ml with a bicarbonate content of 27.4 mEq, whereas ISENBERG and GROSSMAN (1969a) obtained with 3 U/kg of the new Swedish secretin a first hour volume of 283 ml with a mean bicarbonate output of 24 mEq and a more prolonged response which remained near the peak level for 2 hours instead of 1½ hours as in the series of LAGERLÖF et al. DREILING and JANOWITZ (1956) observed after 1 U/kg of Secretin Lilly a return to almost basal level first during the fourth 20 min period.

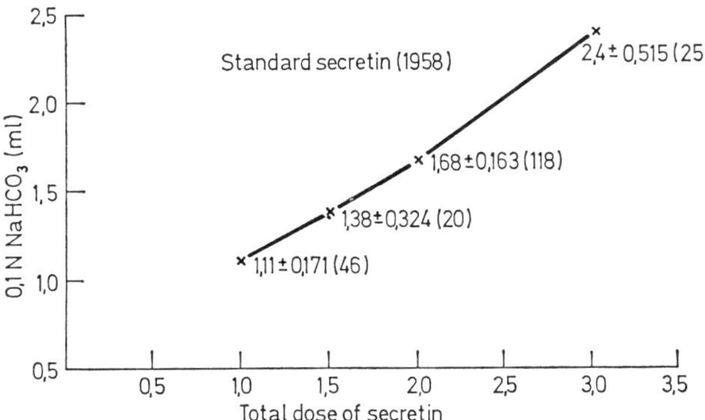

Fig. 41. Relationship between secretin dose injected in the anesthetized cat and the amount of alkali secreted in 15—20 min. The figure 1.68 ml obtained with 2 micrograms corresponds to 420 clinical units (8.400 HCU) per milligram (JORPES and MUTT, 1966b)

However, in the largest series as those of LAGERLÖF (1942), DREILING (1955), DREILING and JANOWITZ (1957, 1962), DAVILA et al. (1961), DREILING, JANOWITZ and PERRIER (1964) and PETERSEN (1969, 1970) one unit/kg of the different brands of secretin, Astra, Lilly, Wyeth or Vitrum gave satisfactory figures for volume and bicarbonate excretion.

Using the Astra preparation, Pancreotest, LAGERLÖF (1942, p. 269) found, in 48 healthy subjects, the mean volume of pancreatic juice collected in 60 minutes to be 202 ± 4 ml (2.2—5.5 ml per kg body weight), the corresponding figure for bicarbonate being 194 ± 6 ml 0.1 N or 97 m Eq/l.

In 1950 DREILING made a statistical study in 172 normal persons of the response in the secretin test with respect to volume and alkalinity of the pancreatic juice after one clinical unit of secretin per kg body weight. The secretins used were delivered by Astra, Sweden, and by the Wyeth Co., Philadelphia, an equal number of persons being treated with each of the two brands. The collecting period was 80 minutes. The frequency distribution curve of the data for people with no pancreatic disorder was essentially symmetrical with a range between 2.0 and 4.4 ml of pancreatic juice per kg body weight, mean 3.57 ± 0.68 ml.

In reporting on 1500 secretin tests performed with Secretin Lilly on patients without pancreatic disease DREILING (1955) (Table 22) and DREILING and JANOWITZ (1957) described the details of the technique and presented the normal ranges for volume, maximal bicarbonate concentration, total bicarbonate output and total amylase secretion during periods of 30, 60 and 80 min after intravenous injection of 1.0 clin. unit/kg of secretin.

The techniques of LAGERLÖF and of DREILING and JANOWITZ are generally accepted, although most workers prefer to use the 60-minute values. Thus this should be the lead to follow in adjusting the strength of the clinical unit of secretin, of which, for practical reasons, it is desirable to give one unit per kg body weight (in infants twice this amount).

Table 22. *Mean values for volume of pancreatic secretion, maximal bicarbonate concentration, and bicarbonate output after intravenous injection of 1 U/kg of Secretin Lilly in patients without pancreatic disease* (DREILING, 1955)

		30 min	60 min	80 min
Volume ml/kg		1.73 ± 0.3	2.72 ± 0.5	3.22 ± 0.5
Range		1.0 – 2.8	1.6 – 4.8	2.0 – 6.2
Max. bicarbonate				
Concentration mEq/l	107.7 ± 0.7			
Range	88 – 137			
Bicarbonate output mEq		11.27 ± 0.10	17.81 ± 0.17	20.83 ± 0.18
Range		6.8 – 16.0	13.2 – 23.7	15.9 – 32.6

Since it was quite evident from the results obtained by LAGERLÖF et al. (1967) and by SARLES et al. (1966) that the potency of the clinical unit of Secretin Vitrum manufactured between 1958 and 1965 did not correspond to that of the Pancreotest preparation and the Secretin Lilly used by the above authors for the elaboration of the secretin test, we decided, when production was taken over by the GIH Research Unit, Karolinska Institutet, Stockholm, to adjust the level of potency to that of their praparations. From the beginning of 1966, batch No. 16611, a 4 times higher level of strenght was therefore applied (GROSSMAN, 1969a). Thereby the secretin test or the combined secretin-CCK test could be performed with 1 U/kg or possibly 2 U/kg, which is a great practical advantage.

In the rat test HEATLEY (1968a) found the later standard to be 6.9 times more potent than the two older ones used in assaying Secretin Vitrum. The pancreatic function tests performed during the last years with the improved potency of the secretin unit (PETERSEN, 1969, 1970) (Fig. 20), are comparable to those of LAGERLÖF (1942) and of DREILING (1955) and DREILING and JANOWITZ (1957). The variations in strength among a number of lots adjusted to the new level of potency were found to be less than 20% (STENING, VAGNE and GROSSMAN, 1968).

II. On the bioassay of cholecystokinin preparations

1. The choice of unit

There is good reason to express the strength of CCK in Ivy dog units (IDU). IVY and coworkers elaborated the first method of assay (IVY and OLDBERG, 1928a, b). When in the 1950's CCK became available in a purified form, IVY and JANECEK (1959) assayed a standard preparation in both dogs and cats. A very strong reason for the use of the Ivy dog unit for measuring the strength of CCK is that an optimal contraction of the human gallbladder is obtained in cholecystography when 1 IDU/kg is administered intravenously. Should this principle have been applied in establishing the international unit for heparin, the last two completely unnecessary zeros could have been avoided.

2. Determination of the Ivy dog unit

The Ivy dog unit is defined as that amount of dry material (in the dose used) which when dissolved in normal saline solution and injected intravenously, during 10 to 15 sec into an anesthetized dog weighing about 15 kg, results in a more or less immediate (1 to 3 min) rise in intra-gallbladder pressure of 1 cm of bile (IVY, KLOSTER, DREWYER and LUETH, 1930). The sample is injected intravenously in the dog when the basal bile pressure is from 7 to 10 cm as measured by means of a glass tube introduced into the gallbladder at the level of the fundus and firmly fixed in situ. There is good proportionality between dose and response within the range of 2 to 6—7 cm increase in pressure. The results are easily reproducible in a given dog, although the individual responses in different animals show great variation. The sensitivity of an animal also varies during the course of an experiment, particularly if the animals are used continuously during the course of 48—72 hours. Frequent doses of a standard sample should therefore be given. The details of the techniques for assaying both secretin and CCK in the anesthetized dog were described by GERSHBEIN, WANG and IVY (1949) and by IVY and JANECEK (1959).

IVY and JANECEK (1959), in assaying the lyophilized dry powder of our cholecystokinin standard in 11 dogs, found 45 μg to be the average dog unit, the strength thus being 22 Ivy dog units per mg. In August 1958 we checked the analysis in our laboratory (JORPES, MUTT and OLBE, 1959) in three anesthetized dogs, two of which were used continuously day and night during the course of 48 hours, and found about 20 units per mg. After adjusting the basal bile pressure to 7—10 cm by adding, when needed, saline solution warmed to 37°C into the glass cannula, there was a good proportionality between dose and response within the range of 2 to 6—7 cm increase in pressure.

The technique of IVY and OLDBERG (1928b) was modified by SNAPE, FRIEDMAN and THOMAS (1948), who recorded the increase in pressure in the cannulated common bile duct in unanesthetized dogs equipped with permanent fistulas of the duodenum and of the stomach. A given dog could be used for up to 2—3 years (SNAPE, FRIEDMAN and SVENSON, 1948). A similar technique using cats under Nembutal anesthesia was applied by HAVERMARK and HULTMAN (1952).

A number of authors applied an *in vitro* technique using *the isolated guinea pig gallbladder and/or strips of the terminal guinea pig ileum* (JUNG and GREENGARD, 1933; ÅGREN, 1939; DOUBILET and IVY, 1938; GERSHBEIN, DENTON and HUBBARD, 1953; HULTMAN, 1955a, b). SEAGER (1939, 1941) used frogs. The preparation to be tested was injected intracardially into the frog and the effect was observed by inspecting the gallbladder in situ.

Almost consistently the authors found that peristaltic contractions of the ileum were induced by the crude preparations available at that time. HULTMAN (1955a) came to the conclusion that these contractions, which still occurred after blocking the action of acetylcholine and histamine stimulation, were due to impurities. They were absent when purified CCK-preparations were used. Furthermore, both preparations, that of the ileum and of the gallbladder from the guinea pig were strongly sensitive to changes in pH, to the salt concentration and to ammonium salts added to the bath, inconveniences not encountered when using the guinea pig gallbladder in situ. The purified CCK containing 22 IDU/mg exerted no substance P-activity on the intestine (HULTMAN, 1955b).

SVATOS (1957) measured the pressure in the guinea pig gallbladder in situ by means of a graduated pipet connected to a cannula introduced into the common bile duct, a technique which evidently functioned satisfactorily. Instead of applying the technique of SVATOS, as recommended for assaying the concentration of urocholecystokinin in the urine, DAL MONTE and coworkers (1964) elaborated a technique of their own. Urine was injected intravenously into a rabbit, the gallbladder of which had been visualized with 7 ml of a 30% solution of a tri-iodoanilide derivative, given intravenously 4 hours in advance. CCK liberation from the duodenum was stimulated by 25 g of Sorbitol taken by mouth in a 50% solution. Ordinarily 3 ml of urine caused a contraction of the rabbit's gallbladder. The mean volume of urine necessary from 15 patients, partially gastrectomized one year earlier was 8.26 (6—12) ml (DAL MONTE et al., 1965).

3. The Ljungberg technique with the guinea pig gallbladder in situ

LJUNGBERG (1964, 1969a), instead of measuring the intra-gallbladder pressure, registered the contraction of the guinea pig gallbladder in situ. A thin suture is tied with a knot, not sewn, to the tip of the fundus of the gallbladder and runs in caudal direction over an easily movable pulley with a weight of about 0.8 g fastened to its free end. The strain-gauge transducer attached to the thread, gives a ten-to thirtyfold magnification of the gallbladder movements. According to the individual sensitivity of the animals, doses of 0.03—0.1 IDU/100 g b.w. are injected through an indwelling cannula in the internal jugular vein, always alternating with a dose of similar strength of the standard preparation. LJUNGBERG recommends a four point assay with 100% variation between the two doses. The method allows even visual discrimination between doses varying by 20—25%. The present authors found the method to be extremely useful both for the analysis of crude preparations and for the assay of pure samples.

4. The Amer and Becvar technique with strips of rabbit gallbladder in vitro

Pointing out that the dog methods are subject to great variation and are not suitable for routine assays on a larger scale and that the *in vitro* methods available are less specific, AMER and BECVAR (1969) devised a new *in vitro* technique using *transverse or oblique strips of the rabbit gallbladder* in an ordinary tissue bath. The transverse muscle of the rabbit gallbladder is much more sensitive to CCK than the guinea pig gallbladder (Fig. 42). It is not responsive to secretin, histamine or

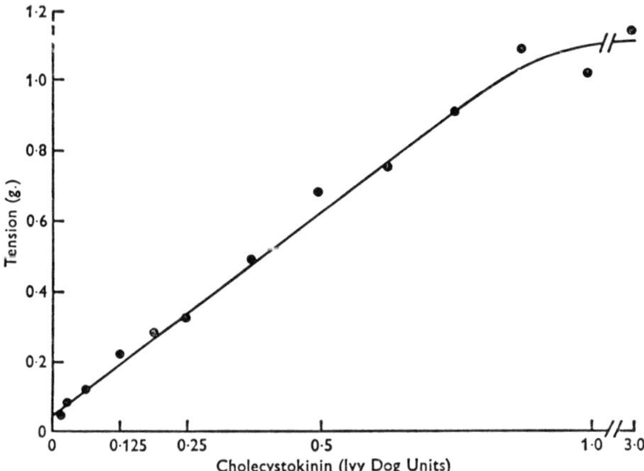

Fig. 42. Effect of increasing doses of cholecystokinin on the tension (measured in g) of a rabbit gallbladder strip. There is a straigt-line relationship between the dose as measured in Ivy dog units and the effect up to 1.0 Ivy dog unit. Bath volume: 25 ml (AMER and BECVAR, 1969)

ammonium salts. The sensitivity of the muscle strips increases with time until a plateau is reached after 5—6 hours. Six hours after preparation, the increase in tension is linear with the dose up to about 1.0 IDU in the 25 ml bath. The method is described as being fast and accurate, suitable for series of assays. Amounts of CCK as small as 0.05 IDU can be accurately assayed.

In determining the relative molar potency of CCK, the synthetic gastrin pentapeptide and the sulfated and desulfated porcine gastrin and caerulein respectively in the three systems: isolated rabbit gallbladder strips (AMER and BECVAR, 1969), isolated guinea pig gallbladder (HULTMAN, 1955a) and guinea pig gallbladder in situ (LJUNGBERG, 1964), AMER (1969) found fairly good agreement among the different systems (Table 18). The isolated guinea pig gallbladder was less sensitive than the isolated rabbit gallbladder strips and frequently showed spontaneous rhythmic contractions. Whereas in the in situ preparation (LJUNGBERG, 1964) there was an immediate response to the injection of the peptides, a lag period, varying in length for the different peptides, was normal in both the *in vitro* systems, twice as long for the isolated guinea pig gallbladder as for the rabbit gallbladder muscle strips. AMER found the lengths of time necessary for the different peptides to reach maximal contractions in the *in vitro* systems to be approximately proportional to their molecular weights.

Similarly ÅGREN (1939) found the effect of CCK on the gallbladder to be considerably slower than that of acetylcholine and of histamine. Cholecystokinin results in a slow rise in tone, which often reaches its maximum 10—15 minutes after injection into the intestinal bath. When acetylcholine is injected, maximal contractions can be recorded after only a few seconds.

5. The assay of "pancreozymin" activity

"Pancreozymin" activity has been measured in cats (BURN and HOLTON, 1948; CRICK, HARPER and RAPER, 1949; JORPES and MUTT, 1966a) in dogs (WANG, GROSSMAN and IVY, 1948; LIN and GROSSMAN, 1956; LIN and ALPHIN, 1962), in rats (LIN and ALPHIN, 1962; DEBRAY et al., 1962a, b) and in rabbits (DORCHESTER, 1959). The technique elaborated by LOVE (1957) for the assay of secretin in rats was further refined by HEATLEY (1968b) for the assay of "pancreozymin" simultaneously with that of secretin in the same animal. Particular attention has to be paid to the procedure of flushing the common bile duct for the quantitative collection of the pancreatic juice. The author found a good straight line dose-response curve up to 0.3 Crick, Harper and Raper units of PZ. Most authors prefer to determine only the protein content of the pancreatic juice.

With the demonstration (MUTT, 1964; JORPES and MUTT, 1966a; MUTT and JORPES, 1968a, b) that "pancreozymin" activity is due to cholecystokinin, its separate assay lost actuality. Taking into account that the enzyme output from the pancreas is under neural influences as well and is strongly influenced by the flushing-out effect of secretin, the "pancreozymin" activity of a preparation is much more difficult to measure than the tonic contraction of the gallbladder stimulated by CCK. The assay will therefore be limited to the determination of the CCK activity on the gallbladder or strips of the gallbladder musculature.

Standard preparations. The crude preparations of CCK are stable for many years when preserved in a dry atmosphere. The selection of a standard is thereby greatly facilitated.

HARPER (1967), however, considered the crude acetone-dried powder of BURN and HOLTON to be unsuitable as a standard for the assay of "pancreozymin" partly because of the contamination with histamine and partly because the secretin present will potentiate the "pancreozymin" effect.

The present authors found both the lyophilized dry powder of CCK containing 22 IDU/mg and further purified samples containing 250—300 IDU/mg to still have full activity after storage at room temperature in ordinary weighing flasks with the exclusion of moisture for 3—4 years as assayed in both dogs and guinea pigs. The secretin content was 30 and 4—6 units per 75 Ivy dogs units of CCK respectively.

6. Urocholecystokinin

Because of the relatively low molecular weight of CCK and the potentiated activity of its C-terminal peptides, CCK or "pancreozymin" activity is to be expected in the urine. In fact the urine from both man and animals contains electrophoretically separable fractions which show such an activity.

The excretion of CCK with the urine under different conditions has been followed by SVATOS and coworkers (SVATOS, 1957, 1959, 1960, 1964; SVATOS and VOKAC, 1960; SVATOS and QUEISNEROVA, 1960; PLESSIER and PLESSIER, 1960). The increase in pressure in the anesthetized guinea pig's gallbladder was measured and expressed in mm bile in the glass cannula inserted in the cystic duct (SVATOS, 1959). In experimental animals duodenectomy was followed by a reduced excretion of CCK (SVATOS, 1959). An increased excretion was observed in man after occlusion of the cystic duct and after cholecystectomy (SVATOS and VOKAC, 1960; PLESSIER and PLESSIER, 1960). In comparing the urinary excretion of CCK in 19 normal persons, 19 patients previously submitted to a Billroth I operation, and 14 patients operated upon according to Billroth II, the response to 50 ml of olive oil taken orally was after 60 and 120 min in the 3 groups 30, 25 and 18 mm, respectively (VOKAC and SVATOS, 1962), a clear indication of the functional insufficiency of the duodenum in the last group of patients.

The atonic state of the gallbladder frequently observed after partial gastrectomy according to Billroth II is accompanied by a reduced liberation of CCK by the functionally impaired duodenum. As a consequence the excretion of urocholecystokinin is reduced (DAL MONTE et al., 1965). A similar reduction in the urocholecystokinin content of the urine occurs in cases with chronic cholecystitis (POPOVA et al., 1967).

References

ABERNETHY, R. J., GILLESPIE, I. E., LAWRIE, J. H., FORREST, A. P. M., PAYNE, R. A., BARABAS, A., JOHNSTON, I. D. A., BURNS, G. P., HOBBS, K. E. F., CLEGG, R. T., DUTHIE, H. L., FITZGERALD, J. D.: Pentagastrin as a stimulant of maximal gastric acid response in man. A multicentre pilot study. Lancet 1967 I, 291—295.

ADLERCREUTZ, E.: Corpus luteum hormone in the treatment of biliary dyskinesia and especially of the postcholecystectomy syndrome. Acta Med. Scand **145,** 15—19 (1953).

— O tratamento médico das disquinésias biliares. Europa Medica **3,** No. 2 (1966).

— JORPES, J. E., MUTT, V., WEGELIUS, C.: L'emploi de la cholécystokinine dans la cholécystographie. Arch. Mal. App. Dig. **46,** 414—418 (1957).

— PETTERSSON, T., ADLERCREUTZ, H., GRIBBE, P., WEGELIUS, C.: Effect of cholecystokinin on duodenal tonus and motility. Acta Med. Scand. **167,** 339—342 (1960).

AFFOLTER, H., PILLER, M., GUBLER, A.: Tierexperimentelle Untersuchungen über die Wirkung von gereinigtem Sekretin und Cholecystokinin-Pankreozymin, sowie von Decholin auf die Gallensekretion. Gastroenterologia **101,** 247—258 (1964).

ÅGREN, G.: Über die pharmakodynamischen Wirkungen und chemischen Eigenschaften des Secretins. Skandinav. Arch. Physiol. **70,** 10—87 (1934).

— On preparation of cholecystokinin. Skandinav. Arch. Physiol. **81,** 234—243 (1939).

— LAGERLÖF, H.: The pancreatic secretion in man after intravenous administration of secretin. Acta Med. Scand. **90,** 1—29 (1936).

ÅGREN, G., LAGERLÖF, H., The biliary response in the secretin test. Acta Med. Scand. **92,** 359—361 (1937).
— — BERGLUND, H.: The secretin test of pancreatic function in the diagnosis of pancreatic disease. Acta Med. Scand. **90,** 224—271 (1936).
— WILANDER, O.: Reinigung von Sekretin. Biochem. Zeitschr. **259,** 365—373 (1933).
ALESSANDRINI, A., PALAGI, L., RAMORINO, MARIA LETIZIA, COLAGRANDE, C.: Contributo alla studio dell'attivita motoria biliare. Ras. Fisiop. Clin. Torano., **33,** 1160—1188 (1961).
ALLEGRI, A., BALDRIGHI, V., MONTEMARTINI, C.: Effetti della colecistochinina sulla dinamica della vie biliari con particolare riguardo al comportamento degli sfinteri colecistico e choledocio. Arch. Sci. Med. (Torino) **104,** 656—675 (1957).
AMER, M. S.: Studies with cholecystokinin. II. Cholecystokinetic potency of porcine gastrins I and II and related peptides in three systems. Endocrinology **84,** 1277—1281 (1969).
— BECVAR, W. E.: A sensitive *in vitro* method for the assay of cholecystokinin. J. Endocr. **43,** 637—642 (1969).
ANASTASI, A., BERNARDI, L., BERTACCINI, G., BOSISIO, G., DE CASTIGLIONE, R., ERSPAMER, V., GOFFREDO, O., IMPICCIATORE, M.: Synthetic peptides related to caerulein. Experientia (Basel) **24,** 771—773 (1968).
— BERTACCINI, G., CEI, J. M., DE CARO, G., ERSPAMER, V., IMPICCIATORE, M.: Structure and pharmacological actions of phyllocaerulein, a caerulein-like nonapeptide. Its occurrence in extracts of the skin of *Phyllomedusa sauvagei* and related Phyllomedusa species. Brit. J. Pharmac. **37,** 198—206 (1969).
— BERTACCINI, G., CEI, J. M., DE CARO, G., ERSPAMER, V., IMPICCIATORE, M., ROSEGHINI, M.: Presence of caerulein in extracts of the skin of *Leptodactylus pentadactylus labyrinthicus* and of *Xenopus laevis*. Brit. J. Pharmacology **38,** 221—228 (1970).
— — ERSPAMER, V.: Pharmacological data on phyllokinin (bradykinyl-isoleucyl-tyrosine O-sulphate) and bradykinyl-isoleucyl-tyrosine. Brit. J. Pharmac. Chemother. **27,** 479—485 (1966).
— ERSPAMER, V.: Caerulein and caerulein-like peptides. In: Proc. 3rd Symp. Europ. Pancreatic Club, Prague July 2—4, 1968, pp. 50—53, edit. by P. FRIC, F. MALIS and R. RONSKY. Czech. Med. Press, Praha, 1970.
— — ENDEAN, R.: Isolation and structure of caerulein, an active decapeptide from the skin of *Hyla caerulea*. Experientia **23,** 699—700 (1967).
— — — Isolation and amino acid sequence of caerulein, the active decapeptide of the skin of Hyla caerulea. Arch. Biochem. Biophys. **125,** 57—68 (1968).
ANDERSSON, S.: Inhibitory effects of acid in antrum-duodenum on fasting gastric secretion in Pavlov and Heidenhain pouch dogs. Acta Physiol. Scand. **49,** 42—56 (1960a).
— Inhibitory effects of hydrochloric acid in antrum and duodenum on gastric secretory responses to test meal in Pavlov and Heidenhain pouch dogs. Acta Physiol. Scand. **49,** 231—241 (1960b).
— Inhibitory effects of hydrochloric acid in the duodenum on gastrin-stimulated gastric secretion in Heidenhain pouch dogs. Acta Physiol. Scand. **50,** 105—112 (1960c).
— Inhibitory effects of hydrochloric acid in antrum and duodenum on histamine-stimulated gastric secretion in Pavlov and Heidenhain pouch dogs. Acta Physiol. Scand. **50,** 186—196 (1960d).
— Gastric and duodenal mechanisms inhibiting gastric secretion of acid. *Handbook of Physiol. Section* **6**, *Vol. II*, pp. 865—878. Amer. Physiol. Soc. Wash. 1967.
— GROSSMAN, M. I.: Effect of vagal denervation of pouches on gastric secretion in dogs with intact or resected antrums. Gastroenterology **48,** 449—462 (1965).
— —Effects of Histalog and secretin on gastroduodenal profile of pH, potential difference, and pressure in man. Gastroenterology **51,** 10—17 (1966).
— NILSSON, G.: pH-dependence of the mechanism in the duodenal bulb inhibiting gastric acid responses to exogenous gastrin. Acta Physiol. Scand. **76,** 182—190 (1969).
— — SJÖDIN, L., UVNÄS, B.: Mechanism of duodenal inhibition of gastric acid secretion. NOBEL Symposium XVI. Frontiers in Gastrointestinal Hormone Research, Stockholm, July 20—21, 1970; (In press) Edit. S. ANDERSSON, Almqvist and Wiksell, Upsala, Sweden, 1972.
— — UVNÄS, B.: Inhibition of gastric secretion by acid in proximal and distal duodenal pouches. Acta Physiol. Scand. **65,** 191—192 (1965).
— — — Effect of acid in proximal and distal duodenal pouches on gastric secretory responses to gastrin and histamine. Acta Physiol. Scand. **71,** 368—378 (1967).
— OLBE, L.: Inhibition of gastric acid response to sham feeding in Pavlov pouch dogs by acidification of antrum. Acta Physiol. Scand. **61,** 55—64 (1964).
— UVNÄS, B.: Inhibition of postprandial gastric secretion in Pavlov pouches by instillation of hydrochloric acid into the duodenal bulb. Gastroenterology **41,** 486—490 (1961).

Antinone, R. L., Bluvas, R., Magee, D. F.: Antral acidity and gastric secretion. Ann. Surg. **166,** 990—994 (1967).
Astwood, E. B., Raben, M. S., Rayne, R. W., Grady, A. B.: Purification of corticotrophin with oxycellulose. J. Am. Chem. Soc. **73,** 2969—2970 (1951).
Aures, D., Johnson, L. R., Way, L. W.: Gastrin-obligatory intermediate for activation of histidine decarboxylase in the rat. Amer. J. Physiol. **219,** 214—216 (1970).
Babkin, B. P.: Die äußere Sekretion der Verdauungsdrüsen. Springer, Berlin, 1914.
— Die Sekretorische Tätigkeit der Verdauungsdrüsen. Handbuch der normalen und pathologischen Physiologie. Edit. Bethe et al. Vol **3** B II, 689—818. Springer, Berlin, 1927.
— Die äußere Sekretion der Verdauungsdrüsen. Sec. Ed. Springer, Berlin, 1928.
— Studies on the pancreatic secretion in skates. Biol. Bull. of the Marine Biol. Laboratory (Woods Hole) **57,** 272—291 (1929).
— Pavlov. A Biography. The University of Chicago Press 1949.
— Secretory mechanism of the digestive glands. Sec. Ed. P. Hoeber, New York, 1950.
— Rubashkin, W. J., Savich, W. W.: Über die morphologischen Veränderungen der Pankreaszellen unter der Einwirkung verschiedener Reize. Arch. mikr. Anat. **74,** 68—104 (1909).
— Savich, W. W.: Zur Frage über den Gehalt an festen Bestandteilen in dem auf verschiedene Sekretionserreger erhaltenen pankreatischen Saft. Z. physiol. Chem. **56,** 321—342 (1908).
— Starling, E. .H: A method for the study of the perfused pancreas. J. Physiol., **61,** 245—248 (1926).
Backlund, V.: Die Verwendung des Cholecystokinins in der Röntgendiagnostik. Der Radiologe **10,** 36—39 (1970).
Baggenstoss, A. H., Power, M. H., Grindlay, J. H.: The extraction of secretin from the intestine of man: absence of secretin in a case of fibrocystic disease of the pancreas. Gastroenterology **11,** 208—220 (1948).
Ball, E. G.: The composition of pancreatic juice and blood serum as influenced by the injection of acid and base. J. Biol. Chem. **86,** 433—448 (1930a).
— The composition of pancreatic juice and blood serum as influenced by the injection of inorganic salts. J. Biol. Chem. **86,** 449—462 (1930b).
— Tucker, H. F., Solomon, A. K., Vennesland, B.: The source of pancreatic juice bicarbonate. J. Biol. Chem. **140,** 119—129 (1941).
Banks, P. A., Rudick, J., Janowitz, H. D., Dreiling, D. A.: Action of antidiuretic hormone on pancreatic exocrine secretion. Surg. Forum **18,** 392—393 (1967).
— — Dreiling, D. A., Janowitz, H. D.: Effect of antidiuretic hormone on pancreatic exocrine secretion. Amer. J. Physiol. **215,** 361—365 (1968).
Banwell, J. G., Northam, B. E., Cooke, W. T.: Secretory response of human pancreas to continuous intravenous infusion of secretin. Gut **8,** 50—57 (1967).
Barabas, A. P., Payne, R. A., Johnston, I. D. A., Burns, G. P.: The effect of vagotomy on gastrin-stimulated gastric-acid secretion in man. Lancet **I**: 118—119 (1966).
Barbezat, G. O., Isenberg, J. I., Grossman, M. I.: Diuretic action of secretin in dog. Proc. Soc. exper. Biol. (N.Y.) **139,** 211—215 (1972).
Barcroft, J., Starling, E. H.: The oxygen exchange of the pancreas. J. Physiol. (London) **31,** 491—496 (1904).
Barlow, T. E., Greenwell, J. R., Harper, A. A., Scratcherd, T.: Factors influencing pancreatic blood flow. In: Blood flow through organs and tissues, edit. by W. H. Bain and A. M. Harper, pp. 469—486. Edinburgh and London, Livingstone 1968.
Baron, J. H., Perrier, C. V., Janowitz, H. D., Dreiling, D. A.: Maximum alkaline (bicarbonate) output of the dog pancreas. Amer. J. Physiol. **204,** 251—256 (1963).
Barrington, E. J. W.: The supposed pancreatic organs of *Petromyzon fluviatilis* and *Myxine glutinosa*. Quart. J. Microscop. Sci. **85,** 391—417 (1945).
— Dockray, G. J.: The effect of intestinal extracts of lampreys *(Lampetra fluviatilis* and *Petromyzon marinus)* on pancreatic secretion in the rat. Gen. Comp. Endocrinol. **14,** 170—177 (1970).
Bauduin, H.: Personal communication (1967).
— Christophe, J., Reuse, J.: Effets de divers acides organiques et de l'acetylcholine sur le métabolism du pancréas de rat *in vitro*. C. R. Soc. Biol. **158,** 917—919 (1964).
— Reuse, J. J.: A propos de l'effet de la secrétine sur la respiration du pancréas de rat *in vitro*. Arch. int. Pharmacodyn. **157,** 224—227 (1965a).
— — Cholinomimétiques, hormones duodénales et échanges respiratoires du pancréas du rat. J. de Physiol. **57,** 550—557 (1965b).
Bayliss, W. M.: Principles of general physiology. Longmans and Green London 1915, p. 706; III ed. 1920, p. 712; IV ed. 1924, p. 912.
— Starling, E. H.: On the causation of the so-called "peripheral reflex secretion" of the pancreas. Proc. Roy. Soc. **69,** 352—353 (1902a).

BAYLISS, W. M., STARLING, E. H., Mechanism of pancreatic secretion. J. Physiol. **28**, 325—353 (1902b).
— — On the uniformity of the pancreatic mechanism in vertebrates. J. Physiol. **29**, 174—180 (1903).
— — The chemical regulation of the secretory process. Croonian Lecture. Proc. Roy. Soc. **73**, 310—322 (1904).
— — Die chemische Koordination der Funktionen des Körpers. Ergebn. d. Physiologie **5**, 664—697 (1906).
BECKER, N. M.: De l'influence des solutions de bicarbonate de soude, de sel marin, d'acide carbonique et de quelques alcalines sur la sécrétion du suc pancréatic. Arch. Sci. Biol. **2**, 433—461 (1893).
BECKER, V.: Histochemistry of the exocrine pancreas. In: Ciba Foundation Symposium on the Exocrine Pancreas, pp. 56—63, edit. by A.V.S. DE REUCK and M. P. CAMERON, CHURCHILL, London 1962.
BEDI, B. S., DEBAS, H. T., GILLESPIE, G., GILLESPIE, I. E.: Effect of bile salts on antral gastrin release. Gastroenterology **60**, 252—262 (1971).
— GILLESPIE, G., GILLESPIE, I. E.: Effects of a specific gastrinantagonist on gastric acid secretion in pouch dogs. Lancet 1967 I, 1240—1243.
— GOVAERTS, J. P., MASTER, S. P., GILLESPIE, I. E.: Inhibition of gastric acid secretion by intravenous cholecystokinin extract. Scand. J. Gastroenterol. **2**, 68—76 (1967).
— — — Secretin and cholecystokinin-pancreozymin in combination in the inhibition of gastric acid secretion. Brit. J. Surg. **56**, 384—385 (1969).
BENJAMIN, B. I., CORTELL, S., CONRAD, M. E.: Bicarbonate induced iron complexes and iron absorption: one effect of pancreatic secretions. Gastroenterology **53**, 389—396 (1967).
BENNETT, A.: Effect of gastrin on isolated smooth muscle preparations. Nature **208**, 170—173 (1965).
— MISIEWICZ, J. J.: The role of gastrin in gastrointestinal motility. Gastroenterology **53**, 680—681 (1967).
— — WALLER, S. L.: Analysis of the motor effects of gastrin and pentagastrin on the human alimentary tract *in vitro*. Gut **8**, 470—474 (1967).
BENNET, J., CHÉRIGIÉ, E., CAROLI, J., DOYON, D., ECONOMOPOULOS, P., PLESSIER, J., STOOPEN, M.: La pancréatographie après stimulation par la sécrétine intra-artérielle. Ann. Radiol. **10**, 422—430 (1967).
BENSLEY, R. R.: Studies on the pancreas of the guinea pig. Amer. J. Anat. **12**, 297—388 (1912).
BERNARD, CL.: Leçons de Physiologie Experimental **2**, 429 (1856a).
— Mémoire sur le pancreas. C. R. Acad. Sci. (Paris) Suppl. **1**, 379—563 (1856b).
— Leçons sur les propriétés physiologiques et les altérations pathologiques des liquides de l'organisme. Paris: Baillière et Fils. 2 vols. (1859).
BERNIER, J. J., LAMBLING, A.: Relations between volume and output of bicarbonate in pancreatic secretion. Ciba Found. Symp. on Exocrine Pancreas, pp. 138—149, edit. by A. V. S. DE REUCK and M. CAMERON. London, Churchill 1962.
BERSON, S. A., WALSH, J. H., YALOW, R. S.: Radioimmunoassay of gastrin in human plasma and regulation of gastrin secretion. In: NOBEL Symposium XVI. Frontiers in Gastrointestinal Hormone Research, Stockholm, July 20—21, 1970; (In Press), edit. by S. ANDERSSON. Upsala: ALMQVIST and WIKSELL 1972.
BERSTAD, A.: Stimulation of gastric secretion of pepsin by secretin in man. Scand. J. Gastroent. **4**, 617—622 (1969).
— PETERSEN, H.: A comparison between the effects of secretin and histamine on the gastric secretion of pepsin in man. Scand J. Gastroenterology **4**, 511—515 (1969).
— — Dose-response relationship of the effect of secretin on acid and pepsin secretion in man. Scand J. Gastroenterology **5**, 647—654 (1970).
— — MYREN, J.: Effect of duodenal acidification on pentagastrin stimulated gastric secretion in man. In Gastrointestinal Hormones and other Subjects. ALFRED BENZON Publication I. pp. 49—54. Edit. E. HESS-THAYSEN. Munksgaard, Copenhagen, 1971.
— — — Effect of secretin on histamine and pentagastrin induced secretion of pepsin in man. Abstr. 4th World Congress of Gastroenterology, p. 244, edit. by P. RIIS, P. ANTHONISEN and H. BADEN, Copenhagen, 1970.
BERTACCINI, G., AGOSTI, A.: Action of caerulein on intestinal motility in man: Gastroenterology. **60**, 55—63 (1971).
— DE CARO, G., ENDEAN, R., ERSPAMER, V., IMPICCIATORE, M.: The actions of caerulein on the smooth muscle of the gastrointestinal tract and gallbladder. Brit. J. Pharmacol. **34**, 291—310 (1968).
— — — — — The action of caerulein on pancreatic secretion of the dog and biliary secretion of the dog and the rat. Brit. J. Pharmacol. **37**, 185—197 (1969).

Bertaccini, G., Endean, R., Erspamer, V., Impicciatore, M.: The actions of caerulein on gastric secretion in the dog and rat. Brit. J. Pharmac. **34**, 311—329 (1968).
Binet, M. E., Jahiel, R.: Le syndrome hépatoendocrinien. Gaz. Med. France **41**, 13—19 (1934).
Birnbaum, D., Hollander, F.: Inhibition of pancreatic secretion by the carbonic anhydrase inhibitor 2-acetylamino-1,3, 4-thiadiazole-5-sulfonamide, Diamox (6063). Amer. J. Physiol. **174**, 191—195 (1953).
Bizard, G., Paris, J.: La cholécystokinine. Lille Med. **5**, 850—857 (1960a).
— — Actions pharmacologiques sur les voies biliaires. Actual. pharmacol., Paris. Masson et Cie, **1** (1960b).
Blair, E. L., Clark, D. G., Harper, A. A., Lake, H. J., Scratcherd, T.: A gastric phase of pancreatic secretion in cats. J. Physiol. (Lond.) **157**, 17 P (1961a).
— Falkner, S., Hellerström, C., Östberg, H., Richardson, D.: Investigation of gastrin activity in pancreatic islet tissue. Acta Pathol. Microbiol. Scand. **75**, 583—597 (1969).
— Farra, Y., Richardson, D. D., Steinbok, P.: The half life of exogenous gastrin in circulation. J. Physiol. (Lond.) **208**, 299—315 (1970).
— Harper, A. A., Lake, H. J.: The pepsin-stimulating effects of gastric and intestinal extracts in cats. J. Physiology (Lond.) **121**, 20—21 P (1953).
— — — Reed, J. D.: Characteristics of response to gastric extracts. J. Physiol. (Lond.) **165**, 81 P (1963).
— — — — Scratcherd, T.: A simple method of preparing gastrin. J. Physiol. (Lond.) **156**, 11—13 P (1961b).
— — Pearson, J. A., Reed, J. D.: Stimulation of pepsin secretion without stimulation of gastric acid secretion, by extracts of intestinal mucosa. J. Physiol. (London) **175**, 60—61 (1964).
— Sherratt, H. S. A., Wood, D. D.: The subcellular distribution of gastrin and secretin activity in the mucosa of the small intestine. Biochem. J. **104**, 54 P (1967).
Blake, C. C. F., Koenig, D. F., Mair, G. A., North, A. C. T., Phillips, D. C., Sarma, V. R.: Structure of hen egg-white lysozyme. A three-dimensional Fourier synthesis at 2 Å resolution. Nature **206** I, 757—761 (1965).
Blasberg, G., Edmunds, R. T., Finby, N.: Effect of cholecystokinin on the normal common duct after cholecystectomy. Surg. Forum **15**, 375—377 (1964).
Bodanszky, Agnes, Ondetti, M. A., Mutt, V., Bodanszky, M.: Synthesis of Secretin. IV. Secondary structure in a miniature protein. J. Amer. Chem. Soc. **91**, 944—949 (1969).
Bodanszky, M.: Synthesis of peptides by aminolysis of nitrophenyl esters. Nature **175**, 685 (1955).
— The secondary-tertiary structure of secretin. In: Nobel Symposium XVI. Frontiers in Gastrointestinal Hormone Research, Stockholm, July 20—21, 1970; (In press), edit. by S. Andersson. Upsala: Almqvist and Wiksell 1972.
— Levine, S. D., Narayanan, V., Ondetti, M. A., von Saltza, M., Sheehan, J. T., Williams, Nina J.: Confirmation by synthesis of secretin sequences. IUPAC Internat. Congress on Chemistry of Natural Products, Stockholm, June 26th—July 2nd 1966a. Section 2C—2.
— Ondetti, M. A., Levine, S. D., Narayanan, V. L., von Saltza, M., Sheehan, J. T., Williams, N. J., Sabo, E. F.: Synthesis of a heptacosapeptide amide with the hormonal activity of secretin. Chemistry and Industry **42**, 1757—1758 (1966b).
— — — Williams, N. J.: Synthesis of secretin. II. The stepwise approach. J. Amer. Chem. Soc. **89**, 6753—6757 (1967).
— Williams, N. J.: Synthesis of secretin. I. The protected tetradecapeptide corresponding to sequence 14—27. J. Amer. Chem. Soc. **89**, 685—689 (1967).
Bodvall, B.: Late results following cholecystectomy in 1930 cases and special studies on post-operative biliary distress. Acta Chir. Scand. Suppl. 329, Stockholm (1964).
Bolgert, M.: Lésions du pancréas et troubles fonctionnels pancréatiques. Diagnostic en clinique par l'épreuve à la sécrétine purifiée. Thèse de Paris 1935 (Masson).
— Dix ans de practique de l'épreuve à la sécrétine dans les affections du pancréas. Acta chir. belg. **47**, (Suppl. 2), 453—458 (1948).
Bossi, R.: La prova colecistocinina. Minerva Medica **52**, 1109—1114 (1961).
Bourde, J., Robinson, L. A., Suda, Y., White, T. T.: Vagal stimulation: I. A technic for repeated stimulation of the vagus on conscious dogs. Ann. Surg. **171**, 352—356 (1970a).
— — — — Vagal stimulation: II. Its effect on pancreatic secretion in conscious dogs. Ann. Surg. **171**, 357—364 (1970b).
Boyden, E. A.: The gallbladder in the cat — its functional periodicity, and its anatomical variation as recorded in 2500 specimens. Anat. Rec. **24**, 388—426 (1923).
— The effect of natural foods on the distension of the gallbladder, with a note on the change in pattern of the mucosa as it passes from distension to collapse. Anat. Rec. **30**, 333—356 (1925).

BOYDEN, E. A.: A study of the behavior of the human gallbladder in response to the digestion of food; together with some observations on the mechanism of the expulsion of bile in experimental animals. Anat. Rec. **33**, 201—239 (1926).

— The choledochoduodenal junction in the cat. Surgery **41**, 773—786 (1957).

BRIDGEWATER, A. B., KUROYANAGI, Y., CHILES, TH., NECHELES, H.: Secretin inactivating enzyme of the liver. Proc. Soc. exp. Biol. (N.Y.) **110**, 852—855 (1962).

— — GEISEL, T., NECHELES, H.: Pancreozymin-cholecystokinin injected by portal and systemic routes. Proc. Soc. exp. Biol. (N.Y.) **112**, 1056—1058 (1963).

BROMER, W. W., SINN, L. G., BEHRENS, O. K.: The amino acid sequence of glucagon V. Location of the amide groups, acid degradation studies and summary of sequential evidence. J. Amer. Chem. Soc. **79**, 2807—2810 (1957).

BROOKS, A. M., AGOSTI, A., BERTACCINI, G., GROSSMAN, M. I.: Inhibition of gastric acid secretion in man by peptide analogues of cholecystokinin. New Engl. J. Med. **282**, 535—538 (1970).

— GROSSMAN, M. I.: Comparison of gastric secretion in conscious dogs and cats. Gastroenterology **52**, 29—34 (1967a).

— — Postprandial pH and neutralizing capacity of the proximal duodenum in dogs. Gastroenterology **59**, 85—89 (1970b).

— — Effect of secretin and cholecystokinin on pentagastrin stimulated gastric secretion in man. Gastroenterology **59**, 114—119 (1970a).

— ISENBERG, J., GROSSMAN, M. I.: The effect of secretin, glucagon and duodenal acidification on pepsin secretion in man. Gastroenterology **57**, 159—162 (1969).

— JOHNSON, L. R., GROSSMAN, M. I.: Effect of secretin on gastric acid secretion stimulated by gastrin II, caerulein and desulfated caerulein. Proc. Soc. exp. Biol. (N.Y.) **131**, 1019—1021 (1969).

— — Effect of combinations of histamine and pentagastrin on gastric secretion in man and dog. Gastroenterology **58**, 470—475 (1970).

BROOKS, F. P.: The secretion of bile. Amer. J. Dig. Dis. N.S. **14**, 343—349 (1969).

BROOMÉ, A., FYRÖ, B.: Gastrin-like activity in different parts of the gastrointestinal tract of the cat. Acta physiol. scand. **74**, 359—367 (1968).

— FYRÖ, B., OLBE, L.: Localization of gastrin activity in the gastric antrum. Acta physiol. scand. **74**, 331—339 (1968).

BROWN, J. C.: Presence of a gastric motor stimulating property in duodenal extracts. Gastroenterology **52**, 225—229 (1967).

— A gastric inhibitory polypeptide. I. The amino acid composition and the tryptic peptides. Canad. J. Biochem. **49**, 255—261 (1971).

— DRYBURGH, J. R.: A gastric inhibitory polypeptide II: the complete amino acid sequence. Canad. J. Biochem. **49**, 867—872 (1971).

— HARPER, A. A., SCRATCHERD, T.: The effect of the vagus on the rate of flow of secretin-stimulated pancreatic juice in the cat. J. Physiol. (Lond.) **166**, 31 P (1963).

— — — Stimulation of pancreatic secretion by oxethazaine-hydrochloride. J. Physiol. (Lond.) **181**, 61—62 P (1965).

— — — Potentiation of secretin stimulation of the pancreas. J. Physiol. (Lond.) **190**, 519—530 (1967).

— MAGEE, D. F.: Inhibitory action of cholecystokinin on acid secretion from Heidenhain pouches induced by endogenous gastrin. Gut **8**, 29—31 (1967).

— MUTT, V., PEDERSON, R. A.: Further purification of a polypeptide demonstrating enterogastrone activity. J. Physiol. (Lond.) **209**, 57—64 (1970).

— PARKES, C. O.: Effect of fundic pouch motor activity of stimulatory and inhibitory fractions separated from pancreozymin. Gastroenterology **53**, 731—736 (1967).

— PEDERSON, R. A.: A multiparameter study on the action of preparations containing cholecystokinin-pancreozymin. Scand. J. Gastroent. **5**, 537—541 (1970).

— — JORPES, E., MUTT, V.: Preparation of highly active enterogastrone. Can. J. Physiol. Pharmacol. **47**, 113—114 (1969).

BROWN, P., GINSBURG, M.: The storage and binding of gastrin. Brit. J. Pharmacol. **35**, 372—373 P (1969).

BRUGSCH, TH., HORSTERS, H.: Cholagoga und Cholagogie. I. Mitteilung. Arch. exp. Pathol. Pharmacol. **118**, 265—291 (1926a).

— — Cholagoga und Cholagogie. II. Mitteilung. Arch. exp. Pathol. Pharmacol. **118**, 292—304 (1926b).

— — Cholagoga und Cholagogie. III. Mitteilung. Arch. exp. Pathol. Pharmacol. **118**, 303—312 (1926c).

BUCHER, G. R., IVY, A. C., GRAY, J. S.: Is histamine able to maintain an augmented pepsin response comparable to that of pilocarpine? Amer. J. Physiol. **132**, 698—706 (1941).

BUCHSTAB, J. A.: The work of the pancreatic gland after section of the vagus and splanchnicus nerves. Thesis. St. Petersburg, 1904 (Russian).
BURN, J. H., HOLTON, P.: The standardisation of secretin and pancreozymin. J. Physiol. (Lond.) **107**, 449—455 (1948).
BUSSOLATI, G., CAPELLA, C., SOLCIA, E., VASSALO, G., VEZZADINI, P.: Ultrastructural and immunofluorescent investigations on the secretin cell in the dog intestinal mucosa. Histochemie **26**, 218—227 (1971).
BUTCHER, R. W., CARLSON, L. A.: Effects of secretin on fat mobilizing lipolysis and cyclic AMP levels in rat adipose tissue. Acta Physiol. Scand. **79**, 559—563 (1970).
CAMERON, A. J., PHILLIPS, S. F., SUMMERSKILL, W. H. J.: Effect of cholecystokinin on motility of human stomach and gallbladder muscle *in vitro*. Clin. Res. **15**, 416—420 (1967).
— — — Effect of cholecystokinin, gastrin, secretin and glucagon on human gallbladder muscle *in vitro*. Proc. Soc. exp. Biol. (N.Y.) **131**, 149—154 (1969).
— — — Comparison of effects of gastrin, cholecystokinin-pancreozymin, secretin, and glucagon on human stomach muscle in vitro. Gastroenterology **59**, 539—545 (1970).
CAPLE, I., HEATH, T.: Regulation of output of electrolytes in bile and pancreatic juice in sheep. Austr. J. biol. Sciences.
CARLSON, A. J., KANTER, A. E., TUMPOVSKI, I.: The question of the stability of secretin. J. Amer. Med. Ass. **70**, 115—119 (1918).
— LEBENSOHN, J. E., PEARLMAN, S. J.: Has secretin a therapeutic value? J. Amer. Med. Ass. **65**, 178—185 (1916).
CARLSON, L. A.: Lipolysis of adipose tissue triglycerides. Regulation, physiological and clinical significance. In Protein and Polypeptide Hormones, pp. 143—149, edit. by M. MARGORELIES. Amsterdam, Excerpta Medica Foundation, 1969.
CAROLI, J., PLESSIER, J., PLESSIER, B.: L'hormone inhibitrice de la cholécystokinine, son rôle en pathologie biliaire et pancréatique. Rev. Franç. D' Étud. Clin. et Biol. **5**, 545—557 (1960).
CASE, R. M., HARPER, A. A., SCRATCHERD, T.: The relationship between bicarbonate and chloride in pancreatic juice. J. Physiol. (Lond.) **182**, 49 P (1966).
— — — Water and electrolyte secretion by the perfused pancreas of the cat. J. Physiol. (Lond.) **196**, 133—149 (1968).
— — — The secretion of electrolytes and enzymes by the pancreas of the anaesthetized cat. J. Physiol. (Lond.) **201**, 335—348 (1969a).
— — — Water and electrolyte secretion by the pancreas. In: The Exocrine Glands, pp. 39—56, edit. S.Y. BOTELHO, F. P. BROOKS and W. B. SHELLEY. Univ. Philadelphia, Pennsylvania Press 1969b.
— — — On the mode of action of secretin and pancreozymin. In: Proc. 3rd Symp. Europ. Pancreatic Club, Prague July 2—4, 1968, pp. 25—33, edit. by P. FRIC, F. MALIS and R. RONSKY, Praha, Czech. Med. Press, 1970.
— LAUNDY, T. J., SCRATCHERD, T.: Adenosine 3',5'-mono-phosphate (cyclic AMP) as the intracellular mediator of the action of secretin on the exocrine pancreas. J. Physiol. (Lond.) **204**, 45—47 P (1969).
CELESTIN, L. R.: Gastrin-like effects of cholecystokinin-pancreozymin. Nature **215**, 763—764 (1967).
CHABROL, E.: Actualités cliniques et thérapeutiques de la patholigie du foie, MASSON et Cie. 1950.
— Pathologie du foi. Études cliniques et biologiques p. 41, MASSON et Cie. 1954.
CHARBON, G. A., SEBUS, J., KOAL, D. S., HOEKSTRA, M. H.: Augmentation by glucagon of histamine-induced gastric secretion. Gastroenterology **44**, 805—809 (1963).
CHARTERS, A. C., DAVIDSON, W. D., ODELL, W. D., THOMPSON, J. C.: Secretory and immunochemical properties of gastrin and pancreozymin-cholecystokinin. Gastroenterology **57**, 156—158 (1969).
CHEY, W. Y.: Pancreozymin-secretin test in pancreatic disease, biliary tract disease, and diabetes mellitus. Thesis, University of Pennsylvania, Philadelphia 1962.
— HITANANT, S., HENDRICKS, J., LORBER, S. H.: Effect of intestinal hormones on human gastric function. Gastroenterology **54**, 1225 (1968).
— — — — Effect of secretin and cholecystokinin on gastric emptying and gastric secretion in man. Gastroenterology **58**, 820—827 (1970).
— — — — Effect of secretin and cholecystokinin on gastric emptying and gastric secretion in man. NOBEL Symposium XVI. Frontiers in Gastrointestinal Hormone Research, Stockholm, July 20—21, 1970; (in press) edit. by S. ANDERSSON. Upsala, ALMQVIST and WIKSELL, 1972.
— KOSAY, S., HENDRICKS, J., BRAVERMAN, S., LORBER, S. H.: Effect of secretin on motor activity of stomach and Heidenhain pouch in dogs. Amer. J. Physiol. **217**, 848—852 (1969).

CHEY, W. Y., KOSAY, S., HENDRICKS, J., LORBER, S. H.: Effect of secretin on the motor function of stomach and Heidenhain pouch and gastric emptying in dogs. Abstr. Proc. XXIV International Congress of Physiological Sciences, August 25—31, 1968, Washington, D.C.
— LEE, H. W., LORBER, S. H.: Role of the liver on the biological actions of secretin. Gastroenterology **58**, 934 (1970).
— LORBER, S. H., KUSAKCIOGLU, O., HENDRICKS, J.: Effect of secretin and pancreozymin-cholecystokinin on motor function of stomach and duodenum. Fed. Proc. **26**, March—April, 383 (1967).
— SIVASOMBOON, B., HENDRICKS, J., LORBER, S. J.: Effects of secretin and cholecystokinin on gastric secretion in rats. Gastroenterology **58**, 1037 (1970b).
CHIRAY, M., BOLGERT, M.: Le diagnostic des affections pancréatiques par l'épreuve à la sécrétine purifiée. Presse méd. **44**, 428—431 (1936).
— JEANDEL, A., SALMON, A.: L'exploration clinique du pancréas et l'injection intraveineuse de sécrétine purifiée. Presse méd. **38**, 977—982 (1930).
— SALMON, A. R., MERCIER, A.: Action of purified secretin on external secretion of pancreas in man. Bull. Mém. Soc. méd. Paris **50**, 1417—1426 (1926).
CHRISTENSEN, B. C.: Studies on the secretin test. Acta Med. Scand. **173**, 315—327 (1963).
CLARKE, S. D., NEILL, D. W., WELBOURN, R. B.: Effect of glucagon on gastric secretion in the dog. Gut **1**, 146—148 (1960).
CLODI, P. H., SCHNACK, H.: The influence of enterohormones (secretin, pancreozymin) on the secretion and composition of bile in the isolated perfused rat liver. Liver Research (J. VANDENBROUCHE et al.). Tijdschr. Gastroenterologie **10b**, 418—422 (1967).
CODE, C. F., WATKINSON, G.: Importance of vagal innervation in the regulatory effect of acid in the duodenum on gastric secretion of acid. J. Physiol. **130**, 233—252 (1955).
COHEN, N., MAZURE, P., DREILING, D. A., JANOWITZ, H. D.: Effect of glucagon on histamine-stimulated gastric secretion in man. Gastroenterology **39**, 48—54 (1960).
COHEN, S., LIPSHUTZ, W.: Hormonal regulation of human lower esophageal sphincter competence: Interaction of gastrin and secretin. J. Clin. Invest. **50**, 449—454 (1971).
COLAGRANDE, C., RAMORINO, M. L., SISTI, P.: Sul impiego della „Colecistocinina" negli esami radiological dell'apparato biliare. Arch. Ital. Mal. Appr. Dig. **27**, 469—481 (1960).
COLWELL, A .R., JR.: Collection of pancreatic juice from rats and consequences of its continued loss. Amer. J. Physiol. **164**, 812—821 (1951).
COMLINE, R. S., HALL, L. W., HICKSON, J. C. D., MURILLO, A., WALKER, R. G.: Pancreatic secretion of the horse. J. Physiol. (London) **204**, 10P—11P (1969).
— HICKSON, J. C. D., MESSAGE, M. A.: Nervous tissue in the pancreas of different species. J. Physiol. (London) **170**, 47—48 P (1964).
COOK, D. L., BIANCHI, R. G.: SC-15396: A new antiulcer compound possessing anti-gastrin activity. Life Sc. **6**, 1381—1387 (1967).
COOKE, A. R.: The glands of Brunner. Handbook of Physiol. Section 6 Vol. II pp. 1087—1095. Amer. Physiol. Soc. Wash. 1967.
— Potentation of acid secretion. Amer. J. Physiol. **216**, 968—973 (1969).
— GROSSMAN, M. I.: Studies on the secretion and motility of Brunner's gland pouches. Gastroenterology **51**, 506—514 (1966).
COZZOLINO, H. J., GOLDSTEIN, F., GREENING, R. R., WIRTS, C. W.: The cystic duct syndrome. J. Amer. Med. Ass. **185**, 920—924 (1963).
CREAN, G. P., MARSHALL, M. W., RUMSEY, R. D. E.: Parietal cell hyperplasia induced by the administration of pentagastrin (ICI 50, 123) to rats. Gastroenterology **57**, 147—155 (1969).
CRICK, J., HARPER, A. A., RAPER, H. S.: On the preparation of secretin and pancreozymin. J. Physiol. (Lond.) **110**, 367—376 (1949).
CRIDER, J. O., THOMAS, J. E.: Secretion of pancreatic juice after cutting the extrinsic nerves. Amer. J. Physiol. **141**, 730—737 (1944).
CRISPIN, J. S., CHOI, Y. W., WISEMAN, D. G. H., GILLESPIE, D. J., LIND, J. F.: A direct manometric study of the canine choledochoduodenal junction. Ann. Surg. **101**, 215—218 (1970).
CULMER, C. U., GRAY, J. S., ADKISON, J. L., IVY, A. C.: On the origin of urogastrone. Science **91**, 148—149 (1940).
CUMMING, J. D., PERCIVAL, H. G.: The effect of glucagon upon gastric secretion and total stomach blood flow. J. Physiol. (London) **191**, 81P—82P (1967).
CUMMINS, A. J., SCHAPIRO, H., MERKER, P. C.: Effect of secretin on gastric motility. Amer. Surg. **32**, 187—189 (1966).
DAHLGREN, S.: The afferent loop syndrome. Acta Chir. Scand. Suppl. **327** (1964).
— Cholecystokinin: Pharmacology and clinical use. Acta Chir. Scand. Suppl. **357**, 256—260 (1966).

Dahlgren. S.: The effect of cholecystokinin on duodenal motility. Acta Chir. Scand. **133**, 403—405 (1967).
— Thorén, L.: Intestinal motility in low small bowel obstruction. Acta Chir. Scand. **133**, 417—421 (1967).
Dale, H. H., Laidlaw, P. P.: A method of preparing secretin. J. Physiol. (Lond.) **44**, 11 (1912).
Dal Monte, P. P., Giro, C., Mazzanti, G.: Proposita di un nuovo metodo di dosaggio biologico dell' urocolecystochinina. Boll. Soc. Ital. Biol. Sperim. **40**, 552—554 (1964).
— — — Verlicchi, G.: L'eliminazione dell' urocolecystochinina nel gastro-resicato par mattia ulcerosa. Boll. Soc. Ital. Biol. Sperim. **41**, 155—156 (1965).
Danhof, I. E.: Mechanism of action of cholecystokinin in the dog. The Physiologist **9**, 164 (1966).
Davidson, W. D., Davies, R. E.: The stomach and duodenum: Gastrin and the duodenal hormones. The actions of hormones on molecular processes, pp. 336—359. Edit. Litwack, G. and D. Kritchevsky, New York, Wiley & Sons, 1964.
— Urushibara, O., Thompson, J. C.: Action of pancreozymin-cholecystokinin on the isolated gastric mucosa of the bullfrog. Proc. Soc. exper. Biol. (N.Y.) **129**, 711—713 (1969a).
— — — Comparison of the effects of human and porcine gastrin on isolated gastric mucosa of the bullfrog. Proc. Soc. exp. Biol. (N.Y.) **130**, 204—206 (1969b).
Davies, R. E.: The mechanism of hydrochloric acid production by the stomach. Ph. D. Thesis, University of Sheffield (1948).
— The mechanism of hydrochloric acid production by the stomach. Biol. Rev. Cambridge Phil. Soc. **26**, 87—120 (1951).
— Harper, A. A., Mackay, I. F. S.: A comparison of the respiratory activity and histological changes in isolated pancreatic tissue. Amer. J. Physiology **157**, 278—282 (1949).
Davila, M., Parrochia, F., Rufin, S., Fuenzalida, S., Gonzalez, I.: Sondeo pancreático con secretina. Resultados en individuos normales.—Sondeo pancreático en la pancreatitis chronica. Rev. Med. Chile **89**, 81, 94—99, 100—103 (1961).
Davis, A. E., Biggs, J. C.: The pancreas and iron absorption. Gut **6**, 140—142 (1965).
— — The pancreas and iron absorption: Current Views. Amer. J. Dig. Dis. N.S. **12**, 293—302 (1967).
Debray, Ch., de la Tour, J., Vaille, Ch., Rozé, Cl., Souchard, M.: Contribution à l'étude de la sécrétion biliaire et pancréatique externe chez le rat. J. Physiol. (Paris) **54**, 459—499 (1962a).
— Vaille, Ch., de la Tour, J., Rozé, Cl., Souchard, M.: Action des sécrétines du commerce sur la sécrétion pancréatique externe du rat. J. Physiol. (Paris) **54**, 549—577 (1962b).
— — — — — Études sur la sécrétion pancréatico-biliaire du rat. Presse Med. **69**, 2601—2603 (1961).
Delaney, J. P., Grim, E.: Drug influences on pancreatic blood flow. Fed. Proc. 23:1 252 (1964).
— — Influence of hormones and drugs on canine pancreatic blood flow. Amer. J. Physiol. **211**, 1398—1402 (1966).
Delezenne, C., Hallion, L., Gayet, R.: Sur le mécanisme de la sécrétion pancréatique. Mise en dérivation d'une anse intestinale et du pancréas sur la circulation carotidienne. Ann. Physiol. Physicochim. biol. **3**, 508—511 (1927).
— Pozerski, E.: Action de l'extrait aqueux d'intestine sur la sécrétine. C. R. Soc. Biol. **56**, 987—989 (1904).
— — Action de l'extrait aqueux d'intestin sur la sécrétine. J. Physiol. Pathol. gén. **14**, 521—529 (1912a).
— — Sur la pre-existence de la sécrétine dans la muqueuse intestinale. J. Physiol. Pathol. gén. **14**, 540—553 (1912b).
Denton, R. W., Gershbein, L. L.: Effect of cholecystokinin concentrates on the isolated heart. Cardiologia, Basel, **49**, Suppl. 1, 59—63 (1966).
— — Ivy, A. C.: Response of human and canine gallbladder to cholecystokinin. J. Appl. Physiol. **2**, 671—679 (1950).
Deutsch, W., Raper, H. S.: Respiration and functional activity. J. Physiol. (London) **87**, 275—286 (1936).
Dhariwal, A. P. S., Schally, A. V., Meyer, J., Sun, D. C. H., Jorpes, J. E., Mutt, V.: Purification of pancreozymin. Gastroenterology **44**, 316—321 (1963).
Dickman, S. R., Holtzer, R. L., Gazzinelli, G.: Protein synthesis in beef pancreas slices: Biochemistry. **1**, 574—580 (1962).
— Morrill, G. A.: Stimulation of respiration and secretion of mouse pancreas *in vitro*. Amer. J. Physiol. **190**, 403—407 (1957).

DICKMAN, S. R.: YANG, J.: Effects of pancreozymin, urecholine and actinomycin D on the metabolism of ribonucleic acid in canine pancreas. Biochem. J. **99,** 56 P—57 P (1966).
DICKSTEIN, S., BIRNBAUM, D.: The mechanism of external pancreatic secretion. Experientia **16,** 365—367 (1960).
DINOSO, V. P., CHEY, W. Y., LORBER, S. H.: Effect of secretin on gastric secretion and motor function of the upper gastrointestinal tract in man. Clinical Research **14,** 295 (1966).
— — HENDRICKS, J., LORBER, S. H.: Intestinal mucosal hormones and motor function of the stomach in man. J. Appl. Physiol. **26,** 326—329 (1969).
DIXON, M. B. F., MOORE, S., STACK-DUNNE, M. P., YOUNG, F. G.: Chromatography of adrenocorticotrophic hormone on ion-exchange columns. Nature **168,** 1044—1045 (1951).
DOLINSKI, I. L.: Influence of acids on the secretion of the pancreatic gland. Arch. de Soc. Biol. St. Petersburg **3,** 399—427 (1894).
DORCHESTER, J. E. C.: Effect of vagotomy on secretin and pancreozymin activity of intestines of albino rats. Amer. J. Physiol. **196,** 847—849 (1959).
— HAIST, R. E.: A method of secretin assay. J. Physiol. (Lond.) **118,** 182—187 (1952a).
— — The secretin content of the intestine in normal and hypophysectomized rats. J. Physiol. (Lond.) **118,** 188—195 (1952b).
DORIGOTTI, L., GLÄSSER, A. H.: Comparative effects of caerulein, pancreozymin and secretin on pancreatic blood flow. Experientia, (Basel) **24,** 806—807 (1968).
DOTEVALL, G., GILLBERG, R., KOCK, N. G., WALAN, A.: Stimulatory and inhibitory effects on gastric secretion in man by glucagon infusion in small doses. In: Abstr. 4th World Congress of Gastroenterology, p. 133, edit. by P. RIIS, P. ANTHONISEN and H. BADEN, Copenhagen, 1970a.
— — — — Gastric secretion of acid and pepsin in man during glucagon infusion in small doses. Gastroenterology **58,** 942 (1970b).
— KOCK, N. G.: The effect of glucagon on intestinal motility in man. Gastroenterology **45,** 364—367 (1963).
— — WALAN, A.: Inhibition of pentagastrin-induced gastric acid secretion in man by glucagon given intravenously. Scand. J. Gastroenterology **4,** 713—716 (1969).
— — — Inhibition of basal gastric acid secretion in man by glucagon given intraportally. Scand. J. Gastroenterology **5,** 391—394 (1970).
— WESTLING, H.: On the effect of glucagon on histamine-induced and spontaneous gastric acid secretion in man. Scand. J. Clin. Lab. Invest., **12,** 489—492 (1960).
DOUBILET, H., IVY, A. C.: The response of the smooth muscle of the gallbladder at various intravesicular pressure to cholecystokinin. Amer. J. Physiol. **124,** 379—390 (1938).
DOUGLAS, M. C., WATTS, M. McK., JABLONSKI, P., OWEN, J. A.: The effect of various gastroduodenal hormones on output of hepatic bile in the isolated perfused porcine liver. Gut **10,** 79 (1969).
DRAGSTEDT, L. R.: The physiology of gastric antrum. In: The Stomach, pp. 124—131, edit. by C. THOMPSON, D. BERKOWITZ and E. POLISH. Grune and Stratton, New York 1967.
— COHATSU, S., GREENLEE, H. B.: Further studies on the question of an inhibitory hormone from the gastric antrum. Arch. Surg. **79,** 10—21 (1959).
— WOODWARD, E. R., OBERHELMAN, H. A., JR., STORER, E. H., SMITH, C. A.: Effect of transplantation of antrum of stomach on gastric secretion in experimental animals. Amer. J. Physiol. **165,** 386—398 (1951).
DREILING, D. A.: The technique of secretin test: normal ranges. J. Mt. Sinai Hosp. **21,** 363—372 (1955).
— Mechanism of pancreatic exocrine secretion. Amer. J. Gastroenterology **52,** 17—29 (1969).
— JANOWITZ, H. D.: The secretion of electrolytes by the human pancreas. Gastroenterology **30,** 382—390 (1956).
— — The laboratory diagnosis of pancreatic disease, the secretin test. Amer. J. Gastroent. **28,** 268—279 (1957).
— — The effect of glucagon on gastric secretion in man. Gastroenterology **36,** 580—581 (1959).
— — The measurement of pancreatic secretory function. In: Ciba Foundation Symposium on the Exocrine Pancreas, pp. 225—252, edit. by A. V. S. DE REUCK and M. P. CAMERON. London. Churchill 1962.
— — Haemmerli, U. P., Marshall, D.: The effect of glucagon on the exocrine pancreatic secretion of man. J. Mount Sinai Hosp. **25,** 240—243 (1958).
— — HALPERN, M.: The effect of a carbonic anhydrase inhibitor, Diamox, on human pancreatic secretion. Gastroenterology **29,** 262—279 (1955).
DREWER, D. A., IVY, A. C.: On the non-ubiquitous occurrence of secretin. Proc. Soc. exp. Biol. Med. **27,** 186—187 (1929).

Dritsas, K. G., Kowalevski, K.: Further studies on *ex vivo* isolated perfused canine stomach: Role of antrum as inhibitor of gastric secretory function. Scand. J. Gastroenterol. **3**, 99–105 (1968).
Duncan, P. R., Harper, A. A., Howat, H. T., Oleesky, S., Varley, H.: The effects of pancreozymin on human subjects. J. Physiol. (London) **111**, 63 P (1950).
– – – – – Tests of gallbladder function in man. Gastroenterologia **78**, 349–353 (1952).
– – – – – Scott, J. E.: The use of cholecystokinetic agent in preparations of pancreozymin to study gallbladder function in man. J. Physiol. (Lond.) **121**, 19–20 P (1953).
Dupré, J.: Effect of route of administration on disposal glucose loads. J. Physiol. (Lond.) **175**, 58–60 P (1964a).
– An intestinal hormone affecting glucose disposal in man. Lancet 1964 II, 672–673.
– Rojas, L., White, J. J., Unger, R. H., Beck, J. C.: Effects of secretin on insulin and glucagon in portal and peripheral blood in man. Lancet 1966 II, 26–27.
– Regulation of the secretions of the pancreas. Ann. Rev. Med. **21**, 299–316 (1970).
Dyck, W. P., Rudick, J., Hoexter, B., Janowitz, H. D.: Influence of glucagon on pancreatic exocrine secretion. Gastroenterology, **56**, 531–537 (1969).
– Texter, E. C., Lasater, J. M., Hightower, N. C.: Influence of glucagon on pancreatic exocrine secretion in man. Gastroenterology **58**, 532–539 (1970).
Edholm, P.: Gallbladder evacuation in the normal male induced by cholecystokinin. Acta Radiol. (Stockholm) **53**, 257–265 (1960).
– Jonson, G., Thulin, L.: Le débit biliaire du foie: Stimulation par la cholécystokinine, la sécrétine et l'alimentation perorale. Path.-Biol. **10**, 447–450 (1962).
Edkins, J. S.: On the chemical mechanism of gastric secretion. Proc. roy. Soc. B **76**, 376 (1905).
– The chemical mechanism of gastric secretion. J. Physiol. (Lond.) **34**, 133–144 (1906).
Ekholm, R., Zelander, T., Edlund, Y.: The ultrastructural organization of the rat exocrine pancreas. J. Ultrastruct. Res. **7**, 73–83 (1962).
Elliott, D. F., Peart, W. S.: The amino acid sequence in a hypertensin. Biochem. J. **65**, 246–254 (1957).
Elwin, C.-E.: Absorption at different pH levels of some gastrin releasing agents. In: Gastrointestinal Hormones and other Subjects pp. 32–36. V Scand. Conf. Gastroenterology. Edit. by E. Hess Thaysen. Munksgaard, Copenhagen, 1971.
– Uvnäs, B.: Distribution and local release of gastrin. In: Gastrin, pp. 69–82, edit. M. I. Grossman, Univ. Calif. Press, Berkeley, 1966.
Emås, S., Billings, A., Grossman, M. I.: Effects of gastrin and pentagastrin on gastric and pancreatic secretion in dogs. Scand. J. Gastroent. **3**, 234–240 (1968).
– Fyrö, B.: Gastrin-like activity in different parts of the gastrointestinal tract of the cat. Acta Physiol. Scand. **74**, 359–367 (1968).
– Grossman, M. I.: Comparison of gastric secretion in conscious dogs and cats. Gastroenterology **52**, 29–34 (1967a).
– – Difference in response between dogs and cats to large doses of gastrin on gastric secretion. Gut **8**, 267–275 (1967b).
Enriquez, E., Hallion, L.: Réflex acid de Pavlov et sécrétine; Méchanism humoral commun. C. R. Soc. Biol. **55**, 233–234 (1903).
Eriksson, S., Sjöquist, J.: Quantitative determination of N-terminal amino acids in some serum proteins. Biochim. Biophys. Acta **45**, 290–296 (1960).
Erlinger, S., Dhumeaux, D., Benhamon, J.-P., Fauvert, R.: La sécrétion biliaire du lapin. Preuves en faveur d'une importante fraction indépendente des sels biliaires. Rev. Franc. Étud. Clin. Biol. **14**, 144–150 (1969).
– Preisig, R.: Les méchanismes de la cholérèse. Rev. Franc. Étud. Clin. Biol. **14**, 117–121 (1969).
Erspamer, V.: The spectrum of biological activity of the caeruleins. In: Nobel Symposium XVI. Frontiers in Gastrointestinal Hormone Research, Stockholm, July 20–21, 1970; (In press), edit. by S. Andersson, Almqvist and Wiksell. Upsala: 1972.
– Anastasi, A.: Structure and pharmacological actions of eledoisin, the active endecapeptide of the posterior salivary glands of eledone. Experientia **18**, 58–59 (1962).
– – Polypeptides active on plain muscle in the amphibian skin. In: Hypotensive Peptides, pp. 63–75, edit. E. G. Erdös, N. Back and F. Sicuteri, Berlin, Springer 1966.
– – Comments. Gastroenterology **54**, 988 (1968).
– – Bertaccini, G., Cei, J. M.: Structure and pharmacological actions of physalaemin, the main active polypeptide of the skin of *Physalaemus fuscumaculatus*. Experientia (Basel) **20**, 489–490 (1964).
– Bertaccini, G., de Caro, G., Endean, R., Impicciatore, M.: Pharmacological actions of caerulein. Experientia (Basel) **23**, 702–703 (1967).

ERSPAMER, V., ROSEGHINI, M., ENDEAN, R., ANASTASI, A.: Biogenic amines and active polypeptides in the skin of Australian amphibians. Nature **212**, 204 (1966).

ERTAN, A., BROOKS, F. P., OSTROW, J. D., ARVAN, D. A., WILLIAMS, D. N., CERDA, J. J.: Effect of jejunal amino acid perfusion and exogenous cholecystokinin on the exocrine pancreatic and biliary secretions in man. Gastroenterology **61**, 686—692 (1971).

FABIAN, M., FORSLING, M. L., IBBITSON, D., JONES, J. J., STONE, D.: The half-time (t ½), clearance, binding and stability of neurohypophysial hormones in human plasma. J. Physiol. (Lond.) **198**, 19—20P (1968).

FALLOISE, A.: Action de l'acide chlorhydrique introduit dans l'intestin sur la sécrétion biliaire. Bull. Class. d. Sciences, Acad. Roy. Belgique, 757—791 (1903).

FARRELL, J. I., IVY, A. C.: Studies on the motility of the transplanted gastric pouch. Amer. J. Physiol. **76**, 227—228 (1926a).

— — Contributions to the physiology of the pancreas. II. The proof of a humoral mechanism for external pancreatic secretion. Amer. J. Physiol. **78**, 325—338 (1926b).

FENG, T. P., HOU, H. C., LIM, R. K. S.: On the mechanism of the inhibition of gastric secretion by fat. Chinese J. Physiol. **3**, 371—378 (1929).

FISHMAN, L.: The purification and structure of secretin. Dissertation, Chemistry Biological. New York Univ. Ph. D. 1957.

— Purification and structure of secretin. Fed. Proc. **18**, 226 (1959).

FLEIG, C.: Réflex de l'acide sur la sécrétion biliaire. C. R. Soc. Biol. **55**, 353—355 (1903).

— Du mode d'action des excitants chimiques des glandes digestives. Arch. internat. de Physiol. **1**, 286—346 (1904).

FLOREY, H. W., HARDING, H. E.: A humoral control of secretion of Brunner's glands. Proc. Roy. Soc. (Biol.) **117**, 68—77 (1935a).

— — The nature of the hormone controlling Brunner's glands. Quart. J. Exp. Physiol. **25**, 329—339 (1935b).

FOGELSON, S. J., BACHRACH, W. H.: Response of Brunner's glands to secretin. Amer. J. Physiol. **128**, 121—123 (1939).

FORELL, M. M.: Bile salts as stimulants of pancreatic secretion. In: NOBEL Symposium XVI. Frontiers in Gastrointestinal Hormone Research, Stockholm, July 20—21, 1970; (In press), edit. by S. ANDERSSON. Upsala: ALMQVIST and WIKSELL 1972.

— OTTE, M., KOHL, H. J., LEHNERT, P., STAHLHEBER, H. P.: The influence of bile and pure bile salts on pancreatic secretion in man. Scand. J. Gastroenterology **6**, 261—266 (1971).

— STAHLHEBER, H.: Gallefluß und Pankreassekretion. Klin. Wschr. **44**, 1184—1189 (1966).

— — SCHOLZ, F.: Galle als Reiz der Enzymsekretion des Pankreas. Deutsch. Med. Wschr. **90**, 1128—1132 (1965).

FRAENKEL-CONRAT, H., HARRIS, J. I., LEVY, A. L.: Terminal and sequence studies in peptides and proteins. In: Methods of Biochemical Analysis **2**, pp. 359—425, edit. by D. GLICK New York, Interscience 1954.

FRANZEN, J.: Beziehungen des Gallenflusses zur Ileozökalregion. Fortschr. Röntgenstrahl. u. Nuklearmedizin **95**, 769—781 (1961).

FREY, E. K., KRAUT, H., WERLE, E.: Das Kallikrein-Kinin-System und seine Inhibitoren, pp. 76—80, Stuttgart, FERDINAND ENKE 1968.

FRIEDMAN, M. H. F.: The significance of the discovery of secretin. Gastroenterology **26**, 795—801 (1954).

— CHENG, L. K.: Pancreatic function in portal cirrhosis. Amer. J. Gastroenterology **35**, 492—498 (1961).

— PINCUS, I. J., THOMAS, J. E., REHFUSS, M. E.: Stimulation of pepsin secretion by means of acid in the intestine. Amer. J. Physiol. **140**, 708—712 (1944).

— SNAPE, V. J.: Comparative effectiveness of extracts of intestinal mucosa in stimulating the external secretions of the pancreas. Fed. Proc. **4** II, 21—22 (1945).

— THOMAS, J. E.: The preparation of secretin. Proc. Soc. exp. Biol. (N.Y.) **73**, 345—348 (1950a).

— — The assay and distribution of secretin. J. Lab. Clin. Med. **35**, 366—372 (1950b).

GAMBLE, W. S.: Impaired pancreozymin (CCK-PZ) secretion after vagotomy and pyloroplasty. J. Lab. Clin. Med. **76**, 871 (1970).

GAYET, R., GUILLAUMIE, M.: Sur les modifications de l'excrétion pancréatique consécutives à l'hyperglycémie des centres encéphaliques. C. R. Soc. Biol. **105**, 373—377 (1930).

GERARD, R. W., STILL, E. U.: Studies on the physiology of secretin. V. The effects on the respiration of the excised pancreas. Amer. J. Physiol. **103**, 232—234 (1933).

GERBER, M. L., HERTZOG, F. J., LEE, Y. P., FIELD, J. B., DRAPANAS, T.: Effect of secretin on visceral hemodynamics and pancreatic function. Surg. Forum 18, 385—387 (1967).

GERRING, E. L.: Some observations on the actions of pure urogastrone. Gut **10**, 1053 (1969).

Gerring, E. L.: The effect of pure urogastrone on gastric secretion in dogs and cats. In: Abstr. 4th World Congress of Gastroenterology, p. 142, edit. by P. Riis, P. Anthonisen, H. Baden, Copenhagen, 1970.
— Haworth, E.: The effect of urogastrone on gastric acid secretion in dogs and cats. Rendic. R. Gastroenterol. **2**, 167—171 (1970).
Gershbein, L. L., Denton, R. W., Hubbard, B. H., Jr.: In vitro assay of cholecystokinin concentrates. J. Appl. Physiol. **5**, 712—716 (1953).
— Krup, M.: The preparation of a potent secretin concentrate. J. Amer. Chem. Soc. **74**, 679—685 (1952).
— Wang, C. C., Ivy, A. C.: Assay of secretin and cholecystokinin concentrates. Proc. Soc. exp. Biol. (N.Y.) **70**, 516—521 (1949).
Gibbs, G. E., Gershbein, L. L.: Presence of secretin in cystic fibrosis of the pancreas. Proc. Soc. exp. Biol. (N.Y.) **74**, 336—337 (1950).
Gillespie, I. E., Clark, D. H., Kay, A. W., Tankel, H. I.: Effect of antrectomy, vagotomy with gastrojejunostomy and antrectomy with vagotomy on the spontaneous and maximal acid output in man. Gastroenterology **38**, 361—367 (1960).
— Grossman, M. I.: Gastric secretion of acid in response to portal and systemic venous injection of gastrin. Gastroenteroly **43**, 189—192 (1962).
— — Potentiation between urecholine and gastrin extracts and between urecholine and histamine in the stimulation of Heidenhain pouches. Gut **5**, 71—76 (1964a).
— — Inhibitory effect of secretin and cholecystokinin on Heidenhain pouch responses to gastrin extract and histamine. Gut, Lond., **5**, 342—345 (1964b).
Gley, E.: Sur les excitants de la sécrétion pancréatique. Classification rationelle de ces substances. J. de Physiol. Pathol. Gen. **14**, 509—520 (1912).
Go, V. L. W., Hoffmann, A. F., Summerskill, W. H. J.: Sites of secretion and effects of pancreatic enzyme output in man. J. Lab. Clin. Med. **72**, 875 (1968).
— — — Pancreozymin: Sites of secretion and effects on pancreatic enzyme output in man. J. Clin. Invest. **48**, 29a—30a (1969).
— — — Pancreozymin bioassay in man based on pancreatic enzyme secretion: potency of specific amino acids and other digestive products. J. Clin. Invest. **49**, 1558—1564 (1970a).
— — — Simultaneous measurements of total pancreatic, biliary, and gastric outputs in man using a perfusion technique. Gastroenterology, **58**, 321—328 (1970b).
Goebell, H., Bode, Ch., Horn, H. D.: Einfluß von Secretin und Pankreozymin auf die Calciumsekretion im menschlichen Duodenalsaft bei normaler und gestörter Pankreasfunktion. Klin. Wschr. **48**, 1330—1339 (1970).
— Horn, H. D., Gossmann, H. H., Bode, Ch.: Calcium excretion in duodenal juice before and after application of secretin and pancreozymin in human. In: Proc. 3rd Symp. Europ. Pancreatic Club, Prague, July 2—4, 1968, pp. 174—182, edit. by P. Fric, F. Malis and R. Ronsky, Praha, Czech. Med. Press, 1970.
— Steffen, Ch., Bode, Ch.: Parallel enhancement of calcium and protein concentration in canine pancreatic juice by pancreozymin. In: Abstr. 4th World Congress of Gastroenterology. p. 540, edit. by P. Riis, P. Anthonisen and H. Baden, Copenhagen, 1970.
van Goidsenhoven, G. E., Henke, W. J., Vacca, J. B., Knight, W. A.: Pancreatic function in cirrhosis of the liver. Amer. J. Dig. Dis. **8**, 160—173 (1963).
Goldner, M. G., Gomori, G.: Alloxan diabetes in the dog. Endocrinology **33**, 297—308 (1943).
Gomori, G.: The distribution of phosphatase in normal organs and tissues. J. Cell. Comp. Physiol. **17**, 71—84 (1941).
Goodhead, B., Himal, H. S., Zanbilowicz: Relationship between pancreatic secretion and pancreatic blood flow. Gut, **11**, 62—68 (1970).
Graaf, R. de: Tractatus anatomico — medicus de succi pancreatici natura et usu. Officina Hackiana. Delft 1671.
Graham, E. A., Cole, N. H.: Roentgenologic examination of the gallbladder. J. Amer. Med. Ass. **82**, 613—614 (1924).
Grall, A.: Le radiocinéma accéléré de l'intestine grêle. Technique d'utilisation de la cholécystokinine. Etude de 170 cas. Dissert. Université de Paris 1967. Service d'Electro-Radiologie. Central Bichat.
Gray, J. S.: The effect of atropine on gastric secretion and its relation to the gastrin theory. Amer. J. Physiol. **120**, 657—662 (1937).
— Culmer, C. U., Wieczorowski, E., Adkison, J. L.: Preparation of pyrogen-free urogastrone. Proc. Soc. exp. Biol. (N.Y.) **43**, 225—228 (1940).
— Wieczorowski, E., Ivy, A. C.: Inhibition of gastric secretion in man with urogastrone. Amer. J. Dig. Dis. **7**, 513—515 (1940).
Gray, W. R.: Dansyl chloride procedure, in Methods in Enzymology **11**, 139—151, edit. by S. P. Colowick and N. O. Kaplan, New York and London, Acad. Press 1967.

GREENGARD, H.: Enzymatic inactivation of cholecystokinin by blood serum. Amer. J. Physiol. **134**, 833—738 (1941).
— Hormones of the gastrointestinal tract. In: The Hormones **1**, 201—254. edit. by G. PINCUS and K. V. THIMANN. New York. Acad. Press. 1948.
— ATKINSON, A. J., GROSSMAN, M. I., IVY, A. C.: The effectiveness of parenterally administered "enterogastrone" in the prophylaxis of recurrences of experimental and clinical peptic ulcer. Gastroenteroly **7**, 625—649 (1946).
— GROSSMAN, M. I., WOOLLEY, J. R., IVY, A. C.: Confirmation of the presence of pancreozymin in duodenal mucosa. Science **99**, 350—351 (1944).
— IVY, A. C.: The isolation of secretin. Amer. J. Physiol. **124**, 427—434 (1938).
— — Purification of pancreozymin and secretin. Fed. Proc. **4**, 26—27 (1945).
— STEIN, I. F.: Assay of secretin. Proc. Soc. exp. Biol. (N.Y.) **46**, 149—151 (1941).
— — IVY, A. C.: Secretinase in blood serum. Amer. J. Physiol. **133**, 121—127 (1941a).
— — — The enzymatic inactivation of cholecystokinin by blood serum. Amer. J. Physiol. **134**, 733—738 (1941b).
— WOLFROM, M. L., NESS, R. K.: The composition of crystalline secretin picrolonate. Fed. Proc. **6**, 115—116 (1947).
GREENLEE, H. B., LONGHI, E. H., GUERRERO, J. D., NELSEN, T. S., EL-BEDRI, A. L., DRAGSTEDT, L. R.: Inhibitory effect of pancreatic secretin on gastric secretion. Amer. J. Physiol. **190**, 396—402 (1957).
GREGORY, H., HARDY, P. M., JONES, D. S., KENNER, G. W., SHEPPARD, R. C.: The antral hormone gastrin. Structure of gastrin. Nature **204**, 931—933 (1964).
GREGORY, R. A.: Secretory Mechanisms of the Gastro-intestinal Tract. Edward Arnold Ltd. London, 1962.
— Isolation and chemistry of gastrin. In: Handbook of Physiol. Section 6 Vol. II pp. 827—834. Wash., Amer. Physiol. Soc. 1967a.
— Enterogastrone — A reappraisal of the problem. In: Gastric Secretion, pp. 469—477, edit. by T. K. SHNITKA, J. A. L. GILBERT and R. C. HARRISON. New York, Pergamon, 1967b.
— TRACY, H. J.: The preparation and properties of gastrin. J. Physiol. **156**, 523—543 (1961).
— — The constitution and properties of two gastrins extracted from hog antral mucosa. Gut **5**, 103—117 (1964).
GREIDER, M., MCGUIGAN, J. E.: A comparison of ulcerogenic tumors of the pancreas with the gastrin cell of normal human pancreas and hog antrum. Amer. J. Path. **59**, No. 3, 76a to 77a (1970).
GRILL, W., PICHLMAIER, H., NEFF, V., STUHLFAUTH, K.: Beitrag zur Motilität der Gallenwege. Münch. med. Wschr. **105**, 130—136 (1963).
GROGAN, R., LUCKHARDT, A. B.: Do pancreatic secretin preparations represent the normal duodenal hormone? Amer. J. Physiol. **68**, 142—143 (1924).
GROSS, B., WITKOP, B.: Selective cleavage of the methionyl peptide bonds in ribonuclease with cyanogen bromide. J. Amer. Chem. Soc. **83**, 1510—1511 (1961).
GROSSMAN, M. I.: The peptic digestion of living tissue. Gastroenterology **8**, 678—679 (1947).
— Gastrointestinal hormones. Physiol. Rev. **30**, 33—90 (1950).
— The physiology of secretin. In: Vitamins and Hormones, **16**, 179—203, edit. by R. S. HARRIS, G. F. MARRIAN and K. V. THIMANN, New York. Acad. Press 1958.
— The glands of BRUNNER. Physiol. Rev. **38**, 675—690 (1958a).
— Pancreatic secretion in the rat. Amer. J. Physiol. **194**, 535—539 (1958b).
— Cholinergic potentiation of the response to gastrin. J. Physiol. (Lond.) **157**, 14—15P (1961).
— Nervous and hormonal regulation of pancreatic secretion. In: Ciba Foundation Symposium Exocrine Pancreas, pp. 208—224, edit. by A. V. S. DE REUCK and M. P. CAMERON. London, Churchill 1962.
— Integration of neural and hormonal control of gastric secretion. Physiologist **6**, 349—357 (1963).
— Treatment of duodenal ulcer with secretin: a speculative proposal. Gastroenterology **50**, 912—913 (1966).
— Review and perspective. In: Gastrin, pp. 325—331, edit. by M. I. GROSSMAN. Berkeley Univ. Calif. Press, 1966.
— Gastrointestinal hormones. Med. Clin. N. Amer. **52**, 1297—1303 (1968).
— Stability of secretin. Gastroenterology **57**, 767 (1969a).
— Potentiation. A reply. Gastroenterology **56**, 815—816 (1969b).
— Proposal: Use the term cholecystokinin in place of cholecystokinin-pancreozymin. Gastroenterology **58**, 128 (1970).
— Spectrum of biological actions of gastrointestinal hormones. In: Nobel Symposium XVI. Frontiers in Gastrointestinal Hormone Research, Stockholm, July 20—21, 1970; (In press), edit. by S. ANDERSSON. Upsala: Almqvist and Wiksell 1972a.

Grossman, M. I.: Hormone-hormone and vagus-hormone interactions on gastric acid secretion. In: Nobel Symposium XVI. Frontiers in Gastrointestinal Hormone Research, Stockholm, July 20—21, 1970; (In press), edit. by S. Andersson. Upsala: Almqvist and Wiksell 1972b.
— Ivy, A. C.: Effect of alloxan upon external secretion of the pancreas. Proc. Soc. exp. Biol. (N.Y.) **63**, 62—63 (1946).
— Janowitz, H. D., Ralston, H., Kim, K. S.: The effect of secretin on bile formation in man. Gastroenterology **12**, 133—138 (1949).
— Wang, C. C., Wang, K. J.: Alkaline phosphatase: Correlation of histochemical demonstrability in pancreatic tissue with presence in pancreatic juice. Proc. Soc. exp. Biol. (N.Y.) **78**, 310—311 (1951).
Gryboski, W. A., Menguy, R.: Effects of secretin on gastric secretion. Amer. J. Dig. Dis. **9**, 87—91 (1964).
Hadorn, B., Johansen, P. G., Anderson, Ch. M.: Pancreozymin secretin test of exocrine pancreatic function in cystic fibrosis and the significance of the result for the pathogenesis of the disease. Can. Med. Ass. J. **98**, 377—385 (1968).
Håkanson, R., Liedberg, G.: The role of endogenous gastrin in the activation of gastric histidine decarboxylase in the rat. Effect of antrectomy and vagal denervation, Europ. J. Pharmacol. **12**, 94—103 (1970).
Hallion, L., Lequex: Sur la présence et la localisation de la sécrétine dans l'intestin du nouveau-né et du foetus humains. C. R. Mém. Soc. Biol. **61**, 33 (1906).
Hammarsten, E.: Secretin of Bayliss and Starling (Edward Gamyliel Janeway Lecture). J. Mt. Sinai Hospital, New York, **6**, 59—67 (1939).
— Ågren, G., Hammarsten, H., Wilander, O.: Versuche zur Reinigung von Sekretin. V. Biochem. Ztschr. **264**, 275—284 (1933).
— Jorpes, E.: Die Einwirkung der Pankreassekretion auf die Alkalireserve im Blute und auf die Wasserstoffionenkonzentration in der Drüse. Acta Med. Scand. **68**, 205—214 (1928).
— — Ågren, G.: Versuche zur Reinigung von Secretin. Biochem. Ztschr. **264**, 272—274 (1933).
— — Lagerlöf, H.: The correlation between secretin dose and pancreatic effect in man. Acta Med. Scand. **92**, 256—266 (1937).
— Wilander, O., Ågren, G.: Versuche zur Reinigung von Secretin. Acta Med. Scand. **68**, 239—247 (1928).
Hanscom, D. H., Jacobson, B. J., Littman, A.: Output of protein after pancreozymin. A test of pancreatic function. Ann. Intern. Med. **66**, 721—726 (1967).
— Littman, A., Pinto, J. V.: Dose-response relationship to pancreozymin in normal subjects and patients with chronic pancreatitis. Gastroenterology **45**, 209—214 (1963).
Hansky, J., Tiscornia, O. M., Dreiling, D. A., Janowitz, H. D.: Maximal secretory capacity of the canine pancreas in response to pancreozymin and secretin. Amer. J. Physiol. **206**, 351—356 (1964).
Hardison, W. G., Norman, J. C.: Effect of bile salt and secretin upon bile flow from the isolated perfused pig liver. Gastroenterology **53**, 412—417 (1967).
— — Electrolyte composition of the secretin fraction of bile from the perfused pig liver. Amer. J. Physiol. **214**, 758—763 (1968).
Harper, A. A.: The effect of extracts of gastric and intestinal mucosa on the secretion of HCl by the cat's stomach. J. Physiol. (Lond.) **105**, 31P (1946).
— Physiologic factors regulating pancreatic secretion. Gastroenterology **36**, 386—391 (1959).
— A gastric phase of pancreatic secretion? Gastroenterology **45**, 279—281 (1963).
— Hormonal control of pancreatic secretion. In: Handbook of Physiology. Section 6, Vol. II, pp. 969—996. Washington, Amer. Physiol. Soc. 1967.
— Blair, E. L., Scratcherd, T.: The distribution and physiological properties of pancreozymin. In: Ciba Foundation Symposium on the Exocrine Pancreas, pp. 168—182, edit. by A. V. S. de Reuck and M. P. Cameron, London. Churchill 1962.
— Kidd, C., Scratcherd, T.: Vago-vagal reflex effects on gastric and pancreatic secretion and gastrointestinal motility. J. Physiol., (Lond.) **148**, 417—436 (1959).
— MacKay, I. F. S.: A comparison of the effects on the pancreas of pancreozymin and of vagal nerve stimulation. J. Physiol. (London) **104**, 27P (1945/46).
— — The effects of pancreozymin and of vagal nerve stimulation upon the histological appearance of the pancreas. J. Physiol. (Lond.) **107**, 89—96 (1948).
— Raper, H. S.: Pancreozymin, a stimulant of the secretion of pancreatic enzymes in extracts of the small intestine. J. Physiol. (Lond.) **102**, 115—125 (1943).
— Reed, J. D., Smy, J. R.: Gastric blood flow in anesthetized cats. J. Physiol. (Lond.) **194**, 795—807 (1968).
— Vass, C. C. N.: The control of the external secretion of the pancreas in cats. J. Physiol. (Lond.) **99**, 415—435 (1941).

Harrison, L. A., Johnson, L. R.: Analysis of gastric secretory inhibition by duodenal acidification. Gastroenterology **58**, 1043 (1970).
Hart, J. C., Clarke, J. S.: The effect of the liver on secretin. Amer. Surgeon **25**, 857—859 (1959).
Hart, W. M., Thomas, J. E.: Bicarbonate and chloride of pancreatic juice secreted in response to various stimuli. Gastroenterology **4**, 409—420 (1945).
Hartley, R. C., Gambill, E. E., Engstrom, G. W., Summerskill, H. J.: Pancreatic exocrine function. Comparison of response to augmented secretin stimulus, augmented pancreozymin stimulus and test meal in health and disease. Amer. J. Digest. Dis. N. S. **11**, 27—39 (1966).
Hauge, C. W., Mark, J. B. D.: Common bile duct motility and sphincter mechanism: I. Pressure measurements with multiple-lumen catheter in dogs. Ann. Surg. **162**, 1028—1038 (1965).
Havermark, P. G., Hultman, E. H.: A method for recording the contractions of the gallbladder in situ. Its application in cholecystokinin determination. Acta Physiol. Scand. **27**, 242—246 (1952).
Heath, T.: Effect of secretin on bile formation in sheep. Quart. J. exp. Physiol. **55**, 301—312 (1970).
Heatley, N. G.: The assay of secretin in the rat. J. Endocrin. **42**, 535—547 (1968a).
— The assay of pancreozymin, and of secretin and pancreozymin simultaneously, in the rat. J. Endocr. **42**, 549—557 (1968b).
Hedner, P.: Effect of the C-terminal octapeptide of cholecystokinin on guinea pig ileum and gallbladder *in vitro*. Acta Physiol. Scand. **78**, 232—235 (1970).
— Persson, H., Rorsman, G.: Effect of cholecystokinin on small intestine. Acta Physiol. Scand. **70**, 250—254 (1967).
— Rorsman, G.: Structures essential for the effect of cholecystokinin on the guinea pig small intestine in vitro. Acta Physiol. Scand. **74**, 58—68 (1968).
— — On the mechanism of action for the effect of cholecystokinin on the choledochoduodenal junction in the cat. Acta Physiol. Scand. **76**, 248—254 (1969).
Heimburg, R. L., von, Hallenbeck, G. A.: Inhibition of gastric secretion in dogs by glucagon given intraportally. Gastroenterology **47**, 531—535 (1964).
Heisig, N.: Pancreatic microcirculation under the influence of adequate secretory stimulation. In: 4th Europ. Confer. Microcirculation, Cambridge 1966, pp. 175—180, edit. by H. Harders. Basle, S. Karger.
— Functional analysis of the microcirculation in the exocrine pancreas. In: Advances in Microcirculation I pp. 89—151, edit. by H. Harders. Basel, New York, S. Karger 1968.
Heitmann, P., Jungreis, A. M., Janowitz, H. D.: Effect of acetazolamide and cholecystokinin on the secretion of pepsin from histamine-stimulated Heidenhain pouches. Gastroenterology **52**, 211—215 (1967).
Henriksen, F. W.: The effect of synthetic secretin on the external pancreatic secretion in dogs. Acta Physiol. Scand. **72**, 433—440 (1968).
— The concept of potentiation. Gastroenterology **57**, 617—618 (1969a).
— Effect of vagotomy or atropine on the canine pancreatic response to secretin and pancreozymin. Scand. J. Gastroent. **4**, 137—144 (1969b).
— Rune, S. J.: Effect of vagotomy on the canine pancreatic secretion after feeding. Scand. J. Gastroent. **4**, 435—440 (1969).
— Worning, M.: The interaction of secretin and pancreozymin on the external pancreatic secretion in dogs. Acta Physiol. Scand. **70**, 241—249 (1967).
— — The mutual influence of gastrin and secretin on the external pancreatic secretion in dogs. Acta Physiol. Scand. **76**, 67—72 (1969).
Hermier, M., Mathieu, M., Fillat, M., Gilly, R., Chazalette, J. P., Cotte, J.: Étude de la fonction pancréatique exocrine dans la mucoviscidose. Rev. Franç. Étud. Clin. Biol. **14**, 867—884 (1969).
Hermon-Taylor, J.: A technique for perfusion of the isolated canine pancreas. Responses to secretin and gastrin. Gastroenterology **55**, 488—501 (1968).
— Beaugie, J. M.: The action of pure natural cholecystokinin-pancreozymin on the isolated perfused canine pancreas and liver. In: Nobel Symposium XVI. Frontiers in Gastrointestinal Hormone Research, Stockholm, July 20—21, 1970; (In press), edit. by S. Andersson. Upsala: Almqvist and Wiksell 1972.
— Code, C. F.: Effect of secretin on small bowel myoelectric activity of conscious healthy dogs. Amer. J. Dig. Dis. N. S. **15**, 545—550 (1970).
Hickson, J. C. D.: The effect of stimulation of the vagus nerves on pancreatic secretion in the pig. J. Physiol. (Lond.) **168**, 24—25P (1963).
— The secretion of pancreatic juice in response to stimulation of the vagus nerves in the pig. J. Physiol. (Lond.) **206**, 275—297 (1970a).

HICKSON, J. C. D.: The secretory and vascular response to nervous and humoral stimulation in the pancreas of the pig. J. Physiol. (Lond.) **206**, 299—322 (1970b).
HIGGINS, G. H., MANN, F. C.: Observations on the emptying of the gallbladder. Amer. J. Physiol. **78**, 339—348 (1926).
HILTON, S. M., JONES, M.: Plasma kinin and functional vasodilatation in the pancreas. J. Physiol. (Lond.) **165**, 35—36P. (1963).
HOKIN, L. E.: Metabolic aspects and energetics of pancreatic secretion. In: Handbook of Physiol. Section 6 Vol. II pp. 935—954, Wash., Amer. Physiol. Soc. 1967.
— HOKIN, M. R.: The actions of pancreozymin in pancreas slices and the role of phospholipids in enzyme secretion. J. Physiol. (Lond.) **132**, 442—453 (1956).
— HOKIN, M. R.: The synthesis and secretion of digestive enzymes by pancreas tissue *in vitro*. In: Ciba Foundation Symposium on the Exocrine Pancreas, pp. 187—207, edit. by A. V. S. DE REUCK and M. P. CAMERON. London, Churchill 1962.
— HUEBNER, D.: Phospholipids and pancreatic acinar cell function. J. Cell. Biol. **33**, 521—530 (1967).
HOKIN, M. R.: The formation of amylase by mouse pancreas *in vitro*. J. Biol. Chem. **219**, 77—83 (1956).
— Studies on chemical mechanisms of the action of neurotransmitters and hormones. II. Increased incorporation of ^{32}P into phosphatides as a second, adaptive response to pancreozymin or acetylcholine in pigeon pancreas slices. Arch. Biochem. Biophysics **124**, 280—284 (1968).
HOLLANDER, F., BIRNBAUM, D.: The role of carbonic anhydrase in pancreatic secretion. Trans. N.Y. Acad. Sci., Ser. 2, **15**, 56—58 (1952).
HOLTON, P., JONES, M.: Some observations on changes in the blood content of the cat's pancreas during activity. J. Physiol. **150**, 479—488 (1960).
HONG, S. S.: Mechanism of gallbladder evacuation. New Med. J. (Korea) **3**, 49—62 (1960).
— MAGEE, D. F.: Pharmacological studies on the regulation of pancreatic secretion in pigs. Ann. Surg. **172**, 41—48 (1970).
— — CREWDSON, F.: The physiological regulation of gallbladder evacuation. Gastroenterology **30**, 625—630 (1956).
— NAKAMURA, M., MAGEE, D. F.: Relationship between duodenal pH and pancreatic secretion in dogs and pigs. Ann. Surg. **166**, 778—782 (1967).
HOUSSAY, B.-A., MOLINELLI, E.-A.: La greffe duodéno-pancréatique et son emploi pour déceler des décharges d'adrenaline et de sécrétine dans le sang. C. R. Mém. Soc. Biol. **97**, 1032—1034 (1927).
— RUBIO, H.-H.: Fonctionnement de la vésicule biliaire graffée au cou. C. R. Soc. Biol. **111**, 453—455 (1932).
HOWAT, H. T.: Pancreatitis. In: Modern Trends in Gastroenterology, edit. by F. A. JONES. London, Butterworth 1952.
HUBEL, K. A., COLBERT, B.: Effect of secretin on bicarbonate secretion in fluid perfusing the rat ileum. Experientia **23**, 337—338 (1967).
HULTMAN, E. H.: A method for the standardization of cholecystokinin in vitro. Acta Physiol. Scand. **33**, 291—295 (1955a).
— The relation between cholecystokinin and substance P. Acta Chem. Scand. **9**, 1042—1044 (1955b).
HUNT, J. N., RAMSBOTTOM, N.: Effect of gastrin II on gastric emptying and secretion during a test meal. Brit. Med. J. **4**, 386—387 (1967).
ISENBERG, J. I., BROOKS, A. M., GROSSMAN, M. I.: Pentagastrin vs Betazole as stimulant of gastric secretion. J. Amer. Med. Ass. **206**, 2897—2898 (1968).
— GROSSMAN, M. I.: Comparison of subcutaneous and intravenous secretin in man. Gastroenterology **56**, 88—91 (1969a).
— — Effect of gastrin and SC 15396 on gastric motility in dogs. Gastroenterology **56**, 450—455 (1969b).
ITOH, Z., LUCIEN, H. W., SCHALLY, A. V.: Inhibitory mechanisms of duodenal hormones (secretin, cholecystokinin/pancreozymin and enterogastrone) on gastrin- or histamine-stimulated gastric secretion in Heidenhain pouch dogs. In: Abstr. 4th World Congress of Gastroenterology, p. 148, edit. P. RIIS, P. ANTHONISEN and H. BADEN, Copenhagen, 1970.
IVY, A. C.: The role of hormones in digestion. Physiol. Rev. **10**, 282—335 (1930).
— The physiology of the gallbladder. Physiol. Rev. **14**, 1—102 (1934).
— The mechanism of gastric secretion. Surgery, **10**, 861—878 (1941a).
— Internal secretions of the gastro-intestinal tract. J. Amer. med. Ass., **117**, 1013—1016 (1941b).
— Motor dysfunction of biliary tract. Am. J. Roentgenol. **57**, 1—11 (1947).
— Gastrointestinal hormones. Oral Surgery **4**, 612—614 (1951).

IVY, A. C.: Cholecystokinin. In: Polypeptides which Stimulate Plain Muscle, pp. 115—119, edit. by J. H. GADDUM. Baltim, Williams & Woreilkins 1955.
— DREWYER, G. E., ORNDOFF, B. H.: Effect of cholecystokinin on human gallbladder. Endocrinology **14**, 343—348 (1930 a).
— FARRELL, J. I.: Contributions to the physiology of gastric secretion. VIII. The proof of a humoral mechanism. A new procedure for the study of gastric physiology. Amer. J. Physiol. **74**, 639—649 (1925).
— — A method for the subcutaneous auto-transplantation of the pancreas. Amer. J. Physiol. **77**, 474—479 (1926).
— — LUETH, H. C.: Contributions to the physiology of pancreas. III. A hormone for external pancreatic secretion. Amer. J. Physiol. **82**, 27—33 (1927).
— FISHER, N. F.: The presence of an insulin-like substance in gastric and duodenal mucosa and its relation to gastric secretion. Amer. J. Physiol. **67**, 445—450 (1924).
— JANECEK, H. M.: Assay of Jorpes-Mutt secretin and cholecystokinin. Acta Physiol. Scand. **45**, 220—230 (1959).
— KLOSTER, G., DREWYER, G. E., LUETH, M. C.: The preparation of a secretin concentrate. Amer. J. Physiol. **95**, 35—39 (1930 b).
— KLOSTER, G., LUETH, H. C., DREWYER, G. E.: On the preparation of "cholecystokinin". Amer. J. Physiol. **91**, 336—344 (1929).
— McILVAIN, G. B.: The excitation of gastric secretion by application of substances to the duodenal and jejunal mucosa. Amer. J. Physiol. **67**, 124—140 (1923—1924).
— OLDBERG, E.: Contraction and evacuation of gallbladder caused by a highly purified "secretin" preparation. Proc. Soc. exp. Biol. (N.Y.) **25**, 113—115 (1927).
— — Contraction and evacuation of the gall bladder by a purified "secretin" preparation. J. Amer. med. Ass. **90**, 445—446 (1928 a).
— — Hormone mechanism for gallbladder contraction and evacuation. Amer. J. Physiol. **86**, 599—613 (1928 b).
— — KLOSTER, G., LUETH, H. C.: A hormone mechanism for gallbladder contraction. Amer. J. Physiol. **85**, 381—383 (1928).
JACOBSON, E. D.: Secretion and blood flow in the gastrointestinal tract. In: Handbook of Physiology. Section 6, Volume II. Alimentary Canal, pp. 1043—1062, edit. by C. F. CODE. Washington, D. C. Amer. Physiol. Soc. 1967.
JACOBY, F.: The pancreas and alkaline phosphatase. Nature **158**, 268—269 (1946 a).
— Differences in localization, by histochemical means, of alkaline phosphatase within the same organ of different experimental animals. J. Physiol. **105**, 19 P (1946 b).
JANOWITZ, H. D.: Pancreatic secretion of fluid and electrolytes. In: Handbook of Physiol. Vol. II Section 6, pp. 925—933, edit. by C. F. CODE. Washington D.C., Amer. Physiol. Soc. 1967.
— COLCHER, H., HOLLANDER, F.: Inhibition of gastric secretion of acid in dogs by carbonic anhydrase inhibitor, 2-acetylamino-1,3,4-thiadiazole-5-sulfonamide. Amer. J. Physiol. **171**, 325—330 (1952).
— DREILING, D.: The pancreatic secretion of fluid and electrolytes. In: Ciba Found. Symp. on the Exocrine Pancreas, pp. 115—137, edit. by A. V. S. DE REUCK and M. P. CAMERON, London, CHURCHILL 1962.
JOHANSEN, P. G., HADORN, B., ANDERSON, C. M.: Effect of secretin on human rectal mucosa in vivo: Nature, **217**, 468 (1968).
JOHNSON, L. R., AURES, D., HÅKANSON, R.: Effect of gastrin on the *in vivo* incorporation of ^{14}C-leucine into protein of the digestive tract. Proc. Soc. exp. Biol. (N.Y.) **132**, 996—998 (1969).
— AURES, D., YUEN, L.: Pentagastrin-induced stimulation of protein synthesis in gastrointestinal tract. Amer. J. Physiol. **217**, 251—254 (1969).
— GROSSMAN, M. I.: Secretin: the enterogastrone released by acid in the duodenum. Amer. J. Physiol. **215**, 885—888 (1968).
— — Effects of fat, secretin and cholecystokinin on histamine-stimulated gastric secretion. Amer. J. Physiol. **216**, 1176—1179 (1969 a).
— — Characteristics of inhibition of gastric secretion by secretin. Amer. J. Physiol. **217**, 1401—1404 (1969 b).
— — Potentiation of gastric acid response in the dog. Gastroenterology **56**, 687—692 (1969 c).
— — Analysis of inhibition of gastric acid secretion by cholecystokinin in dogs. Amer. J. Physiol. **218**, 550—554 (1970 a).
— — Progress in gastroenterology: Intestinal hormones as inhibitors of gastric secretion. Gastroenterology **60**, 120—144 (1970 b).
— JONES, R. S., AURES, D., HÅKANSON, R.: The effect of antrectomy on gastric histidine decarboxylase activity in the rat. Amer. J. Physiol. **216**, 1051—1053 (1969).

JOHNSON, L. R., STENING, G. F., GROSSMAN, M. I.: Effect of sulfation on the gastrointestinal actions cf caerulein. Gastroenterology, **58**, 208—216 (1970).
— TUMPSON, D. B.: Effect of secretin on histamine-stimulated secretion in the gastric fistula rat. Proc. Soc. exp. Biol. (N.Y.) **133**, 125—127 (1970).
JOHNSON, L. P., BROWN, J. C., MAGEE, D. F.: Effect of secretin and cholecystokinin-pancreozymin extracts on gastric motility in man. Gut **7**, 52—57 (1966).
— MAGEE, D. F.: Inhibition of gastric motility by commercial duodenal mucosal extract containing cholecystokinin and pancreozymin. Nature **207**, 1401—1402 (1965a).
— — Cholecystokinin-pancreozymin extracts and gastric motor inhibition. Surg. Gyn. Obstetr. **121**, 557—562 (1965b).
JOHNSON, M., SHERRATT, H. S. A., CASE, R. M., SCRATCHERD, T. (1970). The effect of secretin, pancreozymin and acetylcholine on the concentration of cyclic AMP in cat pancreas. Biochem. J. (London) **120**, 8P—9P (1970).
JOHNSTON, D., DUTHIE, H. L.: Inhibition of histamine stimulated gastric secretion by acid in the duodenum in man. Gut, **7**, 58—68 (1966).
JONES, R. S., BROOKS, F. P.: The pyloric antrum as a mediator of insulin induced choleresis. Physiologist 8, 202—293 (1965).
— — Role of pyloric antrum in choleresis after insulin and feeding. Amer. J. Physiol. **213**, 1406—1408 (1967).
— GEIST, R. E.: HALL. A. D.: Choleretic effects of glucagon and secretin in the dog. Gastroenterology **60**, 64—68 (1971).
— GROSSMAN, M. I.: Choleretic effects of secretin and histamine in the dog. Amer. J. Physiol. **217**, 532—535 (1969).
— — Choleretic effects of cholecystokinin, gastrin II and caerulein in dog. Amer. J. Physiol. **219**, 1014—1018 (1970).
— HALL, A. D.: The effect of glucagon on Brunner's gland secretion in dogs. Proc. Soc. exp. Biol. (N.Y.) **132**, 1159—1161 (1969).
JONES, T. W., HARKINS, H. N.: The mechanism of inhibition of gastric acid secretion by the duodenum. Gastroenterology **37**, 81—86 (1959).
JONSON, G.: Permanent biliary fistulas in the dog. A new method. Part one: Evolution and description of the method. Evidence in plasma of biliary stasis. Plasma cholesterol and phospholipids, bile return and nutrition. Acta Chir. Scand. Suppl. **316**, 1—40 (1963).
Part two: Output of bile, dry matter, phospholipids, bilirubin and alkaline phosphatase activity; bacteriologic findings. Acta Chir. Scand. Suppl. **317**, 1—32 (1963).
— SUNDMAN, L., THULIN, L.: The influence of chemically pure secretin on hepatic bile output. Acta Physiol. Scand. **62**, 287—290 (1964).
JORDAN, P. H., PETERSON, N. D.: Effects of secretin upon gastric secretion. Ann. Surg. **156**, 914—923 (1962).
— DE LA ROSA, C.: Inhibition of gastric secretion by duodenal mucosal extracts. Ann. Surg. **160**, 978—985 (1964).
JORPES, J. E.: The isolation and chemistry of secretin and cholecystokinin. Memorial Lecture. Gastroenterology **55**, 157—164 (1968).
— The ionic mechanisms for accumulation and release of peptide hormones. The release of the gastrointestinal hormones secretin, CCK and gastrin. In: NOBEL Symposium XVI. Frontiers in Gastrointestinal Hormone Research, Stockholm, July 20—21, 1970; (In press), edit. by S. ANDERSSON. Upsala: Almqvist and Wiksell 1972.
— JALLING, O., MUTT, V.: A method for the preparation of gastrin. Biochem. J. **52**, 327—328 (1952).
— MUTT, V.: A new method for the preparation of secretin. Arkiv f. Kemi **6**, 273—276 (1953a).
— — Purification of secretin by freezing out of impurities from methanolic solution at —80°C. Nature **172**, 124 (1953b).
— — On the action of highly purified preparations of secretin and of pancreozymin. Arkiv f. Kemi **7**, 553—559 (1954).
— — On the strength of secretin. Arkiv f. Kemi **8**, 49—51 (1955).
— — Swed. pat. No 156013 (1956).
— — Secretin, pancreozymin and cholecystokinin. Gastroenterology **36**, 377—383 (1959).
— — The gastrointestinal hormones, secretin and cholecystokinin-pancreozymin. Ann. Int. Med. **55**, 395—405 (1961a).
— — On the biological activity and amino acid composition of secretin. Acta Chem. Scand. **15**, 1790—1791 (1961b).
— — The gastrointestinal hormones, secretin and cholecystokinin. In: The Exocrine Pancreas, Ciba Found. Symp. pp. 150—164, edit. by A. V. S. DE REUCK and M. P. CAMERON, London, Churchill 1962.
— — Gastrointestinal hormones. In: The Hormones IV. pp. 365—385, edit. by PINCUS and THIMANN. New York: Acad. Press 1964.

JORPES, J. E.: MUTT, V.: Cholecystokinin and pancreozymin, one single hormone? Acta Physiol. Scand. **66**, 196—202 (1966a).
— — On the biological assay of secretin. The reference standard. Acta Physiol. Scand. **66**, 316—325 (1966b).
— — Secretin. In: Proc. III Symp. Europ. Pancreatic Club Prague 2—4 July 1968, pp. 16—20, edit. by P. FRIC, F. MALIS and R. RONSKY, Praha, Czech. Med. Press 1970a.
— — Cholecystokinin (CCK). Physiologie und klinische Anwendung. Klin. Wschr. **48**, 65—71 (1970b).
— — JONSON, G., SUNDMAN, L.: The effect of secretin on bile flow. Gastroenterology **45**, 786—788 (1963).
— — — THULIN, L., SUNDMAN, L.: Influence of secretin and cholecystokinin on bile flow. In: The Biliary System. A Symposium of the Nato Adv. Study Institute, pp. 293—301, ed. by W. TAYLOR, Oxford, Blackwell 1965.
— — MAGNUSSON, S., STEELE, B.: Amino acid composition and N-terminal amino acid sequence of porcine secretin. Biochem. Biophys. Res. Com. **9**, 275—279 (1962).
— — OLBE, L.: On the biological assay of cholecystokinin and its dosage in cholecystography. Acta Physiol. Scand. **47**, 109—114 (1959).
— — TOCZKO, K.: Further purification of cholecystokinin and pancreozymin. Acta Chem. Scand. **18**, 2408—2410 (1964).
JUNG, F. T., GREENGARD, H.: Response of the isolated gallbladder to cholecystokinin. Amer. J. Physiol. **103**, 275—278 (1933).
KAESS, H., BRECH, W., SCHLIERF, G.: Der Einfluß von Glukagon auf die exokrine und endokrine Pankreasfunktion. Klin. Wschr. **46**, 1314—1315 (1968).
KAHLSON, G.: The nervous and humoral control of gastric secretion. Brit. Med. J. **II**, 1091—1095 (1948).
KAMIONKOWSKI, M., GROSSMAN, S., FLESHLER, B.: The inhibitory effect of secretin on broth-stimulated gastric secretion in human subjects. Gut **5**, 237—240 (1964).
KAVIN, H., CARLTON, R. W., JACOBS, P., GREEN, R., TORRANCE, J. D., BOTHWELL, T. H.: Effect of exocrine pancreatic secretion on iron absorption. Gut, **8**, 556—564 (1967).
KAY, A. W.: Memorial Lecture. An evaluation of gastric acid secretion tests. Gastroenterology **53**, 834—844 (1967).
KELLY, K. A., WOODWARD, E. R., CODE, CH. F.: Effect of secretin and cholecystokinin on canine gastric electrical activity. Proc. Soc. exp. Biol. (N.Y.) **130**, 1060—1063 (1969).
KENNEDY, J. A., HALLENBECK, G. A.: The pancreas and gastric secretion: Failure of pancreatectomy to prevent inhibition of gastric secretion by secretin. Gut **4**, 58—60 (1963).
KIM, S. K.: Small intestine transit time in the normal small bowel study. Amer. J. Roentgenol. **104**, 522—524 (1968).
KISSELER, B., LEISTNER, G. H., BARTH, E.: Zur Darstellung des Pankreas im Roentgenbild. Fortschr. Röntgenstrahlen u. Nuklearmed. **100**, 309—318 (1964a).
— — — A new method for the roentgenologic opacification of the pancreas. Radiology **83**, 6—11 (1964b).
— — — KUSTER, H. H.: Die Röntgendiagnostik der Pankreaserkrankungen. Deutsch. Med. Wschr. **90**, 422—424 (1965).
KIYOHARA, K.: Action de la sécrétine sur la respiration des tissus de certains organes. C. R. Soc. Biol. **116**, 1166—1168 (1934).
KNODELL, R. G., TOSKES, P. P., REBER, H. A., BROOKS, F. P.: Significance of cyclic AMP in the regulation of exocrine pancreatic secretion. Experientia **26**, 515—517 (1970).
KOCK, N. G., DARLE, N., DOTEVALL, G.: Inhibition of intestinal motility in man by glucagon given intraportally. Gastroenterology **53**, 88—91 (1967).
KOKAS, E., BRUNSON, W. D.: Gastric secretion inhibition in chickens. The Physiologist **12**, 272 (1969).
— PHILLIPS, J. L., Jr., BRUNSON, W. D., Jr.: The secretory activity of the duodenum in chickens. Comp. Biochem. Physiol. **22**, 81—90 (1967).
KOMAROV, S. A.: Gastrin. Proc. Soc. exp. Biol. (N.Y.). **38**, 514—516 (1938).
— Studies on gastrin. I. Methods of isolation of a specific gastric secretagogue from the pyloric mucous membrane and its chemical properties. Revue Canad. Biol. **1**, 191—205 (1942a).
— Studies on gastrin. II. Physiological properties of the specific gastric secretagogue of the pyloric mucous membrane. Revue Canad. Biol. **1**, 377—401 (1942b).
KONTUREK, S. J.: The effect of secretin on gastric acid secretion and peptic ulcers induced by pentagastrin in cats with intact or resected duodenum. Amer. J. Dig. Dis. **13**, 874—881 (1968).
— Comparison of pancreatic responses to natural and synthetic secretins in conscious cats. Amer. J. Dig. Dis. **14**, 557—565 (1969).

Konturek, S. J.: Pancreatic dose-response curves to intravenous secretin in man. Gastroenterology **58**, 828—832 (1970).
— Dabrowski, A., Adamczyk, B., Kulpa, J.: The effect of secretin, gastrin-pentapeptide and histamine on gastric acid and hepatic bile secretion in man. Amer. J. Dig. Dis. N. S. **14**, 900—907 (1969).
— Dubiel, J., Gabrys, B.: Effect of acid infusion into various levels of the intestine on gastric and pancreatic secretion in the cat. Gut **10**, 749—753 (1969).
— Gabrys, B., Dubiel, J.: Effect of exogenous and endogenous secretin on gastric and pancreatic secretion in cats. Amer. J. Physiol. **217**, 1110—1113 (1969).
— — Effect of large doses of gastrin I on pepsin secretion. Proc. Soc. exp. Biol. (N.Y.) **119**, 443—444 (1965b).
— Grossman, M. I.: Effect of perfusion of intestinal loops with acid fat or dextrose on gastric secretion. Gastroenterology **49**, 481—489 (1965a).
— — Localization of the mechanism for inhibition of gastric secretion by acid in intestine. Gastroenterology **49**, 74—78 (1965b).
— Oleksy, J.: Potentiation between pentapeptide (ICI 50,123) and histamine in the stimulation of gastric secretion in man. Gastroenterology **53**, 912—917 (1967).
— Tasler, J., Obtulovicz, W.: Localization of the endogenous release of secretin in the dog. In: Abstr. 4th World Congress of Gastroenterology, p. 233, edit. by P. Riis, P. Anthonisen and H. Baden, Copenhagen 1970.
— — — Localization of secretin release by acid in small intestine of the dog. Amer. J. Physiol. **220**, 124—127 (1971).
Kosaka, T., Lim, R. K. S.: On the mechanism of the inhibition of gastric secretion by fat. The role of bile and cystokinin. Chinese J. Physiol. **4**, 213—220 (1930a).
— — Demonstration of the humoral agent in fat inhibition of gastric secretion. Proc. Soc. exp. Biol. (N.Y.), **27**, 890—891 (1930b).
— — Ling, S. M., Liu, A. C.: On the mechanism of the inhibition of gastric secretion by fat. A gastric inhibitory agent obtained from the intestinal mucosa. Chinese J. Physiol. **6**, 107—128 (1932).
Køster, K. H., Rødbro, P., Petersen, H. J.: Comparative effects of tetragastrin and histamine on acid and intrinsic factor secretion in man. Scand. J. Gastroent. **3**, 23—35, 1968.
— Faber, V., Rødbro, P.: Comparative effects of tetragastrin and histamine on pepsin secretion in man. Scand. J. Gastroent. **3**, 106—109 (1968).
Kraintz, L.: The effect of vasopressin on salivation. The Physiologist **3**, 97 (1960).
Krawitt, E. L., Zimmerman, G. R., Clifton, J. A.: Location of secretin in dog duodenal mucosa. Amer. J. Physiol. **211**, 935—938 (1966).
Kudrewecki, W. W.: Materiale zur Physiologie der Bauchspeicheldrüse. Diss. 1890. St. Petersburg.
Kulka, R. G., Sternlicht, E.: Enzyme secretion in mouse pancreas mediated by adenosine-3'5'-cyclic phosphate and inhibited by adenosine-3'-phosphate. Proc. Nat. Acad. Sc. **61**, 1123—1128 (1968).
Kunitz, M.: Formation of trypsin from crystalline trypsinogen by means of enterokinase. J. Gen. Physiol. **22**, 429—446 (1939a).
— Purification and concentration of enterokinase. J. Gen. Physiol. **22**, 447—450 (1939b).
Kuznetsova, E. K.: Characteristics of blood supply of the pancreas during different phases of its activity. Fed. Proc. **22** II No. 1 T 99-T 104 (1963a).
— External pancreatic secretion in response to humoral stimuli in acute radiation sickness. Med. Radiol. **8**, 23—28 (1963b).
la Barre, J.: La Sécrétine, son role physiologique, ses propriétés therapeutiques. Masson, Paris 1936.
— Goffin, R.: A propos de l'hypersécrétion biliaire consécutive à l'administration de sécrétine où à l'injection intraduodénale d'acide chlorhydrique dilué. Arch. Internat. de Physiol. **44**, 444—458 (1937).
Lagerlöf, H.: The secretin test of pancreatic function. Quart. J. Med. **32**, (N. S. 8) 115—126 (1939).
— Pancreatic function and pancreatic disease studied by means of secretin. Macmillan Co., New York, 1942 and Acta Med. Scand. Suppl. 128 (1942).
— Pancreatic secretion: pathophysiology. In: Handbook of Physiology. Section 6. Alimentary Canal Vol. II, pp. 1027—1042, edit. by C. F. Code, Baltimore, William and Wilkins 1967.
— Ek, S. Y., Nyberg, A.: The duodenal secretion in man as a function of secretin dose and secretin inactivation. Gastroenterology **43**, 174—180 (1962).
— Schütz, H. B., Holmén, S.: A secretin test with high doses of secretin and correction for incomplete recovery of duodenal juice. Gastroenterology **52**, 67—77 (1967).
— Welin, G.: Pancreatic secretion after secretin during insulin hypoglucemia and after graded amounts of secretin. Acta Med. Scand. **91**, 397—408 (1937).

LAKE, M.: Diagnostic value of secretin test, including report of 19 operated or autopsied cases with anatomical studies of pancreas. Amer. J. Med. **3**, 18—30 (1947).
LALOU, S.: Recherches sur la sécrétine. Paris 1912.
LASTER, L., WALSH, J. H.: Enzymatic degradation of C-terminal tetrapeptide amide of gastrin by mammalian tissue extracts. Fed. Proc. **27**, 1328—1330 (1968).
LÁSZLO, B. W., GÖRGEY, E.: Die Behandlung biliärer Dyskinesien mit Gelbkörper-Hormon. Münch. Med. Wschr. **102**, 231—234 (1960).
LAZARUS, N. R., VOYLES, N. R., DEVRIM, S., TANESE, T., RECANT, L.: Extra-gastrointestinal effects of secretin, gastrin and pancreozymin. Lancet 1968 II, 248—250.
LEDRUT, J., ALECHINSKY, G.: Absence de spécificité des sécrétines de raie et de porc. Arch. Internat. de Physiol. **37**, 329—335 (1933).
— UNGAR, G.: Action de la sécrétine chez *l'Octopus Vulgaris*. Arch. Intern. Physiol. (Paris) **44**, 205—211 (1937).
LEE, T. H., LERNER, A. B., BUETTNER-JANUSCH, V.: On the structure of human corticotropin. J. Biol. Chem. **236**, 2970—2974 (1961).
— — — Melanocyte-stimulating hormones from sheep pituitary glands. Biochim. Biophys. Acta. **71**, 706—709 (1963).
LEGGE, J. W., MORIESON, A. S., ROGERS, G. E., MARGINSON, M. A.: The chromatography and counter-current distribution of secretin. Austral. J. Exp. Biol. **35**, 569—582 (1957).
LEHNERT, P., STAHLHEBER, H., FORELL, M. M., DOST, F. H., FRITZ, H., HÜTZEL, M., WERLE, E.: Bestimmung der Halbwertzeit von Secretin. Klin. Wschr. **47**, 1200—1204 (1969).
— — — — — — — Bestimmung der Halbwertzeit von Cholecystokinin. Z. Physiol. Chem. **351**, 983—989 (1970).
LEROY, J., MORISSET, J. A., WEBSTER, P. D.: Dose-related response of pancreatic synthesis and secretion to cholecystokinin-pancreozymin. J. Lab. Clin. Med. **78**, 149—157 (1971).
LESCUT, J.-CH.: Sur l'emploi de la cholécystokinine dans le radiodiagnostic des affections des voies biliaires. Thèse. Clin. Mal. App. Dig., Lille, France, 1963.
LEURET, F., LASSAIGNE, J. L.: Recherches physiologiques et chimiques pour servir à l'histoire de la digestion, pp. 141—142, Huzard, Paris, 1825.
LE VEEN, H. H., BOREK, B.: Role of liver metabolism of gastrin in gastric secretion. Fed. Proc. **28**, No 2, 718 (1969).
LICK, R. F., WELSCH, K. H., HART, W., BRÜCKNER, W., BALSER, D., GÜRTNER, T.: On the secretory function of the stomach after injection of histamine, gastrin and synthetic tetrapeptide into the systemic and portal circulation. Ztschr. Gastroent. **5**, 7—12 (1967).
LIEDBERG, G.: The effect of vagotomy on gallbladder and duodenal pressure during rest and stimulation with cholecystokinin. Acta Chir. Scand. **135**, 695—700 (1969).
LIM, R. K. S., IVY, A. C., MCCARTHY, J. E.: Contributions to the physiology of gastric secretion. I. Gastric secretion by local (mechanical and chemical) stimulation. Quart. J. exp. Physiol., **15**, 13—23 (1925).
— MOZER, P.: Does vagus excitation liberate pyloric gastrin? Fed. Proc. **10**, 84 (1951).
LIN, T. M., ALPHIN, R. S.: Cephalic phase of gastric secretion in the rat. Amer. J. Physiol. **192**, 23—26 (1958).
— — Comparative bio-assay of secretin and pancreozymin in rats and dogs. Amer. J. Physiol. **203**, 926—928 (1962).
— GROSSMAN, M. I.: Dose-response relationship of pancreatic enzyme stimulants: pancreozymin and metacholine. Amer. J. Physiol. **186**, 52—56 (1956).
— IVY, A. C.: Relation of secretin to the parasympathetic mechanism for pancreatic secretion. Amer. J. Physiol. **189**, 361—368 (1957).
— SPRAY, G. F.: Effect of glucagon on gastric HCl secretion. Gastroenterology **54**, 1254 (1968).
— — Effect of pentagastrin, cholecystokinin, caerulein and glucagon on the choledochal resistance and bile flow of conscious dog. Gastroenterology **56**, 1178 (1969).
LJUNGBERG, S.: Biologisk styrkebestämning av cholecystokinin. Svensk Farm. Tidskr. **68**, 351—354 (1964).
— Biological assay of cholecystokinin in guinea-pig gallbladder in situ. Acta Pharmaceutica Suecica **6**, 599—606 (1969a).
— Some pharmacological properties of cholecystokinin. Acta Pharmaceutica Suecica **6**, 607—612 (1969b).
LONGHI, E. H., GREENLEE, H. B., BRAVO, J. L., DELGADILLO, J., DRAGSTEDT, L. R.: Question of an inhibitory hormone from the gastric antrum. Amer. J. Physiol. **191**, 64—70 (1957).
LORBER, S. H., CHEY, W. Y., DINOSO, V., HENDRICKS, J., KOSAY, S.: Effect of secretin and cholecystokinin on gastric motility. In: NOBEL Symposium XVI. Frontiers in Gastrointestinal Hormone Research, Stockholm, July 20—21, 1970, (In press), edit. by S. ANDERSSON. Upsala, Almqvist and Wiksell 1972.

Lorber, S. H.: Chey, W. Y., Lewi, Z.: Effect of secretin an motor activity in the main stomach. Gastroenterology **48**, 866 (1965).
Love, J. W.: A method for the assay of secretin using rats. Quart. J. exp. Physiol. **42**, 279—284 (1957).
— Bass, D. D., Ustach, T. J., Schuster, M. M.: The hormonal control of Brunner's gland secretion and duodenal motility in the dog. J. Surg. Res. **10**, 395—403 (1970).
— Walder, A. I., Bingham, C.: Effect of natural and synthetic secretin on Brunner's gland secretion in dogs. Nature (Lond.) **219**, 731—732 (1968).
Lucas, K., Magee, D. F., Nakajima, S., Veith, N.: Pancreozymin/cholecystokinin a physiological mediator of gastric secretory inhibition of duodenal origin. Experientia (Basel) **24**, 570—571 (1968).
Lucien, H. W., Itoh, Z., Sun, D. C. H., Meyer, J., Carlton, N., Schally, A.: The purification of enterogastrone from porcine gut. Arch. Biochem. Biophys. **134**, 180—184 (1969).
Luckhardt, A. B., Barlow, O., Weaver, M.: Note on a rapid and simple method of preparing a highly active secretin solution. Amer. J. Physiol. **76**, 182—235 (1926).
— Blonder, E.: Vasodilatins are not responsible for the secretagogue action of pancreatic secretin preparations. Amer. J. Physiol. **68**, 142 (1924).
Lueth, H. C., Kloster, G.: The effect of purified secretin on bile flow from the liver. Amer. J. Physiol. **85**, 389—415 (1928).
Lyon, B. B. V.: Diagnosis and treatment of diseases of the gallbladder and biliary ducts. J. Amer. Med. Ass. **73**, 980—982 (1919).
Mackowiak, R., Friedman, M. H. F., Horn, J.: Effect of pancreotrophic agents on pancreatic blood flow. Gastroenterology **52**, 1106 (1967).
Magee, D. F., Nakajima, S.: Stimulatory action of secretin on gastric pepsin secretion. Experientia (Basel) **24**, 689—690 (1968).
— — Is secretin enterogastrone? Experientia (Basel) **25**, 1051 (1969).
— — Odori, Y.: On potentiation. Gastroenterology **55**, 648—649 (1968).
— Nakamura, M.: Action of pancreozymin prepararations on gastric secretion. Nature **212**, 1487—1488 (1966).
Makhlouf, G. M., Blum, A. L.: An assessment of models for pancreatic secretion. Gastroenterology **59**, 896—908 (1970).
— — McManus, J. P. A., Card, W. I.: Action of the pentapeptide (ICI 50, 123) on gastric secretion. Gastroenterology **51**, 455—465 (1966).
— — — Comparative effects of gastrin II and histamine on pepsin secretion in man Gastroenterologie **52**, 787—791 (1967).
Maltesos, C., Watson, R. H.: Durchblutung und Sekretion des Pankreas bei humoraler Anregung. Pflüg. Arch. ges. Physiol. **241**, 516—523 (1939).
Manzke, E.: Inaugural dissertation, Kiel 1959.
Marchis-Mouren, G., Reggio, H.: Effect of carbamylcholine, pancreozymin and secretin on pancreatic enzyme synthesis in the rat. In: Proc. 3rd Symp. Europ. Pancreatic Club, Prague, July 2—4, 1968, pp. 86—96. edit. by P. Fric, F. Malis and R. Ronsky, Praha, Czech. Med. Press 1970.
Marks, I. N.: Changes in the icteric index of the duodenal aspirates after the injection of secretin and pancreozymin. Gastroenterology **37**, 73—80 (1959).
— Komarov, S. A., Shay, H.: Influence of cholinergic stimuli on gastric secretory responses to histamine in the dog. Am. J. Digest. Dis. **11**, 122—141 (1966).
Matsuo, J.: On the secretion of pancreatic juice. J. Physiol. **45**, 447—458 (1912—1913).
McDonald, J. K., Callihan, P. X., Zeitman, B. B., Ellis, S.: Inactivation and degradation of glucagon by dipeptidyl aminopeptidase I (Cathepsin C) of rat liver. J. Biol. Chem. **244**, 6199—6208 (1969).
McGuigan, J. E.: Gastric mucosal intracellular localization of gastrin by immunofluorescence. Gastroenterology **55**, 315—327 (1968).
— Immunological determination of gastrin in tissues and blood. In: Nobel Symposium XVI. Frontiers in Gastrointestinal Hormone Research, Stockholm, July 20—21, 1970; (In press), edit. by S. Andersson. Upsala: Almqvist and Wiksell 1972.
— Greider, M. H.: Correlative immunochemical and light microscopic studies of the gastrin cell of the antral mucosa. Gastroenterology **60**, 223—236 (1971).
— Jaffe, B. M., Newton, W. T.: Immunochemical measurement of endogenous gastrin release and circulation. Gastroenterology **56**, 1181 (1969).
— Trudeau, W. L.: Immunochemical measurement of elevated levels of gastrin in the serum of patients with pancreatic tumors of the Zollinger-Ellison variety. New Eng. J. Med. **278**, 1308—1313 (1968).
McIlrath, D. C., Hallenbeck, G. A.: Comparison of gastric inhibitory properties of two secretin preparations. Amer. J. Physiol. **206**, 1077—1080 (1964).

McIntyre, N., Holdsworth, C. D., Turner, D. S.: New interpretation of oral glucose tolerance. Lancet 1964, II, 20—21.
— Turner, D. S., Holdsworth, C. D.: Intestinal factors and insulin secretion. Diabetologia **1**, 73 (1965).
— — — Comparative effects of gastrin II and histamine on pepsin secretion in man. Gastroenterology **52**, 787—791 (1967).
Meldolesi, J.: Effect of caerulein on protein synthesis and secretion in guinea pig pancreas. Brit. J. Pharmac. **40**, 721—731 (1970).
Mellanby, J. M.: Mechanism of pancreatic digestion; function of secretin. J. Physiol. **60**, 85—91 (1925).
— Mechanism of pancreatic secretion. Lancet **211**, 215—218 (1926a).
— The secretion of pancreatic juice. J. Physiol. (Lond.) **61**, 419—435 (1926b).
— Bile salts and secretin as cholagogues. J. Physiol. (Lond.) **64**, 331—340 (1927).
— The isolation of secretin — its chemical and physiological properties. J. Physiol. (Lond.) **66**, 1—18 (1928).
— Secretin. Proc. Roy. Soc. Biol., London, **111**, 429—436 (1932).
— Huggett, A. St. G.: The relations of secretin formation to the entrance of acid chyme into the small intestine — the properties of secretin. J. Physiol. (Lond.) **61**, 122—130 (1926).
— Suffolk, F. S.: Enterohepatic circulation of the bile salts in the cat. Proc. R. Soc. Biol. **126**, 287—302 (1938/1939).
Mentzner, S. H.: Anomalous bile ducts in man. Based on a study of comparative anatomy. J. Amer. Med. Ass. **93**, 1273—1278 (1929).
Mering, J., von, Minkowski, O.: Diabetes mellitus nach Pankreasexstirpation. Arch. f. Exper. Pathol. u. Pharmakol. **26**, 372—387 (1889/1890).
Mett, S. G.: Zur Innervation der Bauchspeicheldrüse. Diss. 1889. St. Petersburg.
Meyer, J. H., Grossman, M. I.: Comparison of D- and L-phenylalanine as pancreatic stimulants. Gastroenterology **58**, 1046 (1970a).
— — Complexities of hormonal control of the pancreas by intestinal chyme. In: Abstr. 4th World Congress of Gastroenterology. p. 234, edit. by P. Riis, P. Anthonisen and H. Baden, Copenhagen, 1970b.
— Way, L. W., Grossman, M. I.: Pancreatic bicarbonate response to various acids in the duodenum of dogs. Amer. J. Physiol. **219**, 964—970 (1970a).
— — — Pancreatic response to acidification of various lengths of proximal intestine in the dog. Amer. J. Physiol. **219**, 971—977 (1970b).
Michlin, S. J., Heymberg, V. G., Pavlova, Z. M.: On the role of the microflora in the destruction of enterokinase and phosphatase in the large intestine of the rabbit. Vaprosyi Med. Chim. **4**, 8—14 (1958).
Minkowski, O.: Untersuchungen über den Diabetes mellitus nach Exstirpation des Pankreas. Arch. f. exp. Path. Pharm. **31**, 85—189 (1893).
— Bemerkungen über den Pankreasdiabetes. Zur Abwehr gegen Eduard Pflüger. Arch. f. exper. Pathol. u. Pharmak. **53**, 331—338 (1905).
Monod, E.: Action entéro-kinétique de la cécékine. Arch. Mal. Appar. dig. **53**, 607—608 (1964).
Moody, A. J., Markussen, J., Fries, A. S., Steenstrup, C., Sundby, F.: The insulin releasing activities of extracts of pork intestine. Diabetologia **6**, 135—140 (1970).
Moreland, H. J., Johnson, L. R.: Effect of vagotomy on pancreatic secretion stimulated by endoegnous and exogenous secretin. Gastroenterology **58**, 1047 (1970).
Morin, G., Besancon, F., Grall, A., Jouve, R., Debray, Ch.: Technique d'accélération du transit du grêle. Arch. Mal. Appar. Dig. **54**, 1285—1290 (1965).
— — — Debray, Ch., Jouve, R., Garat, J.-P.: La cholécystokinine appliquée au radiodiagnostique de l'intestine grêle: nouvelle technique de radiocinématographie complète en quelques minutes, avec 62 observations. Entretiens de Bichat, Radiologie 247—250 (1966).
Morisset, J. A., Webster, P. D.: In vitro and in vivo effects of pancreozymin, urecholine, and cyclic AMP on rat pancreas. Amer. J. Physiol. **230**, 202—208 (1971).
Morley, J. S.: Gastrin and gastrin analogues. In: Proc. 3rd Symp. Europ. Pancreatic Club, Prague, July 2—4, 1968. pp. 36—41, edit. by P. Fric, F. Malis and R. Ronsky, Praha. Czech. Med. Press 1970.
— Structure-activity relations in GI hormones. In: Nobel Symposium XVI. Frontiers in Gastrointestinal Hormone Research, Stockholm, July 20—21, 1970; (In press), edit. by S. Andersson. Upsala: Almqvist and Wiksell 1972.
— Tracy, H. J., Gregory, R. A.: Function relationships in the active C-terminal tetrapeptide sequence of gastrin. Nature (Lond.) **207**, 1356—1359 (1965).

MORRIS, A. I., BESWICK, F. B., HOWAT, H. T., MORLEY, J. S.: Action of gastrin and gastrin analogues on cat stomach and pancreas. In: Proc. 3rd Symp. Europ. Pancreatic Club, Prague, July 2—4, 1968, pp. 42—49, edit. by P. FRIC and R. RONSKY, Praha, Czech. Med. Press 1970.
MORRIS, T. Q., SARDI, G., BRADLEY, S. E.: Character of glucagon induced choleresis. Fed. Proc. **26**, 774 (1967).
MORTIMER, B., IVY, A. C.: An attempt to repeat the Mellanby procedure for the isolation and purification of secretin. Amer. J. Physiol. **91**, 220—224 (1929).
MURAT, J. E., WHITE, T. T.: Stimulation of gastric secretion by commercial cholecystokinin extracts. Proc. Soc. exp. Biol. (N.Y.) **123**, 593—594 (1966).
MUTT, V.: Electrophoretic purification of highly active secretin preparations. Arkiv f. Kemi **14**, 275—278 (1959a).
— Chromatography of secretin on carboxymethyl cellulose. Acta Chem. Scand. **13**, 1247—1248 (1959b).
— Preparation of highly purified secretin. Arkiv f. Kemi **15**, 69—74 (1959c).
— On the preparation of secretin. Arkiv f. Kemi **15**, 75—95 (1959d). (Thesis.)
— Behaviour of secretin, cholecystokinin and pancreozymin to oxidation with hydrogen peroxide. Acta Chem. Scand. **18**, 2185—2186 (1964).
— JORPES, J. E.: Secretin: isolation and determination of structure (abstr.). Proc. I. U. P. A. C. Fourth International Congress on the Chemistry of Natural Products, June 26—July 2, 1966, Stockholm, Sweden. Section 2C—3.
— — Contemporary developments in the biochemistry of the gastrointestinal hormones. In: Recent Progress in Hormone Research, **23**, 483—495, edit. by G. PINCUS, N.Y., Acad. Press 1967a.
— — Isolation of aspartyl-phenylalanine amide from cholecystokinin-pancreozymin. Biochem. Biophys. Res. Com. **26**, 392—397 (1967b).
— — Secretin, Cholecystokinin. In Internat. Symp. on the Pharmacol. of Hormonal Polypeptides and Proteins. (Milan, Italy, Sept. 14—16, 1967). pp. 569—580, New York, Plenum Press 1968a.
— — Structure of porcine cholecystokinin-pancreozymin. I. Cleavage with thrombin and with trypsin. Eur. J. Biochem. **6**, 156—162 (1968b).
— — Hormonal polypeptides of the upper intestine, Biochem. J.**125**, 57P—58P (1971)
— — MAGNUSSON, S.: Structure of porcine secretin. The amino acid sequence. Eur. J. Biochem. **15**, 513—519 (1970).
— MAGNUSSON, S., JORPES, J. E., DAHL, E.: Structure of porcine secretin. I. Biochemistry **4**, 2358—2362 (1965).
— SÖDERBERG, U.: On the assay of secretin. Arkiv f. Kemi **15**, 63—68 (1959).
NAHRWOLD, D. L., COOKE, A. R., GROSSMAN, M. I.: Choleresis induced by stimulation of the gastric antrum. Gastroenterology **52**, 18—22 (1967).
NAITO, S., IWATA, R., SAITO, T.: Etude sur la cholécystokinine, son mode d'action sur la contraction de la vésicule biliaire. Presse Méd. **55**, 2688—2689 (1963).
NAKAJIMA, S., MAGEE, D. F.: Influences of duodenal acidification on acid and pepsin secretion of the stomach in dogs. Amer. J. Physiol. **218**, 545—549 (1970a).
— — Inhibitory action of cholecystokinin-pancreozymin on gastric pepsin secretion. Experientia (Basel) **26**, 159 (1970b).
— — Inhibition of exocrine pancreatic secretion by glucagon and D-glucose given intravenously. Can. J. Physiol. Pharmacol. **48**, 299—305 (1970c).
— NAKAMURA, M., MAGEE, D. F.: Effect of secretin on gastric acid and pepsin secretion in response to various stimuli. Amer. J. Physiol. **216**, 87—91 (1969).
NAKAMURA, M., NAKAJIMA, S., MAGEE, D. F.: Action of pancreozymin preparations on gastric acid secretion. Gut **9**, 405—410 (1968).
NARDI, G. L., GREEP, J. M., CHAMBERS, D. A., MCCRAE, C., SKINNER, D. B.: Physiologic peregrinations in pancreatic perfusion. Annals of Surgery **158**, 830—839 (1963).
NECHELES, H.: Effects of glucagon on external secretion of the pancreas. Amer. J. Physiol. **191**, 595—597 (1957).
— HANKE, M. E., FANTL, E.: Preparation and assay of inhibitor of gastric secretion and motility from normal human urine. Proc. Soc. exp. Biol. (N.Y.) **42**, 618—619 (1939).
— LIM, R. K. S.: Isolation of gastric and pancreatic secretory excitants from the circulation by vivi-dialysis. Chinese Journ. Physiol. **2**, 415 (1928).
— OGAWA, T., CHILES, TH., LEVINSON, M.: Effect of secretin given into portal or peripheral vein. Proc. Soc. exp. Biol. (N.Y.) **102**, 110—112 (1959).
— SPORN, J., WALKER, L.: Effect of glucagon on gastrointestinal motility. Amer. J. Gastroenterology. **45**, 34—39 (1966).
NEWTON, G. G. F., LOVE, J. W., HEATLEY, N. G., ABRAHAM, E. P.: Purification of secretin. Biochem. J. **71**, 6P. (1959).

NILSSON, A.: Gastrointestinal hormones in the holocephalian fish *Chimaera monstrosa* (L.). Comp. Biochem. Physiol. **32**, 387–390 (1970).
NILSSON, G.: Effect of acid in the duodenal bulb on gastric secretory responses to sham feeding. Acta Physiol. Scand. **77**, 308–315 (1969).
— YALOW, R. S., BERSON, S. A.: Distribution of gastrin in the gastrointestinal tract of human, dog, cat and hog. In: NOBEL Symposium XVI. Frontiers in Gastrointestinal Hormone Research, Stockholm, July 20–21, 1970; (In press), edit. by S. ANDERSSON. Upsala: Almqvist and Wiksell 1972.
NILSSON, S., STATTIN, S.: Gallbladder emptying during the normal menstrual cycle. Acta Chir. Scand. **133**, 648–652 (1967).
OBERHELMAN, H. A., Jr., WOODWARD, E. R., ZUBIRAN, M. J., DRAGSTEDT, L. R.: Physiology of the gastric antrum. Amer. J. Physiol. **169**, 738–748 (1952).
ODORI, Y., MAGEE, D. F.: Cholecystokinin-pancreozymin as a physiological mediator of gastric acid inhibition. Pflügers Arch. Eur. J. Physiol. **318**, 287–293 (1970).
OKADA, S.: On the secretion of bile. J. Physiol. (Lond.) **49**, 457–482 (1914–1915).
OLBE, L.: The gastrin mechanism in cephalic phase of canine gastric acid secretion. Thesis, Karolinska Institutet, Stockholm, 1964a.
— Potentiation of sham feeding response in Pavlov pouch dogs by subthreshold amounts of gastrin with and without acidification of denervated antrum. Acta Physiol. Scand. **61**, 244–254 (1964b).
— Effect of resection of gastrin releasing regions on acid response to sham feeding and insulin hypoglycaemia in Pavlov pouch dogs. Acta Physiol. Scand. **62**, 169–175 (1964c).
— RIDLEY, P. T., UVNÄS, B.: Effects of gastrin and histamine on vagally induced acid and pepsin secretion in antrectomized dogs. Acta Physiol. Scand. **72**, 492–497 (1968).
OLIVER, G., SCHÄFER, E. A.: On the physiological actions of extracts of pituitary body and certain other glandular organs. J. Physiol. (Lond.) **18**, 277–279 (1895).
OLMSTED, J. M. D., OLMSTED, E. H.: CLAUDE BERNARD. SCHUMAN, New York 1952.
ONDETTI, M. A.: Synthesis of secretin. Recent progress in hormone research **23**, 496–499, edit. by G. PINCUS. New York. Acad. Press 1967.
— NARAYANAN, V. L., VON SALTZA, M., SHEEHAN, J. T., SABO, E. F., BODANSZKY, M.: The synthesis of secretin. III. The fragment-condensation method. J. Amer. Chem. Soc. **90**, 4711–4716 (1968a).
— PLUŠČEC, J., SABO, E. F., SHEEHAN, J. T., WILLIAMS, N.: Synthesis of cholecystokinin-pancreozymin. I. The C-terminal dodecapeptide. J. Amer. Chem. Soc. **92**, 195–216 (1970a).
— RUBIN, B., ENGEL, S. L., PLUŠČEC, J., SHEEHAN, J. T.: Cholecystokinin-pancreozymin: recent developments. Amer. J. Digest. Dis. **15**. 149–156 (1970b).
— SHEEHAN, J. T., BODANSZKY, M.: Synthesis of gastrointestinal hormones. In: Pharmaccology of Hormonal Polypeptides and Proteins pp. 18–31. Edit. N. BACK, L. MARTINI, R. PAOLETTI. Advances in exper. Med. and Biol. Vol. 2. New York, Plenum Press. 1968b.
— — PLUŠČEC, J.: Recent advances in the synthesis of gastrointestinal hormones. In: Peptides: chemistry and biochemistry (Proc. First Amer. Peptide Symposium, Yale Univ., 1968), edit. by B. WEINSTEIN and S. LANDE, p. 181–190. New York. Marcel Dekker, Inc., 1970.
PALADE, G. E.: Functional changes in the structure of cell components. In: Subcellular Particles. New York: Ronald Press Co. 1959.
PALLIN, B., SKOGLUND, S.: On the nervous regulation of the biliary system in the cat. Acta Physiol. Scand. **51**, 187–192 (1961).
— — Neural and humoral control of the gallbladder-emptying mechanism in the cat. Acta Physiol. Scand. **60**, 358–362 (1964).
PARIS, J., ROBELET, A., SALEMBIER, Y., DU BOIS, R.: Étude expérimentale des effets de la cholécystokinine sur les voies biliaires soumises à l'action des substances morphiniques. Rev. Int. Hepat. **12**, 1071–1091 (1962).
PARK, C. Y., PAE, Y. S., HONG, S. S.: Radiological studies on emptying of human gallbladder. Ann. Surg. **171**, 294–299 (1970).
PASSARO, E. J., GILLESPIE, I. E., GROSSMAN, M. I.: Potentiation between gastrin and histamine in stimulation of gastric secretion. Proc. Soc. exp. Biol. (N.Y.) **114**, 50–52 (1963).
— GROSSMAN, M. I.: Studies of the gastric phase of pancreatic secretion. Gastroenterology **44**, 864–865 (1963).
— — Effect of vagal innervation on acid and pepsin response to histamine and gastrin. Amer. J. Physiol. **206**, 1069–1076 (1964).
PAVLOV, I. P.: Beiträge zur Physiologie der Absonderung. Zbl. Physiol. **2**, 137–138 (1888).
— Lectures on the Work of the Principal Digestive Glands. St. Petersburg, 1897. (Russian.)
— Secretory work of the stomach in hunger. Proc. Soc. Russ. Physicians, St. Petersburg, **65**, Sept., 1897–98. (Russian.)
— Die Arbeit der Verdauungsdrüsen, p. 156. J. F. Bergmann, Wiesbaden, 1898.

PAVLOV, I. P.: Das Experiment als zeitgemäße und einheitliche Methode medizinischer Forschung. Lecture given to the memory of S. P. Botkin. J. F. Bergmann, Wiesbaden, 1900.
— Le travail des glandes digestives, Masson et Cie, Paris, 1901.
— Die äußere Arbeit der Verdauungsdrüsen und ihr Mechanismus. Nagels Handbuch d. Physiol. d. Menschen, **2**, 666. Braunschweig, F. Vieweg & Sohn 1907.
— The Work of the Digestive Glands. Translated by W. Thompson. 2nd ed., London, C. Griffin & Co., 1910.
PENAU, H., SIMONNET, H.: Sécrétine duodénale et insuline. Bull. Soc. Chim. Biol. **7**, 17—25 (1925).
PERKS, A. M., SCHAPIRO, H., WOODWARDS, E. R.: The influence of antidiuretic hormone on pancreatic secretion. Acta Endocrin. **45**, 340—348 (1964).
PERMAN, G., BONERA, E.: The secretin test in patients with haemochromatosis. Acta Med. Scand. **175**, 787—790 (1964).
PETERSEN, H.: The effect of secretin on the basal gastric acid secretion in man. Scand. J. Gastroenterology **4**, 609—616 (1969).
— The effect of pure natural secretin on the bicarbonate secretion into the duodenum in man. Scand. J. Gastroenterology **5**, 105—112 (1970).
— BERSTAD, A., MYREN, J.: Effect of secretin on histamine and pentagastrin stimulated secretion of acid in man. In: Abstr. 4th World Congress of Gastroenterology. p. 137, edit. by P. RIIS, P. ANTHONISEN and H. BADEN, Copenhagen 1970.
— — — Effect of pentagastrin on pancreatic secretion in man. In Gastrointestinal Hormones and other Subjects. ALFRED BENZON Publication I. pp. 72—73. Edit. E. HESS-THAYSEN. Munksgaard, Copenhagen, 1971.
PFEIFFER, E. F., FRANK, M., FUSSGÄNGER, R., GOBERNA, R., HINZ, M., RAPTIS, S.: Gastrointestinal hormones and islet function. In: NOBEL Symposium XVI. Frontiers in Gastrointestinal Hormone Research, Stockholm, July 20—21, 1970; (In press), edit. by S. ANDERSSON. Upsala: Alm qvist and Wiksell 1972.
— TELIB, M., AMMON, J., MELANI, F., DITSCHUNEIT, H.: Direkte Stimulierung der Insulin-Sekretion *in vitro* durch Sekretin. Deutsch. med. Wschr. **90**, 1633—1669 (1965).
— SCHRÖDER, K. E., RAPTIS, S.: Alimentary polypeptides and insulin secretion. In: Rep. 3rd Symp. Europ. Pancreatic Club, Prague 2nd—4th July 1968, pp. 54—64, edit. by P. FRIC, F. MALIS and R. RONSKY, Praha, Czech. Med. Press 1968.
PINCUS, I. J., FRIEDMAN, M. H. F., THOMAS, J. E., REHFUSS, M. E.: A quantitative study of the inhibitory effect of acid in the intestine and gastric secretion. Amer. J. Dig. Dis. **11**, 205—208 (1944).
— THOMAS, J. E., LACHMANN, P. O.: The effect of vagotomy on the secretion of pancreatic juice after ingestion of various food-stuffs. Fed. Proc. **7**, 94 (1948).
PISSIDIS, A. G., BOMBECK, C. T., MERCHANT, F., NYHUS, L. M.: Hormonal regulation of bile secretion: A study in the isolated perfused liver. Surgery **66**, 1075—1084 (1969).
PLESSIER, J.: Confrontation des actions cholécystokinétiques et cholérétiques de la cholécystokinine, du sorbitol, de l'huile d'olive et du sulfate de magnésie. Path.-Biol. **8**, 1201—1210 (1960).
— DOYON, D., BENETT, J., STOOPEN, M., ECONOMOPOULOS, P., CHÉRIGIÉ, E., CAROLI, J.: Effet de la sécrétine intra-artérielle en angiographie coeliaque (Artériographie couplée avec le tubage duodénal). Arch. Franc. Mal. Appar. Dig. **57**, 307—315 (1967).
— MARSICO, G.: La cholécystokinine. Son emploi en cholécystographie, radiomanométrie et cinématographie biliaire. Ann. Radiol. **3**, 801—810 (1960).
— NAJEAN, Y., ECONOMOPOULOS, P.: Le rôle du pancréas dans l'absorption duodéno-jéjunale du fer. Rev. Med-Chir. Maladies du Foie **42**, 115—128 (1967).
— PLESSIER, B.: Dosage biologique de l'urocholécystokinine selon la méthode de Svatos. Arch. Mal. App. Digest. **49**, 1601—1610 (1960).
— WETTENDORFF, P., PLESSIER, B., COHEN, J.: L'atonie vésiculaire chez la femme et le cobaye gravides. Essai d'explication par le dosage biologique des hormones digestives. Ann. Biol. Clin. **19**, 843—850 (1961).
PLUŠČEC, J., SABO, E. F., SHEEHAN, J. T., WILLIAMS, N., KOCY, O., ONDETTI, M. A.: Synthesis of analogs of the C-terminal octapeptide of cholecystokinin-pancreozymin. Structure-activity relationship. J. Med. Chem. **13**, 349—352 (1970).
POPIELSKI, L. B.: The secretory-inhibitory nerves of the pancreatic gland. Thesis, St. Petersburg, 1896. (Russian.)
— Über das peripherische reflektorische Nervencentrum des Pankreas. Pflüg. Arch. ges. Physiol. **86**, 215—246 (1901).
— Über die physiologische Wirkung und chemische Natur des Sekretins. Zentralblatt f. Physiol. **19**, 801—805 (1906).
— Die Sekretionstätigkeit der Bauchspeicheldrüse unter dem Einfluß von Salzsäure und Darmextrakt (des sogenannten Sekretins). Pflüg. Arch. ges. Physiol. **120**, 451—491 (1907).

POPIELSKI, L. B.: Über den Charakter der Sekretionstätigkeit des Pankreas unter dem Einfluß von Salzsäure und Darmextrakt. Pflüger's Arch. ges. Physiol. **121**, 239—264 (1907—1908).
POPOVA, E. A., ZYCHOVA, A. A., FIOLETOVA, A. A., GOLTYAKOVA, T. V.: Urocholecystokinin in diagnosis of extrahepatic biliary ducts. Ther. Archiv, **39**, 37—40 (1967).
POTT, J. T., Jr., NIALL, H. D., KEUTMANN, H. T., BREWER, H. B., Jr., DEFTOS, L. J.: The amino acid sequence of porcine thyrocalcitonin. Proc. Nat. Acad. Sci. **59**, 1321—1328 (1968).
PRATT, C. L. G.: The influence of secretin on gastric secretion. J. Physiol. (Lond.) **98**, 1—2P (1940).
PREISIG, R., BUCHER, H., STIRNEMANN, H., TAUBER, J.: Postoperative choleresis following bile obstruction in man. Rev. Franc. Étud. Clin. Biol. **14**, 151—158 (1969).
— COOPER, H. L., WHEELER, H. O.: The relationship between taurocholate secretion rate and bile production in the unanesthetized dog during cholinergic blockade and during secretin administration. J. Clin. Invest. **41**, 1152—1162 (1962).
PRESHAW, R. M.: Integration of nervous and hormonal mechanisms for external pancreatic secretion. In: Handbook of Physiology. Section 6: Alimentary Canal. Vol. II: Secretion. pp. 997—1005, edit. by C. F. CODE, Washington, Amer. Physiol. Soc. 1967.
— Duodenal acidification and the release of secretin. In: Exocrine Glands, 247—252, edit. by S. Y. BOTELHO, F. P. BROOKS, and W. B. SHELLEY. Philadelphia, Univ. Penn. Press 1969.
— ADASHEK, K., COOKE, A. R., GROSSMAN, M. I.: Failure of Urecholine to potentiate the pancreatic response to exogenous stimuli. Proc. Soc. exp. Biol. (N.Y.) **119**, 1040—1044 (1965).
— COOKE, A. R., GROSSMAN, M. I.: Stimulation of pancreatic secretion by a humoral agent from the pyloric gland area of the stomach. Gastroenterology **49**, 617—622 (1965a).
— — — Pancreatic secretion induced by stimulation of the pyloric gland area of the stomach. Science **148**, 1347—1348 (1965b).
— — — Quantitative aspects of response of canine pancreas to duodenal acidification. Amer. J. Physiol. **210**, 629—634 (1966).
— GROSSMAN, M. I.: Stimulation of pancreatic secretion by extracts of the pyloric gland area of the stomach. Gastroenterology **48**, 36—44 (1965a).
— — Comparison of subcutaneous and intravenous administration of pancreatic stimulants. Amer. J. Physiol. **209**, 803—810 (1965b).
QUIGLEY, J. P., ZETTLEMAN, H. J., IVY, A. C.: Factors in the gastric motor inhibition by fats. Amer. J. Physiol. **108**, 643—651 (1934).
RAMIREZ, M., FARRAR, J. T.: The effect of secretin and cholecystokinin-pancreozymin on the intraluminal pressure of the jejunum in the unanesthetized dog. Amer. J. Dig. Dis. N.S. **15**, 539—544 (1970).
— HUBEL K. A., CLIFTON, J. A.: Intestinal factors affecting pancreatic exocrine secretion in the rat. Amer. J. Physiol. **211**, 260—263 (1966).
RAMORINO, MARIA LETIZIA, COLAGRANDE, C., MONTI, G., SISTI, P.: Effetti della colecistocinina su l'apparato biliare extraepatico e sul duodeno. Arch. Ital. Mal. App. Dig. **27**, 403—432 (1960).
RAWLS, J. A., WISTRAND, P. J., MAREN, TH. H.: Effects of acid-base changes and carbonic anhydrase inhibition on pancreatic secretion. Amer. J. Physiol. **205**, 651—657 (1963).
RAZIN, E., FELDMAN, M. G., DREILING, D. A.: The hormonal regulation of thoracic ductal lymph flow. The effect of secretin and related hormones on the thoracic ductal flow and composition in dogs. J. Surg. Res. **2**, 320—331 (1962).
REBER, H. A., WOLF, CH. J.: Micropuncture study of pancreatic electrolyte secretion. Amer. J. Physiol. **215**, 34—40 (1968).
— — LEE, S. P.: Role of the main duct in pancreatic electrolyte secretion. Surg. Forum **20**, 382—384 (1969).
REDFORD, M., SAVAGE, L. E., SCHOFIELD, B.: The blocking of gastrin release. J. Physiol. (Lond.) **162**, 61—62P (1962).
— SCHOFIELD, B.: The effect of local anesthesia of the pyloric antral mucosa on acid inhibition of gastrin-mediated acid secretion. J. Physiol. (Lond.) **180**, 304—320 (1965).
RIDDERSTAP, A. S.: Action of secretin on exocrine pancreatic secretion in vitro. PFLÜGERS Arch. **311**, 205—208 (1969).
— BONTING, S. L.: Enzyme secretion by the isolated rabbit pancreas: absence of relation with the Na-K activated ATPase. Studies on Na-K activated ATPase, XXVII. PFLÜGERS Arch. **313**, 53—61 (1969a).
— — Cyclic AMP and enzyme secretion by the isolated rabbit pancreas. Pflügers Arch. **313**, 62—70 (1969b).
— — Na-K-activated adenosine triphosphatase and pancreatic secretion in the dog. Amer. J. Physiol. **216**, 547—554 (1969c).

Robert, A., Stout, Th. J., Dale, J. E.: Production by secretagogues of duodenal ulcers in the rat. Gastroenterology **59,** 95—102 (1970).

Robinson, R. M., Harris, K., Hlad, C. J., Eiseman, B.: Effect of glucagon on gastric secretion. Proc. Soc. exp. Biol. (N.Y.) **96,** 518—520 (1957).

Robison, G. A., Butcher, R. W., Sutherland, E. W.: Cyclic AMP. Annual Rev. Biochem. **37,** 149—174 (1968).

Rodbell, M., Birnbaumer, L., Pohl, S. L.: Adenyl cyclase in fat cells. III. Stimulation by secretin and the effects of trypsin on the receptors for lipolytic hormones. J. Biol. Chem. **245,** 718—722 (1970).

Rogers, G. E.: Enzymatic inactivation of secretin. Nature **167,** 771—772 (1951).

Rosenbusch, G., Cen, M.: Zöliakographie mit Sekretin. Fortschr. Gebiet der Röntgenstrahlen **110,** 639—651 (1969).

Ross, G.: Cardiovascular actions of glucagon and secretin. Brit. J. Pharmacol. **37,** 528P (1969).

Rothman, S. S.: Electrolyte secretion from the isolated rabbit pancreas: Fed. Proc. **23,** 439 (1964a).

— Exocrine secretion from the isolated rabbit pancreas. Nature **204,** 84—85 (1964b).

— Transport of protein by pancreatic acinar cells. Random or selective. In The Exocrine Glands. pp. 169—185, edit. by S. Y. Botelho, F. P. Brooks and W. B. Shelley. Philadelphia, Univ. Pennsylvania Press. 1969.

— The release of cholecystokinin-pancreozymin: The effects of duodenal perfusion of various amino acids. In: Nobel Symposium XVI. Frontiers in Gastrointestinal Hormone Research, Stockholm, July 20—21, 1970; (In press), edit. by S. Andersson. Upsala: Almqvist and Wiksell 1972.

— Brooks, F. P.: Electrolyte secretion from rabbit pancreas in vitro. Amer. J. Physiol. **208,** 1171—1176 (1965a).

— — Pancreatic secretion *in vitro* in "Cl′-free", "CO_2-free" and low-Na^+ environment. Amer. J. Physiol. **209,** 790—796 (1965b).

— Wells, H.: Enhancement of pancreatic enzyme synthesis by pancreozymin. Amer. J. Physiol. **213,** 215—218 (1967).

Rous, P., McMaster, P. D.: Physiological causes for the varied character of stasis bile. J. Exp. Med. **34,** 75—95 (1921).

Rozé, Cl., Feldmann, D.: Mécanisme de l'action cholérétique de la pancréozymine chez le rat. C. R. Acad. Sci. Paris **272,** 988—991 (1971).

Rubin, B., Engel, S. L.: Some biological characteristics of cholecystokinin (CCK-PZ) and synthetic analogs. In: Nobel Symposium XVI. Frontiers in Gastrointestinal Hormone Research, Stockholm, July 20—21, 1970; (In press), edit. by S. Andersson. Upsala: Almqvist and Wiksell 1972.

— — Drungis, A. M., Dzelzkalns, M., Grigas, E. O., Waugh, M. H., Yiacas, E.: Cholecystokinin-like activities in guinea pigs and in dogs of the C-terminal octapeptide (SQ 19, 844) of cholecystokinin. J. Pharmaceut. Sci. **58,** 955—959 (1969a).

— — Grigas, E. O., Yiacas, E., Gold, B. I.: Gallbladder contracting activities of octapeptide analogs of the C-terminal sequence of cholecystokinin (CCK). The Pharmacologist **11,** 277 (1969b).

Rubin, W.: Phospholipids and pancreatic acinar cell function. Gastroenterology **53,** 1000—1002 (1967).

Rudman, D., del Rio, A. E.: Lipolytic activity of synthetic porcine secretin. Endocrinology **85,** 214—217 (1969).

Rune, S. J., Worning, H.: Endogenous releasable secretin in man. Abstr. 4th World Congress of Gastroenterology. Edit. P. Riis, P. Anthonisen and H. Baden, Copenhagen, 1970, p. 232.

Rutherford, W.: On the physiological actions of drugs on the secretion of bile. Trans. Roy. Soc. of Edinburgh **29,** 133—263 (1880).

Sacks, J., Ivy, A. C., Burgess, J. P., Vandolah, E.: Histamine as the hormone for gastric secretion. Amer. J. Physiol. **101,** 331—338 (1932).

Sahba, M. M., Morisset, J. A., Webster, P. D.: Synthetic and secretory effects of cholecystokinin-pancreozymin in the pigeon pancreas. Proc. Soc. exper. Biol. (N.Y.) **134,** 728—732 (1970).

Samols, E., Marri, G., Marks, V.: Promotion of insulin secretion by glucagon. Lancet II, 415—416 (1965a); ref. in: S + Tyler + Marri + Marks.

Sandblom, P.: Function of human gallbladder studied in connection with blood transfusions and after stomach operations. Acta Radiol. **14,** 249—258 (1933).

— Voegtlin, W. L., Ivy, A. C.: The effect of cholecystokinin on the choledochoduodenal mechanism (sphincter of Oddi). Amer. J. Physiol. **113,** 175—180 (1935).

SARLES, H., PREZLIN, G., SOUVILLE, C., FIGARELLA, C.: Action des doses croissantes de sécrétine sur le pancreas humain. La capacité sécrétoire maximum. Rev. Franc. Étud. Clin. Biol. **11**, 294—298 (1966).
SAVICH, V. V.: The role which the pyloric part plays in the secretion of pepsin by the glands of the fundus (Russian). J. russe Physiol. **4**, 165 (1922).
— ZELIONY, G.: Zur Physiologie des Pylorus. Pflügers Arch. Physiol. **150**, 128—138 (1913).
SCHALLY, A. V., REDDING, T. W., LUCIEN, H. W., MEYER, J.: Enterogastrone inhibits eating by fasted mice. Science **157**, 210—211 (1967).
SCHAPIRO, H., RAGLAND, J. B., SHERMAN, R., WRUBLE, L. D.: A study of a patient with an external pancreatic fistula. Amer. J. Dig. Dis. N.S. **12**, 1029—1035 (1967).
— WOODWARD, E. R.: Inhibition of secretin mechanism with local anesthetics. Amer. Surg. **31**, 139—141 (1965).
SCHOFIELD, B.: Vagal release of gastrin and its inhibition. XXII Internat. Congr. Physiol. Sciences Leiden, 1962. Vol. I Part 1 pp. 352—353. Internat. Congr. Series No 47. Excerpta Med. Found.
SCHRAMM, M.: Secretion of enzymes and other macromolecules. Ann. Rev. Biochem. **36**, 307—320 (1967).
SCHUCHER, R., HOKIN, L. E.: The synthesis and secretion of lipase and ribonuclease by pigeon pancreas slices. J. Biol. Chem. **210**, 551—557 (1954).
SCHULMAN, J. L., CARLETON, J. L., WHITNEY, G., WHITEKORN, J. C.: Effect of glucagon on food intake and body weight in man. J. Appl. Physiol. **11**, 419—421 (1957).
SCHULZ, I.: Micropuncture studies of the pancreas of the rabbit. In: Non-Insulin-Producing Tumors of the Pancreas. Internat. Symp. Erlangen, July 16—17, 1968, on Modern Aspects on Zollinger-Ellison-syndrome and Gastrin. pp. 100—108, edit. by L. DEMLING and R. OTTENJANN, Stuttgart, G. Thieme. 1969.
— YAMAGATA, A., WESKE, M.: Micropuncture studies on the pancreas of the rabbit. Pflügers Arch. **308**, 277—290 (1969).
SCHWYZER, R., SIEBER, P.: Die Totalsynthese des β-corticotropins. Helv. Chim. Acta **49**, 134—158 (1966).
SCRATCHERD, T.: Electrolyte composition and control of biliary secretion in the cat and rabbit. In: The Biliary System. Symposium Nato Advanced Study Institute. pp. 515—529, ed. by W. TAYLOR, Oxford, Blackwell Scientif. Publications 1965.
— CASE, R. M.: The action of cyclic AMP, methyl xanthines and some prostaglandins on pancreatic exocrine secretion. In: NOBEL Symposium XVI. Frontiers in Gastrointestinal Hormone Research, Stockholm, July 20—21, 1970; (In press), edit. by S. ANDERSSON. Upsala: Almqvist and Wiksell 1972.
SEAGER, L. D.: Contractions of frog gallbladder and its use as an assay method. Proc. Soc. exp. Biol. (N.Y.) **41**, 326—327 (1939).
— Further studies on a frog method for assaying gallbladder contracting substances. Proc. Soc. exp. Biol. (N.Y.) **47**, 257—260 (1941).
SEWING, K. F., GORINSKY, P. D., LEMBECK, F.: Failure of "antigastrin" (SC-15396) to inhibit gastric acid and pepsin secretion in anaesthetized gastric fistula cats. Naunyn Schmiedeberg Arch. Pharm. exp. Pathol. **261**, 89—92 (1968).
SHAY, H., GERSHON-COHEN, J., FELS, S. S.: A self regulatory duodenal mechanism for gastric acid control and an explanation for the pathologic gastric physiology in uncomplicated duodenal ulcer. Amer. J. Dig. Dis. **9**, 124—128 (1942).
SHEPOVALNIKOV, N. P. The physiology of the intestinal juice. Thesis. St. Petersburg, 1899. (Russian.)
SHIPP, J. C., HANENSON, I. B., WINDHAGER, E. E., SCHATZMANN, H. J., WHITTEMBURY, G., YOSHIMURA, H., SOLOMON, A. K.: Single proximal tubules of the necturus kidney. Methods for micropuncture and microperfusion. Amer. J. Physiol. **195**, 563—569 (1958).
SHLYGIN, G. K.: The importance of determining enterokinase and alkaline phosphatase for the assessment of the state of human intestines. Clin. Chim. Acta **1**, 421—433 (1956).
SHOEMAKER, W. C., VAN ITALLIE, T. B., WALKER, W. F.: Measurement of hepatic glucose output and hepatic blood flow in response to glucagon, Amer. J. Physiol. **196**, 315—318 (1959).
SIRCUS, W.: The intestinal phase of gastric secretion. Quart. J. exp. Physiol. **38**, 91—99 (1953).
— Studies on the mechanism in the duodenum inhibiting gastric secretion. Quart. J. exp. Physiol. **43**, 114—133 (1958).
SJÖDIN, L.: Hormonal effects on vagally stimulated gastric secretion in Pavlov pouch dogs. In Gastrointestinal Hormones and other Subjects. ALFRED BENZON Publication I. pp. 21—23. Edit. E. HESS-THAYSEN. Munksgaard, Copenhagen, 1971.
SJÖHOLM, I.: Enzymatic inactivation of oxytocin. Acta Chem. Scand. **18**, 889—898 (1964).
— YMAN, L.: Preparation of highly purified oxytocinase (cystine aminopeptidase) from retroplacental serum. Acta Pharmaceutica Suecica **3**, 377—388 (1966).

SJÖHOLM, I., YMAN, L.: Degradation of oxytocine, lysine-vasopressin, angiotensin II and angiotensin-II-amide by oxytocinase. Acta Pharmaceutica Suecica **4**, 65—76 (1967).
SKILLMAN, J. J., SILEN, WM., HARPER, H. A.: Role of the liver in secretin inactivation. Amer. J. Physiol. **202**, 347—348 (1962).
SLAYBACK, J. B., SWENA, E. M., THOMAS, J. E., SMITH, L. L.: Secretory response of the pancreas to topical anesthetic block of the small bowel. Surg. Forum **17**, 351—353 (1966).
— — — — The pancreatic secretory response to topical anaesthetic block of the small bowel. Surgery **61**, 591—595 (1967).
SMITH, A. M.: Congenital absence of gallbladder. Virgin. Med. Monthly **91**, 497—501 (1964).
SMITH, A. N., HOGG, D.: Effect of gastrin II on the motility of the gastrointestinal tract. Lancet **1**, 403—404 (1966).
SNAPE, W. J., FRIEDMAN, M. H. F., SWENSON, P. C.: Correlation between the cholecystogram and the secretin test for gallbladder function. Amer. J. Med. Sc. **216**, 188—194 (1948).
— — THOMAS, J. E.: The assay of cholecystokinin and the influence of vagotomy on the gall bladder response. Gastroenterology **10**, 496—501 (1948).
SOKOLOV, A.: Zur Analyse der Abscheidungsarbeit des Magens bei Hunden. Thesis. St. Petersburg. 1904. (Russian) Quoted by Lawrow (1904) in *Jahresber. Fortschr. Tier-Chem.* **34**, 469—470, and by Babkin, B. P. *Secretory mechanisms of the digestive glands*, p. 467, 2nd Edition. New York, Paul B. Hoeber 1950.
SOLOMON, A. K.: Electrolyte secretion in the pancreas. Fed. Proc. **11**, 722—731 (1952).
SOLOMON, S. P., SPIRO, H. M.: The effects of glucagon and glucose on the human stomach. Amer. J. Dig. Dis. N.S. **4**, 775—786 (1959).
SPERBER, I.: Secretion of organic anions in the formation of urine and bile. Pharmacol. Rev. **11**, 109—134 (1959).
SPINGOLA, L. J., GROSSMAN, M. I.: Bioassay of secretin. In: Methods in Investigative and Diagnostic Endocrinology, Section 4, Peptide Hormones, edited by ROSALYN YALOW and S. A. BERSON. Amsterdam, North Holland Publishing Company 1972.
— MEYER, J. H., GROSSMAN, M. I.: Potentiated pancreatic response to secretin and endogenous cholecystokinin (CCK). Clin. Res. **18**, 175 (1970).
STARLING, E. H.: The chemical correlation of the functions of the body. The chemical control of the function of the body. Croonian Lecture I, Lancet II, 338—341 (1905a).
— The chemical correlation of the functions of the body. The chemical reflexes of the alimentary tract. Croonian Lecture II, Lancet II, 423—425 (1905b).
— The chemical correlation of the functions of the body. The chemical reflexes of the alimentary tract. Croonian Lecture III, Lancet II, 501—503 (1905c).
— Recent advances in the physiology of digestion. London. A. Constable & Co, 1906.
— Die Anwendung des Sekretins zur Gewinnung von Pankreassaft. Abderhalden Handbuch d. biochem. Arbeitsmethoden *VII*, 65—73, 1913.
STATE, D.: Inhibition of gastrin release. In: Abstr. XXII Internat. Congr. Physiol. Sciences, Leiden 1962. Vol. I, Part 1, pp. 348—350. Internat. Congr. Series No 47, Exerpt. Med. Found.
STENING, G. F.: A modification of a chronic pancreatic fistula in the dog. Brit. J. Surg. **56**, 308—310 (1969).
— GROSSMAN, M. I.: Stimulating Brunner's gland secretion. Lancet 1968, **I**, 1435.
— — Gastrin related peptides as stimulants of pancreatic and gastric secretion. Amer. J. Physiol. **217**, 251—254, 262—266 (1969a).
— — Hormonal control of Brunner's glands. Gastroenterology **56**, 1047—1052 (1969b).
— — Potentiation of cholecystokinetic action of cholecystokinin (CCK) by secretin. Clin. Res. **17**, 528 (1969c).
— JOHNSON, L. R., GROSSMAN, M. I.: The effect of secretin on acid and pepsin secretion in cat and dog. Gastroenterology **56**, 468—475 (1969b).
— — — Effect of cholecystokinin and caerulein on gastrin- and histamine-evoked gastric secretion. Gastroenterology **57**, 44—50 (1969a).
— VAGNE, M., GROSSMAN, M. I.: Relative potency of commercial secretins. Gastroenterology **55**, 687—689 (1968).
STEPP, W.: On the preparation of secretin. J. Physiol. **43**, 441—448 (1911—1912).
STILL, E. U.: Studies on the physiology of secretin. I. On the preparation and isolation. Amer. J. Physiol. **91**, 405—408 (1930).
— Secretin. Physiol. Rev. **11**, 328—357 (1931).
— BENNETT, A. L., SCOTT, V. B.: A study of the metabolic activity of the pancreas. Amer. J. Physiol. **106**, 509—523 (1933).
— MCBEAN, J. W., RIES, F. A.: Studies on the physiology of secretin. IV. Effect on the secretion of bile. Amer. J. Physiol. **99**, 94—100 (1931).
STIRNEMANN, H., BUCHER, H., PREISIG, R.: Gallenbildung bei Patienten mit Gallengangsverschluß. Einfluß des Sekretinmechanismus. Langenbecks Arch. Chir. **325**, 1152—1159 (1969).

STUNKARD, A. J., VAN ITALLIE, T. B., REIS, B. B.: The mechanism of satiety: Effect of glucagon on hunger contractions in man. Proc. Soc. exp. Biol. (N.Y.) **89**, 258—261 (1955).
SUGAWARA, K., ISAZA, J., CURT, J., WOODWARD, E. R.: Effect of secretin and cholecystokinin on gastric motility. Amer. J. Physiol. **217**, 1633—1638 (1969).
— — WOODWARD, E. R.: Effect of gastrin on gastric motor activity. Gastroenterology **57**, 649—658 (1969).
— — Pancreozymin-secretin test. The combined study of serum enzymes and duodenal contents in the diagnosis of pancreatic disease. Gastroenterology **38**, 570—581 (1960).
SUN, D. C. H., SHAY, H.: Pancreozymin secretin test. The combined study of serum enzymes and duodenal contents in the diagnosis of pancreatic disease. Gastroenterology **38**, 570 —581 (1960).
SUTHERLAND, E. W., ØYE, I., BUTCHER, R. W.: The action of epinephrine and the role of the adenyl cyclase system in hormone action. Recent Prog. Horm. Res. **21**, 263—646 (1965).
— ROBISON, G. A., BUTCHER, R. W.: Some aspects of the biological role of adenosine 3',5'-monophosphate (cyclic AMP). Circulation **37**, 279—306 (1968).
SVATOS, A.: Pancreozymin activity of urine. Naturwissenschaften **45**, 523—524 (1957).
— Cholecystokinin activity of urine. Science **129**, 566—567 (1959).
— Urocholecystokinin. Cas. Lek. Cesk. **99**, 1146—1150 (1960).
— Effect of intravenous administration of pancreozymin on the uropancreozymin concentration in urine. Cesk. Physiol. **13**, 62—66 (1964).
— BARTOS, V., BRZEK, V.: The concentration of cholecystokinin in human lymph and serum. Arch. Int. Pharmacodyn. **149**, 515—520 (1964).
— JELINEK, V.: Gastrointestinal hormones; titration of secretin in rats. Cesk. Physiol. **6**, 220—223 (1957).
— KOZLIK, V.: VERISOVA, Z.: Titration of secretin on small laborato y animals. Cesk. Physiol. **9**, 90—91 (1960).
— PADR, Z.: Hormony Trávícího Ustrojí. Státní Zdravotniké Nakladatelství, Praha 1957.
— QUISNEROVÁ, M.: Comparative electrophoretic study of pancreozymin and uropancreozymin. Gastroenterologia **94**, 290—294 (1960).
— VOKAC, V.: The serum cholecystokinin and urine urocholecystokinin concentration in patients with dysfunction of the gallbladder, with hydrops of the gallbladder and in cholecystectomised patients. Rev. Czech. Med. **6**, 204—211 (1960).
— — Effect of intravenous administration of pancreozymin on the uropancreozymin concentration in urine. Physiol. Bohemoslov **13**, 62—66 (1964).
SVENSSON, S.-O., EMÅS, S.: Effect of cholecystokinin on histamine and pentagastrin stimulated acid secretion in conscious cats. In: Abstr. 4th World Congress of Gastroenterology, p. 139, edit. by P. RIIS, P. ANTHONISEN and H. BADEN, Copenhagen, 1970.
SWEETING J. G.: The effect of glucagon on bile and pancreatic juice. Gastroenterology **54**, 1276 (1968).
TAKÁCS, L.: Versuche mit Sekretin. I and II. Z. ges. exp. Med. **57**, 527—531 (1927), ibid. **57**, 532—536 (1927).
— Untersuchungen mit Sekretin. Z. ges. exp. Med. **60**, 424—429 (1928a).
— Versuche mit Sekretin. IV. Der Einfluß des Sekretins auf die Gallenabsonderung und auf die diabetische Acidose. Z. ges. exp. Med. **62**, 114—117 (1928b).
— Über die Reindarstellung des Sekretins. Z. ges. exp. Med. **63**, 553—556 (1928c).
TANKEL, H. J., HOLLANDER, F.: The relation between pancreatic secretion and local blood flow: A Review. Gastroenterology **32**, 633—641 (1957).
TANTURI, C., IVY, A. C., GREENGARD, H.: Secretin is a true cholagogue. Amer. J. Physiol. **120**, 336—339 (1937).
TAYLOR, D. A., MACKEN, K. L., FIORE, A. S.: Angiographic visualization of the secretin-stimulated pancreas. Radiology **87**, 525—526 (1966).
THOMAS, J. E.: The maximal acidity of the intestinal contents during digestion. Amer. J. Dig. Dis. **7**, 195—197 (1940).
— An improved cannula for gastric and intestinal fistulas. Proc. Soc. exp. Biol. (N.Y.) **46**, 260—261 (1941).
— The external secretion of the pancreas. American Lecture Series. Springfield, Ill.: Charles C Thomas 1950.
— The normal and pathological physiology of the external secretion of the pancreas. Acta Gastro-Enterologica Belgica, **15**, 811—819 (1952a).
— Physiology of the external secretion of the pancreas. Trans. New York Ac. Sci. Ser. II**14**, 310—313 (1952b).
— Neural regulations of pancreatic secretion. In: Handbook of Physiol. Section 6, Vol. II, Alimentary Canal, pp. 955—968, edit by C. F. Code, Amer. Physiol. Soc. Wash. 1967.
— CRIDER, J. O.: A quantitative study of acid in the intestine as a stimulus for the pancreas. Amer. J. Physiol. **131**, 349—356 (1940).

THOMAS, J. E., SWENA, E. M.: The effect of local anesthetics applied to the intestinal mucosa on the response of the pancreas to intestinal stimuli. Fed. Proc. **22,** 664 (1963).
THOMPSON, J. C.: The question of an antral chalone. In: Gastrin, pp. 193—228, edit. by M. I. GROSSMAN, Los Angeles, University of California Press 1966.
— REEDER, D. D., DAVIDSON, W. D., CHARTERS, A. C., BRÜCKNER, W. L., LEMMI, C. A. E., MILLER, J. H.: Effect of hepatic transit of gastrin, pentagastrin, and histamine measured by gastric secretion and by assay of hepatic vein blood. Ann. Surg. **170,** 493—505 (1969).
— — — — — — — Effect of hepatic transit of gastrin, pentagastrin, and histamine measured by gastric secretion and by assay of hepatic vein blood. In: Abstr. 4th World Congress of Gastroenterology, p. 198, edit. by P. RIIS, P. ANTHONISEN and H. BADEN, Copenhagen, 1970.
— — — JACKSON, B. M., CLENDINNEN, B. G.: Studies on metabolism of gastrin. In: NOBEL Symposium XVI. Frontiers in Gastrointestinal Hormone Research, Stockholm, July 20—21, 1970; (In press), edit. by S. ANDERSSON. Upsala: Almqvist and Wiksell 1972.
TIBBLIN, S., KOCK, N. G., SCHENK, W. G., Jr.: The mechanism by which the hemodynamic effects of glucagon are evoked. In: Abstr. 4th World Congress of Gastroenterology, p. 533, edit. by P. RIIS, P. ANTHONISEN and H. BADEN, Copenhagen, 1970.
TIGERSTEDT, R., BERGMAN, P. G.: Niere und Kreislauf. Skand. Archiv f. Physiologie **8,** 223—271 (1898).
TINKER, J., COX, A. G.: Gallbladder function after vagotomy. Brit. J. Surg. **56,** 779—782 (1969).
TISCORNIA, O. M., JANOWITZ, H. D., DREILING, D. A.: The effect of alloxan upon canine exocrine pancreatic secretion. Amer. J. Gastroenterol. **49,** 328—340 (1968).
TOMENIUS, J., BACKLUND, V., JORPES, J. E., MUTT, V.: Cholecystokinin in roentgenologic examination of the biliary tract. Röntgenblätter **11,** 145—157 (1958).
— — Cholecystokinin vid röntgenundersökning av gallvägarna. Nord. Med. **61,** 46—47 (1959).
TONKICH, A.: Zur Physiologie des Pankreas. Pflügers Arch. Physiol. **206,** 525—553 (1924).
TORSOLI, A., RAMORINO, MARIA LETIZIA, COLAGRANDE, C., DEMAIO, G.: Experiments with cholecystokinin. Acta Radiol. Stockholm **55,** 193—206 (1961a).
— — PALAGI, L., COLAGRANDE, C., BASCHIERI, I., RIBOTTA, S., MARINOSCI, M.: Observations roentgen-cinématographiques et électronmanométriques sur la motilité des voies biliaires. Sem. Hôp. Paris **37,** 790—802 (1961b).
TRACY, H. J., GREGORY, R. A.: Physiological properties of a series of synthetic peptides structurally related to gastrin I. Nature **204,** 935—938 (1964).
TUMPSON, D. B., JOHNSON, L. R.: Effect of secretin and cholecystokinin on the response of the gastric fistula rat to pentagastrin (33835). Proc. Soc. exp. Biol. (N.Y.) **131,** 186—188 (1969).
TUPPY, H.: The influence of enzymes on neurohypophyseal hormones and similar peptides. In Handbuch der experimentellen Pharmakologie XXIII, p. 67, edit. by O. EICHLER, A. FARAH, H. HERKEN, and A. D. WELCH. Berlin, Heidelberg, Springer 1968.
UDÉN, R.: Effect of secretin in celiac and superior mesenteric angiography **8,** 497—513 (1969).
ULLRICH, K. J., THURAU, K.: Technische Hilfsmittel bei der Punktion von Nierentubuli und Blutkapillaren. Leitz-Mitt. Wiss. u. Techn. Bd II/3, S. 85 (1962).
UNGER, R. H.: The gastrointestinal hormones as modifiers of islet cell hormone function. NOBEL Symposium XVI. Frontiers in Gastrointestinal Hormone Research, Stockholm, July 20—21, 1970; (In press), edit. by S. ANDERSSON. Upsala: Almqvist and Wiksell 1972.
— EISENTRAUT, A. M., MCCALL, M. S., MADISON, L. L.: Glucagon antibodies and an immunoassay for glucagon. J. Clin. Invest. **40,** 1280—1289 (1961).
— KETTERER, H., EISENTRAUT, A., DUPRÉ, J.: Effect of secretin on insulin secretion. Lancet **1966 II,** 24—26 (1966).
— — DUPRÉ, J., EISENTRAUT, A. M.: The effects of secretin, pancreozymin and gastrin upon insulin and glucagon secretion in anesthetized dogs. J. Clin. Invest. **46,** 630—645 (1967).
UVNÄS, B.: The part played by the pyloric region in the cephalic phase of gastric secretion. Acta Physiol. Scand. 4, Suppl. 13 (1942).
— Is the secretion of pepsin hormonally controlled? Acta Physiol. Scand. **15,** 438—445 (1948).
— Mechanism of gastrin release. In: Abstr. XXII Internat. Congr. Physiol. Sciences **1,** 342—347 (1962).
— Gastrin and vagus. In: Proc. Internat. Un. Physiol. Sciences Vol. VI, pp. 189—190· 24 Internat. Congr. Washington 1968.
— Role of duodenum in inhibition of gastric acid secretion. Scand. J. Gastroenterology **6,** 113—125 (1971).

UVNÄS, B., ÅBORG, C.-H., BERGENDORFF, A.: Storage of histamine in mast cells. Evidence for an ionic binding of histamine to protein carboxyls in the granule heparin-protein complex. Acta Physiol. Scand. **78**, Supplement No 336, pp. 1—26 (1970).
— EMÅS, S., FYRÖ, B., SJÖDIN, L.: The interaction between vagal impulses and gastrin in the control of gastric acid secretion. Amer. J. Digest. Dis. N.S. **11**, 103—112 (1966).
VAGNE, M.: Contribution à l'étude physio-pharmacologique des hormones gastrointestinales. Thèse. Université de Lyon. Section de Pharmacie, 1969.
— Les hormones gastro-intestinales. I. La gastrine. Pathol. Biol. (Paris) **18**, 887—904 (1970a).
— ANDRE, CL.: The effect of secretin on gastric emptying in man. Gastroenterology **60**, 421—424 (1971).
— DESCOS, L., MARTIN, P.: La sécrétion bicarbonatée maximum du pancréas humain. C. R. Soc. Biol. **163**, 1403—1406 (1969).
— GROSSMAN, M. I.: Comparison of intravenous and subcutaneous secretin. Gastroenterology **54**, 907—912 (1968a).
— — Cholecystokinetic potency of gastrointestinal hormones and related peptides. Amer. J. Physiol. **215**, 881—884 (1968b).
— STENING, G. F., BROOKS, F. P., GROSSMAN, M. I.: Synthetic secretin: comparison with natural secretin for potency and spectrum of physiological actions. Gastroenterology **55**, 260—267 (1968).
— GROSSMAN, M. I.: Gastric and pancreatic secretion in response to gastric distension in dogs. Gastroenterology **57**, 300—310 (1969).
WAITMAN, A. M., DYCK, W. P., JANOWITZ, H. D.: Effect of secretin and acetazolamide on the volume and electrolyte composition of hepatic bile in man. Gastroenterology **56**, 286—294 (1969).
WAKIM, K. G.: Reassessment of the source, mode and locus of action of antidiuretic hormone. Amer. J. Med. **42**, 394—411 (1967).
WALEY, S. G., WATSON, J.: The action of trypsin on polylysine. Biochem. J. **55**, 328—337 (1953).
WALTHER, A. A.: Die sekretorische Arbeit der Bauchspeicheldrüse. Diss. St. Petersburg, 1897.
VANDERPOOL, D., KLINGENSMITH, W., OLES, P.: Congenital absence of the gallbladder. Amer. Surgeon **30**, 324—333 (1964).
WANG, C. C., GROSSMAN, M. I.: Physiological determination of release of secretin and pancreozymin from intestine of dogs with transplanted pancreas. Amer. J. Physiol. **164**, 527—544 (1951).
— — IVY, A. C.: Effect of secretin and pancreozymin on amylase and alkaline phosphatase secretion by the pancreas in dogs. Amer. J. Physiol. **154**, 358—368 (1948).
WARNES, T. W., HINE, P., KAY, G.: The action of secretin and pancreozymin an small intestinal alkaline phosphatase. In: Abstr. 4th World Congress of Gastroenterology, p. 131, edit. by P. RIIS, P. ANTHONISEN and H. BADEN, Copenhagen, 1970.
WASTELL, C., RUDICK, J., DREILING, D. A.: Diffusion of bicarbonate across pancreatic duct epithelium. Surg. Forum **17**, 339—341 (1966).
— — — Bicarbonate-chloride exchange across pancreatic duct epithelium in dogs. Amer. J. Gastroenterol. **52**, 99—110 (1969).
WAY, L. W.: The concept of potentiation. A reply. Gastroenterology **57**, 619—622 (1969).
— The effect of secretin on acid secretion in response to cholinergic stimuli. Clin. Res. **18**, 175 (1970).
— Effect of cholecystokinin and caerulein on gastric secretion in cats. Gastroenterology **60**, 560—565 (1971).
— DIAMOND, J. M.: The effect of secretin on electrical potential differences in the pancreatic duct. Biochim. Biophys. Acta **203**, 298—307 (1970).
— GROSSMAN, I.: Pancreatic stimulation by duodenal acid and exogenous hormones in conscious cats. Amer. J. Physiol. **219**, 449—454 (1970).
— JOHNSON, L. R., GROSSMAN, M. I.: Comparison of pancreatic response to portal and systemic venous administration of secretin, cholecystokinin and caerulein. Fed. Proc. **28** (2), 274 (1969).
WEAVER, M. M.: Distribution of pancreatic secretin in the gastrointestinal tract. Amer. J. Physiol. **82**, 106—112 (1927).
— Studies on the visceral vasomotor responses to intravenous injection of purified pancreatic secretin. Amer. J. Physiol. **85**, 410—411 (1928).
— LUCKHARDT, A. B., KOCH, F. C.: Preparation of potent vasodilatin free pancreatic secretin. J. Amer. Med. Ass. **87**, 640—645 (1926).
WEBSTER, P. D.: Comparison of metabolic and secretory effects of methacholine and pancreozymin on the pancreas. Gastroenterology **56**, 1267 (1969a).
— Hormonal control of pancreatic acinar cell metabolism. In: The Exocrine Glands. pp. 153—169, edit. by S. Y. BOTELHO, F. P. BROOKS and W. B. SHELLEY. Philadelphia: Univ. Pennsylvania Press 1969b.

WEMSTER, P. D., GUNN, L. D., TYOR, M. P.: Effect of in vivo pancreozymin and metacholien on pancreatic lipid metabolism. Amer. J. Physiol. **211**, 781—785 (1966).
— TYOR, M. P.: Effect of intravenous pancreozymin on amino acid incorporation *in vitro* by pancreatic tissue. Amer. J. Physiol. **211**, 157—160 (1966).
VEGA, R. E., APPERT, H. E., HOWARD, J. M.: Effects of secretin in stimulating the output of amylase and lipase in the thoracic duct of the dog. Annals of Surgery **166**, 995—1001 (1967).
WEINSTEIN, B.: On the relationship between glucagon and secretin. Experientia **24**, 406—408 (1968).
VENABLES, C. W., RUDICK, J., KARK, A., DREILING, D. A.: Effects of commercial pancreozymin preparation (Cecekin) and gastrin pentapeptide upon acid and pepsin secretion in gastric fistula dogs. J. Surg. Research **9**, 55—60 (1969).
WERNER, B.: Invärtesmedicinska synpunkter på pankreasfunktionen. Nord. Med. **55**, 169—170 (1956).
— MUTT, V.: The pancreatic response in man to the injection of highly purified secretin and of pancreozymin. Scand. J. Clin. Lab. Invest. **6**, 228—236 (1954).
WERTHEIMER, E.: Sur le méchanisme de la sécrétion pancréatique. C. R. Soc. Biol. **54**, 472—474 (1902a).
— Sur le mode d'association fonctionelle du pancréas avec l'intestin. C. R. Soc. Biol. **54**, 474—476 (1902b).
— De l'action des acides et du chloral sur la sécrétion biliaire. C. R. Soc. Biol. **55**, 286—287 (1903).
— DUVILLIER, E.: Sur l'absorption de la sécrétine. C. R. Soc. Biol. **68**, 535—537 (1910).
— LEPAGE, L.: Sur les fonctions réflexes des ganglions abdominaux du sympathique dans l'innervation sécrétoire du pancréas. J. Physiol. Path. Gén. **3**, 335—348 (1901a).
— — Sur les fonctions réflexes des ganglions abdominaux du sympathique dans l'innervation sécrétoire du pancréas. J. Physiol. Pathol. Gén. **3**, 363—374 (1901b).
— — Sur l'association réflexe du pancréas avec l'intestin grêle. J. Physiol. Path. Gén. **3**, 689—702 (1901c).
— — Sur l'association réflexe du pancréas avec l'intestin grêle. J. Physiol. Path. Gén. **3**, 708—718 (1901d).
— — Des réflexes ganglionnaires chez les animaux chloroformés. J. Physiol. Pathol. Gén. **4**, 1061—1070 (1902).
WHEELER, H. O.: Inorganic ions in bile. In: The Biliary System. Symposium Nato Advanced Study Institute, pp. 481—493, edit. by W. TAYLOR, Oxford. Blackwell Scientif. Publications 1965.
— MANCUSI-UNGARO, P. L.: Role of bile ducts during secretin choleresis in dogs. Amer. J. Physiol. **210**, 1153—1159 (1966).
— RAMOS, O. L.: Determination of flow and composition of bile in the unanesthetized dog during constant infusion of sodium taurocholate. J. Clin. Invest. **39**, 161—170 (1960).
WHITAKER, L. R.: The mechanism of the gallbladder. Amer. J. Physiol. **78**, 411—436 (1926).
— MILLIKEN, G.: A comparison of sodium tetrabrom- and sodium tetraiodophenolphthalein in gallbladder radiography. Surg. Gyn. Obstet. **40**, 17—21 (1925).
WILANDER, O., ÅGREN, G.: Standardisierung von Sekretin. Biochem. Zeitschr. **250**, 489—495 (1932).
WILHELMJ, C. M., O'BRIEN, F. T., HILL, F. C.: The inhibitory influence of the acidity of the gastric contents on the secretion of acid by the stomach. Amer. J. Physiol. **115**, 429—440 (1936).
— MCCARTHY, H. H., HILL, F. C.: Acid inhibition of the intestinal and intragastric chemical phases of gastric secretion. Amer. J. Physiol. **118**, 766—774 (1937a).
— FINEGAN, R. W., HILL, F. C.: The physiological control of gastric acidity. Amer. J. digest. Dis. **4**, 547 (1937b).
— MCCARTHY, H. H., HILL, F. C.: Acid inhibition and the cephalic (psychic) phase of gastric secretion. Amer. J. Physiol. **120**, 619—623 (1937c).
VOKAC, V., SVATOS, A.: Die Ausscheidung von Urocholezystokinin bei Patienten nach Magensektion. Dtsch. Zeitschr. f. Verdauungs- u. Stoffwechselkrankheiten **21**, 213—216 (1962).
VOLBORTH, G. W.: The presence of secretin in the intestinal juice. Amer. J. Physiol. **72**, 331—336 (1925).
WOODS, L. P.: Secretin inhibition of gastric hydrochloric acid in human beings. Surg. Forum **16**, 315—317 (1965).
WOODWARD, E. R., LYON, S. E., LANDOR, J., DRAGSTEDT, L. R.: The physiology of the gastric antrum; experimental studies on isolated antrum pouches in dogs. Gastroenterology **27**, 766—785 (1954).
— DRAGSTEDT, L. R.: Role of pyloric antrum in regulation of gastric secretion. Physiol. Rev. **40**, 490—504 (1960).

WORMSLEY, K. G.: The action of secretin on the secretion of enzymes by the human pancreas. Scand. J. Gastroent. **3**, 183—188 (1968a).
— Gastric response to secretin and pancreozymin in man. Scand. J. Gastroenterology **3**, 632—636 (1968b).
— Response to secretin in man. Gastroenterology **54**, 197—209 (1968c).
— Response to secretin and pancreozymin in man. J. Physiol. (Lond.) **203**, 53P—54P (1969a).
— A comparison of the response to secretin, pancreozymin and a combination of these hormones, in man. Scand. J. Gastroent. **4**, 413—417 (1969b).
— The response to infusion of a combination of secretin and pancreozymin in health and disease. Scand. J. Gastroent. **4**, 623—632 (1969c).
— GROSSMAN, M. I.: Inhibition of gastric acid secretion by secretin and by endogeneous acid in the duodenum. Gastroenterology **47**, 72—81 (1964).
— MAHONEY, M. P., KAY, G.: Gastric response to subcutaneous injection of a gastrin like pentapeptide. Gut **8**, 475—481 (1967).
— — NG, M.: Effects of a gastrin-like pentapeptide (ICI 50, 123) on stomach and pancreas. Lancet **1966 I**, 993—996.
YALOW, R. S., BERSON, S. A.: Assay of plasma insulin in human subjects by immunological methods. Nature **184**, 1648—1649 (1959).
— — Size and charge distinctions between endogenous human plasma gastrin in peripheral blood and heptadecapeptide gastrins. Gastroenterology **58**, 609—615 (1970).
— — State of endogenous gastrin in blood and tissues. In: NOBEL Symposium on Frontiers in Gastrointestinal Hormone Research. (In press), edit. by S. ANDERSSON, Upsala, Almqvist and Wiksell: 1972.
— — Immunoassay of endogenous plasma insulin in man. J. Clin. Invest. **39**, 1157—1195 (1960a).
— — Plasma insulin concentrations in nondiabetic and early diabetic subjects determined by a new sensitive immuno-assay technique. Diabetes **9**, 254—260 (1960b).
— BLACK, H., VILLAZON, M., BERSON, S. A.: Comparison of plasma insulin levels following administration of tolbutamide and glucose. Diabetes **9**, 356—362 (1960).
YAMASHINA, I.: Studies on enterokinase. I Purification and general properties. Arkiv f. Kemi **7**, 539—543 (1955).
— Studies on enterokinase. II The further purification. Arkiv f. Kemi **9**, 225—229 (1956a).
— The action of enterokinase on trypsinogen. Acta Chem. Scand. **10**, 739—743 (1956b).
— The action of enterokinase on trypsinogen. Biochem. Biophys. Acta **20**, 433—434 (1956c).
YANG, J., DICKMAN, S. R.: Effects of pancreozymin, urecholine and actinomycin D on the metobalism of ribonucleic acid in canine pancreas. Biochem. J. **100**, 548—555 (1966).
YMAN, L.: Studies on human serum aminopeptidases. Some properties of oxytocinase, human serum aminopeptidase A and leucine aminopeptidase and their purification from retroplacental serum. Acta Pharmaceut. Suecica, **7**, 75—86 (1970).
ZAJTCHUCK, R., AMATO, J. J., PALOYAN, E., BAKER, R. J.: Inhibition of pancreatic exocrine secretion by glucagon. Surg. Forum **18**, 410—411 (1967).
ZATERKA, S., GROSSMAN, M. I.: The effect of gastrin and histamine on secretion of bile. Gastroenterology **50**, 500—505 (1966).
ZELIONY, G. P., SAVICH, V. V.: On the mechanism of gastric secretion. (Russian). Proc. Med. Soc. St. Petersburg Jan.—May 1911/12.
— — Sur la sécrétion de la pepsine. C. R. Soc. Biol. **77**, 50—52 (1914).
ZIEVE, L., MULFORD, B.: Secretion of pancreatic enzymes. III. Response of patients with cirrhosis to secretin and pancreozymin. Amer. J. Dig. Dis. N.S. **12**, 303—309 (1967).
ZUNZ, E., LA BARRE, J.: Hyperinsulinémie consécutive à l'injection de solution de sécrétine nonhypotensive. C. R. Soc. Biol. **98**, 1435—1438 (1928).

Chapter II

The Synthesis of (Porcine) Secretin

A. Introduction

MIKLOS BODANSZKY

With 6 Figures

The elucidation of structure and the synthesis of oxytocin (VINCENT DU VIGNEAUD et al., 1953) marks the beginning of a new era in the chemistry of peptide hormones. Soon it became obvious that the synthetic approach to peptide hormones and their analogs can serve several purposes. Proof by synthesis can be provided for the correctness of proposed amino acid sequences, the relationships between structure and hormonal activities can be studied through synthetic hormone analogs and biologically important materials can be made available for medicine in high purity and practically unlimited quantities. Finally, one should admit that beyond these rational reasons, the synthesis of molecules of unusual size and complexity is challenging enough to tempt the peptide chemists into arduous and laborious endeavors.

An impressive series of peptide hormones were synthesized within a few years: vasopressin, angiotensin, the melanocyte-stimulating hormones, corticotropins, bradykinin, gastrin, thyrocalcitonin, and a most remarkable accomplishment, insulin. It is rather surprising therefore that a hormone known since the earliest years of this century, the factor for which the word "hormone" was coined, has not become the subject of synthetic experimentation. The obvious reason for this delay lies in the hard fact that for more than half a century secretin resisted the vigorous attempts of many investigators and has not been obtained in pure form. Only as late as 1961 was the isolation of secretin reported from the Karolinska Institutet by Professor J. Erik JORPES and Dozent Viktor MUTT (JORPES and MUTT, 1961). Their efforts, of many years, requiring tremendous amounts of hog intestines, the employment of a combination of refined separation and fractionation techniques, led to a fruitful conclusion. The delicate molecule of secretin, a peptide containing 27 amino acid constituents, was isolated in pure form and in quantities which were sufficient for structural studies. These studies, again in the hands of MUTT, JORPES and their associates, revealed the amino acid composition (JORPES, MUTT, MAGNUSSON and STEELE, 1962), partial sequences (MUTT, MAGNUSSON, JORPES and DAHL, 1965) and finally the full sequence of the amino acid constituents of secretin (MUTT and JORPES, 1966) (Fig. 1).

His-Ser-Asp-Gly-Thr-Phe-Thr-Ser-Glu-Leu-Ser-Arg-Leu-Arg-
1 2 3 4 5 6 7 8 9 10 11 12 13 14
Asp-Ser-Ala-Arg-Leu-Gln-Arg-Leu-Leu-Gln-Gly-Leu-Val-NH_2
15 16 17 18 19 20 21 22 23 24 25 26 27

Fig. 1

In 1964 the structural studies had advanced far enough to allow the proposal of a tentative sequence. During a visit to the Karolinska Institute in the last days of August, 1964, this author had the privilege of being informed prior to publication about the tentative structure of secretin. Upon his return to the U. S., the synthetic effort suggested by JORPES and MUTT was immediately started at the Squibb Institute for Medical Research. Within a month or two, a synthetic hexapeptide amide, corresponding to the carboxyl terminal tryptic fragment of the hormone, was sent to Stockholm where Dr. MUTT compared it with the natural material and found them to be indistinguishable from each other. A similar comparison was made on the carboxyl terminal tridecapeptide, a thrombic fragment, and again the natural and the synthetic preparations were found to be identical in all respects. There were two minor revisions made in the N-terminal part of the sequence, but the above comparisons showed that for the carboxyl terminal half of the molecule the first tentative structure needed no correction and could be considered as final. These reassuring results gave new impetus to the work of the Squibb group and a few months later, early in 1966, a synthetic sample, (BODANSZKY et al., 1966) a rather crude preparation, was sent from New Brunswick to Stockholm. The biological activity it revealed led to elated transatlantic telephone conversations.

All three attempted synthetic pathways, only two of them successful, will be reported in the following pages, because this may give a more truthful rendering of the experimental effort. Also, this will indicate the double purpose of the synthesis: to close a glorious chapter of more than 60 years of secretin research and to explore the ways and means, tactics and strategies toward the synthesis of long peptide chains, like those of proteins.

B. Strategies

An already classical approach to the building of long peptide chains is the condensation of fragments. For the preparation of an octapeptide, two tetrapeptide derivatives can be coupled, each in turn synthesized by linking appropriate dipeptides to each other. Such schemes were and are still successfully applied in the synthesis of most peptide hormones. This strategy requires the minimum number of steps and, at least in principle, if the calculations are based on the amounts of the starting amino acids, should give the highest overall yields. However, since coupling of peptides generally involves racemization of the C-terminal acid of the protected peptide used as acylating agent, the fragments to be linked to each other have to be prepared through stepwise synthesis, starting from the C-terminus of each peptide with the addition of single protected amino acids. For the coupling of peptides only the azide method (CURTIUS, 1902), indeed the oldest known procedure, can be used without the risk of racemization. Unfortunately, the azide method can yield many byproducts; thus while racemization is avoided the products often contain, instead of diastereo-isomers, other undesired materials.

To gain more freedom in the choice of coupling methods, the long chains to be synthesized are "dissected" into fragments in such a way that these segments should have proline or glycine as C-terminal acids, because proline is quite resistant to racemization, and glycine has no center of asymmetry. As shown in the more detailed discussion of the fragment condensation approach, secretin is not eminently suitable for such dissection of its sequence: it contains only two glycine moieties in moderately advantageous positions, and no proline residue.

Although "a priori" it would be an attractive procedure, the building of long peptide chains in the way of stepwise addition of amino acids starting with the N-terminal acid is not possible with the presently available coupling methods. While the suitably masked amino acids are protected not only against unwanted acylation, but against racemization as well, this protection does not function when protecting groups and activated carboxyl groups do not belong to the same amino acid, and this is the case in peptides. Therefore the only stepwise procedure which can be envisaged at this time is the one in which the C-terminal amino acid is the starting point of the synthesis. This "stepwise strategy from the C-terminus" seemed to be impractical for considerable time and only with the advent of the active ester method of coupling could it be considered for the synthesis of long chains. After the introduction of nitrophenyl esters of protected amino acids (Bodanszky, 1955), the stepwise strategy was proposed (Bodanszky, 1960), and used first for the preparation of oxytocin (Bodanszky and du Vigneaud, 1959), and later for the vasopressins (Bodanszky, Meienhofer and du Vigneaud, 1960), and many of their analogs. A combination of the stepwise approach with fragment condensation was applied in the synthesis of larger peptides such as β-corticotropin (Schwyzer and Sieber, 1966).

The use of the entirely stepwise approach received new impetus with the introduction of the solid phase technique (Merrifield, 1963). The possibility of mechanization and automation of peptide synthesis based on the entirely stepwise strategy was predicted as early as 1960 (Bodanszky, 1960). The prediction turned into reality only when the technical execution of peptide synthesis on a solid support was ingeniously developed in the Rockefeller Institute (Merrifield, 1963).

The synthesis of the "first hormone" was considered to be an objective important enough to warrant simultaneous attack by all the three discussed approaches: solid phase synthesis, entirely stepwise synthesis through isolated intermediates, and synthesis by fragment condensation.

C. Attempted Synthesis of Secretin on a Solid Support

The Merrifield method (Fig. 2) scored a number of remarkable successes. Its far-reaching possibilities were first demonstrated in the synthesis of bradykinin (Merrifield, 1964). This was soon followed by a spectacular synthesis of angiotensin (Marshall and Merrifield, 1965). The most noteworthy accomplishment so far in this area is represented by the synthesis of the individual insulin chains (Merrifield, 1966). Needless to say that the community of peptide chemists was not left unimpressed and these results led to wide acclaim and great expectations. The expectations, however, were not completely fulfilled. The solid phase method obviously needs some improvements.

For the elimination of some minor shortcomings of this technique, several suggestions were made (Bodanszky and Sheehan, 1964). Improvements in the formation of the ester bond between the first amino acid and the resin, replacement of the "overactivating" dicyclohexylcarbodiimide method by the less drastic acylation with active esters, resulted also in increased possibilities of monitoring the completion of the acylations (Bodanszky and Sheehan, 1966). In the incorporation of glutamine and especially of asparagine the use of active esters instead of carbodiimide coupling is quite imperative. The hydroxyamino acids serine and threonine can be left with their hydroxyl functions unprotected only if active esters are used and certainly not with carbodiimides as coupling reagents. All these partial corrections did not provide a remedy for a serious limitation of the solid phase synthesis: the completed peptide chain can be removed from the solid support as an acid but not always in the form of a peptide amide.

Many biologically important peptides (oxytocin, vasopressin, vasotocin, gastrin, secretin, physalaemin, eledoisin, etc.) have an amino acid amide as their C-terminus: therefore, this problem cannot be belittled. In an early model experiment (BODANSZKY and SHEEHAN. 1964), the protected C-terminal tripeptide sequence of oxytocin, benzyloxycarbonyl-L-prolyl-L-leucylglycine was built up on the solid support and the peptide was separated from the resin by treatment with a methanolic solution of ammonia. The product, the protected tripeptide amide, was obtained in moderate yield, but the experiment was still somewhat encouraging. On the other hand, while this tripeptide had glycine as its C-terminal amino acid, in secretin valine is in the same position and it is well known that steric hindrance by the isopropyl side chain of valine is quite noticeable in the aminolysis and ammonolysis of valine esters. Therefore first the ammonolysis of benzyloxycarbonyl-L-valine-resin ester was examined. In about a day all the protected amino acid was removed from the resin, but only about one fifth of the product turned out to be the desired amide, the major portion was found to be benzyloxycarbonyl-L-valine methyl ester. Seemingly, the steric hindrance prevails more in ammonolysis than in transesterification. Of course this gave no serious reason for concern since by prolonged ammonolysis the methyl ester could be converted into the desired amide. In the next experiment the protected C-terminal hexapeptide sequence of secretin, L-leucyl-L-leucyl-L-glutaminylglycyl-L-leucyl-L-valine, was built up on the MERRIFIELD resin. In the synthesis of this sequence p-nitrophenyl esters of the protected amino acids were applied for acylation and the completion of each coupling was ascertained by the determination (UV absorption) of p-nitrophenol in the filtrate. The unreacted excess of the active ester was determined similarly. The protected hexapeptide on the resin was treated with methanolic ammonia. This time all the material was isolated as methyl ester, and practically no amide was found. The amide, however, could be made by a prolonged exposure of the protected hexapeptide methyl ester to ammonia in methanol. Obviously the combined hindering effects from the valine side chain, the resin matrix and the peptide chain led to this result (BODANSZKY and SHEEHAN, 1966).

Since it still seemed to be possible to continue the synthesis in this manner, the stepwise lengthening of the peptide was continued until the tridecapeptide sequence, tert-butyloxycarbonyl-β-benzyl-L-aspartyl-0-benzyl-L-seryl-L-alanyl-nitro-L-arginyl-L-leucyl-L-glutaminyl-nitro-L-arginyl-L-leucyl-L-leucyl-L-glutaminylglycyl-L-leucyl-L-valine attached to the resin by an ester bond was prepared. In this case the chain withstood many vigorous attempts and could not be removed by ammonolysis or ester exchange. That the peptide was indeed present on the polymeric support was shown by its removal with hydrobromic acid in acetic acid, but this treatment resulted of course in a peptide acid and not in the peptide amide which is necessary for the synthesis of secretin. At this point our attempt to synthesize secretin on a solid support had to be abandoned.

D. Synthesis of Secretin by the Stepwise Approach (Through Isolated Intermediates)

In most respects this synthesis (BODANSZKY and WILLIAMS, 1967; BODANSZKY, ONDETTI, LEVINE and WILLIAMS, 1967) was based on the synthesis of oxytocin by the stepwise nitrophenyl ester method (BODANSZKY and DU VIGNEAUD, 1959). The first amide bond was produced by the ammonolysis of benzyloxycarbonyl-L-valine p-nitrophenyl ester. The protecting group was removed from the resulting amide by treatment with hydrobromic acid in glacial acetic acid and the next amino acid L-leucine was introduced via benzyloxycarbonyl-L-leucine p-nitrophenyl ester. The chain was lengthened in the same manner until the C-terminal hexapeptide amide, L-leucyl-L-leucyl-L-glutaminyl-glycyl-L-leucyl-L-valinamide was in hand. All the intermediates so far were secured in excellent yield and in crystalline form. The next amino acid was applied as benzyloxycarbonyl-L-arginine 2,4-dinitrophenyl ester (BODANSZKY and ONDETTI, 1966). The nitroguanidine derivative was chosen as the protected form of arginine because the nitro group can be removed by hydrogenolysis, a rather mild operation. The sensitivity of secretin to sodium in liquid ammonia was unknown and therefore the tosyl-protection of arginine could not be considered. The different side chain protecting groups were selected in such a way that all should be removed in a single step by hydrogenolysis at the completion of the synthetic procedure. These considerations, the nitro protecting group on the arginine moieties introduced some limitation in the choice of methods of activation: the p-nitrophenyl ester of benzyloxycarbonyl-(and of t-butyloxycarbonyl)-nitro-L-arginine is difficult to prepare and is unstable (BODANSZKY and SHEEHAN, 1960). The 2,4-dinitrophenyl esters are more suitable intermediates; they still show some shortcomings, e. g. they are readily hydrolysed by traces of water that is often present in the commonly used solvent, dimethylformamide. The L-threonine residues were also incorporated through 2,4-dinitrophenyl esters. The hydroxyl group of L-serine, the side chain carboxyl groups of the glutamic acid and aspartic acid residues were all protected by benzyl groups.

The protected hendecapeptide derivative benzyloxycarbonyl-L-alanyl-nitro-L-arginyl-L-leucyl-L-glutaminyl-nitro-L-arginyl-L-leucyl-L-leucyl-L-glutaminyl-glycyl-L-leucyl-L-valinamide was the last intermediate that was prepared with benzyloxycarbonyl (BERGMANN and ZERVAS, 1932) as aminoprotecting group. Since the nitro group on the arginine residues had to be kept intact all the way during the chain lengthening procedure, hydrogenolysis could not be applied for the removal of the benzyloxycarbonyl protection. The only remaining practical method, treatment with hydrobromic acid in acetic acid leads to a partial 0-acetylation of the serine residues. Therefore when in the preparation of the protected dodecapeptide a derivate of L-serine had to be chosen, 0-benzyl-L-serine was protected on its amino function not by the benzyloxycarbonyl but by tert. butyloxycarbonyl grouping (MCKAY and ALBERTSON, 1957; ANDERSON and MCGREGOR, 1957; SCHWYZER, SIEBER and KAPPELER, 1959), because the latter can be removed by a comparatively mild treatment with acids, e.g. with trifluoroacetic acid at room temperature within a few minutes. Of course the tert. butyloxycarbonyl protection had to be applied throughout the rest of the lengthening of the chain, except in the addition of the N-terminal amino acid, histidine. For the preparation of the last protected intermediate, the heptacosapeptide derivative N-benzyloxycarbonyl-L-histidyl-0-benzyl-L-seryl-β-benzyl-L-aspartyl-glycyl-L-threonyl-L-phenylalanyl-L-threonyl-0-benzyl-L-seryl-γ-benzyl-L-glutamyl-L-leucyl-0-benzyl-L-seryl-nitro-L-arginyl-L-leucyl-nitro-L-arginyl-β-benzyl-L-aspartyl-0-benzyl-L-seryl-L-alanyl-nitro-L-arginyl-L-leucyl-L-glutaminyl-nitro-L-arginyl-L-leucyl-L-leucyl-L-glutaminyl-glycyl-L-leucyl-L-valinamide the benzyloxycarbonyl group needs no selective removal. It is lost during the hydrogenolysis used for the removal of the benzyl protecting groups from the amino acid side chains. Therefore the histidine residue could be attached to the partially protected hexacosapeptide as benzyloxycarbonyl-L-histidine azide (HOLLEY and SONDHEIMER, 1954), or as bisbenzyloxycarbonyl-L-histidine p-nitrophenyl ester.

Without going into technical details, it still seems to be of interest to mention some general features in the execution of the synthesis. The protected peptides were dissolved in a small volume of trifluoroacetic acid. After about fifteen minutes at room temperature most of the trifluoroacetic acid was removed in vacuo and the amino-deprotected peptides were isolated from the residue by trituration with ether, filtration and washing the precipitate with ether. The trifluoroacetates thus obtained were white, nonhygroscopic solids. They were easy to handle and showed correct analytical values for nitrogen and fluorine. For the next step in the lengthening of the chain the trifluoroacetates were dissolved in dimethylformamide, the solutions were made slightly alkaline with triethylamine and the active ester of the next (protected) amino acid was added. The reactions were carried out at room temperature and the end of the acylation was observed by spotting a very small sample of the mixture on filter paper and testing with ninhydrin. A negative test indicates that the amino component (the already existing part of the chain to be lengthened) was completely acylated by the newly added amino acid. Normally, a few hours are sufficient for the completion of an acylation reaction. For practical reasons, however, the mixtures often were left to stand at room temperature overnight. The protected intermediates frequently separated as crystalline solids turning the reaction mixture into a semi-solid mass. For isolation ethyl acetate was added to the mixture, the insoluble peptide filtered, washed with ethyl acetate and dried. The simplicity of this procedure makes it questionable whether the solid phase techniques could be more convenient (except in the case of automation) than the entirely stepwise synthesis with active esters through isolated intermediates. The scheme of the synthesis of secretin according to this strategy is shown in Fig. 2.

The average yield in the lengthening of the chain by one amino acid was 94%. The fully protected intermediates were isolated in reasonably pure form, most of them were crystalline with correct values in elemental and amino acid analysis. Neither the analysis nor examinations by paperchromatography did reveal a subtle heterogeneity that was detected later in some intermediates, and which will be discussed below. Most of the intermediates were used without purification, but some preparations of the hydrobromide of the amino-deprotected hendecapeptide S_{17-27} were recrystallized from methanol and in some instances the protected tetradecapeptide derivative S_{14-27} was purified by countercurrent distribution in a system of butanol-pyridine-acetic acid and water.

The most characteristic feature of the synthesis by the entirely stepwise strategy is the use of excess acylating agent in a systematic manner. The excess, small in the first few steps, was gradually raised until near the end of the chain lengthening procedure about threefold excess was applied. The amounts of the acylating active esters were so calculated that their initial concentration at the start of the reaction should be at least 0.1 molar. In this way the reactions become pseudounimolecular, and some intramolecular side reactions can be suppressed. This seems to be the only solution to the problem of bimolecular reactions with reactants in low concentration, a problem particular to the synthesis of peptides of considerable length (Bodanszky and Bodanszky, 1967; Bodanszky, 1968).

The danger of racemization was not overlooked either during the chain lengthening procedure nor during the removal of protecting groups. The use of protected amino acids (rather than protected peptides) with a urethane type amino-protecting group prevents racemization by the azlactone mechanism (Bodanszky and Ondetti, 1966). Reversible β-elimination, a less common cause of racemization, had to be considered mainly in connection with the introduction of the 0-benzyl-L-serine residues. By avoiding an excess of base this type of

Val-NH_2
Leu-Val-NH_2
Gly-Leu-Val-NH_2
Gln-Gly-Leu-Val-NH_2
Leu-Gln-Gly-Leu-Val-NH_2
Leu-Leu-Gln-Gly-Leu-Val-NH_2
Arg-Leu-Leu-Gln-Gly-Leu-Val-NH_2
Gln-Arg-Leu-Leu-Gln-Gly-Leu-Val-NH_2
Leu-Gln-Arg-Leu-Leu-Gln-Gly-Leu-Val-NH_2
Arg-Leu-Gln-Arg-Leu-Leu-Gln-Gly-Leu-Val-NH_2
Ala-Arg-Leu-Gln-Arg-Leu-Leu-Gln-Gly-Leu-Val-NH_2
Ser-Ala-Arg-Leu-Gln-Arg-Leu-Leu-Gln-Gly-Leu-Val-NH_2
Asp-Ser-Ala-Arg-Leu-Gln-Arg-Leu-Leu-Gln-Gly-Leu-Val-NH_2
Arg-Asp-Ser-Ala-Arg-Leu-Gln-Arg-Leu-Leu-Gln-Gly-Leu-Val-NH_2
Leu-Arg-Asp-Ser-Ala-Arg-Leu-Gln-Arg-Leu-Leu-Gln-Gly-Leu-Val-NH_2
Arg-Leu-Arg-Asp-Ser-Ala-Arg-Leu-Gln-Arg-Leu-Leu-Gln-Gly-Leu-Val-NH_2
Ser-Arg-Leu-Arg-Asp-Ser-Ala-Arg-Leu-Gln-Arg-Leu-Leu-Gln-Gly-Leu-Val-NH_2
Leu-Ser-Arg-Leu-Arg-Asp-Ser-Ala-Arg-Leu-Gln-Arg-Leu-Leu-Gln-Gly-Leu-Val-NH_2
Glu-Leu-Ser-Arg-Leu-Arg-Asp-Ser-Ala-Arg-Leu-Gln-Arg-Leu-Leu-Gln-Gly-Leu-Val-NH_2
Ser-Glu-Leu-Ser-Arg-Leu-Arg-Asp-Ser-Ala-Arg-Leu-Gln-Arg-Leu-Leu-Gln-Gly-Leu-Val-NH_2
Thr-Ser-Glu-Leu-Ser-Arg-Leu-Arg-Asp-Ser-Ala-Arg-Leu-Gln-Arg-Leu-Leu-Gln-Gly-Leu-Val-NH_2
Phe-Thr-Ser-Glu-Leu-Ser-Arg-Leu-Arg-Asp-Ser-Ala-Arg-Leu-Gln-Arg-Leu-Leu-Gln-Gly-Leu-Val-NH_2
Thr-Phe-Thr-Ser-Glu-Leu-Ser-Arg-Leu-Arg-Asp-Ser-Ala-Arg-Leu-Gln-Arg-Leu-Leu-Gln-Gly-Leu-Val-NH_2
Gly-Thr-Phe-Thr-Ser-Glu-Leu-Ser-Arg-Leu-Arg-Asp-Ser-Ala-Arg-Leu-Gln-Arg-Leu-Leu-Gln-Gly-Leu-Val-NH_2
Asp-Gly-Thr-Phe-Thr-Ser-Glu-Leu-Ser-Arg-Leu-Arg-Asp-Ser-Ala-Arg-Leu-Gln-Arg-Leu-Leu-Gln-Gly-Leu-Val-NH_2
Ser-Asp-Gly-Thr-Phe-Thr-Ser-Glu-Leu-Ser-Arg-Leu-Arg-Asp-Ser-Ala-Arg-Leu-Gln-Arg-Leu-Leu-Gln-Gly-Leu-Val-NH_2
His-Ser-Asp-Gly-Thr-Phe-Thr-Ser-Glu-Leu-Ser-Arg-Leu-Arg-Asp-Ser-Ala-Arg-Leu-Gln-Arg-Leu-Leu-Gln-Gly-Leu-Val-NH_2
1 2 3 4 5 6 7 8 9 10 11 12 13 14 15 16 17 18 19 20 21 22 23 24 25 26 27

Fig. 2. The entirely stepwise strategy

racemization can be kept at a minimum. Triethylamine used for the liberation of the free amines from their salts was added to the reaction mixture until a weak alkaline reaction was seen on a piece of wet universal indicator paper held closely above the surface of the solution. This technique allows a rather accurate determination of the amount of tertiary base needed. The hindered amine, ethyldiisopropyl amine can prevent racemization that is not caused by azlactone formation (Bodanszky and Bodanszky, 1967a; Bodanszky and Bath, 1968), but at the time of the first synthesis of secretin this was not yet known.

The possible presence of diastereoisomers in the product was examined by digestion of the purified synthetic material with trypsin and leucine aminopeptidase. No evidence for racemization was found: no D-amino acid containing peptides could be detected and quantitative amino acid analysis of the enzymic digests gave the expected ratios of the component amino acids. Since these enzymic degradations were performed on the purified product, the possibility that racemization to some minor extent did occur and the undesirable diastereoisomers were removed in the purification, cannot be excluded. The crude synthetic material was certainly not pure. It showed a potency of about 1000—2000 clinical units per mg. while pure secretin contains about 4000 to 5000 units per mg. The byproducts were removed during purification that was based on the methods developed for the isolation of secretin from porcine intestines (JORPES and MUTT, 1961). Countercurrent distribution (CRAIG, 1968) in a butanol-phosphate buffer (pH 7) system followed by adsorption on alginic acid and elution with dilute hydrochloric acid led to substantial purification and trace impurities were eliminated by chromatography on a diethylaminoethyl-Sephadex G 25 column in acetate cycle. The synthetic hormone was eluted as the acetate salt and could be secured in solid form by lyophilization. The thus purified synthetic material is indistinguishable from pure preparations of natural porcine secretin when compared on paperchromatograms or electropherograms. Also no difference could be detected in the degradation products when natural and synthetic preparations were hydrolyzed with trypsin or thrombin in parallel experiments. A careful comparison of the qualitative and quantitative hormonal spectra completed the identification (VAGNE et al., 1968).

The nature of the byproducts in the crude preparations was not left without attention. One of the main concerns, the possibility of an aspartyl-aminosuccinyl-β-aspartyl rearrangement was in the focus of this investigation. A sample assaying only about 1000 units per mg. was degraded by trypsin and the five peptides S_{1-12} (b), S_{13-14} (d), S_{15-18} (a), S_{17-21} (c) and S_{22-27} (e) (MUTT, MAGNUSSON, JORPES and DAHL, 1965) were separated. Digestion with leucine aminopeptidase gave the expected molar ratios of amino acids in peptide "a" (S_{15-18}) and therefore no rearrangement of the aspartyl residue in position 15 could be assumed. On the other hand, when the N-terminal hexapeptide (S_{1-6}) was secured from a chymotryptic digest and was further degraded with leucine aminopeptidase the subsequent amino acid analysis suggested a partial rearrangement of the aspartyl residue in position 3. These findings offer some explanation for the lower activity of the crude synthetic preparations and might also explain the instability of secretin under certain conditions (e.g., in the attempted purification by countercurrent distribution in a butanol-pyridine acetic acid-water system). The aspartyl-glycyl sequence is probably more susceptible to the here described rearrangement than other aspartyl sequences, because the aminosuccinyl residue contains an N-diacyl group and it is well known (WIELAND and HEINKE, 1956; KOPPLE and RENICK, 1958) that among amino acids only glycine shows distinct readiness for the formation of N-diacyl derivatives. It should be emphasized that the complete digestibility with trypsin and leucine aminopeptidase of the *purified* synthetic preparations clearly shows that these do not contain aminosuccinyl or β-aspartyl residues.

The complete agreement between the physiological, physical and chemical properties of the synthetic and natural preparations of the hormone, together with the unambiguous nature of the synthetic procedure, which leaves no doubt about the sequence of amino acids in the intermediates and in the final product, serves as unequivocal evidence for the correctness of the structure proposed by MUTT and JORPES (1966) for porcine secretin.

E. Synthesis of Secretin by Fragment Condensation

Porcine secretin contains no proline and its two glycine residues are near to the two ends of the chain and do not allow a favorable "dissection" of the molecule. The fragments were selected, therefore, with the consideration that their C-terminal acid should not be one which is easily racemized.

The first plan for the fragment condensation synthesis of the hormone (ONDETTI et al., 1968) is shown in Fig. 3.

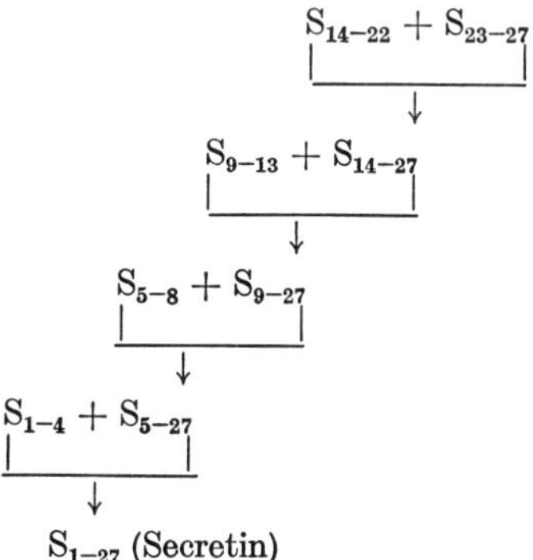

Fig. 3. Scheme of planned fragment condensation synthesis of secretin

The attempted condensation of S_{14-22} with S_{23-27} gave no practical results. During these attempts the desired tetradecapeptide derivative corresponding to sequence S_{14-27} became available through the stepwise approach described earlier. The plan therefore was accordingly changed and the first condensation step, the coupling of S_{14-22} to S_{23-27} was omitted. Synthesis of the S_{1-4}, S_{5-8} and S_{9-13} fragments is summarized in Fig. 4.

For the addition of S_{9-13} to the partially protected tetradecapeptide S_{14-27} the azide method of coupling was selected to avoid racemization of its C-terminal leucine. The next fragment used for the lengthening of the chain, S_{5-8}, had a serine residue at its C-terminal and this once more made it necessary to choose the azide procedure. In the last condensation step, the joining of S_{1-4} to the tricosapeptide derivative S_{5-27} racemization was out of the question since the N-terminal tetrapeptide sequence ends with a glycine residue. Nevertheless, the azide method was utilized again because, in exploratory experiments coupling with the aid of N,N-carbonyldiimidazole (STAAB, 1957; ANDERSON and PAUL, 1960) or 5-phenylisoxazolium-3-sulfonate (WOODWARD, OLOFSON and MAYER, 1961) and even the application of the mixed anhydrid procedure (WIELAND and BERNHARD, 1951) led to complicated mixtures.

In the execution of the azide method the elegantly simple conditions proposed by MEDZIHRADSZKY (1960) were followed. In order to ensure complete acylation and therefore full utilization of the more valuable amino components, a considerable excess of the protected peptide azide was added to the reaction mixtures, usually in several portions. In the first coupling step (S_{9-13} to S_{14-27}) the excess peptide material could be easily removed by extraction of the crude product (after removal of the tert. butyloxycarbonyl protecting group) with water. In the subsequent couplings (S_{5-8} to S_{9-27} and S_{1-4} to S_{5-27}) more elaborate purification procedures such as countercurrent distribution and ion exchange chromotography were needed for purification. In the linking of the azide from S_{9-13} to S_{14-27} the latter could be present either in partially protected or in fully deprotected form. In the last two condensation reactions all the protecting groups were removed from the amino components before acylation. The yields in these condensation steps were quite different in each case: 80% in the first, 50% in the second and 33% in the final coupling. The calculation of an overall yield is not warranted since such a single figure cannot express the significant sacrifices on those protected intermediates which were used in excess.

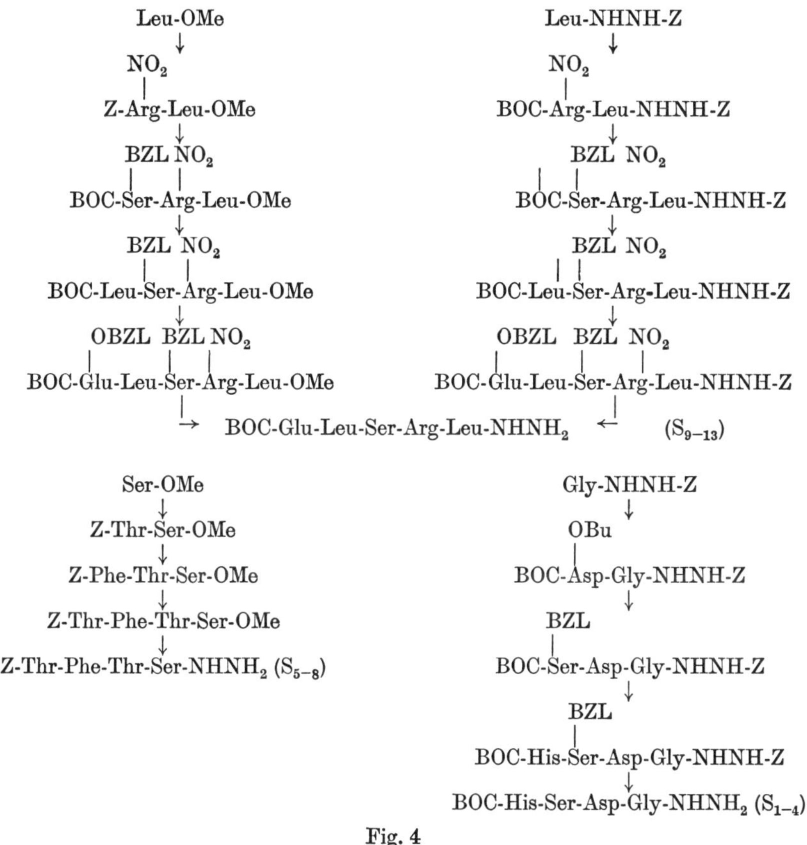

Fig. 4

The synthesis by fragment condensation followed, in a sense, a "stepwise" pattern as seen in Fig. 3. The systematic use of excess acylating agent is also a concept which originates from the stepwise strategy.

After the completion of the heptacosapeptide chain the tert. butyloxycarbonyl group was removed from the N-terminal amino acid by a brief treatment at room temperature with trifluoroacetic acid. The crude product was purified by countercurrent distribution and ion exchange chromatography as described in connection with the product obtained by stepwise synthesis. In all the already discussed physical, chemical and physiological tests the purified product was found to be indistinguishable from natural porcine secretin and also from the synthetic hormone prepared by the entirely stepwise strategy.

F. The Conformation of Secretin

The question, whether peptide hormones possess a certain architecture, a preferred conformation, raises itself rather naturally. It follows from our present knowledge of enzymes and other proteins with highly specific functions, that their architecture is a prerequisite for the specificity in their biological activities. In the case of hormones such a requirement is far from being obvious. They could even without possessing a particular conformation, develop one during the process of attachment to the receptor site. Nevertheless in some hormones the existence of a more or less defined geometry can be postulated from their covalent structure: the 20 membered ring lends considerable rigidity to the molecules of oxytocin, vasopressin and vasotocin and the three disulfide bridges introduce a serious limitation to the freedom of conformation in insulin. No such limitations can be assumed in single chain peptide hormones and unless the more subtle forces of hydrogen bonding and side chain interactions determine their geometry, corticotropin, bradykinin, angiotensin, gastrin, cholecystokinin-pancreozymin, caerulein, etc., should exist as random coils.

It is rather difficult to visualize, that any of the presently available techniques could give a definite answer to the question of conformation to oligopeptides. While the frequently heard objection to the X-ray chrystallographic description of protein architecture, that it is valid only for the solid state and not in solution, is probably not serious, such an objection could easily be raised in the case of smaller, single chain peptides. No drastic conformational change can be expected during crystallization of a highly complex, globular protein. A small, single chain, however, could undergo serious changes on crystallization, due to packing forces. Therefore, if and when X-ray crystallographic evidence for the architecture of peptide hormones will be forthcoming, it will have to be treated with certain reservation. At this time most of the peptide hormones are available only as amorphous solids. Their lack of readiness to crystallize is suggestive in itself. This could be the consequence of a conformational freedom absent in globular proteins, many of which were obtained in crystalline form.

Conformational analysis of proteins by means of rotational spectra has obvious limitations. The information deduced from spectral evidence can at best give some general description of the molecule, such as helix content, some types of folding, or perhaps the presence of cyclic areas. Nevertheless the examination of optical rotatory dispersion spectra is still the principal method of investigation for peptides and proteins not available in the crystalline form necessary for X-ray studies.

The identity of the optical rotatory dispersion (ORD) and circular dichroism (CD) spectra of natural and synthetic secretin contributed to the already substantial evidence supporting the structure proposed by MUTT and JORPES (1966). Moreover, these showed a striking resemblance to those of egg-lysozyme (PHILLIPS, 1966) and thus suggested a peptide chain with a low but definite helix content. In order to locate the helical part of the molecule the rotational spectra of peptides corresponding to partial sequences (S_{22-27}, S_{15-27}, S_{14-27}, S_{9-27}, S_{5-27}, S_{1-9} and S_{1-14}) were also studied (BODANSZKY, ONDETTI, MUTT and BODANSZKY, 1968).

The ORD and CD spectra of the C-terminal hexa-, trideca- and tetradecapeptides show with increasing chain length some increase in the values at their maxima and minima, but these spectra are not significantly different from those of peptides that are present as random coils. In the case of the nonadecapeptide S_{9-27} both the wavelength and the values of the Cotton effects are similar to those of a peptide with a low helix content. These characteristics are even more pronounced in the spectra of the tricosapeptide S_{5-27}. There is almost no additional change when the chain is further lengthened to the complete sequence (S_{1-27}) of secretin.

The absence in S_{14-27} and then the rather dramatic emergence of indication for a helical portion in S_{9-27} and even more in S_{5-27} suggest that this helical stretch lies between positions 5 and 14. Since no major difference can be found between the spectra of S_{5-27} and those of secretin, one has to assume that the N-terminal sequence S_{1-4} lies outside of the helical region. An inspection of the ORD and CD spectra of the N-terminal peptides S_{1-6} and S_{1-14} brought a disturbing contradiction into the picture: no helicity could be deduced from these spectra for the N-terminal half of the molecule.

This serious discrepancy was resolved and the harmony in the interpretation of the experimental data restored when the distribution of non-polar side chains was brought into consideration. Such hydrophobic resides are found in positions 6, 10, 13, 19, 22, 23, 26 and 27. From these the positions 6, 10 and 13 are in the region where a helix was suggested by the spectra of the C-terminal peptides. According to PERUTZ, KENDREW and WATSON (1965), hydrophobic residues are located on one side of helical stretches and helices are stabilized by hydrophobic bonds formed between the non polar side chains and an adjacent second hydrophobic region of the molecule. The absence of water in such hydrophobic pockets eliminates the competition of water molecules in the formation of hydrogen bonds and leads to a stabilization of the intrachain hydrogen bridges (KAUZMANN, 1964). Such a stabilizing effect is indeed badly needed in a helical stretch consisting of only two turns, which is probably the shortest helix that can exist as a preferred conformation. In secretin one such very short helix can be postulated; calculations based on the values of the rotational spectra do not allow a longer one. The assumption was made that the chain undergoes a general folding in such a way that the accumulation of amino acids carrying hydrophobic side chains (in positions 22, 23, 26, 27) comes close to the short helical region. This assumption removes the contradiction created by the rotational spectra of the N-terminal peptides: in these the stabilizing C-terminal positions are not present and thus the helix cannot exist. A schematic representation of the secondary structure that follows from these considerations is shown in Fig. 5.

That the distribution of non-polar amino acid residues is indeed meaningful and therefore the above assumptions are not arbitrary is illustrated by the distribution of hydrophobic side chains in the peptide hormone glucagon. It is well known that 14 of the amino acids of secretin are identical with 14 residues of glucagon in identical positions of the amino acid sequence. Secretin contains 8, glucagon 9 amino acids with hydrophobic side chains. Most of these non polar residues are not identical amino acids in the two sequences, yet they occupy identical positions as shown in Fig. 6. There cannot be much doubt that this remarkable analogy in the distribution of hydrophobic side chains is meaningful and has a conformation determining effect.

The biological activity of secretin is probably dependent on secondary structure. The hydrophobic pocket created by the side chains of the amino acids in positions 6, 10, 13 on one side and 22, 23, 26 and 27 on the other forms an "inside" of the molecule. The amino acids of the N-terminal nonhelical portion and those in the helix but opposite to positions 6, 10, 13 are on the "outside" and should be in contact with the receptor site. These assumptions might be useful guidelines in the planning of secretin analogs with altered (e.g., more selective), hormonal spectrum. The inactivation of secretin by thrombin, which cleaves between

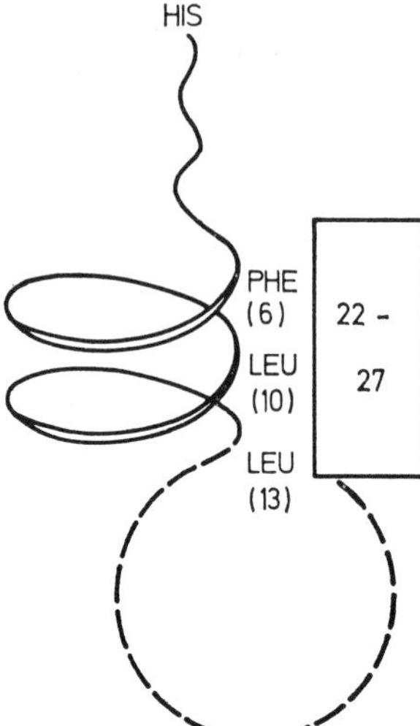

Fig. 5. A schematic representation of the proposed conformation of secretin. This figure intends to show that there is a helical portion in the region between amino acids 6 and 13 but does not want to state the exact length of the helix. In the demonstration of the stabilization through folding of the chain and formation of a hydrophobic pocket the C-terminal sequence 22—27, rich in amino acids with hydrophobic side chain, is represented as a block to indicate the uncertainties, e.g., in the direction of the chain. An inspection of a model of secretin assembled from space filling (CPK) atomic models suggests that the side chain of leucine (26) is sandwiched between the side chains of phenylalanine (6) and leucine (10) and similarly the side chain of leucine (23) lies between those of leucine (10) and leucine (13). Of course, these suggestions can be considered only as possibilities and not as evidence

His-Ser-Asp-Gly-Thr-*Phe*-Thr-Ser-Glu-*Leu*-Ser-Arg-*Leu*-Arg-Asp-Ser-*Ala*-Arg-*Leu*-*Leu*-Gln-Gly-*Leu*-*Val*-NH_2
His-Ser-Gln-Gly-Thr-*Phe*-Thr-Ser-Asp-*Tyr*-Ser-Lys-*Tyr*-Leu-Asp-Ser-Arg-Arg-*Ala*-Gln-Asp-*Phe*-*Val*-Gln-*Try*-*Leu*-*Met*-Asp-Thr
1 2 3 4 5 6 7 8 9 10 11 12 13 14 15 16 17 19 19 20 21 22 23 24 25 26 27 28 29

Fig. 6. Amino acids with non polar side chains in secretin and glucagon

residues 14 and 15 (Mutt, Magnusson, Jorpes and Dahl, 1965) is in full harmony with the above picture and the latter is corroborated also by the importance for activity of the N-terminal histidine residue.

G. Conclusions

The synthesis of porcine secretin by two different routes served more than one purpose. The sequence proposed by Mutt and Jorpes (1966) was confirmed.

The hormone was made available for medical purposes in quantities unlimited by the supply of animals at one given location. The synthetic routes are sufficiently unequivocal and the yields are practical enough to permit the preparation of analogs which in turn can shed light on the relationships between structure and hormonal activity. Thus the first chapter of secretin research, encompassing more than half a century, was closed and a new one was opened.

The scope of the entirely stepwise strategy and the principle of excess acylating agent found clear demonstration. The synthesis of a chain containing twenty-seven amino acids (the longest synthesized so far entirely stepwise through isolated, well defined intermediates) provided an excellent opportunity for a comparison of the two principal strategies of peptide synthesis. The availability of the intermediates of the synthesis in pure form prompted the examination of their rotational spectra which together with the spectra of the hormone itself led to the postulation of a three-dimensional arrangement of the peptide chain. This is the first study in which the secondary structure of a peptide could be deduced by an "anatomy" of the sequence. The relationship between this preferred conformation and hormonal activity gradually emerges and the arbitrary distinction between proteins and peptides is reduced to the rather trivial difference in size: the absence of secondary structure in peptides as a distinguishing mark cannot be maintained. Secretin therefore is indeed a miniature protein.

The difficulties encountered in these syntheses, especially the sequence dependent aspartyl-aminosuccinyl rearrangement serve as warning against complacency. Peptide synthesis is still not a routine operation, it cannot be done without experience and expertise. Nevertheless, these successful syntheses of porcine secretin should be looked upon as good auspices for even more ambitious endeavors, for the synthesis of proteins.

References

Anderson, G. W., McGregor, A. C.: L-butyloxycarbonylamino acids and their use in peptide synthesis. J. Amer. Chem. Soc. **79**, 6180—6183 (1957).

— Paul, R.: N,N[1]-carbonyldiimidazole, a new reagent for peptide synthesis. J. Amer. Chem. Soc. **80**, 4423 (1958).

Bodanszky, A., Ondetti, M. A., Mutt, V., Bodanszky, M.: Synthesis of secretin. IV. Secondary structure in a miniature protein. J. Amer. Chem. Soc. **91**, 944—949 (1969).

Bodanszky, M.: The principle of excess in the synthesis of secretin. In Prebiotic and Biochemical Evolution, ed. by A. P. Kimball and J. Oró. North-Holland Publishing Co., Amsterdam, 1971, p. 217—222.

—: Synthesis of peptides by aminolysis of nitrophenyl esters. Nature **175**, 685 (1955).

—: Stepwise synthesis of peptides by the nitrophenyl-ester method. Ann. N.Y. Acad. Sci. **88**, 655—664 (1960).

— Bath, R.: Hindered amines in peptide synthesis. Synthesis of 7-glycine-oxytocin. Chem. Comm. **1968**, 766—767.

— Bodanszky, A. A.: From peptide synthesis to protein synthesis. Amer. Sci. **55**, 185—196 (1967).

— —: Racemization in peptide synthesis. Mechanism-specific models. Chem. Comm. **1967a**, 591—593.

— du Vigneaud, V.: A method of synthesis of long peptide chains using a synthesis of oxytocin as an example. J. Amer. Chem. Soc. **81**, 5688—5691 (1959).

— Meienhofer, J., du Vigneaud, V.: Synthesis of lysine-vasopressin by the nitrophenyl ester method. J. Amer. Chem. Soc. **82**, 3195—3198 (1960).

— Ondetti, M. A.: Peptide synthesis. New York: Interscience Publishers 1966.

— — Levine, S. D., Williams, N. J.: Synthesis of secretin. II. The stepwise approach. J. Amer. Chem. Soc., **89**, 6753—6757 (1967).

— — — Narayanan, V. L., von Saltza, M., Sheehan, J. T., Williams, N. J., Sabo, E. F.: Synthesis of a heptacosapeptide amide with the hormonal activity of secretin. Chem. and Ind. **1966**, 1757—1758.

Bodanszky, M., Sheehan, J. T.: Active esters and resins in peptide synthesis. Chem. and Ind. **1964,** 1423—1424.
— —: Active esters and resins in peptide synthesis. Chem. and Ind. **1966,** 1597—1598.
— Williams, N. J.: Synthesis of secretin. I. The protected tetradecapeptide corresponding to sequence 14—27.J. Amer. Chem. Soc. **89,** 685—689 (1967).
Craig, L. C., in Alexander, P., Block, R. J., Ed.: A laboratory manual of analytical methods of protein chemistry, Vol. 1. New York: Pergamon 1960.
Curtius, T.: Synthetische Versuche mit Hyppurazid. Ber. **35,** 3226—3228 (1902).
Du Vigneaud, V., Ressler, C. H., Swan, J. M., Roberts, C. W., Katsoyannis, P. G., Gordon, S.: The synthesis of an octapeptide amide with the hormonal activity of oxytocin. J. Amer. Chem. Soc., **75,** 4879—4880 (1953).
Holly, R. W., Sondheimer, E.: The synthesis of L-histidyl peptides. J. Amer. Chem. Soc. **76,** 1326—1328 (1954).
Jorpes, J. E., Mutt, V.: On the biological activity and amino acid composition of secretin. Acta Chem. Scand. **15,** 1790—1791 (1961).
— — Magnusson, S., Steele, B. B.: Amino acid composition and N-terminal amino acid sequence of porcine secretin. Biochem. biophys. Res. Commun. **9,** 275—279 (1962).
Kauzmann, W.: The three dimensional structures of proteins. Biophys. J. **4** (2), 43—54 (1964).
Kopple, K. D., Renick, R. J.: Formation of an N-acylamide in peptide synthesis. J. Org. Chem. **23,** 1565—1567 (1958).
Marshall, G. R., Merrifield, R. B.: Synthesis of angiotensins by the solid-phase method. Biochemistry **4,** 2394—2401 (1965).
McKay, F. C., Albertson, N. F.: New amine-masking groups for peptide synthesis. J. Amer. Chem. Soc. **79,** 4686—4690 (1957).
Medzihradszky, K.: Communication at the 3rd European Peptide Symposium, Basle, 1960, cf. M. Zaoral, Coll. Czechoslov. Chem. Comm. **30,** 1853 (1965).
Merrifield, R. B.: Solid Phase Peptide Synthesis. II. The synthesis of bradykinin. J. Amer. Chem. Soc. **86,** 304—305 (1964).
—: Solid phase peptide synthesis. I. The synthesis of a tetrapeptide. J. Amer. Chem. Soc. **85,** 2149—2154 (1963).
— Marglin, A.: Progress in solid phase peptide synthesis — the synthesis of bovine insulin. Proc. 8th European Peptide Symposium (Noordwijk, 1966). Amsterdam: North Holland Publishing Co. 1967, pp. 85—90.
Mutt, V., Jorpes, J. E.: Lecture, Presented at the 4th International Symposium on the Chemistry of Natural Products, Stockholm, Sweden, 1966; cf. Mutt, V., Jorpes, J. E.: Contemporary developments in the biochemistry of the gastrointestinal hormones. Recent Progress in Hormone Research, **23,** 483—495 (1967); also, Mutt, V., Jorpes, J. E.: Secretin, cholecystokinin, in pharmacology of hormonal polypeptides and proteins. New York: Plenum Press 1968, pp. 569—580.
— Magnusson, S., Jorpes, J. E., Dahl, E.: Structure of porcine secretin. I. Degradation with trypsin and thrombin. Sequence of the tryptic peptides. The C-terminal residue. Biochemistry **4,** 2358—2362 (1965).
Ondetti, M. A., Narayanan, V. L., von Saltza, M., Sheehan, J. T., Sabo, E. F., Bodanszky, M.: The synthesis of secretin. III. The fragment condensation approach. J. Amer. Chem. Soc. **90,** 4711—4716 (1968).
Phillips, D. C.: The three-dimensional structure of an enzyme molecule. Scientific American **215** (November), 78—90 (1966).
Perutz, M. F., Kendrew, J. C., Watson, H. C.: Sturcture and function of haemoglobin II. Some relations between polypeptide chain configuration and amino acid sequence. J. Mol. Biol. **13,** 669—678 (1965).
Schwyzer, R., Sieber, P.: Die Totalsynthese des β-Corticotropins. Helv. Chim. Act. **49,** 134—158 (1966).
— — Kappeler, H.: Zur Synthese von N-t-Butyloxycarbonyl-Aminosäuren. Helv. Chim. Acta. **42,** 2622—2624 (1959).
Staab, H. A.: Reaktionsfähige Heterocyclische Diamide der Kohlensäure. Ann. **609,** 75—83 (1957).
Vagne, M., Stening, G. F., Brooks, F. P., Grossman, M. I.: Synthetic secretin: Comparison with natural secretin for potency and spectrum of physiological actions. Gastroenterology **55,** 260—267 (1968).
Wieland, Th., Bernhard, H.: Über Peptid-Synthesen. 3. Die Verwendung von Anhydriden aus N-Acylierten Aminosäuren und Derivaten Anorganischer Säuren. Ann. Chem. **572,** 190—194 (1951).
— Heinke, B.: Über Peptid-Synthesen. 13. Verwendung von Phosphoroxychlorid bei der Methode der Gemischten Anhydride. Ann. **599,** 70—80 (1956).
Woodward, R. B., Olofson, R. A., Mayer, H.: A new synthesis of peptides. J. Amer. Chem. Soc. **83,** 1010—1012 (1961).

Chapter III

The Secretory Process in the Pancreatic Exocrine Cell: Morphologic and Biochemical Aspects

James D. Jamieson

With 16 Figures

The exocrine pancreatic cell synthesizes large quantities of specific digestive enzymes which it transports, concentrates and stores in zymogen granules, and finally discharges into the duct system of the gland in response to physiologic stimuli initiated by feeding. The purpose of this chapter is to briefly review some of the recent findings of our laboratory concerning the pathway, timetable, and metabolic requirements for the intracellular transport and discharge of secretory proteins from the resting exocrine cell; much of the earlier work in this field has been extensively reviewed by Palade et al. (1962). In a later section, the effects of secretogogues in modulating the overall process will be considered in detail since this is of particular relevance to the topic of this volume. Several recent reviews have dealt extensively with the biochemistry of secretion (Schramm, 1967) and with the interrelationship between the induction of zymogen granule discharge and rates of resynthesis of secretory proteins (Webster, 1969), and changes in phospholipid (Hokin, 1969) and nucleic acid metabolism (Webster, 1969).

A. Route and Timetable of Intracellular Transport in Resting Exocrine Cells

The general structural features of the exocrine pancreatic cell and the main steps involved in the secretory process are illustrated in Fig. 1a which is a diagramatic representation of the cell. An electron micrograph of a comparable region of an exocrine cell is shown in Fig. 1b. The secretory process begins with the synthesis of exportable proteins in association with polysomes attached to the outer, or cytoplasmic aspect of the cisternae of the rough endoplasmic reticulum (RER) (step 1). From this site, according to the studies of Redman, Siekevitz, and Palade (1966), and Redman and Sabatini (1966), nascent polypeptides destined for export are vectorially transferred, during the course of their growth, across the limiting membrane of the cisternae and segregated upon completion of synthesis in the cisternal cavity (step 2). This process does not require energy (other than that involved in peptide bond formation), is uninfluenced by secretogogues (Redman, 1967), but depends on chain termination and is determined by the structural relationship of the ribosome to the cisternal membrane. (Blobel and Sabatini, 1970; Sabatini and Blobel, 1970).

From here, the secretory proteins move through the tortuous channels of the RER from where they eventually reach the zymogen granules at the cell apex (step 5). Here their presence has been reliably ascertained by the studies of GREENE, HIRS and PALADE (1963) and KELLER and COHEN (1961) who showed unequivocally that the complement of secretory proteins in zymogen granules is identical to that found in the pancreatic juice.

As noted in the diagram, transport of secretory proteins from the RER to zymogen granules involves a number of different types of transport operations (steps 2—4), mediated by membrane bounded compartments of the cell, all of which are concerned with the directed movement of proteins centripetally through the cell. Over the past few years, studies conducted in our laboratory have been concerned primarily with defining the route and timetable of transport of secretory

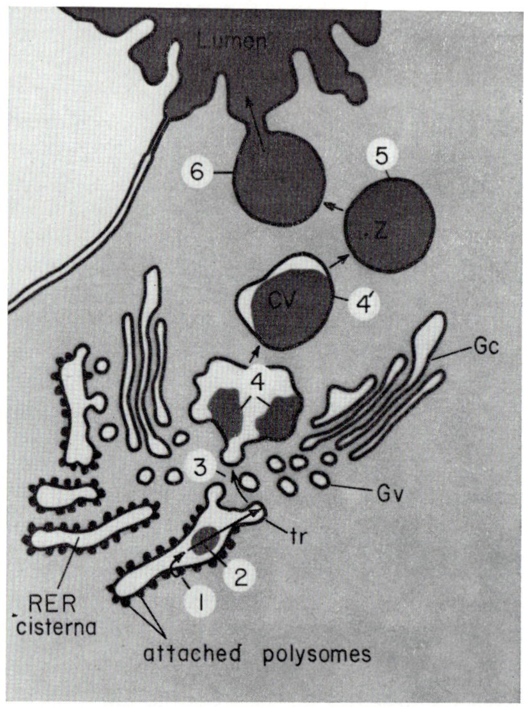

Fig. 1a. Diagrammatic representation of a pancreatic exocrine cell. Only those cell organelles involved in the synthesis, intracellular transport, and discharge of secretory proteins are indicated. They include attached polyribosomes; cisternae of the rough endoplasmic reticulum (*RER*); transitional elements of the RER (*tr*); smooth-surfaced vesicles of the Golgi periphery (*Gv*); Golgi cisternae (*Gc*); condensing vacuoles (*CV*); zymogen granules (*Z*); and the acinar lumen. The steps of the secretory process discussed in the text are indicated (1—6)

proteins over this segment of the pathway (CARO and PALADE, 1964; JAMIESON and PALADE, 1967a, 1967b). The initial radioautographic studies of CARO and PALADE (1964) and VAN HEYNINGEN (1964) had clearly indicated that labeled secretory proteins become closely associated with elements of the Golgi complex in the course of their passage through the cell, in particular with small smooth surfaced vesicles located in the periphery of the Golgi region (step 3). However, while these studies strongly implicated the Golgi elements in this part of the transport sequence, the results could not be interpreted unambiguously for two reasons. First, since the studies were conducted on whole animals following in vivo administration of labeled amino acids, it was not possible to obtain a sufficiently short pulse labeling of secretory proteins to clearly follow the progress of the wave of labeled proteins through the cell, expecially in relation to step 3 which is rapid. Second, due to the limitations of the radioautographic technique, it was not possible to determine whether the labeled proteins were in transit through the cell within the content to the elements of the Golgi complex or if they were

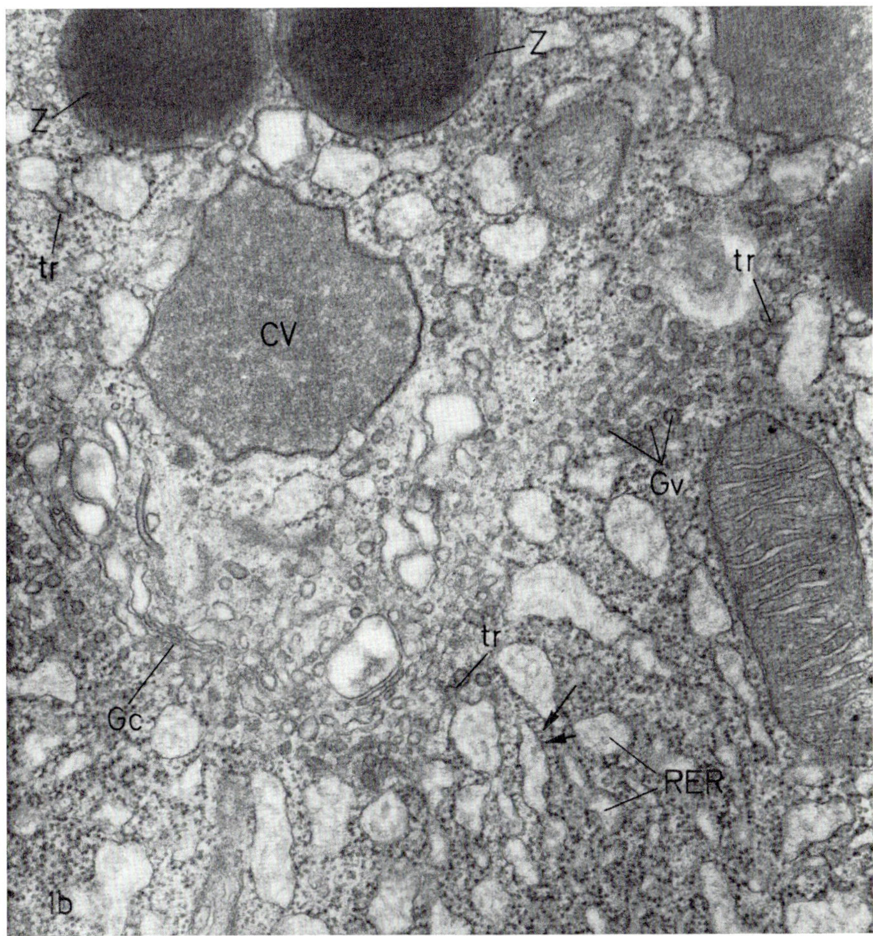

Fig. 1b. Electron micrograph of a thin section cut through the Golgi region of a guinea pig pancreatic exocrine cell. Shown are attached ribosomes (arrows); rough ER cisternae (*RER*); transitional ER elements (*tr*); Golgi cisternae (*Gc*) and vesicles (*Gv*); a condensing vacuole (*CV*) with a scalloped, somewhat irregular profile and content of low electron density; and mature zymogen granules (*Z*) identified by their spherical shape and content of high electron density. Note the unit membranes delimiting the RER cisternae, Golgi elements, and zymogen granules. × 31,000. (From Jamieson and Palade, 1967a)

associated with the surrounding cytoplasmic matrix. To circumvent these limitations, we developed an in vitro system of guinea pig pancreatic slices (Jamieson and Palade, 1967a) whose secretory proteins can be pulse labeled with radioactive amino acids for times sufficiently short (~3 min) to provide the necessary time resolution for following the progress of the wave of labeled proteins through the cell during subsequent chase incubation in the presence of a large excess of

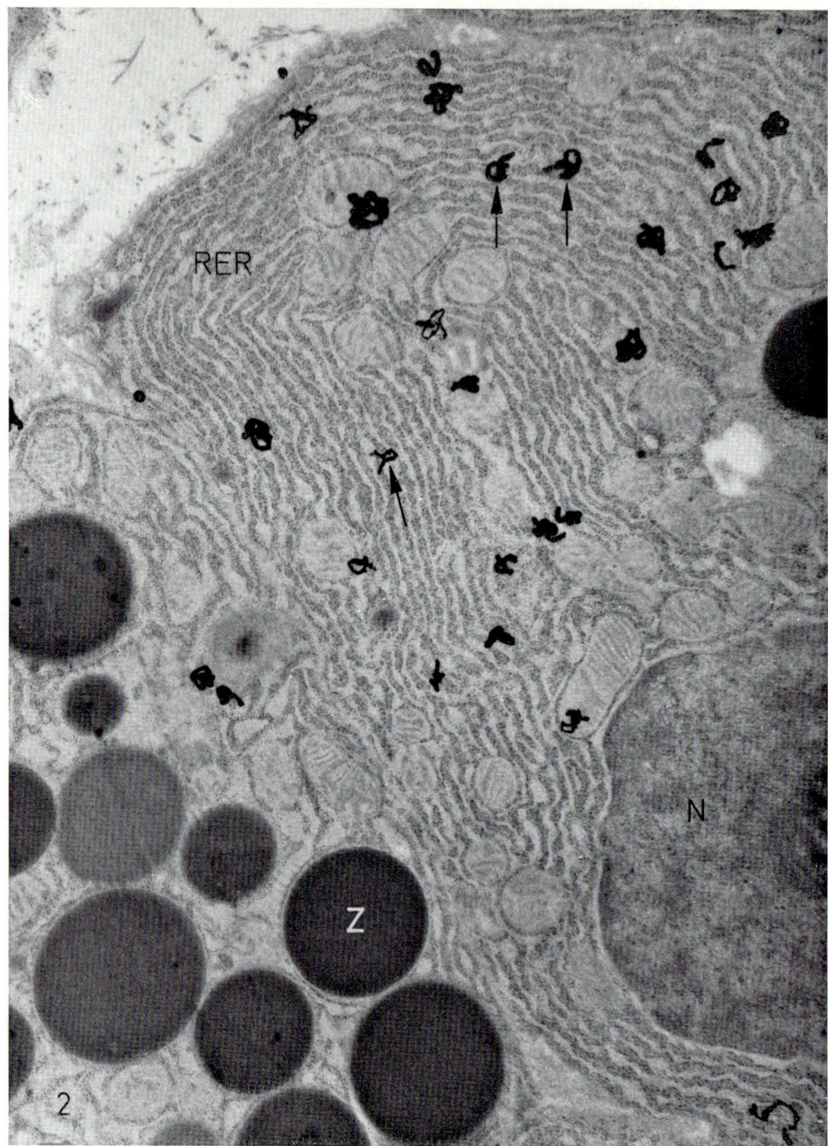

Fig. 2. Electron microscopic radioautogram of a pancreatic exocrine cell pulse-labeled *in vitro* for 3 min with L-leucine-^{3}H. At this time the radioautographic grains (arrows) mark labeled proteins associated with elements of the rough endoplasmic reticulum (*RER*). Other elements of the cell are largely unlabeled at the end of the pulse. *N*, nucleus; *Z*, zymogen granule. × 14,000. (From Jamieson and Palade, 1967b)

unlabeled amino acids. In addition, the slices can be subjected to cell fractionation procedures in which all of the subcellular elements involved in protein transport can be isolated and accounted for. This technique provides the necessary spatial resolution for the definition of the role of subcellular organelles in transport, especially in regard to the question of the movement of secretory proteins through the cell sap as mentioned above. The cell fractions isolated include rough microsomes derived from fragmented and resealed elements of the RER; smooth microsomes derived largely from the vesicles and cisternae of the Golgi complex; a total zymogen granule fraction consisting primarily of zymogen granules with a smaller population of co-sedimenting condensing vacuoles; and a final supernatant fraction which represents in part the soluble cytoplasmic matrix.

By the complementary use of electron microscopic radioautography and cell fractionation techniques applied to the slices at the end of the pulse labeling with leucine-^{3}H and during subsequent chase incubation periods spanning a complete secretory wave lasting ~80 min, we have been able to reconstruct the secretory route as described below and illustrated by the radioautograms and cell fractionation data given in Figs. 2—8 (JAMIESON and PALADE, 1967a, b).

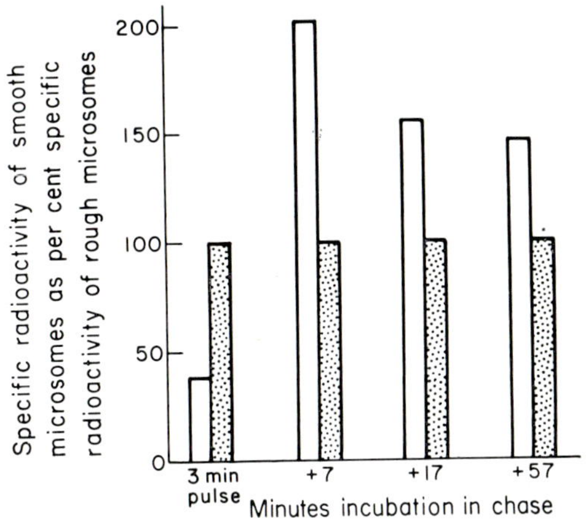

Fig. 3. Distribution of labeled proteins between rough microsomes (derived from elements of the RER) and smooth microsomes (from Golgi peripheral elements) at the end of a 3 min pulse-labeling with L-leucine-^{14}C and during subsequent chase incubation in a large excess of L-leucine-^{12}C for times up to 57 min. Open bars: smooth microsomes; stippled bars: rough microsomes. Note that at the end of the pulse the relative specific radioactivity of secretory proteins is highest in the rough fraction and that during a 7 min chase the ratio reverses, the relative specific activity of labeled proteins in the smooth fraction being maximal at this time. With continued chase incubation the relative specific activity of the smooth fraction progressively declines coincident with transport of labeled proteins to condensing vacuoles (Fig. 5). (From JAMIESON and PALADE, 1967a)

Following segregation in the RER cisternae (Fig. 2), the secretory proteins move through this space to the transitional elements of the RER (part rough and part smooth surfaced ER cisternae abutting on the Golgi periphery). From here the secretory proteins enter the smooth surfaced vesicles of the Golgi periphery (Figs. 3, 4) (possibly as a result of pinching off of the transitional elements filled with secretory product) which in turn ferry them to condensing vacuoles centrally located in the Golgi complex (steps 3—4; Fig. 5). The condensing vacuoles eventually are transformed into zymogen granules (steps 4, 5; Fig. 6) as a result of the progressive filling and concentration of their content. Finally the mature zymogen granules move to the cell surface where their bounding membrane fuses with that of the apical plasmalemma resulting in release of the granule content into the duct lumen by exocytosis (step 6; Fig. 7). Our results lead to the general conclusion that secretory proteins, following initial segregation in the cisternal spaces of the RER, remain within and are transported through

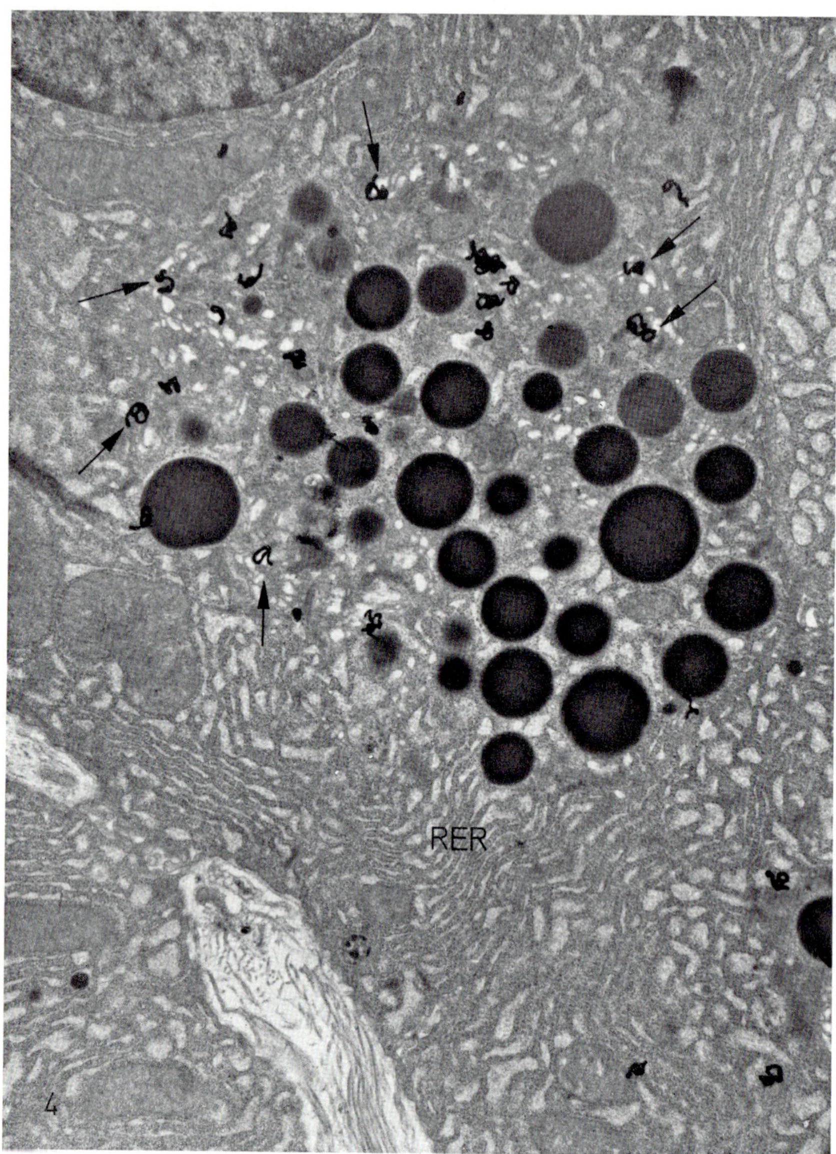

Fig. 4. Radioautogram of an exocrine cell following 7 min chase incubation *in vitro*. Label mainly marks small smooth-surfaced vesicles and cisternae of the Golgi peripheral region (arrows) at this time. Labeled proteins have drained during the chase from the rough cisternae (*RER*), which are generally unlabeled in this micrograph. × 14,000. (From JAMIESON and PALADE, 1967b)

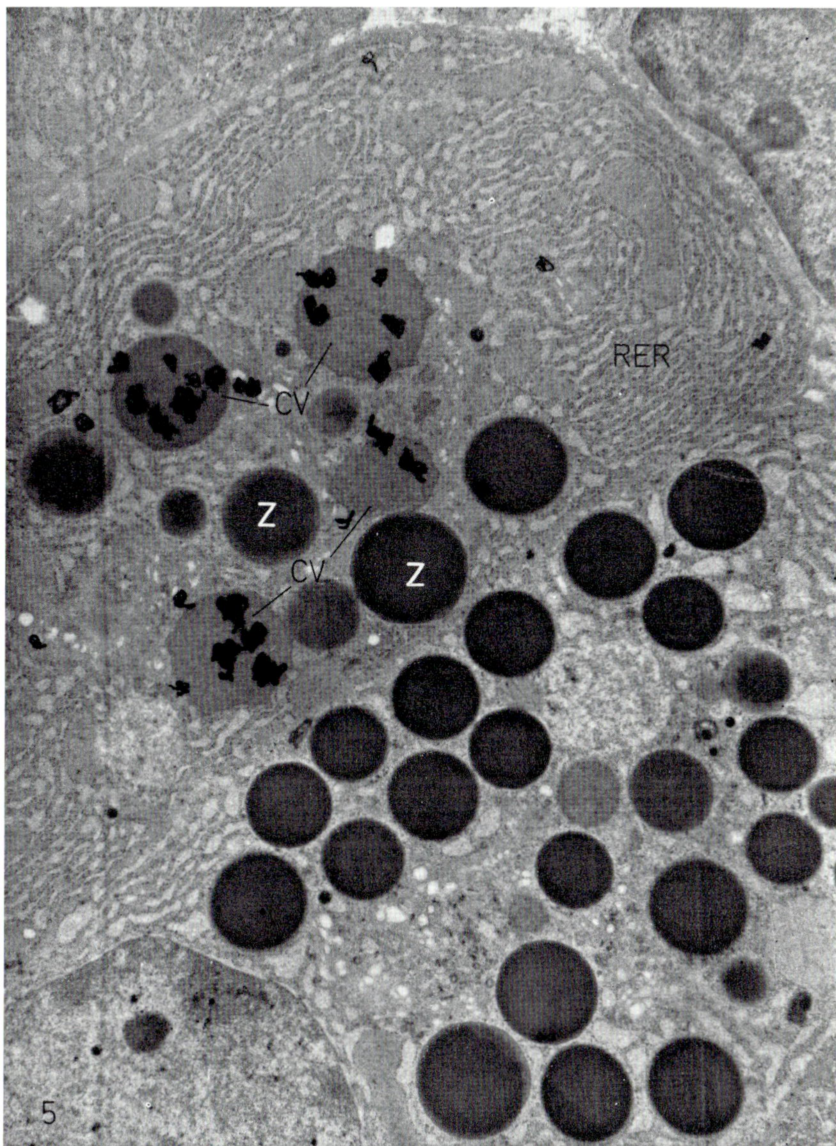

Fig. 5. Radioautogram of an exocrine cell after 37 min chase incubation. At this time labeled proteins have reached condensing vacuoles (*CV*) of the Golgi complex where they become highly concentrated. The labeled proteins have not yet reached the zymogen granules (*Z*). × 10,000. (From JAMIESON and PALADE, 1967b)

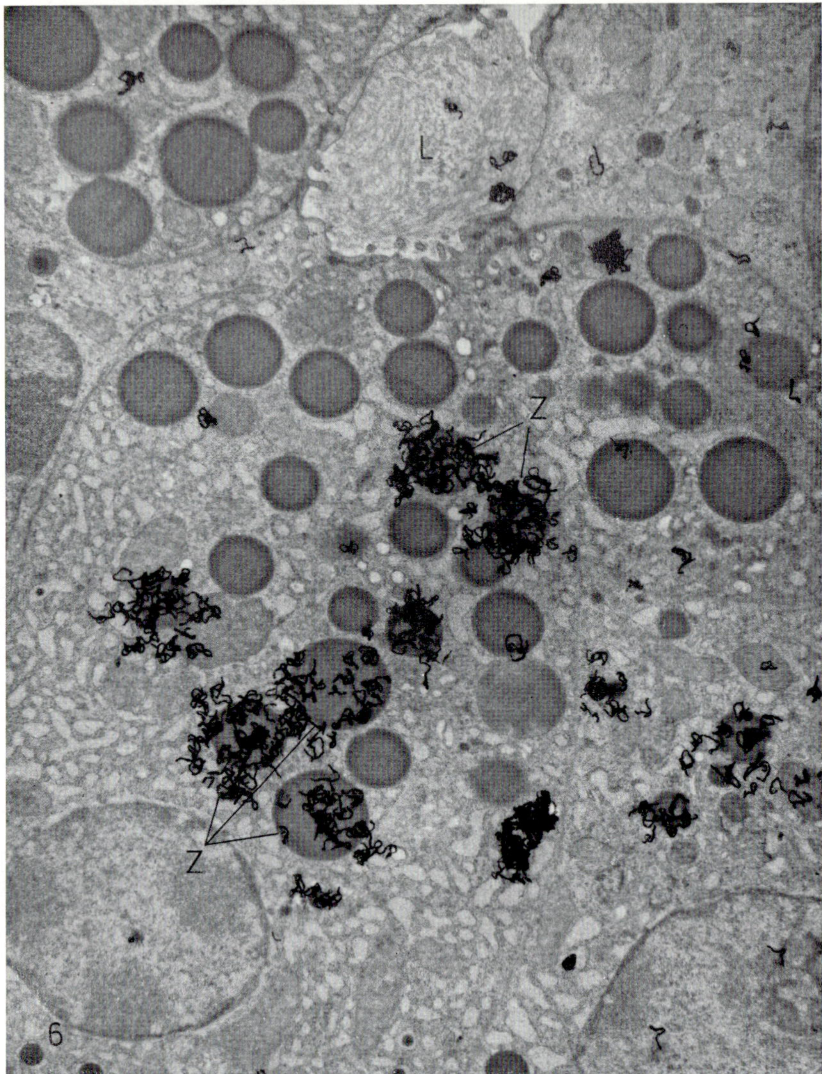

Fig. 6. Radioautogram of an exocrine cell at the end of an 80 min chase period. By now the labeled secretory proteins have been transported to zymogen granules (*Z*) at the cell apex. The acinar lumen (*L*) contains discharged proteins, some of which are radioactive. × 14,000

the cell in association with membrane-bounded compartments until their final discharge into the duct system of the gland. At no time did we find evidence for the transport of secretory proteins through the cell sap (e.g. Fig. 8), an alternative transport pathway proposed in the past by others (e.g., REDMAN and HOKIN, 1959; LAIRD and BARTON, 1958; and MORRIS and DICKMAN, 1960). In our scheme, which most likely applies to the majority of cells which temporarily store their secretory products in storage granules prior to discharge, the secretory proteins need penetrate a membrane only once — at the time of synthesis on attached polysomes. In any alternative scheme, at least two, and possibly more, membrane

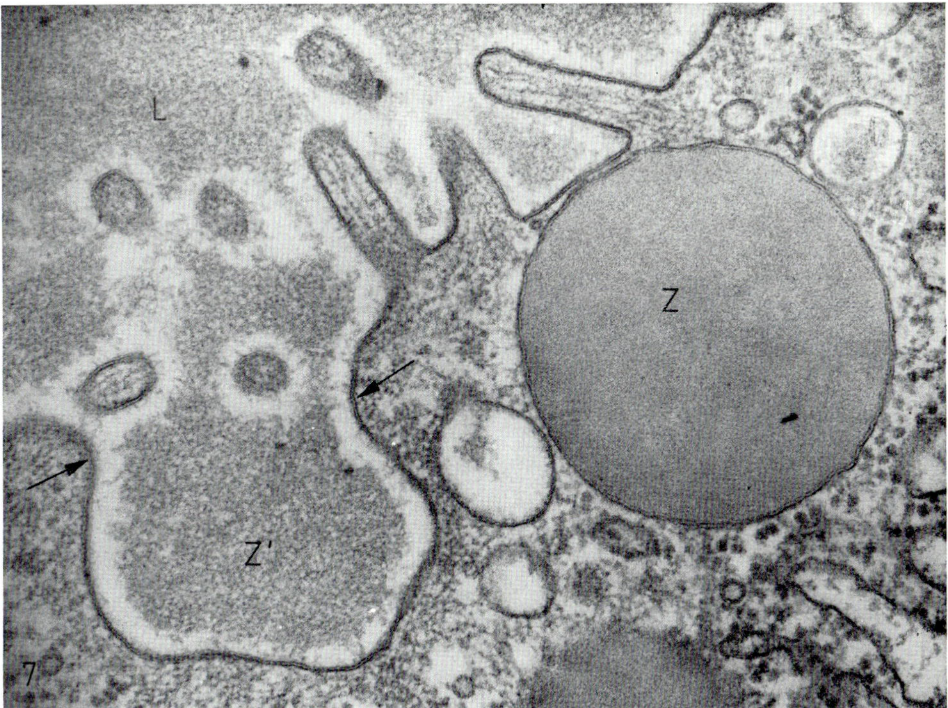

Fig. 7. Electron micrograph of a thin section through the apical region of an exocrine cell. One granule (*Z*) has closely approached the apical plasmalemma where its unit membrane will fuse with that of the cell surface. A second granule (Z^1) has completed the fusion process, and has discharged its content into the acinar lumen (*L*). After fusion the granule membrane has become continuous with that of the cell surface at the points indicated by arrows. ×10,000. (Micrograph courtesy of Dr. George E. Palade)

crossings must be made. In addition, membrane segregation during intracellular transport ensures that the cytoplasmic matrix is protected from the digestive hydrolases, several of which are active as synthesized and which would be potentially dangerous to the cell.

B. Metabolic Requirements for Intracellular Transport over the RER-Condensing Vacuole-Pathway (steps 2-4)

Since we now had a reasonable understanding of the route and kinetics of intracellular transport in the exocrine cell, it was of interest to study the metabolic requirements of the process with two main questions in mind. First, is intracellular transport of secretory proteins obligatorily coupled to continued protein synthesis or does it require ongoing synthesis of exportable proteins or other specific, non-exportable proteins such as couplers, carriers, etc.; and second, what are the energy requirements (if any) for intracellular transport.

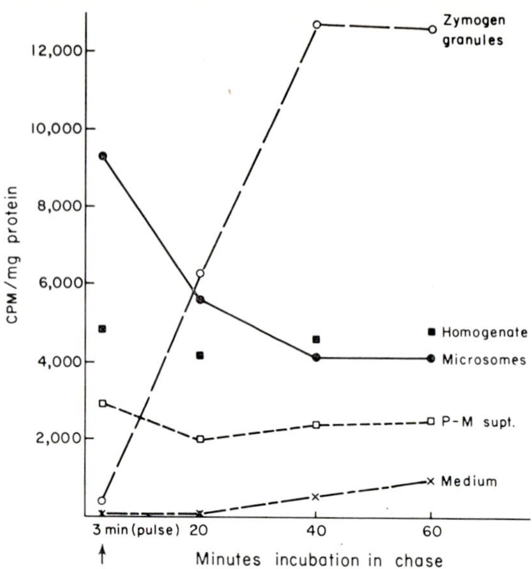

Fig. 8. Distribution of radioactive proteins among cell fractions from pancreatic slices pulse-labeled for 3 min with L-leucine-^{14}C and incubated subsequently in chase medium for up to 60 min. Note that the specific radioactivity of proteins in the homogenate and postmicrosomal supernatant remains constant during the chase. Labeling of the zymogen granule fraction at 20 and 40 min of chase is accounted for mainly by labeled condensing vacuoles recovered in the fraction at these times (see also Figs. 5 and 9), whereas the labeled proteins of this fraction at 60 min are accounted for mainly by labeled zymogen granules (e.g. Fig. 6). The decrease in specific radioactivity of the total microsomal fraction with time is paralleled by drainage of label from the RER cisternae (see Fig. 3 and the radioautograms in Figs. 2—6). (From JAMIESON and PALADE, 1967b)

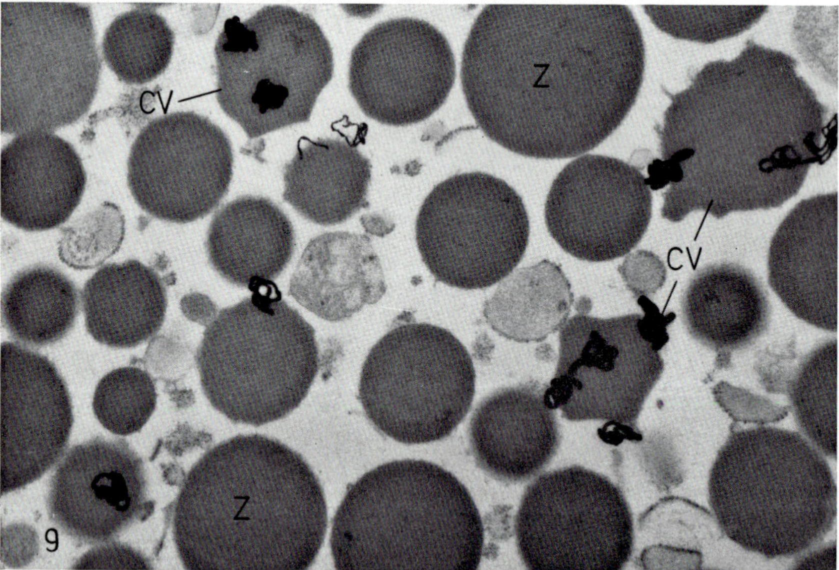

Fig. 9. Electron microscopic radioautogram of the zymogen granule pellet isolated from slices after 37 min chase incubation post-pulse. The majority of labeled structures in the pellet at this time are condensing vacuoles (*CV*), identifiable in the pellet as in the cell (Fig. 5) by their morphologic characteristics. Zymogen granules (*Z*) remain unlabeled at this time. × 10,000. (From JAMIESON and PALADE, 1967b)

To study these problems we have devised a simple assay for transport over this segment of the pathway (JAMIESON and PALADE, 1968a). This assay is based on the finding that following a 3 min pulse-labeling with leucine-^{3}H, ~50% of the labeled proteins migrate during a 37 min chase period to condensing vacuoles (e.g., Fig. 5) which are recovered, upon cell fractionation, in the common zymogen granule pellet (Fig. 9). Here they can be detected by their characteristic morphologic appearance and by their content of labeled secretory proteins at the time mentioned. The end point of the assay consists simply of determining the amount of labeled proteins accumulated in the granule fraction during a standard 37 min chase incubation period.

To examine the first question, we have used this assay to study the effect on intracellular transport of cycloheximide, a potent inhibitor of protein synthesis. The results of this experiment, given in Fig. 10, indicate that at doses of cyclo-

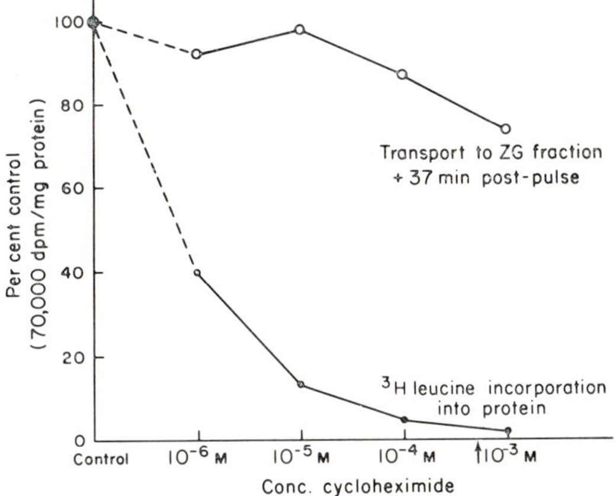

Fig. 10. Effect of cycloheximide on intracellular transport of pulse-labeled proteins to the zymogen granule fraction during 37 min chase incubation with the indicated concentrations of the drug. The effect of cycloheximide on incorporation of leucine-^{3}H into protein is also shown and was determined in a separate experiment. (From JAMIESON and PALADE, 1968a)

heximide which block synthesis by > 95% transport proceeds with an efficiency of 75—80% of that of control, unblocked slices. The small depression of transport which occurs with the highest doses of cycloheximide is most likely related to the concomitant and proportional depression of O_2 uptake by the treated slices. The data indicate that movement of secretory proteins through the RER cisternae does not depend on the maintenance of a concentration gradient which by mass action propels the proteins to the next compartment, for with cycloheximide treatment delivery from attached polysomes practically ceases but nevertheless the pool of labeled proteins continues to drain to elements of the Golgi complex including its condensing vacuoles.

Since intracellular transport could be uncoupled from protein synthesis, it was possible to examine separately, in the uncoupled state, the energy requirements of the pathway using a number of well known metabolic inhibitors. Previously this would not have been possible since potentially the metabolic blockers to be used would also inhibit protein synthesis by virtue of limiting the energy supply of the cell.

For these studies, the same cell fractionation assay for transport as described above was used. In all cases, the compounds and conditions to be tested were

Table 1a. *Effect of temperature and glycolytic inhibitors on intracellular transport*

Post-pulse incubation conditions	Gas phase	Additions (M/liter)	Reincubation conditions	Relative specific activity	Specific activity dpm/mg protein
37 min, 37°	O_2	—	—	100.0	80.000
37 min, 27°	O_2	—	—	26.3	
37 min, 17°	O_2	—	—	7.5	
37 min, 4°	O_2	—	—	1.1	
37 min, 4°	O_2	—	37 min, 37°	57.0	
37 min, 37°	O_2	—	—	100.0	45.000
37 min, 37°	O_2	$F^- 10^{-3}$	—	106.0	
37 min, 37°	O_2	$F^- 10^{-2}$	—	99.0	

Table 1b. *Effect of nitrogen, cyanide and2,4- dinitrophenol on intracellular transport*

Post-pulse incubation conditions	Gas phase	Additions (M/liter)	Reincubation conditions	Relative specific activity %	Specific activity dpm/mg protein
37 min, 37°	O_2	—	—	100	80.000
37 min, 37°	N_2	—	—	12	
37 min, 37°	N_2	—	37 min, 37° O_2	70	
37 min, 37°	O_2	—	—	100	90.000
37 min, 37°	O_2	$CN^- 5\times10^{-5}$	—	98	
37 min, 37°	O_2	$CN^- 1\times10^{-4}$	—	90	
37 min, 37°	O_2	$CN^- 4\times10^{-4}$	—	28	
37 min, 37°	O_2	$CN^- 5\times10^{-4}$	—	22	
37 min, 37°	O_2	$CN^- 7\times10^{-4}$	—	10	
37 min, 37°	O_2	$CN^- 1\times10^{-3}$	—	2	
37 min, 37°	O_2	$CN^- 5\times10^{-4}$	37 min, 37° no CN^-	111	
37 min, 37°	O_2	—	—	100	47.000
37 min, 37°	O_2	DNP 1×10^{-5}	—	116	
37 min, 37°	O_2	DNP 1×10^{-4}	—	67	
37 min, 37°	O_2	DNP 5×10^{-4}	—	20	
37 min, 37°	O_2	DNP 1×10^{-3}	—	10	
37 min, 37°	O_2	DNP 5×10^{-4}	37 min, 37° no DNP	80	

Sets of pancreatic slices were pulse-labeled for 3 min with L-leucine-^3H and incubated in chase medium for 37 min with the indicated additions, including 0.5 mM cycloheximide. In reversal experiments, the slices were reincubated after 37 min chase for a further 37 min under the indicated conditions. At the termination of the assay, zymogen granule fractions were isolated from the slices and the protein radioactivity contained therein determined and compared to that in fractions from control, untreated slices. (JAMIESON and PALADE, 1968b)

applied to the assays immediately at the end of pulse labeling and were continuously present for the 37 min chase period. Further, to ensure a stable and uniform baseline for transport, all assays contained cycloheximide. As seen in Table 1 and Fig. 11 (see also JAMIESON and PALADE, 1968b) transport is an enzymatic process, being inhibited by low temperature (the Q_{10} of the process is $\sim$4); does not depend on aerobic glycolysis for an energy source; but is strongly inhibited by any condtion which interferes with mitochondrial energy production. Except in the case of Antimycin A, transport inhibition was reversible upon removal of the blocker.

While these results indicated that movement of secretory proteins from the RER to condensing vacuoles requires energy, most likely as ATP produced by mitochondrial respiration, this part of the pathway involves several transport operations (i.e., steps 2—4 in Fig. 1). And because of the limitations of the fractionation assay we can only conclude that the energy requiring site is located proximal to the condensing vacuoles. Consequently to better define this site, radioautographic and cell fractionation procedures were applied to slices treated for short times postpulse with the respiratory inhibitor, Antimycin A. Without giving the details here (see JAMIESON and PALADE, 1968b) the experiments led to the conclusion that the most proximal energy-requiring site on the pathway is most likely located at the level of the transitional elements of the RER: in the presence of the blocker labeled proteins move through the RER spaces where

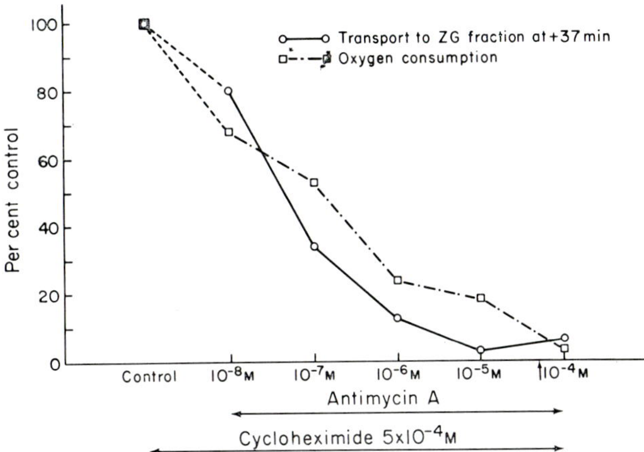

Fig 11. Effect of various concentrations of Antimycin A on transport of labeled proteins to the zymogen granule fraction during a 37 min chase period post-pulse. All assays contained a standard dose of cycloheximide to uniformly inhibit protein synthesis by >95%. Note that O_2 consumption by the slices is depressed in parallel with inhibition of intracellular transport. (From JAMIESON and PALADE, 1968b)

they appear to accumulate at the transitional elements but further migration to the elements of the Golgi complex is prevented. Apparently the cell is provided with a lock or valve at this level whose opening is energy-dependent and which functions to connect two membrane bounded compartments — the cisternae of the RER and that represented by the condensing vacuole. The net result of the functioning of the valve is the active transport of macromolecules in bulk from one compartment to another. This type of active transport differs from active transport in the usual sense where molecules or ions are transported across a membrane.

C. Metabolic Aspects of Condensing Vacuole Transformation

The next step in the secretory process (step 4 in Fig. 1) consists of the maturation of condensing vacuoles into zymogen granules which, as we have already mentioned, results from the progressive filling and concentration of their content. According to our previous studies, this step, like those immediately preceeding it does not require continued protein synthesis (JAMIESON and PALADE, 1968a).

Previously we had assumed that condensing vacuole conversion might result from the extrusion of water and electrolytes from the initially dilute solution of proteins in the vacuole content into the cell sap, this possibly being mediated by ion pumps similar to those found in plasma membranes (i.e., a Na^{+} —K^{+} ATPase). However, recent results (JAMIESON and PALADE, 1971) indicate that the conversion process is not severely interfered with by metabolic inhibitors which block the earlier steps of transport and zymogen granule discharge by > 95%, nor is it interfered with by ouabain treatment at doses (10^{-4}M) far in excess of those required to maximally inhibit ATPases of the type we originally proposed. Since these results rule out the participation of energy consuming ion pumps in conversion, other hypothesis to explain the results were considered. One such possibility which we examined was that secretory proteins, upon segregation into

Table 2. *Effect of resuspending media on release of labeled proteins from zymogen granule fractions*

Chase	Suspending media			
incubation time	0.3 M sucrose pH 4.8	Water pH 4.7	0.2 M $NaHCO_3$ pH 8.4	0.5% Na DOC pH 7.2
	% dpm released			
20 min	11.2 ± 0.6	50.6 ± 1.4	87.2 ± 1.3	86.6
80 min	16.5 ± 0.1	30.2 ± 1.1	87.3 ± 1.2	89.8

Sets of pancreatic slices were pulse-labeled for 4 min with L-leucine-^{3}H and incubated in chase for a further 20 or 80 min to allow labeled proteins to be transported primarily to condensing vacuoles (20 min set) or zymogen granules (80 min set). Labeled zymogen granule fractions were isolated from the slices at the two times by differential centrifugation and resuspended in the indicated fluids. After a 5 min incubation at 0°, the resuspensions were centrifuged (190.000 × g for 20 min) to sediment cell particulates and the proportion of labeled proteins released to the cleared supernatant determined. The data include the standard error of the mean.

condensing vacuoles, might form large osmotically inactive aggregates. To examine this possibility, slices were pulse labeled for 3 min as usual and incubated in chase medium for either 20 min or 80 min to allow labeled proteins to be transported to condensing vacuoles (e.g., Fig. 5) or zymogen granules (e.g., Fig. 6) respectively. At these times the slices were fractionated to yield total zymogen granule pellets, and the pellets were resuspended in the solutions indicated in Table 2. After a brief incubation at 0° the resuspensions were centrifuged to sediment unlysed particles and the percent labeled proteins liberated was determined. From the results, it is clear that osmotic shock results in the net liberation of ~27% of the content of prelabeled condensing vacuoles and only ~11% of the content of prelabeled zymogen granules. Treatment of the suspensions with either mild base or deoxycholate releases the majority of the content of both labeled structures. Base-induced lysis has previously been employed by GREENE et al. (1963) to release the content of zymogen granules and presumably acts by causing swelling of the granule content followed by mechanical rupture of the limiting membrane; deoxycholate effects granule lysis by dissolving its limiting membrane. Our results are thus consistent with the notion that secretory proteins are present in the granule content in a form exerting low osmotic pressure and are in line with evidence presented earlier by HOKIN (1955) and BURWEN and ROTHMAN (1970). The reactions leading to aggregate formation are presently unknown but may result from ionic or other non-covalent interactions between secretory proteins or between these proteins and other molecules in the vacuole content such as divalent cations, matrix substances, etc.

D. Studies on Zymogen Granule Discharge

Finally we have reexamined the metabolic requirements for the last step (no. 6 in Fig. 1) in the secretory process — the discharge of the zymogen granule content into the acinar lumen. Although a number of earlier biochemical studies had indicated that secretory proteins can be discharged in vitro from slices of exocrine glands (pancreas and parotid) by the application of appropriate stimulating agents (HOKIN and HOKIN, 1962; SCHRAMM, 1967), and that discharge induction requires respiratory energy, these results could not be interpreted unambiguously since they were obtained under conditions of continuing protein synthesis and intracellular transport, both processes which also require energy. In order to clarify this problem, we have investigated discharge from pancreatic slices under conditions independent of protein synthesis and of the preceding steps of intracellular transport.

I. Radioassay for Zymogen Discharge

In order to study zymogen discharge, we have developed a simple radioassay for the process based on the radioautographic finding shown earlier (Fig. 6) which indicated that up to ~65% of the labeled proteins synthesized during a short pulse with leucine-^{3}H are transported to zymogen granules at the cell apex during a subsequent 80 min chase period. If at this time we add to the incubation medium a secretogogue such as a cholinergic agent (carbamylcholine or acetylcholine) or the natural stimulant, pancreozymin, the slices respond by rapidly discharging labeled proteins to the medium. As Fig. 12 shows, discharge begins without a lag, and is sustained at a linear rate for the duration of the assay, usually lasting 30—60 min. Although the discharge of enzymatic activity (e.g., amylase) parallels the output of labeled proteins, the background levels of enzymatic activity are ~20% whereas the corresponding figure for labeled proteins is only ~5%. In

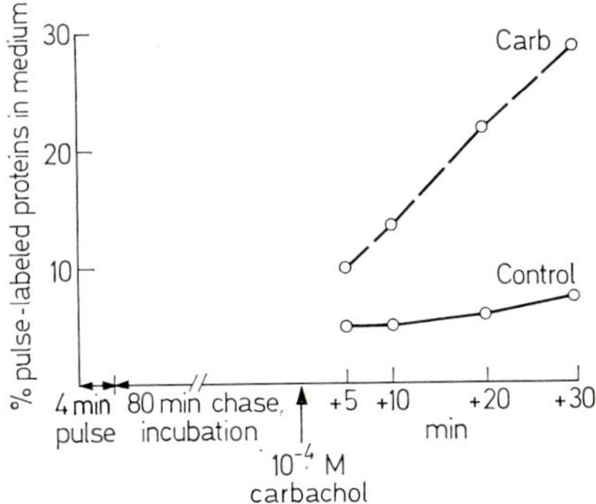

Fig. 12. Kinetics of discharge of pulse-labeled proteins to the incubation medium in response to carbamylcholine (10^{-4} M). Sets of slices were pulse labeled for 4 min with L-leucine-^{3}H and incubated for 80 min in chase medium. At this time the secretogogue was added and the % of pulse-labeled proteins discharged to the medium determined at the times indicated up to 30 min. Controls received no drug

addition to high sensitivity, the radioassay is selective in that it detects only those polypeptides synthesized during the pulse and transported to their storage sites in zymogen granules during the chase. Consequently, the assay is not influenced by preformed enzymes stored in the duct system of the gland which contribute to at least part of the high backgrounds noted for enzyme assays.

Assumptions Involved in the Interpretation of the Radioassay

1. Source of Discharged Proteins

The validity of the assay rests on a number of assumptions. First, we assume that the labeled proteins appearing in the medium are derived from the zymogen granule content. In support of this is the observation that during stimulation the population of zymogen granules seen in the unstimulated cells by microscopy progressively decreases and is finally depleted after 3 hr of in vitro stimulation (Figs. 13a and 13b). Further, as would be expected the number of zymogen granules harvested from the slices by cell fractionation is decreased during stimulation. And as will be seen later, since discharge induction does not lead to any systematic increase in the levels of soluble labeled proteins in the cell sap, we are reasonably confident that the discharged labeled proteins do not derive from molecules extruded directly through the plasma membrane from the cell sap as has been proposed on a number of occasions by others.

2. Effect of Secretogogues on Rates of Protein Synthesis and of Intracellular Transport

The second assumption made is that the secretogogues primarily affect discharge without concurrently accelerating either the rate of protein synthesis or of intracellular transport. To determine if discharge induction changes the rate of incorporation of amino acids into proteins, the following experiments were performed. Sets of pancreatic slices were incubated for various times in the presence or absence of carbamylcholine or pancreozymin in media supplemented with a complete set of amino acids including leucine which was supplied as the tritiated isotope at the indicated concentrations. The results of this experiment, expressed as mμmoles leucine incorporated/mg slice DNA, are given in Fig. 14 and show that so long as the leucine level in the medium is maintained at greater than 0.04 mM, the secretogogues have little effect on protein synthesis which proceeds at a nearly linear rate for 3 hr. If carrier leucine is omitted from the medium and the amino acid supplied only in trace amounts (0.09 μM) incorporation is sustained for only 2 hr and ceases thereafter most likely due to exhaustion of the endogenous pool of leucine in the tissue. The results also show that the absolute concentration of leucine in the medium determines the net incorporation of this amino acid; the dependency of incorporation on concentration for the other 20 amino acids normally present in the medium has not been explored. We should point out that since up to 45% of the labeled proteins synthesized during 3 hr incubation with the secretogogues are discharged to the medium, the incorporation data have been calculated from the protein radioactivity recovered in the slices plus medium. Our results are in accord with the observations of Hokin and Hokin (1962) and Dickman et al. (1962) which indicated that secretogogues do not accelerate protein synthesis when applied to slices in vitro but are at variance with the results of other workers (reviewed by Webster, 1969).

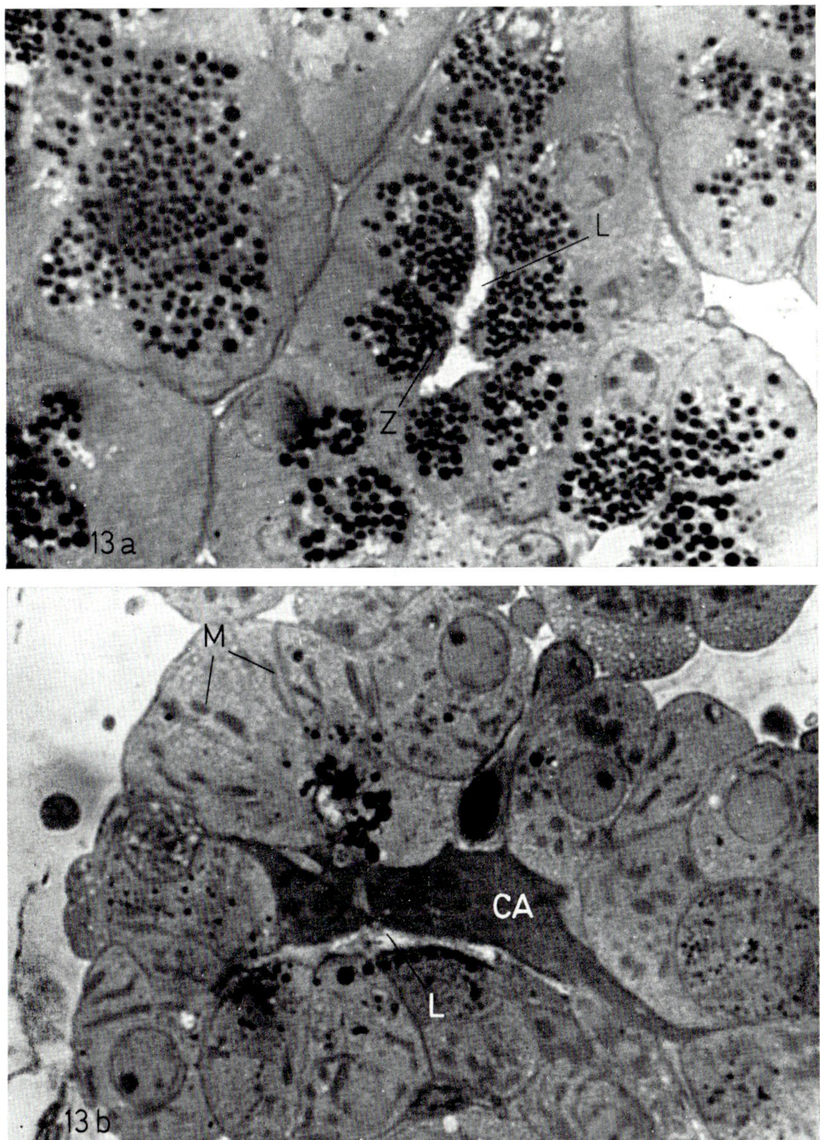

Fig. 13a. 0.5 μ-thick Epon section through a pancreatic slice incubated for 3 hr in control medium. Note the large population of zymogen granules (*Z*) in the apices of the cells, and the outline of the acinar lumen (*L*). × 1,100

Fig. 13b. 0.5 μ section through a pancreatic slice from the same gland as in Fig. 13a but incubated for 3 hr in medium containing 0.01 mM carbamylcholine. The majority of the cells are depleted of their complement of zymogen granules. *L*, acinar lumen; *CA* centroacinar cells; *M*, mitochondria. × 1,100

The latter studies demonstrated that zymogen discharge initiated in vivo is followed by enhanced incorporation of amino acids administered either to the intact animal or to slices incubated subsequently in vitro. While the cause of the discrepancy between the results obtained in vivo or in vitro is still unclear, it may stem from the fact that exocrine cells stimulated in vivo can be expected to lose a large part of their total protein content due to zymogen granule discharge. This would result in an artificially high protein specific radioactivity. To correct for this, incorporation data should be normalized to a more constant denominator such as the DNA content of the tissue.

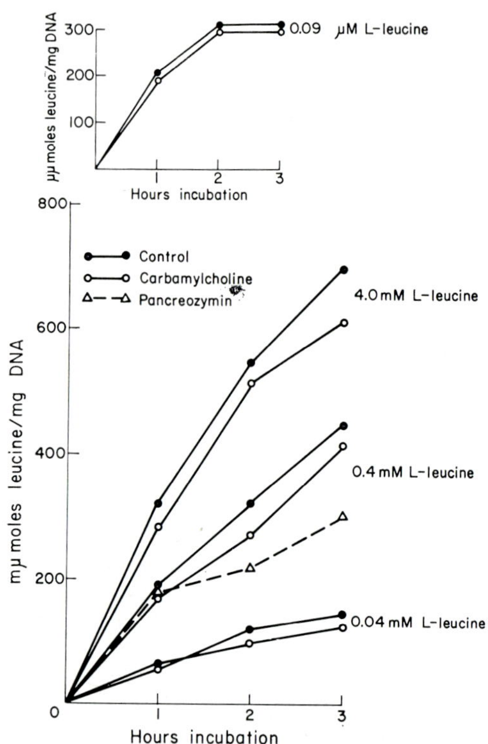

Fig. 14. Effect of 0.01 mM carbamylcholine or 10 units/ml pancreozymin on incorporation of L-leucine-^{3}H into proteins in slices incubated in media containing various concentrations of L-leucine. The results are expressed as mμmoles leucine incorporated/mg slice DNA and are based on TCA-precipitable protein radioactivity recovered in slices plus incubation medium. Controls received no drugs. The insert shows incorporation kinetics in slices incubated with trace amounts of L-leucine-^{3}H. In addition to the indicated concentrations of leucine, all media contained a complete set of 20 other unlabeled amino acids. (From JAMIESON and PALADE, 1967a)

As mentioned above, the validity of the assay also depends on demonstrating that secretogogues do not accelerate intracellular transport of secretory proteins into zymogen granules. To determine this point, we measured the efficiency of transport over the RER-condensing vacuole pathway in slices stimulated for 37 min post-pulse with either carbamylcholine or pancreozymin. As before, transport efficiency was assessed by determining the accumulation of labeled proteins in the total zymogen granule fraction; in addition, an estimate was made of the efficiency of drainage of the RER compartment by measuring comparatively the rate of decrease of radioactivity in the total microsomal fractions derived from control and stimulated slices. This fraction, according to our previous studies (JAMIESON and PALADE, 1967a) consists primarily of rough microsomes. The results, shown in Table 3, indicate that discharge stimulation accelerates neither the rate of accumulation of labeled proteins in the zymogen granule fraction (i.e., into condensing vacuoles recovered in the fraction at this time), nor the rate of egress of proteins from the RER cisternae. The latter finding remains true even in slices stimulated for several hours past the time of complete loss of the zymogen granule population. (Parenthetically, we should point out that such hyperstimulated cells continue to synthesize and transport net amounts of secretory proteins at rates approaching that of resting cells thus confirming the longstanding observations of LIN and GROSSMAN (1956) which indicated that the

Table 3. *Effect of secretogogues on intracellular transport of secretory proteins*

Pulse L-leucine-^{3}H	Conditions	Chase incubation in 2 mM leucine-^{1}H						
		% Amylase in incubation medium[a]	Distribution of radioactivity					
			Microsomal fraction		Zymogen granule fraction		Postmicrosomal supernatant	
			dpm/U amylase	% dpm	dpm/U amylase	% dpm	dpm/U amylase	% dpm
3 min	0 min (pulse)	—	8500	32.4	206	0.8	2730	17.5
3 min	37 min (control)	12.0	4350	14.8	5100	12.0	1550	11.7
3 min	37 min, 0.1 mM carbamylcholine	22.2	6670	19.2	4280	6.7	2400	12.0
3 min	37 min, 10 U/ml pancreozymin	20.6	6150	15.2	4100	8.6	1480	12.0

[a] Amylase in medium × 100/amylase in medium + homogenate.

Sets of pancreatic slices were pulse labeled with leucine-^{3}H for 3 min, and then incubated in chase media with the indicated additions for 37 min. At the end of the pulse, and after 37 min chase incubation, the slices were homogenized, fractionated by differential centrifugation, and the radioactivity of proteins in the microsomal and zymogen granule fractions and in the postmicrosomal supernatant determined. Radioactivity data are expressed as % dpm recovered in the fractions relative to the starting homogenate or as specific radioactivity based on amylase measured in the fractions. The data show relative rather than total changes of radioactivity in cell fractions with time since only the postmicrosomal supernatant was completely recovered in our fractionation scheme; recovery of the microsomal and zymogen granule fractions can be estimated to be ~30% each

pancreas is capable of sustained output of digestive enzymes in the face of chronic stimulation.) The table also indicates that discharge induction does not lead to any systematic increase in either the total or specific radioactivity of proteins in the post-microsomal supernatant. Since this fraction represents in part the soluble cell sap, the finding indicates that discharge stimulation does not result in the preferential movement of secretory proteins through the cytoplasmic matrix, and rules out the long standing notion (REDMAN and HOKIN, 1959; LAIRD and BARTON, 1958; MORRIS and DICKMAN, 1960) that secretory proteins are only stored in zymogen granules during periods of starvation but are usually transferred along a non-particulate pathway during secretogogue action.

The above data, plus the finding that discharge stimulation does not accelerate the rate of protein synthesis (at least in the guinea pig pancreatic slice system) would suggest that secretory stimuli primarily affect the final discharge step and apparently do not, by a feedback mechanism, influence the preceding steps of the secretory process.

E. Metabolic Requirements for Zymogen Granule Discharge

Having established the basic premises of the discharge assay, we can now return to the question of the metabolic requirements for zymogen granule release. As in the studies on intracellular transport, the first facet which we examined was whether or not zymogen discharge was coupled to continued protein synthesis. For this purpose cycloheximide, at a concentration sufficient to block protein synthesis by $> 95\%$, was introduced into the assay at the end of the pulse and was present continuously both during the granule prelabeling period and the subsequent test period with secretogogues added. The results (Fig. 15 and Table 4)

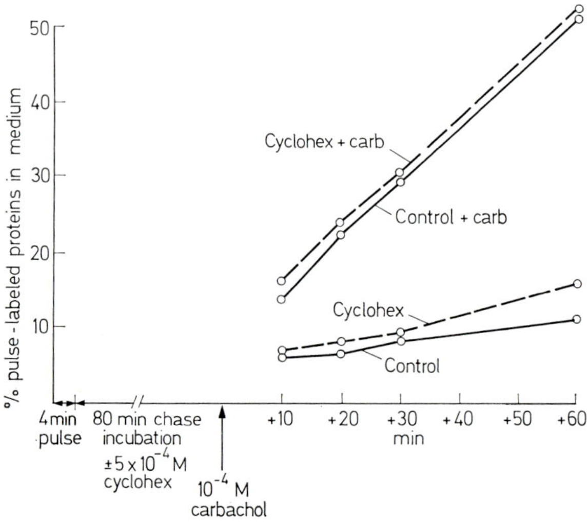

Fig. 15. Effect of cycloheximide on carbamylcholine-induced discharge of labeled proteins. Slices were pulse-labeled and incubated in chase medium as for Fig. 12, except that the indicated flasks contained 0.5 mM cycloheximide which was added immediately post-pulse and was present in the assays for up to 4 hr of incubation

show clearly that the inhibitor is without effect on induced discharge even though continuously present in the assay for 4 hr. Evidently discharge, like the preceding steps of intracellular transport, does not require the continued synthesis either of secretory proteins or of specific proteins such as carriers, couplers, etc., at least over the period of treatment with the inhibitor examined here which encompasses a complete secretory cycle lasting ~80—90 min. In particular, the data would suggest that the cell does not require the synchronized or parallel synthesis of membrane proteins for the containers involved in transport and discharge and supports the initial suggestion of PALADE (1959) that the cell most likely reutilizes extensively its intracellular membranes or their macromolecular components during the secretory process. As he originally proposed, membrane contributed to the cell surface during zymogen granule discharge may be reinternalized for use again in the packaging process, so maintaining the membrane balance of the cell. This particular aspect of the secretory process is discussed in detail by JAMIESON and PALADE, 1971.

Table 4. *Effect of metabolic inhibitors on induced discharge*

Pulse leucine-^{3}H	Chase conditions 80 min with 2 mM leucine-'H	Assay conditions 30 min with 2 mM leucine-'H			% dpm in medium at 30 min
	Cycloheximide 0.5 mM	Cycloheximide 0.5 mM	Secretogogue	Test compound	
4 min	—	—	—	—	5.5
4 min	—	—	pancreoz.[a]	—	36.1
4 min	+	+	—	—	7.6
4 min	+	+	pancreoz.	—	34.4
4 min	+	+	pancreoz.	0.05 mM Anti A	6.3
4 min	+	+	—	—	10.5
4 min	+	+	carbachol[b]	—	38.3
4 min	+	+	carbachol[b]	10 mM NaF	44.5
4 min	+	+	carbachol[b]	0.1 mM IA	29.8
4 min	+	+	carbachol[b]	95% N_2, 5% CO_2	8.1
4 min	+	+	carbachol[b]	1 mM DNP	10.5
4 min	+	+	carbachol[b]	1 mM NaCN	16.5

[a] 10U/ml pancreozymin. [b] 0.1 mM carbamylcholine.

Sets of pancreatic slices were pulse-labeled for 4 min with L-leucine-^{3}H, then incubated in chase medium with the indicated additions to prelabel zymogen granules. Following this the secretogogues and test compounds were added to the assays for a further 30 min, at the end of which time the percent of labeled proteins appearing in the medium was determined and compared to that from stimulated but unblocked slices

Table 5. *Requirements for protein synthesis, energy and effect of secretogogues on the secretory process*

	Step in secretory process				
	(1) Attached polysomes	(2) RER cisternae	(3) Golgi peripheral region (includes transitional elements)	(4+5) Condensing vacuole maturation (zymogen granules)	(6) Discharge
Protein synthesis	+	—	—	—	—
Energy	+	—	+	±	+
Secretogogues	—	—	—	—	+

Again, since discharge could be uncoupled from protein synthesis, it was possible to examine independently the energy requirements for secretogogue action using a number of well known metabolic inhibitors. In each case, the inhibitors were applied to the assay at the time of addition of the secretogogue and were continuously present for a standard 30 min test period. Cycloheximide was also included in the assay to provide a uniform level of inhibition of protein synthesis. The results, summarized in Table 4 and Fig. 16, show that, as for the case of intracellular transport, induced discharge is dependent exclusively on energy derived from oxidative phosphorylation. As seen in Fig. 16, metabolic inhibition blocks induced discharge within 5 min and is apparently without effect on the background levels of radioactivity extruded from control unstimulated slices at least over a 20 min period. This type of discharge from control slices presumably represents passive leakage to the medium from slices damaged during preparation and incubation. We should mention, however, that if unstimulated slices are incubated for longer times (i.e., up to 5 hr post-pulse), up to 20% of the pulse labeled proteins appear in the medium. Recent experiments show that the majority of this long term resting secretion can be blocked by conditions which inhibit respiration suggesting that it corresponds to the so called starvation secretion noted by BAXTER (1931) and others to occur from the unstimulated gland in vivo. Since atropine does not antagonize resting discharge in vitro over these long incubation times, we assume that it is triggered by endogenous digestive hormones present in the tissues (? pancreozymin).

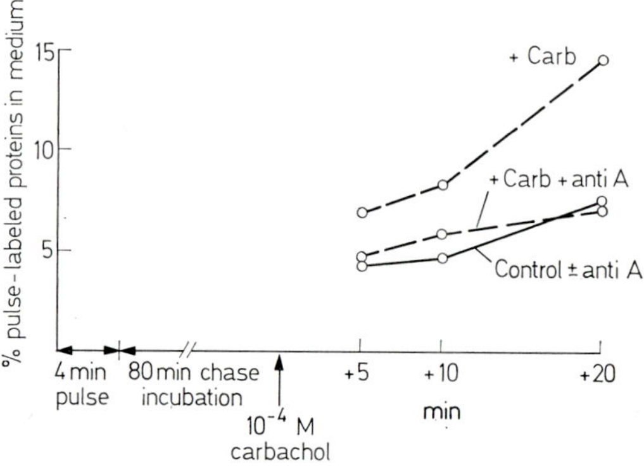

Fig. 16. Effect of Antimycin A on induced discharge. The assay is identical to that shown in Figs. 12 and 15. Antimycin A (0.05 mM) was added together with carbamylcholine at the end of the 80 min preincubation period and was present for the next 20 min of incubation. All flasks contained 0.5 mM cycloheximide

While the mechanism by which secretogogues mediate discharge and the exact site at which energy is consumed in the process are still largely unknown, it is clear that zymogen discharge involves movement of the granule to the cell apex followed by fusion of the granule membrane with that of the cell surface (PALADE, 1959). Both of these events likely require energy which could be utilized either for granule propulsion or be related to fusion and fission of cellular membranes and the concomitant reorganization and/or synthesis of membrane components.

Finally we should mention that the source of oxidizable substrates needed to support both intracellular transport and discharge appears to consist primarily of endogenous stores of fatty acids derived, most likely, from neutral lipid droplets commonly seen in close association with mitochondria in exocrine cells (JAMIESON and PALADE, 1968b).

Summary

In order to put the contents of this chapter in perspective, a summary table (5) is included in which the activity of secretogogues and metabolic inhibitors on the individual steps of the secretory process is indicated. Evidently the studies to date on the exocrine cell leave unanswered many important questions concerning the molecular mechanisms operative in the various transport steps in the secretory process but they at least provide a basis for further work on the subject.

References

Baxter, S. G.: Continuous pancreatic secretion in the rabbit. Amer. J. Physiol. **96**, 343—348 (1931).

Blobel, G., Sabatini, D. D.: Controlled proteolysis of nascent polypeptides in rat liver cell fractions. I. Location of the polypeptides within ribosomes. J. Cell Biol. **45**, 130—145 (1970).

Burwen, S. J., Rothman, S. S.: Protein recapture, osmotic behaviour, and selective ion sensitivity in zymogen granules. Fed. Proc. **29**, 1124 (1970).

Caro, L. G., Palade, G. E.: Protein synthesis, storage, and discharge in the pancreatic exocrine cell. J. Cell Biol. **20**, 473—495 (1964).

Dickman, S. R., Holtzer, R. L., Gazzinelli, G.: Protein synthesis in beef pancreas slices: Biochemistry. **1**, 574—580 (1962).

Greene, L. J., Hirs, C. H. W., Palade, G. E.: On the protein composition of bovine pancreatic zymogen granules. J. Biol. Chem. **238**, 2054—2070 (1963).

van Heyningen, H. E.: Secretion of protein by the acinar cells of the rat pancreas, as studied by electron microscopic radioautography. Anat. Rec. **148**, 488—497 (1964).

Hokin, L. E.: Isolation of zymogen granules of dog pancreas and a study of their properties. Biochim. biophys. Acta (Amst.) **18**, 379—388 (1955).

—: Dynamic aspect of phospholipids during protein secretion. Intern. Rev. Cytol. **23**, 187—208 (1968).

— Hokin, M. R.: The synthesis and secretion of digestive enzymes by pancreas tissue *in vitro*. In: The Exocrine Pancreas. London: J. and A. Churchill Ltd. 1962.

Jamieson, J. D., Palade, G. E.: Intracellular transport of secretory proteins in the pancreatic exocrine cell. I. Role of the peripheral elements of the Golgi complex. J. Cell Biol. **34**, 577—596 (1967a).

— —: II. Transport to condensing vacuoles and zymogen granules. J. Cell Biol. **34**, 597—615 (1967b).

— —: III. Dissociation of intracellular transport from protein synthesis. J. Cell Biol. **39**, 580—588 (1968a).

— —: IV. Metabolic requirements. J. Cell Biol. **39**, 589—603 (1968b).

— —: Condensing vacuole conversion and zymogen granule discharge in pancreatic exocrine cells: metabolic studies. J. Cell Biol. **48**, 503—522 (1971)

Keller, P. J., Cohen, E.: Enzymic composition of some cell fractions of bovine pancreas. J. Biol. Chem. **236**, 1407—1413 (1961).

Laird, A. K., Barton, A. D.: Protein synthesis in rat pancreas. II. Changes in intracellular distribution of pancreatic amylase during the secretory cycle. Biochim. biophys. Acta (Amst.) **27**, 12—15 (1958).

Lin, T. M., Grossman, M. I.: Dose response relationship of pancreatic enzyme stimulants: pancreozymin and metacholine. Amer. J. Physiol. **186**, 52—56 (1956).

Morris, A. J., Dickman, S. R.: Biosynthesis of ribonuclease in mouse pancreas. J. Biol. Chem. **235**, 1404—1408 (1960).

Palade, G. E.: Functional changes in the structure of cell components. In: Subcellular Particles. New York: Ronald Press Co. 1959.

— Siekevitz, P., Caro, L. G.: Structure, chemistry and function of the pancreatic exocrine cell. In: The Exocrine Pancreas. London: J. and A. Churchill Ltd. 1962.

Redman, C. M.: Studies on the transfer of incomplete polypeptide chains across rat liver microsomal membranes *in vitro*. J. Biol. Chem. **242**, 761—768 (1967).

— Hokin, L. E.: Phospholipid turnover in microsomal membranes of the pancreas during enzyme secretion. J. Biophys. Biochem. Cytol. **6**, 207—214 (1959).

— Sabatini, D. D.: Vectorial discharge of peptides released by puromycin from attached ribosomes. Proc. nat. Acad. Sci. (Wash.) **56**, 608—615 (1966).

— Siekevitz, P., Palade, G. E.: Synthesis and transfer of amylase in pigeon pancreatic microsomes. J. Biol. Chem. **241**, 1150—1158 (1966).

Sabatini, D. D., Blobel, G.: Controlled proteolysis of nascent polypeptides in rat liver cell fractions. II. Location of the polypeptides in rough microsomes. J. Cell Biol. **45**, 146—157 (1970).

Schramm, M.: Secretion of enzymes and other macromolecules. Ann. Rev. Biochem. **36**, 307—320 (1967).

Wesbter, P. D.: Hormonal control of pancreatic secretion. In: Exocrine Glands. Philadelphia: University of Pennsylvania Press 1969.

Chapter IV

The Secretin Test

MAURICE J. ZIMMERMAN, DAVID A. DREILING and HENRY D. JANOWITZ

With 7 Figures

Aided by Grant AM-03889 from the National Institute of Arthritis and Metabolic Diseases, National Institutes of Health.

A. General Introduction

Secretin and pancreozymin are two hormones extractable from the mucosa of the upper small intestine which cause the pancreas to secrete water and bicarbonate and enzymes respectively.

I. Secretin

BAYLISS and STARLING (1902), in a now famous experiment, discovered that an acid extract of intestinal mucosa stimulated pancreatic secretion. They named this substance secretin, and about two years later the term hormone was introduced, for the first time. Various preparations were made available over the years, of greater or lesser purity, but the final purification of secretin was not achieved until 1961 (JORPES and MUTT). They (JORPES et al. 1962; MUTT and JORPES, 1966, 1968a; JORPES, 1968) showed that secretin was a polypeptide containing 27 amino acids, composed of 11 amino acids. Absent from the polypeptide chain were cystine, methionine, tyrosine, tryptophan, proline, isoleucine and lysine. The exact composition is Ala 1-Arg 4- Asp 2- Glu 3-Gly 2- His 1- Leu 6- Phe 1- Ser 4- Thr 2- Val 1. The N-terminal sequence is histidyl-seryl-aspartyl. Valine occurs at the carboxyl-terminal in the form of its amide. In two of the glutamic acid residues, the gammacarboxyls are also amidated. BODANSZKY et al. (1969), achieved final synthesis of secretin in 1969. They proposed that secretin was a single chain polypeptide with a helical structure between residues 5 and 13 of the molecule. The entire chain of 27 residues appears to be necessary for activity. In contrast to the other gastrointestinal tract hormones, no active fragment has yet been found. The molecular weight is 3055.

Various preparations of secretin have been available through the years, prepared by different laboratories in several countries. The extraction methods and potency have varied and are difficult to compare with one another (JORPES, 1970, personal communication). He states that it is impossible to make any accurate statements concerning the potency of Pancreotest, Astra, Södertälje, Sweden; Secretin Byla, Paris, Secretin Wyeth, Philadelphia, and Secretin Lilly. The previously popular Hammarsten cat unit equals about 1/16 to 1/20 of what is described as 1 clinical unit, which is the same as the Ivy dog threshhold dose. Between 1958 and 1965, a purer preparation of secretin was prepared under JORPES and MUTT's direction by the Vitrum Laboratories in Sweden. Twenty of the old Hammarsten cat units were then made equal to 1 Vitrum unit. This standard was unstable, and production was discontinued. Production of secretin then continued at the Karolinska Institute beginning with lot No. 16611, and the potency of the clinical unit was increased fourfold. This potency has been maintained through the date of this writing (1970, lot No. 17012). The current unit of secretin produced at the Karolinska Institute probably equals that of the old Pancreotest unit with which Lagerlöf (1942) elaborated the secretin test of pancreatic function. There is no significant variation from one lot to another of the newer secretin preparations. STENING et al. (1968) performed a bioassay of the potency of 4 batches of GIH secretin and compared them with Boots secretin, in chronic fistula dogs. The batches of GIH secretin differed by less than 20% in potency. A similar variation was found in the Boots secretin. However, it was found that 1 clinical unit of GIH secretin was 8 to 9 times greater than 1 Crick, Harper, Raper units of Boots secretin. KONTUREK (1969) thinks the ratio is 1/10. Beginning with 1966 (lot No. 16611), the GIH secretin contained pure, not purified secretin with a content of 3500 units/mgm during the summer and 4000 units/mgm during the winter. GROSSMAN (1969) found a 50% loss of activity of lyophilized secretin powder at −20 °C in 6 months in a rubber stoppered vial. This applied to porcine secretin made by Vitrum during the period 1962—1965. Since 1966, when all glass vials are used, and with 1 mgm cysteine HCl added, activity has been retained for over 1 year at −20 °C.

II. Pancreozymin-Cholecystokinin

Following the discovery of secretin by BAYLISS and STARLING (1902), MELLANBY (1928) attempted an alcohol extraction of duodenal mucosa, using bile acids as an adsorbing surface. The adsorbed substance contained secretin activity. HARPER and RAPER (1943) postulated that a hormone eliciting an enzyme response from the pancreas would have been extracted by the same solvents as secretin, but since MELLANBY's secretin caused no enzyme response, they examined the supernatant. HARPER and RAPER (1943) examined the small intestines of the pig, dog and cat, and extracted a substance which on intravenous injection caused an increase in secretion of enzymes by the pancreas, but no increase in volume of pancreatic juice. The substance was named pancreozymin, and was tested in anesthetized cats against a background of secretin. Pancreozymin was found to be thermostable, acid stable, and dialyzable by cellophane. They showed further that the response of the pancreas to pancreozymin was unaffected by section of either the vagus or splanchnic nerves or atropine-induced vagal blockade. No vasodilator or hypoglycemic effects could be attributed to the substance.

JORPES and MUTT (1962) had improved the extraction methods of pancreozymin so that they were producing the most powerful preparation at that time, about 600 times as potent as the original CRICK, HARPER, RAPER preparation. Currently produced in Stockholm, the preparation (Cecekin) has both cholecystokinetic and pancreozyminic activity. This preparation is about 10% pure (JORPES, personal communication, 1970), and has 250—300 Ivy dog units/mgm. In the beginning the label unfortunately stated activities in terms of Ivy dog units of cholecystokinin and CRICK, HARPER, RAPER units of pancreozymin, since there are 4 CHR pancreozymin units to 1 Ivy dog unit of cholecystokinin. The Ivy dog unit of CCK in Cecekin has approximately the same potency as that in CCK-PZ manufactured at the GIH Research unit at the Karolinska Institute. Different lots do not differ by more than 15% from one another. It is not universally held that the Swedish preparation of CCK-PZ is the most potent, since WORMSLEY (1969) claims that the CRICK, HARPER, RAPER unit in Boots pancreozymin is 3 to 4 times as potent as the GIH unit.

Pancreozymin is a single chain polypeptide containing 33 amino acids, in which the C-terminal sequence resembles that of gastrin (MUTT and JORPES, 1967, 1968b, c; ONDETTI et al., 1970). In regard to pancreatic enzyme secretion, the C-terminal octapeptide was tested, in urethane-anesthetized dogs receiving an intravenous infusion of secretin at the rate of 2 clinical units/kg/hr. The rapid intravenous injection of the octapeptide evoked an immediate, transient dose-related increase in the protein output of the pancreas. The potency of the C-terminal octapeptide as compared to CCK-PZ was 16,000 Ivy dog units/mgm. Further studies (MUTT and JORPES, 1968c; ONDETTI et al., 1970) indicated that the C-terminal peptide sequence displayed the biologic activities of the whole molecule.

B. The Secretin Test of Pancreatic Function

I. Physiologic Effects of Secretin

Pancreatic juice is clear and colorless, isoosmotic with plasma, and the osmolality is independent of rate of flow. The juice appearing in the duodenum consists of water, electrolytes, and a protein mixture of digestive enzymes. The fluid is of low viscosity, alkaline at a pH of about 8.3, and contains Na^+, K^+, HCO_3^- and Cl^- as the major cationic and anionic constituents. Lesser concentrations of Ca^{++} (ZIMMERMAN et al., 1967), as well as Zn^{++}, HPO_3^{--} and SO_4^{--} are present. Sodium and potassium concentrations in the dog as measured by JOHNSTON and BALL (1930), were for sodium $[Na^+] = 154 \pm 7$ and $[K] = 4.8 \pm 0.9$ m-mol/kgm. H_2O. SOLOMON (1952) recapitulated existing data for serum and pancreatic juice of dogs as follows:

	Serum	Juice m-mole/kgm H_2O
Cl	117.8 ± 4.8	variable
Total CO_2	28.3	154 ± 10
Na	153.1 ± 3.2	154 ± 7
K	5.1 ± 0.3	4.8 ± 0.9
H_2O	92.4%	98%

DREILING and JANOWITZ (1956) found Na^+ varied between 139—143 mEq/L and K^+ between 6—9 mEq/L in human juice obtained at duodenal intubation. Magnesium is present in small amounts approximating 0.5 mEq/L, while calcium concentration is lower than in plasma water (ZIMMERMAN et al., 1967). The anionic composition is dependent on rate of secretion. The chief ions are bicarbonate and chloride which have a reciprocal relationship to each other. Bicarbonate concentration varies between 25 and 150 mEq/L and chloride concentration varies inversely with the bicarbonate. The sum of the concentrations of bicarbonate and chloride approximate 150 mEq/L, but under certain conditions, and for as yet unexplained reasons, the sum of bicarbonate and chloride concentrations may exceed 150 mEq/L (PERRIER et al., 1964). DREILING and JANOWITZ (1959) studied the bicarbonate-flow relationships in man and have demonstrated a curvilinear relationship when rate of secretion is plotted against maximum bicarbonate concentration (Fig. 1). For further details on variations in electrolyte composition and cellular sites of secretion of electrolytes, the reader is referred to the recent article by JANOWITZ (1967).

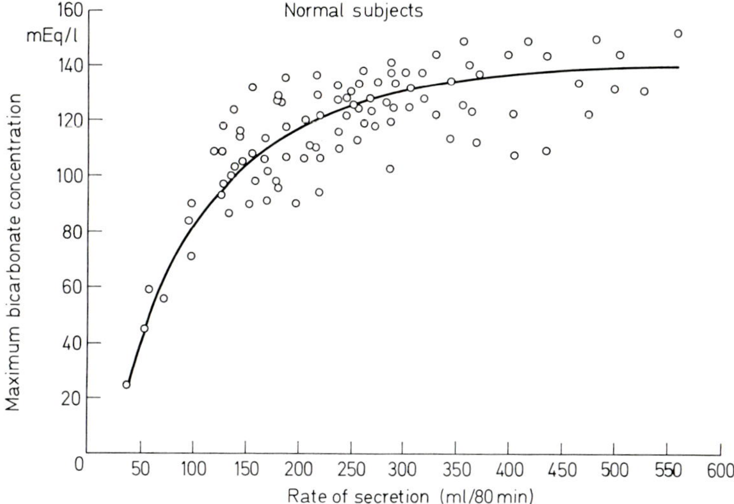

Fig. 1. Relationship between maximum bicarbonate concentration and rate of secretion in 65 subjects without pancreatic disease (DREILING and JANOWITZ, 1962)

In addition to the secretion of fluid and electrolytes in response to a secretin stimulus, there is an initial outpouring of pancreatic digestive enzymes, which has been termed a "wash-out" phenomenon of preformed pancreatic enzymes. Secretin, unlike pancreozymin, is not a pancreatic protein secretagogue, and the enzyme content of pancreatic juice following a secretin stimulus soon falls to low concentrations.

II. Historical

Determination of the secretory capacity of the pancreas should give information regarding the mass of functioning tissue. In theory, at least, there should be a relationship between diminished secretory capacity (function) and organic damage to secretory glands. LIM et al. (1923) demonstrated a method for quantitative recovery of duodenal juice in humans by introduction of two REHFUSS tubes simultaneously, one in the stomach and the other in the duodenum. ÅGREN and LAGERLÖF (1936) improved on this method by combining two tubes in one. Initial attempts at recovering duodenal contents following a secretin stimulus were performed by the French (CHIRAY et al., 1926), but a single lumened tube was used with no means of removing saliva and gastric juice. It is well known that acid gastric juice acts as a stimulant for the release of secretin from the duodenal mucosa. Following the initial use of the double-lumened tube by ÅGREN and LAGERLÖF, numerous European and American workers performed secretin tests (DIAMOND and SIEGEL, 1940; LAKE, 1947) and DREILING and HOLLANDER (1948; 1950) collected large groups of data beginning with the monumental work of LAGERLÖF (1942).

III. Methodology of the Secretin Test at Mount Sinai Hospital

DREILING (1955) has described in great detail his method of performing a secretin test of pancreatic function. In brief, the test is performed in the fasting state, usually early in the morning. The patients have usually been fasting following the evening meal of the previous day. Otherwise food retained in the stomach may induce the endogenous release of secretin and invalidate the test. A double-lumen tube is swallowed by the patient, usually without oral or pharyngeal topical anesthesia. The tube itself is radio-opaque to facilitate fluoroscopic visualization, and in addition, a small metal "olive" is present at the duodenal end to facilitate passage through the pylorus. The tube is constructed so that a sufficient number of drainage holes are available at the duodenal end, and a large number are available to drain the stomach, in which the tube lies along the lesser curvature. Following the entry of the tube into the stomach, the patient is fluoroscoped, any kinks in the tube are straightened out, and the tip is manipulated towards the pylorus. Frequently, one of the next few antral peristaltic waves will carry the "olive" past the pylorus into the duodenum to the ligament of Treitz. If the duodenal tip fails to pass the pylorus spontaneously during the initial fluoroscopy, the patient is placed in bed either flat on his back or lying on his right side. Both outlets (gastric and duodenal) are attached to gentle Gomco suction until bile appears in the duodenal aspirate. Usually this means that the tube has passed into the duodenum, although it is not a certainty. At this point, the patient is taken back to the fluoroscopy room to confirm passage of the tube as described above.

After the tube is in proper position, and excess slack has been taken up, the patient is taken back to bed and is allowed to lie comfortably on his back. Both gastric and duodenal tubes are attached to suction until a clear, alkaline, non-turbid secretion is obtained from the duodenal tube. Following this, a 20 minute control period is taken. After the control period a submaximal dose of secretin is given intravenously, 1 clinical unit/kgm. The secretin is injected slowly over a period of at least 2 minutes. Post-secretin specimens are collected simultaneously from the stomach and duodenum for 80 minutes, 4 twenty minute samples being sufficient for the stomach, but the duodenal specimens are collected in 10, 10, 10, 10, 20, and 20 minute samples.

The gastric specimens are examined for volume, pH, biliary pigment concentration (icteric index) and guaiac reaction. The pH is determined directly with hydrion paper. Free and total acid are determined by titration. Volume, pH and biliary pigment concentration are important indices of duodenal regurgitation into the stomach and are heralded by sudden increases of gastric volumes, the appearence of bile in the stomach and sudden increases in pH, since secretin, per se, should inhibit gastric secretion as first observed by Dragstedt (GREENLEE et al., 1957).

The individual duodenal specimens are analyzed for volume, pH, bicarbonate concentration, enzyme concentration, icteric index, guaiac reaction, and when indicated, the specimens can be collected on ice, centrifuged and sent for cytological examination if carcinoma of the pancreas is strongly suspected. Cytology is not routinely performed. The duodenal pH is an index of gastric contamination of duodenal contents and is of importance, since the entry of gastric acid into the duodenum neutralizes that bicarbonate which has been secreted, inactivates pancreatic enzymes, and also liberates secretin endogenously from the duodenal mucosa. A drop of duodenal pH to below 7.0 is indicative of gastric contamination.

The volume, bicarbonate concentration, and enzyme secretion characterize the response of the pancreas to secretin. At our laboratory, the bicarbonate concentration is measured in each duodenal specimen in a Van Slyke apparatus. Volume is measured directly in a graduated cylinder. Since the pancreatic enzymes have been shown to be secreted in parallel (BAXTER, 1935), it is only necessary to determine the amylase concentration, and this is done by a modification of the Somogyi method (SOMOGYI, 1941).

The bile pigment response to secretin is best studied by determining the icteric index on each individual duodenal specimen. The characteristic normal and abnormal responses are seen in Figure 2.

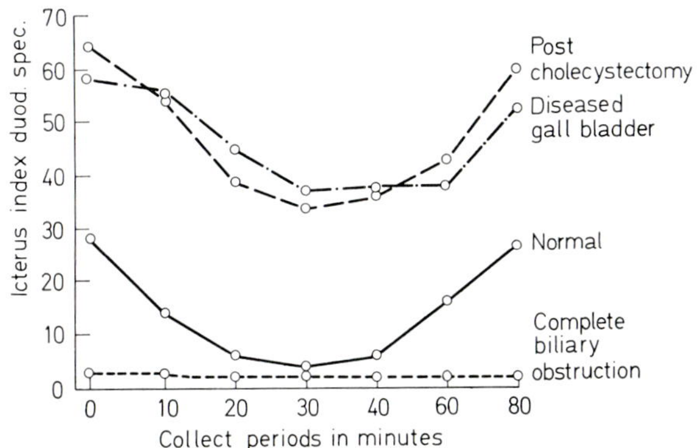

Fig. 2. The biliary pigment response in the secretin test as indicated by serial duodenal icterus index following the administration of secretin to patients with normal gall bladder function, with non-functioning gall bladders (or post-cholecystectomy), and with complete biliary obstruction (DREILING et al., 1964)

IV. Variants of the Secretin Test

The method of performing the secretin test at other institutions varies in some detail from author to author. LAGERLÖF (1942) collected 60 minute post-secretin samples as did Goldstein and co-workers (GOLDSTEIN et al., 1964) and DIAMOND et al. (1940). WENGER and RASKIN (1958) collected 3 ten minute specimens for a total of 30 minutes.

All authors currently use a double-lumened tube. DREILING and JANOWITZ (1962) tried to measure the loss of duodenal juice from duodenum to jejunum in standard secretin tests by means of a triple-bore tube, one opening of which ended in the jejunum. In 16 patients, none of whom retched, only 2 — 12 ml of juice were recovered from the jejunum in 80 minutes. Analysis of bilirubin and amylase showed that these aspirates represented jejunal rather than duodenal juice. In two patients who retched, 69 and 113 ml were recovered, respectively, in 80 minutes. SARLES (1965) and LAGERLÖF (1967) attempted to secure a better separation between gastric and duodenal juice by use of an air-inflated rubber bag in the antral region of the stomach, but the presence of a balloon in the antral region of the stomach may stimulate the antral release of gastrin and thus stimulate enzyme release by the pancreas.

V. The Submaximal Secretin Test: Normal Results

Following an injection of 1 unit of secretin/kgm in the normal subject, there is a rapid, brisk increase in pancreatic flow. Somewhere between 100 and 300 ml of pancreatic juice may be collected during an 80 minute period. Destruction of the pancreatic parenchyma by disease processes, or obstruction of a main pancreatic duct will reduce the volume flow. The concentration of bicarbonate ion in the pancreatic juice rises and falls in a parabolic fashion (see Fig. 3), but more

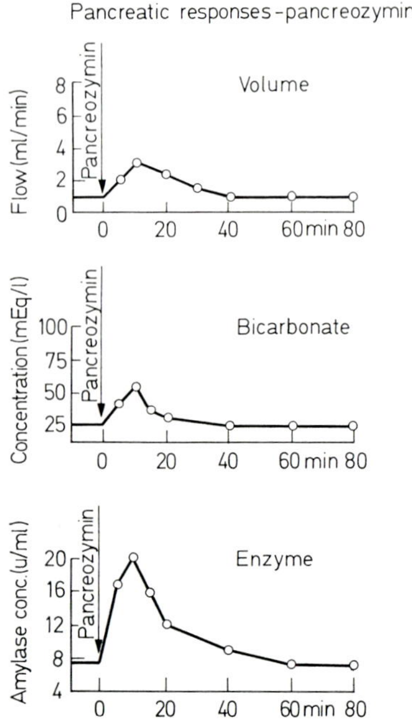

Fig. 3. Pancreatic responses obtained with duodenal drainage in man following intravenous administration of secretin (Dreiling and Janowitz, 1962)

slowly than does the volume rate. In normal human pancreatic juice sampled via a duodenal tube, bicarbonate concentrations as high as 140 mEq/L may be found. One of the hallmarks of chronic inflammatory disease of the pancreas is its inability to secrete a juice of high bicarbonate content. Enzyme concentration in the pancreatic juice after the intravenous administration of secretin begins at a plateau level, but soon falls to extremely low levels, since the enzyme present is being diluted by the sudden outpouring of large volumes of pancreatic juice. Secretin is not a stimulus for pancreatic enzyme secretion. Although the enzyme concentration, per se, is not of great importance in the interpretation of this test, the total enzyme secretion (output) is. It is frequently reduced both in chronic inflammatory and neoplastic ductal obstruction of the pancreas.

Ågren and Lagerlöf (1936) described a secretin test using a double lumened tube and collecting gastric and duodenal juice after injecting 0.1 to 0.5 mgm/kgm of a secretin preparation containing 10—25 cat units/mgm. They described the results in 14 normal cases and compared them with a number of pathologic cases, in seven of which a pancreatic disorder was present. The pancreatic juice was collected for 80 minutes and comparisons were made with regard to volume, amylase, trypsin, and highest bicarbonate concentration. A lowered amount of amylase and total volume was seen in cases of pancreatic lithiasis, cancer and chronic pancreatitis. In acute pancreatitis, only an isolated decrease in the amount of amylase was noted. These findings were confirmed by others (DIAMOND and SIEGEL, 1940; COMFORT and OSTERBERG, 1940).

LAGERLÖF (1942) studied 33 healthy, normal adults under the age of 35 years, including 18 men and 15 women. A second group included 12 men and 3 women hospitalized for reasons other than gastrointestinal disorders. All individuals were noted to have free hydrochloric acid in their gastric aspirate. The following was noted:

1. There was a spontaneous secretion which varied between 1 and 27 ml, with a mean of 11 ml in 20 minutes.

2. One clinical unit (16 Hammarsten cat units) was injected intravenously/kgm.

3. The volume varied between 95 and 266 ml in 60 minutes in 18 healthy men with a mean of 186 $\pm$ 12ml. For 12 hospitalized male patients without abdominal symptoms the range was 116 to 253 ml, with a mean of 175 $\pm$12 ml. Since there was close agreement between these two groups, the figures were combined and the mean volume was 181.7 $\pm$8.6 ml. The 15 healthy women had a duodenal juice volume which varied between 105 and 146 ml, with a mean of 126.3 $\pm$3.5 ml. The difference between the means for men and women was 48 $\pm$10 and was felt to be significant.

4. Bicarbonate secretion (output) was measured. In the healthy male group it varied between 82 and 301 ml of N/10 bicarbonate solution. The corresponding figures for the groups of hospitalized males was 120 to 257 ml. Combination of the data from the two groups gave an average of 175 $\pm$10 ml. Results in the healthy women varied between 84 and 143 ml, while in the female patients it varied between 165 and 182 ml. Combination of all the data from females resulted in a mean of 121 $\pm$6 ml. The difference between the means for men and women was significant.

5. Enzyme secretion was measured. This included estimation of amylase, trypsin and lipase. No sex variation was noted in regard to enzyme secretion. Mean amylase secretion was 637 $\pm$29 units. Mean trypsin secretion for males and females combined was 87.7 $\pm$5.4 units. Mean lipase secretion for both sexes together was 179 $\pm$17 units.

6. The secretin test was performed in individuals with gastric achylia and achlorhydria and no significant differences from normals were found in regard to volume of duodenal juice, bicarbonate, amylase and trypsin outputs.

DIAMOND and SIEGEL (1940) reported on 130 secretin tests in 104 individuals using a double-lumened tube. Twenty-four individuals were thought to be normal, and 80 were labeled "pathologic." A continuous intravenous infusion of Astra secretin was administered at the rate of 150 ml/hr (0.75 mgm/kgm). Basal levels were noted to be reattained by the end of 80 minutes. They described 80 minute volumes ranging from 150—250 ml, a characteristic biliary pigment response, bicarbonate concentrations in the normal individuals which ranged from 90—130 mEq/L, as well as total amylase outputs which ranged between 300—1200 units in 1 hour. Comparison between normals and patients with pancreatic disease led these authors to believe that a diminished enzyme secretion was the earliest manifestation of pancreatic disease, and that diminished volume and bicarbonate concentrations were later manifestations.

DREILING and HOLLANDER (1950) attempted to measure the range of secretory output in normal individuals in response to a single-dose injection of Wyeth secretin, given in a submaximal dose of 1 unit/kgm. One hundred seventy-two patients were studied, all of whom were free of pancreatic disease. Eighty-one patients had the above dose of Wyeth secretin administered, and statistical data were derived by combination of this group with earlier results obtained in 91 normals using 1 unit/kgm of an earlier Wyeth secretin preparation as well as with Astra secretin. As has been described previously (Dreiling and Hollander, 1950), 80 minute collection periods were used, as was a double-lumen tube. Based on this group, the following critical lower limits of normal were established (see Tables 1, 2, 3).

Table 1. *Summary of secretin-test data in 1824 patients without evidence of pancreatic disease* (Dreiling *and* Janowitz, *1962*)

	Total volume ml./kg.	Maximum HCO_3^- mEq/l.	Total amylase u./kg.
Observed range	1·9—7·4	81—152	5·1—56·2
Mean value	3·7	111	22·3
Percentage in abnormal range	3%	3%	4%
Mean normal series	3·2	108	14·9
Lower limit normals	2·0	90	6·0

Table 2. *Secretin-test data of 113 patients with acute pancreatitis and of 296 patients with chronic pancreatitis (*Dreiling *and* Janowitz *1962)*

	Total volume ml./kg.	Maximum HCO_3^- mEq/l.	Total amylase u./kg.
Acute — 113			
Observed range	0·5—4·5	72—132	0·2—26·8
Mean value	2·4	93	9·7
Percentage in normal range	76%	67%	58%
Chronic — 296			
Observed range	0·4—17·1	28—96	0·3—24·1
Mean value	2·7	57	7·1
Percentage in normal range	73%	4%	62%
Mean normal series	3·2	108	14·9
Lower limit normals	2·0	90	6·0

Table 3. *Secretin-test data of 204 patients with cancer of the head of the pancreas, of 76 patients with cancer of the body of the pancreas, and of 29 patients with cancer of the tail of the pancreas (*Dreiling *and* Janowitz *1962)*

	Total volume ml./kg.	Maximum HCO_3^- mEq/l.	Total amylase u./kg.
Head — 204			
Observed range	0·3—2·3	48—148	1·4—14·2
Mean value	1·3	83	5·6
Percentage in normal range	5%	78%	73%
Body — 76			
Observed range	1·1—3·9	83—142	2·8—21·2
Mean value	1·7	93	6·9
Percentage in normal range	41%	95%	91%
Tail — 29			
Observed range	1·9—5·7	93—132	3·6—34·5
Mean value	3·7	109	20·6
Percentage in normal range	97%	100%	97%
Mean normal series	3·2	108	14·9
Lower limit normals	2·0	90	6·0

for total volume: 2.0 ml/kgm or greater: mean 3.2 ml/kgm
for maximum bicarbonate concentration: 90 mEq/L or greater: mean 108 mEq/L
for total amylase secretion: 6.0 units/kgm or greater: mean 14.2 units/kgm

The above data was derived by taking the mean ± 2 standard deviations. It is interesting to note that the calculated lower limits of normal are similar to data derived earlier (LAGERLÖF, 1942), with a different secretin preparation.

DREILING and JANOWITZ (1957) published a summary of a thorough analysis of 1500 secretin tests performed by them using various secretin preparations. Using statistical techniques they classified disorders of the pancreas into two general patterns: (1) A qualitative defect (volume of pancreatic secretion is sustained but the bicarbonate response and to a lesser degree, the enzyme secretion, is diminished) characteristic of chronic inflammatory disease of the pancreas; and (2) a quantitative deficiency in which there tends to be a reduced volume with maintenance of maximum bicarbonate concentration as well as enzyme secretion. The quantitative deficiency was most often associated with major ductal obstruction as seen in neoplastic disease of the pancreas. In advanced neoplastic or chronic inflammatory disease, both quantitative and qualitative defects may be seen.

WENGER and RASKIN (1958) described their results using 1 unit/kgm of Lilly secretin, a double-lumen tube and a 30 minute collection period, divided into 3 ten-minute specimens. In their normals, pancreatic juice volume exceeded 1.1 ml/kgm in 30 minutes, and in at least 1 specimen, the bicarbonate concentration was greater than 90 mEq/L. The authors felt that measurement of enzyme secretion was of no value.

COMFORT and OSTERBERG (1940) described a test with secretin alone, as well as with the addition of acetylbetamethylcholine chloride (Mecholyl). In 14 normal subjects secretin alone was administered on 20 occasions to 13, while secretin plus Mecholyl was administered in 22 experiments to 10 individuals. Secretin alone caused a large increase in pancreatic volume, a juice of high pH, as well as a reduction in enzyme concentration. The only change attributable to Mecholyl was a prolonged increase in enzyme output.

GOLDSTEIN et al. (1964) gave Lilly secretin to 69 control subjects in a single intravenous dose of 1 unit/kgm, and collected the juice for 60 minutes. Their data follow:

total 1 hour volume	65 — 325 ml	mean 187 ml
1 hour vol/kgm	0.92 — 5.20	mean 2.92 ml/kgm/hr
bicarbonate concentration (mEq/L)	64.5 — 130.0	mean 97.6

Enzyme data were not analyzed for this group of patients.

PETERSEN (1970) recently used pure natural secretin (GIH Research Unit, Stockholm) in 26 healthy individuals in various doses, intravenously as a single shot. A double-lumened LAGERLÖF tube was used, good separations of gastric and duodenal contents were obtained, and there was no regurgitation of duodenal contents into the stomach. Duodenal juice was collected in 20 minute samples for 1 hour in some cases and for two hours in others, after a basal collection period of 1 hour. He noted a marked variability in volume of duodenal juice as well as bicarbonate output during the basal period. No significant sex difference was seen. Although various dosages of secretin were injected, it is interesting to observe the responses to 1 clinical unit/kgm.

Table 4. *The duodenal juice collected after an intravenous injection of one clinical unit of pure natural secretin per kg body weight* (Petersen *1970*)

			The first post-secretin hour			The second post-secretin hour		
			Females n = 11	Males n = 15	Difference	Females n = 6	Males n = 8	Difference
Volume	ml	range	151—300	179—418		21—193	87—305	
		mean	218	282	p< 0.01	107	189	NS
		SD	49	60		72	83	
		VC	22%	21%		68%	44%	
	ml/kg	range	2.6—5.2	2.3—5.7		0.4—33	1.1—4.0	
		mean	3.6	3.8	NS	1.8	2.5	NS
		SD	0.8	0.9		1.1	1.1	
		VC	22%	24%		63%	45%	
Peak bicarbonate concentration	mEq/l	range	88—116	90—124		74—111	83—112	
		mean	101	103	NS	93	99	NS
		SD	9	9		17	12	
		VC	9%	8%		18%	12%	
Bicarbonate output	mEq	range	12.1—26.9	13.0—42.3		1.3—17.4	5.2—30.6	
		mean	19.0	25.7	p< 0.02	9.8	17.4	NS
		SD	4.6	7.1		7.1	8.5	
		VC	24%	28%		73%	49%	
	mEq/kg	range	0.22—0.45	0.17—0.58		0.02—0.28	0.07—0.42	
		mean	0.32	0.34	NS	0.16	0.24	NS
		SD	0.07	0.10		0.11	0.12	
		VC	23%	30%		70%	50%	

SD: standard deviation VC: coefficient of variation NS: not significant

During the first post-secretin hour, the volume of duodenal contents was significantly different between males and females, but this sex difference disappeared when the results were expressed on a weight basis (Table 4). The outputs of bicarbonate were nearly constant during the first post-secretin hour, while in the second post-secretin hour, the bicarbonate outputs were about 61% of those during the first hour. Despite the fact that the volume of duodenal contents was falling during the second hour, the peak bicarbonate concentration remained relatively high. Bicarbonate outputs were significantly correlated to body weight and thus were different for males and females. When bicarbonate outputs were thus expressed on a weight basis, the sex difference disappeared. Peterson noted no relationship between the concentration of bicarbonate and volume of duodenal contents when the data were analyzed for the first five 20 minute post-secretin periods. During the time from 100 to 120 minutes post-secretin, a positive correlation between volume and bicarbonate concentration was observed.

Petersen compared his results using pure natural secretin with data observed by many others using earlier secretin preparations of variable purity (Table 5). His values for volume and bicarbonate output were 30 to 60% higher, and the response to secretin was prolonged. Prior authors (Ågren and Lagerlöf, 1936; Diamond et al., 1939; Dreiling, 1955) had felt that the response to 1 clinical unit of secretin persisted for 60—100 minutes, while Peterson has observed relatively high bicarbonate output and volumes for two or more hours. This would seem to indicate that the effect of pure natural secretin is stronger than earlier preparations.

VI. The Maximal Secretory Response of the Pancreas to Secretin

From the foregoing it can be seen that various authors, using different preaprations of secretin (though generally at a 1 unit/kg dose), have obtained variable

Table 5. *The mean secretory response per collection time to different secretin preparations in control materials* (PETERSEN *1970)*

First author	Year	Secretin prep.	Secretin dose cl.u./kg	No. of controls	Coll. time min	Volume ml	Volume ml/kg	Bicarbobate output mEq	Bicarbobate output mEq/kg
Ågren	(1) 1936	Astra	1	15	80		3.8		
Diamond	* 1940	Astra	1.5	24	80	169	2.6		
Dreiling	(9) 1950	Astra	1	91	80	204	3.6		
Lagerlöf	* 1942	Astra	1	33	60	200	3.0	19.0	0.28
Lake	* 1947	Astra	1	18	60	186	3.4	14.6	
Dornberger	* 1948	Astra	1	18	40	123		14.8	
Gross	* 1950	Astra	1	10	40	78		6.8	
Friedman	(12) 1949	Wyeth	1.1	22	60	143			
Dreiling	(9) 1950	Wyeth	1	88	80	191	3.2		
Pfeffer	(23) 1952	Lilly	1	10	80	151	2.0		
Rosenberg	(26) 1966	Lilly	1	103	80	219	3.7	19.2	0.33
Dreiling	(10) 1955	Lilly	1	123	60	165	2.7	17.8	
Sun	* 1957	Lilly	80 cl.u.	20	60	164	2.5		
Wenger	(33) 1958	Lilly	1	108	30		2.0		
Sun	(29) 1960	Boots	80 cl.u.	25	60		2.5		
Sun	(28) 1963	Boots	80 cl.u.	68	60	191	2.8		
Tandon	(30) 1965	Boots	80 cl.u.	21	60	195	3.4		
Chey	(5) 1966	Boots	80 cl.u.	47	60	165	2.7		
Burton	(3) 1960	Boots	1.7	21	30	135		11.4	
Christensen	* 1963	Vitrum	1	15	80		2.8	14.5	
Forell	(11) 1964	Vitrum	1	39	80		3.2		
Gülzow	* 1965	Vitrum	75 cl.u.	12	80	193	2.7		
Cathalan	(4) 1961	Vitrum	1	60	60	166			
Lagerlöf	(16) 1962	Vitrum	1	15	60		2.8		
Perrier	(19) 1964	Vitrum	1	45	60	166			
Hartley	* 1965	Vitrum	1	10	60	118	1.9	7.9	0.13
Plessier	(24) 1966	Vitrum	1	121	40	100			
Creutzfeldt	(7) 1964	Vitrum	1	60	30	113		11.0	
The presented material		Pure natural	1	26	80	316	4.7	28.7	0.43
					60	250	3.6	22.4	0.33

volume and bicarbonate responses. It has not been felt that these differences were real, but merely represented the variable degrees of purity of the preparations used, as well as the fact that the pancreas was not being stimulated to its maximum. Failure to elicit a "normal" volume or bicarbonate response in a particular case may merely signify a lack of recruitment of a sufficient number of pancreatic secretory cells. Since the purpose of doing a secretin test is to assess pancreatic secretory capacity, and thus attempt to relate secretory capacity to structural change, it has been hoped that a maximal stimulus of pancreatic secretory capacity would be more valuable, much as has been expected in regard to assessment of the secretory capacity of the parietal cells of the stomach (KAY, 1953).

BARON et al. (1963), studied the maximum bicarbonate output of chronic pancreatic fistula dogs in response to single injections of secretin as well as to continuous intravenous infusion of secretin. In dogs, a maximum bicarbonate output was attained for Vitrum secretin in doses of 7.5 to 12.5 units/kgm for single injections, and for 4—16 units/minute for intravenous infusions. When supramaximal doses were given as a single injection, or when intravenous infusions were maintained for periods of greater than 30—90 minutes, the concentration of bicarbonate fell, while the volume was still at relatively high levels. They, too, noted the typical inverse relationship between concentrations of bicarbonate and chloride. In their study, the most reproducible measurement was the maximum bicarbonate output in the pancreatic juice during the first 15 minutes after a single injection of secretin.

HARTLEY et al. (1965) used Vitrum secretion in healthy human volunteers. Mean values for volume and bicarbonate increased for all indivudials when the dose of secretin was increased from 1 to 2 clinical units/kgm. Some individuals had a further augmentation of secretory response when the dose was increased from 2 to 3 clinical units/kgm, but most had a diminution of response when the dose was raised from 3 to 4 clinical units/kgm. HARTLEY felt that 2 units/kgm was the dose necessary to elicit a maximal response in the human, in contrast to BARON's data in dogs (BARON et al., 1963).

PERRIER (1966), using Vitrum secretin, attempted to determine the dose required for maximal secretion. A definite sex variation was noted in regard to volume. All normal subjects had bicarbonate concentrations greater than 100 mEq/L, while all patients with pancreatic disease had bicarbonate concentrations below 70 mEq/L. There was a "no mans land" for concentrations of bicarbonate between 76 — 80 mEq/L. PERRIER noted that the maximum bicarbonate output in the first 15 minutes after secretin was the same in his group of humans both for single intravenous injections as well as for continuous intravenous infusions, and seems to be related to the weight of the pancreas. He, too, noted that supramaximal doses can have an inhibitory effect. In PERRIER's hands, and using Vitrum secretin, it was found that with a continuous intravenous secretin infusion, and in a steady state, 4 — 8 units/kgm/hour elicited a maximal bicarbonate response, and that similar levels could be obtained with 2 units/kgm in a single dose.

LAGERLÖF's newer data (1967) do not agree with that of HARTLEY or PERRIER. LAGERLÖF tested humans with a double-lumen tube with correction for the dead-space of the tube, as well as by using radioactive vitamin B_{12} as a marker. In some tests, PEG was used as a dilution indicator. Maximum volume outputs were obtained with 7.5 units/kgm of Vitrum secretin, which was taken to be the maximal dose. Bicarbonate output did not rise significantly, however, when 7.5 units/kgm were used as compared with the response to 1 unit/kgm. Amylase production in 60 minutes was the same as that obtained with the much less potent preparations used during the years 1935 — 1942. Similar results were obtained in regard to lipase and trypsin production.

BANWELL et al. (1967), tried to determine the maximal response of the human pancreas to continuous intravenous infusion of Vitrum secretin at various rates. The population studied included 7 normals, and others with various forms of chronic pancreatic, biliary and miscellaneous disorders. Secretin was infused at rates between 1 and 18 units/minute, and maximal responses were obtained at infusion rates between 4 — 6 units/minute. The authors felt that there was a relationship between maximum pancreatic response and body weight in the normal. Inspection of their data led them to believe that in regard to maximal volume and bicarbonate output, the coefficient of variation was least when the results were expressed in relation to body weight.

PASCAL et al. (1968) used continuous intravenous infusions of Boots secretin, and found maximal responses at 3 units/kgm-hour. Of the different parameters which were measured (volume, bicarbonate output, maximal and mean lipase outputs), the measurement of bicarbonate output showed the least variability.

WORMSLEY (1968) concurs in the supposition that measurement of the maximum bicarbonate response can be used as a guide to the detection of an impaired bicarbonate secretory capacity in chronic pancreatitis. He used Boots secretin both in single intravenous injections and intravenous infusions. Maximum responses were obtained when the continous infusion was given at 10 units/kgm-hour, and in this dose range was greater than for single intravenous injections.

PETERSEN (1970) using pure natural secretin (GIH Research Lab), tested 26 healthy individuals at dose rates for single intravenous injections of 0, 0.04, 0.2, 1, and 5 units/kgm. Near maximal responses were obtained with 1 clinical unit/kgm. Both the magnitude and duration of the bicarbonate response increased with increasing doses of secretin (Fig. 4). The secretion of bicarbonate was signi-

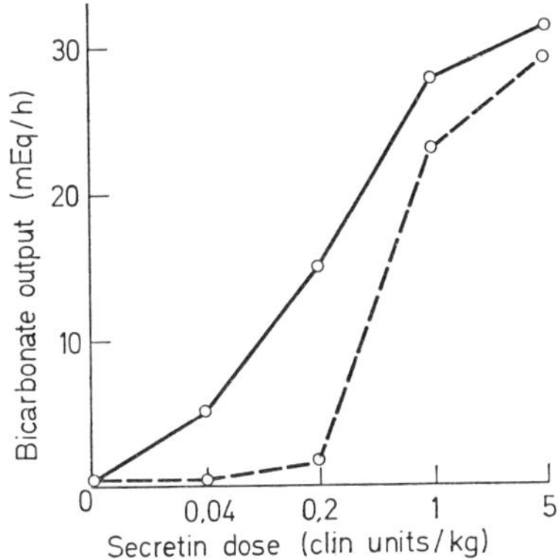

Fig. 4. The mean bicarbonate outputs from three individuals in the first (unbroken line) and in the second (dotted line) hour after intravenous injection of graded doses of pure natural secretin. The doses of secretin are plotted on a logarithmic scale and the '0' dose is dealt with as if it were 0.008 clinical units/kg body weight. The broken vertical lines indicate the range in secretin dose/kg body weight when 75 clinical units are administered to persons weighing between 37.5 and 150 kg (PETERSEN, 1970)

ficantly correlated to the logarithm of the administered dose of secretin. The relationship was approximately linear in dose ranges of 0.04 and 1 unit/kgm, while between 1 and 5 units/kgm, the response was nonlinear.

VII. The Effect of Age and Sex on Pancreatic Secretion

DEBRAY et al. (1962) noted in rats that there was little variation in pancreatic secretion between males and females. ROSENBERG et al. (1966) reanalyzed prior data from The Mount Sinai Hospital for secretin tests using 1 unit of Lilly secretin/kgm, and found little variability in regard to volume or peak bicarbonate concentration when the results in 41 males and 62 females were contrasted. In addition, it was noted that there was very little decline in pancreatic secretory capacity with age in contrast to the situation in the human stomach.

VIII. Effect of Route of Administration of Secretin

It had been formerly held that secretin would be an effective stimulant of pancreatic secretion only if given intravenously. PRESHAW and GROSSMAN (1965) compared the subcutaneous and intravenous administration of secretin Vitrum in dogs with a chronic pancreatic fistula as well as a chronic gastric fistula. In their hands, both crude as well as highly purified secretin (Vitrum) were weak stimulants of pancreatic secretion when given by the subcutaneous route, whereas both preparations gave large responses when given intravenously. A pancreozymin preparation (Cecekin), on the other hand, was an effective stimulant of pancreatic protein secretion by both the subcutaneous and intravenous routes. Gastrin, when tested in the same dogs, was a more effective stimulant of pancreatic secretion when given subcutaneously than intravenously. Later work by the same authors in dog and man (VAGNE and GROSSMAN, 1968; ISENBERG and GROSSMAN, 1969) disagreed with their earlier data. They then found that then available preparations of purified secretin were effective in dogs by both the intravenous and subcutaneous routes, but that higher doses were necessary when secretin was given by the subcutaneous route. Using GIH secretin in 5 normal males, they found that the pancreatic response over a 3 hour period was the same after 3 units/kgm given either subcutaneously or intravenously. The volume flow and bicarbonate output remained at nearly peak levels after secretin by either route. In the dog, however, the pancreatic response after intravenous secretin was more transient than in man. We are not aware of the use of this route for clinical testing.

IX. Results with Synthetic Secretin Preparations

Synthetic secretin preparations are currently becoming available. Insufficient time has elapsed for sufficient number of tests to have been performed, but some animal data are available.

KONTUREK (1969) compared dose responses in conscious cats between synthetic secretin, GIH secretin, and Boots secretin. The cats were equipped with chronic duodenal fistulas. The dose response curves were similar for synthetic and GIH secretin. Boots secretin was found to be 10 times less potent on a unit for unit basis than either of the other two preparations.

VAGNE et al. (1968) compared synthetic secretin with pure natural porcine secretin for potency as well as for the following physiological activities:

1. Stimulation of pancreatic flow and bicarbonate output in pancreatic fistula dogs.
2. Stimulation of biliary flow and bicarbonate output in biliary fistula dogs.
3. Inhibition of gastrin-stimulated gastric acid secretion in gastric fistula dogs.
4. Inhibition of gastric motility in dogs with innervated antral pouches.

Synthetic secretin, as originally prepared, was less potent than purified natural secretin. The newer preparation exactly equalled natural secretin on weight for a weight basis in its capacity to stimulate pancreatic flow. 0.1 microgram of either preparation stimulated a volume flow of 14 ml in 15 minutes.

X. Cytology

In addition to the information obtained from analysis of the duodenal contents for volume, bicarbonate, enzyme content and icteric index, the fluid can be subjected to cytological analysis. Various authors have reported a high incidence of positive smears for carcinoma cells (LEMON and BYRNES, 1949; MCNEER and EWING, 1949; RUBIN et al., 1953). RASKIN et al. (1958) were impressed by results obtained by combination of cytologic and secretory methods where the choice lay between chronic pancreatitis and pancreatic carcinoma. In their series of 199 patients, they felt that there was an 86% accuracy for the combined test.

In our laboratory (NEIBURGS et al., 1962; DREILING et al., 1960), cytological examination was felt to be a useful adjunct to the secretin test. In over 350 studies, a correct diagnosis was made in a high percentage of those cases eventually proved to have cancer of the pancreas. Particularly in lesions of the tail of the pancreas, where secretory data are frequently normal, cytological examination can be of value.

XI. Results of the Secretin Test in Inflammatory and Neoplastic Disease

Analysis of test data from large numbers of patients with various pancreatic disorders leads one to classify the various abnormal secretory patterns into five general categories of abnormality: (1) Total secretory deficiency; (2) quantitative secretory deficiency; (3) qualitative secretory deficiency; (4) isolated enzyme deficiency; and (5) discordant secretory deficiency.

Total secretory deficiency of volume, bicarbonate and enzyme is observed in patients with large tumors of the head of the pancreas which obstruct all excretory ducts, but can also be seen in the end stages of advanced chronic pancreatitis.

Qualitative deficiency, which is a low volume flow with a normal bicarbonate concentration and normal enzyme concentration is seen in carcinomatous obstruction of excretory ducts, usually in the head of the pancreas, but sometimes in the body of the pancreas as well.

Quantitative deficiency, which is a normal volume flow with low bicarbonate concentrations, is characteristic of chronic pancreatic inflammatory disease.

Isolated enzyme deficiency accompanied by normal volume flow and normal bicarbonate concentration is relatively rarely encountered and may be seen in a variety of nutritional and metabolic pancreatic fibrotic processes.

The pattern of discordant secretion with a high volume flow (flow rates 10.5 to 17.1 ml/kgm/80 min), normal enzyme secretion and low maximal bicarbonate concentration has been observed in pancreatic hemochromatosis.

In *acute pancreatitis* the secretin test is of little value. Paralleling the histologic repair of the gland during the first week of the illness, the functional capacity of the gland returns, and the secretin test is usually normal at this time. During the really acute phases of the illness, the patient is too ill to undergo the duodenal intubation and other procedures related to the performance of the test. In some patients in whom secretin tests have been performed during an episode of acute pancreatitis, depression of volume, bicarbonate and enzyme may be observed. Completely normal pancreatic secretion has been observed within three days following an episode of acute pancreatitis in a patient who was ill enough to be in clinical shock at the onset (Dreiling and Janowitz, 1962).

In *chronic pancreatitis* the chief defect is the inability of the gland to secrete a juice with a high bicarbonate concentration (Figure 5). It is only in the most advanced cases that there is a diminution of volume or enzyme secretion. The average maximal bicarbonate concentration in a large series of patients with chronic pancreatitis observed by Dreiling and Janowitz (1961) was 57 mEq/L. Only 4% of the group of 250 patients had bicarbonate values within the normal range. There is a wide variation of volume and enzyme data, but about two-thirds of the group had normal flow and enzyme secretion. In those rather rare instances of chronic pancreatitis accompanied by extensive pancreatic calcinosis, depression of volume and enzyme secretion are observed in addition to the bicarbonate defect.

In *carcinoma of the pancreas* the defects apparent on the secretin test depend on the degree and site of the pancreatic ductal obstruction as well as on the extent of the parenchymal damage. In tumors of the head of the pancreas, where one or both major pancreatic ducts are obstructed, the greatest deficits of volume flow are observed. In the Dreiling and Janowitz series (1962), the mean volume flow was 1.3 ml/kgm/80 minutes. Only 5% of a group of 204 patients had normal volume responses.

Tumors of the pancreatic body affect volume flow to a lesser extent. The mean volume flow in 76 patients with cancer of the body of the pancreas was 1.7 ml/kgm/80 minutes, and 41% of this group had normal volume responses. Carcinoma of the tail of the pancreas cannot anatomically obstruct a major pancreatic duct. The mean volume flow in a group of 29 patients was 3.7 ml/kgm/80 minutes. Only 1 patient in this group had a low volume response.

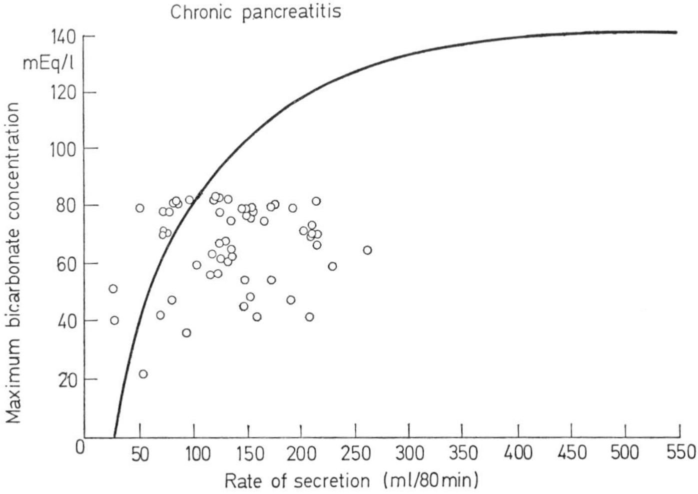

Fig. 5. Relationship between maximum bicarbonate concentration and rate of secretion in 61 subjects with chronic pancreatitis (DREILING and JANOWITZ, 1962)

The bicarbonate and enzyme secretion tends to be normal in all forms of darcinoma of the pancreas. Only in those situations where there is truly extensive cestruction or associated inflammatory change does bicarbonate and enzyme secretion fall.

The bile pigment response observed during the secretin test has been mentioned earlier (see Fig. 2). The actual response seen is a resultant of the hydrocholeretic properties of secretin itself, the patency of the biliary tract, the pancreatic volume response, and the presence of a functioning gall bladder. In the normal situation with a normal pancreatic response to secretin and a normally functioning gall bladder *in situ*, bile disappears from the duodenal drainage as the test proceeds, and this is observed by a fall in the icteric index. In those patients who have previously been subjected to cholecystectomy, or who have nonfunctioning gall bladders, the icteric index remains high during the test, i.e., bile remains in the duodenum throughout the test. The complete absence of bile in the duodenum throughout the test indicates total obstruction of the common bile duct.

C. Secretin-Pancreozymin Tests of Pancreatic Function

I. Historical

Pancreozymin, the presence of which was postulated for years, was discovered by HARPER and RAPER (1943). They were able to extract a substance from the small intestines of the pig, dog, and cat which on intravenous injection caused an increased secretion of enzymes from the pancreas, but which had little effect on the flow of pancreatic juice (Fig. 6). The substance was named pancreozymin. This crude extract was tested in anesthetized, cannulated cats in whom a constant intravenous injection of secretin had been given to cause a continuous flow of pancreatic juice. The authors showed that the response of the pancreas was unaffected by splanchnic or vagus section or atropine. The longitudinal distribution of pancreozymin in the small intestine was similar to that of secretin. GO et al. (1969) confirmed the occurrence of pancreozymin in duodenum and jejunum, but not ileum, and noted the release by isotonic solutions of amino acids.

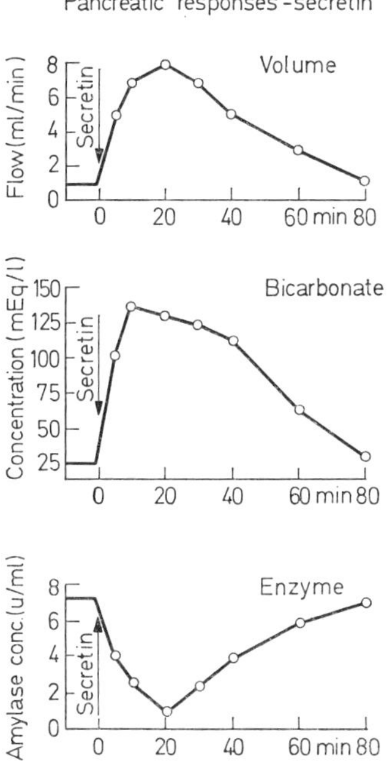

Fig. 6. Pancreatic responses obtained with duodenal drainage in man following intravenous administration of pancreozymin (DREILING and JANOWITZ, 1962)

The action of pancreozymin in man was found to be the same as in cats by members of the same group (DUNCAN et al., 1950). The duodenal contents were examined in healthy humans after an intravenous injection of pancreozymin extract, 30 minutes after a single dose secretin injection given intravenously. Lipase, amylase, trypsinogen and bile content were increased in the duodenal aspirate after the pancreozymin injection, but not after the prior secretin injection. Similar results were obtained by WERNER and MUTT (1954) using a more purified pancreozymin extract. In 3 infant humans who were tested, the enzyme output in the duodenal aspirate increased 20-fold following pancreozymin administration.

It was felt that the availability of a preparation with the known properties of pancreozymin would allow for the assessment not only of the electrolyte secretory properties of the pancreas, but also of its ecbolic function. From the theoretical point of view it was anticipated that whereas secretin, a stimulant to volume and bicarbonate flow might provide an estimation of ductal obstruction, that pancreozymin, a stimulant of enzyme production would more readily disclose evidence of acute or chronic parenchymal inflammation. A combination of secretin and pancreozymin ought to allow for an earlier diagnosis of acute pancreatitis, and might be of value in differentiating pancreatitic parenchymal destruction from extensive malignant ductal obstruction.

Various groups have attempted to assess pancreatic function with combinations of secretin and pancreozymin. The preparations of secretin and pancreozymin have varied in purity and dosage, the sequence of administration of secretin and pancreozymin, as well as the collection times, and the time interval between administration of secretin and pancreozymin have varied. Strict comparison between data from one group to another is difficult.

II. The Secretin-Pancreozymin Test

BURTON et al. (1960a), used a sequence of administration of both hormones which involved giving secretin intravenously, followed in 30 minutes by intravenous pancreozymin, after a 20 minute basal collection period. The dose given of each hormone was 1.7 units/kgm. Two allergic reactions were noted in 301 secretin injections, while 38 allergic reactions were observed after 295 administrations of pancreozymin. A double-lumened tube was first passed, and volume, bicarbonate concentration, amylase, trypsin and lipase content measured, along with measurements of the icteric index.

BURTON noted, as had others, that measurements of the 3 enzymes were unnecessary, since the enzymes are secreted in parallel. In the series of normals, volume increased after administration of secretin alone, and this effect had been dissipated by the end of 50 minutes. Following the administration of pancreozymin 30 minutes after the secretin, there was a second rise in volume, and gall bladder bile appeared in the duodenum. After the injection of secretin, the concentration and output of the three enzymes increased, and then fell to low levels (wash-out). A second peak of enzyme concentration and output was noted after the pancreozymin injection. In some instances BURTON and his co-workers substituted a second injection of secretin for pancreozymin and a second rise in volume was observed without a second rise in enzymes. In 21 normal patients tested in this manner by BURTON, he noted a greater variability of enzyme output than for volume and bicarbonate, but the variability was less when secretin and pancreozymin were given than for secretin alone. Seventeen patients with cancer of the pancreas were tested. In general, there was a decreased volume of duodenal contents. The concentration of bicarbonate and enzymes were decreased, especially in the post-pancreozymin specimens. However, in some patients with cancer of the pancreas, bicarbonate concentration and volume were normal, but the enzyme secretion was low. Fourteen patients recovering from an episode of acute pancreatitis had essentially normal tests, as in the standard secretin test. Fifteen patients with chronic pancreatitis were tested. Decreased volumes and bicarbonate concentrations were observed, and there was a diminution of enzyme secretion in the post-secretin collections, which became more noticeable in the post-pancreozymin stimulated specimens. BURTON felt that mild degrees of functional impairment on the basis of chronic pancreatitis may be manifested by a poor enzyme response which is most marked in the post-pancreozymin period. He also felt that in cancer of the pancreas, the diminution in the post-pancreozymin output of enzyme is a more sensitive index of impaired pancreatic function than the lowered volume or bicarbonate. It is not clear from analysis of the BURTON data that the addition of pancreozymin widened the scope of the standard secretin test.

The dose response curves to pancreozymin were measured by HANSCOM and LITTMAN (1963) in 13 normals and 11 patients with chronic relapsing pancreatitis. Samples were aspirated via a double-lumen tube. Vitrum secretin was infused via a constant infusion pump at the rate of 1.5 units/kgm-hour. An initial "wash-out" dose of 1.5 units Boots pancreozymin/kgm was given. A second dose of pancreozymin was given in doses varying from 0.37 to 3.0 units pancreozymin/kgm. These doses were given in a randomized order, and specimens collected for 45 minutes. It was found that in the normal, protein output in the duodenum was linearly related to the logarithm of the dose of pancreozymin. They noted that patients with chronic pancreatitis had significantly lowered protein output responses at all dose levels.

The secretin-pancreozymin sequence was utilized by MARKS and BANK (MARKS and TOMPSETT, 1958; BANK et al., 1963). Their methodology included the passage of two tubes, one terminating in the stomach, the other in the third part of the duodenum. After collection of duodenal juice for 10 minutes, 1 unit of Boots secretin/kgm was given intravenously and specimens were collected for 60 minutes in two 10 minute and two 20 minute collection periods. Following this, 1.5 units of Boots pancreozymin/kgm were given intravenously, and the juice was collected for a further 20 minutes. The volume, pH, bicarbonate concentration, icteric index, amylase, trypsin and lipase concentrations were determined. In their initial report on 50 tests in 48 patients, the earliest abnormal finding was a diminution in amylase secretion. In their later report (BANK et al., 1963), which included tests on 37 normals and 36 patients with chronic pancreatitis, they concluded that a mean amylase concentration below 1.9 LAGERLÖF units/ml was indicative of pancreatic disease. Bicarbonate concentrations below 60 mEq/L were diagnostic of pancreatic disease. Bicarbonate concentrations in the range between 60 – 67 mEq/L were suggestive of pancreatic disease if the patients in addition had abnormal glucose tolerance tests and/or steatorrhea.

In distinction to the above reports, DREILING and JANOWITZ (1962) utilized the secretin-pancreozymin sequence in 55 patients at The Mount Sinai Hospital. Secretin was given intravenously in doses of 1 unit/kgm, and 40 minutes later 100 clinical units of pancreozymin were given, irrespective of body wieght. The total collection time of 80 minutes was kept, so that a fair comparison could be made with their earlier, larger series of standard secretin tests. A detailed analysis of these tests could not be made since many unsatisfactory results were noted. In 12 of the 55 tests, the enterokinetic action of pancreozymin caused displacement of the tube beyond the ligament of Treitz. There was regurgitation of duodenal contents into the stomach, and gastric contamination of the duodenal contents. In addition, because the post-secretin data was the result of a 40 rather than an 80 minute collection period, there was greater variability. The data for volume and bicarbonate represented the results of an 80 minute collection period based on combined stimulation after secretin and pancreozymin. It is not known what proportion of the volume of duodenal contents is contributed by the biliary tract, but it may significant. That portion of the volume which is derived by pancreozymin stimulation depends on whether the gall bladder is intact. In regard to bicarbonate, surprisingly high concentrations were observed following pancreozymin. The mean was 60 mEq/L with a range of 24 – 108 mEq/L. In 2 patients with chronic pancreatitis, normal maximum bicarbonate concentrations were observed following pancreozymin, but not following the initial secretin injection.

WORMSLEY (1969) demurs, however, and feels that the secretin-pancreozymin test as performed by him is a satisfactory and reproducible stimulant of the secretion of bicarbonate and pancreatic enzymes.

He tested a series of normal adults, as well as some with biliary tract disease, acute pancreatitis following subsidence of the acute attack, hemochromatosis, and chronic pancreatitis. The methodology involved passage of a double-lumened tube, and a separate tube was placed in the antrum of the stomach. All subjects received a continuous intravenous infusion of secretin (0.25 clinical units/kgm-hour. Pancreozymin (4 CRICK-HARPER-RAPER units/kgm-hour) was added to the secretin infusion after 40 minutes, and was increased to 16 U/kgm-hour after a further 40 minutes. Both the secretin and pancreozymin preparations were obtained from the GIH laboratory in Stockholm.

The addition of pancreozymin increased the rate of secretion into the duodenum in all subjects, and the volume response was greater at the 16 unit than the 4 unit/kgm-hour dose level. The volume was significantly lower in pancreatic carcinoma and chronic pancreatitis. The concentration of bicarbonate increased in 8 of 20 normal and duodenal ulcer subjects when 4 units/kgm-hour pancreozymin was added to secretin. The output of bicarbonate in response to 16 units pancreozymin/kgm-hour was significantly greater than to 4 units/kgm-hour. The output of bicarbonate in patients with chronic pancreatitis and pancreatic carcinoma was significantly less than normal. The concentration of trypsin in response to 4 units/kgm-hour pancreozymin was significantly greater than the concentration of trypsin during the last 20 minutes of the secretin infusion alone in the normal and duodenal ulcer groups. The concentration of trypsin remained unchanged in 6 of the 20 normal and duodenal ulcer subjects on increasing the dose rate of pancreozymin, but increased further in the other 14 individuals. In patients with chronic pancreatitis, the values were abnormally low when low flow rates were taken into account. In pancreatic carcinoma, the trypsin concentrations were lower than normal. The output of trypsin was greater in response to 16 units than to 4 units/kgm-hour pancreozymin in 16 of the 20 normal and duodenal ulcer subjects, and also increased in most of the subjects with chronic pancreatitis and pancreatic carcinoma, although in chronic pancreatitis and pancreatic carcinoma, the actual outputs were significantly lower than in normals.

WORMSLEY feels that his test is more advantageous than the standard secretin test in two respects: (1) The combined infusion of secretin and pancreozymin in this dose schedule produced fewer side reactions than larger doses of secretin alone, and (2) that the infusion of the combined hormones provides a criterion of specific pancreatic function as well as a measure of the digestive capacity of an individual. WORMSLEY feels that it is essential to have information about the capacity of the pancreas to secrete digestive enzymes, and that this is not provided by secretin alone. Furthermore, he feels that the combined test is more discriminatory than the secretin test, since in this study patients with pancreatic carcinoma showed a more severe loss of the capacity to secrete enzymes than bicarbonate, while the reverse was true in patients with chronic pancreatitis.

III. The Pancreozymin-Secretin Test

SUN and SHAY (1960), SUN (1963a; 1963b), reversed the order of administration of secretin and pancreozymin, giving pancreozymin first, and secretin 10 minutes later. Ninety units of Boots pancreozymin were given intravenously after a 20 minute basal collection period, and the duodenal contents were collected for 10 minutes. Then 80 units of Boots secretin were given intravenously and the duodenal contents were aspirated for a further 60 minutes. In applying the test to 68 normals, it was found that the least scatter of duodenal contents data occured in the 60 minute post-secretin collection period, in regard to volume and maximum bicarbonate concentration, while amylase output showed least variability in the total 70 minute collection period. When the test was applied to various individuals with disorders of pancreatic function, the following was found: In acute pancreatitis there was too great an overlap in all parameters to be discriminatory. In chronic pancreatitis, all patients had lowered volumes, bicarbonate concentrations and enzyme outputs. In neoplasms of the pancreas, the findings were similar to those in chronic pancreatitis, and could not be regarded as discriminatory.

Utilizing the same sequence of pancreozymin followed by secretin, CHOI and co-workers (1967) attempted to improve the diagnostic accuracy of measurement of duodenal enzymes by measuring the maximum trypsin concentration and output against a substrate of p-toluene-sulfonyl-L-arginine methyl ester. Twenty controls and 12 with pancreatitis were tested. After a 20 minute basal collection period, 75 units of Cecekin were given intravenously irrespective of body weight and duodenal contents were collected for 10 minutes. Then secretin 1 unit/kgm was given and the duodenal contents were collected for another 10 minute period. Maximal trypsin concentrations and outputs were measured. The authors felt that measurement of these two enzyme parameters improved the diagnostic accuracy of the test.

DREILING and JANOWITZ (1962), at The Mount Sinai Hospital, studied 308 patients with the pancreozymin-secretin sequence. One hundred units of pancreozymin, regardless of body weight, were given intravenously, followed in 20 minutes by a standard dose of secretin (1 clinical unit/kgm). The authors felt that administration of pancreozymin prior to secretin obviated the drug-induced intestinal motility, provided that the tube is initially placed more proximal than its eventual ideal position.

Utilizing this test in 156 patients without pancreatic disease, DREILING and JANOWITZ felt that the pancreozymin data displayed too great a variability, with coefficients of variation ranging between 40 and 60%, to allow for the establishment of statistically valid normal ranges. This variability was not improved by reduction of the data to a weight basis. The variability of the data in response to pancreozymin is probably due to the following: (1) Pancreozymin is not a stimulus to volume flow; (2) the pancreozymin collection period of 20 minutes is quite short; (3) the contributions of volume and bicarbonate by the liver depends on gall bladder function and biliary tract patency; and (4) the commercially available pancreozymin is contaminated by variable amounts of secretin. The secretin response data in normal individuals revealed variations of the same order of magnitude as in the standard secretin test in regard to volume and bicarbonate. It was apparent that the prior injection of pancreozymin did not interfere with the pancreatic response to secretin, but that the ecbolic effect of pancreozymin persisted after the 20 minute collection period.

The test was applied to 20 subjects recovering from an attack of acute pancreatitis, 76 patients with chronic pancreatitis, and 56 patients with pancreatic carcinoma. In patients with acute pancreatitis, statistical differences from normals were observed only in the enzyme data following secretin and pancreozymin. In chronic pancreatitis, the statistically significant finding was a lowered bicarbonate concentration both after secretin and pancreozymin. In pancreatic cancer, only the volume data were statistically significant, while enzyme and bicarbonate data were not. It is thus seen, that there is a great overlap in the post-pancreozymin data, especially for enzyme measurements which did not improve over that seen with secretin alone. DREILING and JANOWITZ concluded that the addition of pancreozymin to the standard secretin test did not significantly improve the overlap of enzyme secretory data nor did it furnish additional diagnostic accuracy above that obtainable with the standard secretin test. The authors suggested that a reduction in scatter of data might be obtained by the development of maximum pancreatic secretory tests for both electrolyte and enzyme secretion, and/or by administration of secretin and pancreozymin on a weight basis. While this has not yet been performed in humans, some data is available from dog studies (Hansky et al., 1964). In 9 dogs with chronic pancreatic fistulae, the authors found that pancreozymin given in doses of 0.5 to 2.0 units/kgm-minute as a continuous infusion or 10—25 units/kgm as a single injection would elicit a maximum enzyme response. Injection of 5—15 units/kgm of pancreozymin elicited a maximum response when that hormone was combined with 8 units/kgm of secretin (maximal dose of secretin in dogs). Utilizing stimulation by pancreozymin and secretin, the authors published the following maximal data:

15 minute mean volume 25.7 ml
amylase 364 units
bicarbonate output 3.15 mEq

Similar studies have not yet been performed in humans.

D. Serum Enzyme Tests in the Diagnosis of Pancreatic Disease

Opinion is unified regarding the value of serum enzyme determination in acute pancreatic disease, but is still divided regarding their importance in cancer of the pancreas and chronic pancreatitis. If enzyme levels in cancer of the pancreas and chronic pancreatitis were truly diagnostic, and if the overlap between the diseases were low, then it would obviously be easier to diagnose these ailments by blood tests without going through tedious and troublesome duodenal intubation with the analysis of a large number of specimens.

Based on the fact that elevated lipase and/or amylase levels were noted sporadically in cases of cancer of the pancreas and chronic pancreatitis, Popper and Necheles (1943) devised a test of pancreatic function in dogs which involved the subcutaneous injection of a parasympathomimetic drug, Mecholyl, together with eserine sulfate. They noted a rise of serum amylase and lipase levels in normal dogs, but no rise in dogs with pancreatic atrophy (status post-duct ligation). When the authors administered an intravenous infusion of secretin, normal dogs had no rise in serum lipase, but elevated lipase levels were observed in obstructed, though non-atrophic glands. This response disappeared within 30—45 days following duct ligation, presumably when pancreatic atrophy had taken place.

Under normal circumstances most of the circulating serum amylase is of hepatic origin, while the lipase is derived from the pancreas. In acute pancreatitis, the contribution to serum amylase by the pancreas increases. The enzymes are felt to pass from the acini via the lymphatics or the portal vein to the general circulation, and are then excreted by the kidney (Howat, 1964).

Because of the evanescent changes in blood enzyme levels in chronic pancreatic disease, various methods have been tried to increase the sensitivity of the test, and to prolong the responses by the addition of various drugs.

1. Drugs designed to stimulate the flow of pancreatic juice-secretin.

2. Drugs designed to stimulate the production of pancreatic enzymes-pancreozymin and parasympathomimetic drugs.

3. Drugs which cause obstruction of the pancreatic duct system-morphine
4. Various combinations of the above.

In general, two patterns of response are noted. In the first, a stimulus of a drug causes a rise in serum enzymes in normal patients, and a failure of the rise is considered indicative of pancreatic secretory insufficiency. The second general pattern is that in which a drug stimulus causes no serum enzyme change in normal individuals, but there is a significant rise in patients with pancreatic disease with an obstructed duct system. The first response is seen in normal individuals given morphine, and the second is noted when secretin alone is given to patients with cancer of the pancreas. The interpretation of results becomes more difficult and complex as more drugs are added.

Provocative tests are based on the assumption that in a pancreas free of ductal obstruction, neither stimulation of flow nor enzyme output will cause elevation of serum enzyme levels, whereas in a gland with obstruction of the duct, either stimulus will cause a rise of serum enzymes, which depends on how much functioning pancreatic parenchyma remains. The serum enzyme level, then is the resultant of two opposing forces, the degree of ductal obstruction, which tends to raise serum enzyme levels, and the extent of pancreatic parenchymal damage which tends to lower serum enzyme levels.

In a series of 192 patients investigated by DREILING and RICHMAN (1954) with various combinations of secretin, Mecholyl, urecholine and morphine, the serum enzyme levels could not be correlated with the state of pancreatic function as determined either by operation or standard secretin test (Fig. 7). The overlap of data was too great to allow for a diagnosis to be established.

BURTON et al. (1960b) revived interest in serum enzyme tests by their publication of responses to a new evocative test of pancreatic function which did not include the use of morphine. Two hundred and thirteen evocative tests were performed during a secretin-pancreozymin test with a double-lumened tube in place. Serial amylase and lipase levels were measured in serum at 2, 4, 6, and 24 hours following administration of the secretin and pancreozymin stimuli. Control bloods were drawn. Secretin and pancreozymin were each given in doses of 1.7 units/kgm in a single intravenous dose. In 51 normal individuals, amylase and lipase levels failed to rise on serial enzyme determinations. In 36 patients with carcinoma of the pancreas, in 16 of which the tumor was located in the head, an early rise of serum lipase was observed after the secretin injection, but was especially seen after the pancreozymin injection. In 44 patients with pancreatitis comprising 20 patients recovering from acute pancreatitis and 24 with chronic pancreatitis, the authors observed changes similar to those seen in cancer of the pancreas. The test thus was capable of discerning pancreatic disease but was not really discriminatory for the type of disease.

HOWAT (1962a) feels that the test of BURTON et al. (1960b) is of value, and is sensitive in the early stages of both cancer and chronic pancreatitis before there is too severe a degree of parenchymal destruction. HOWAT (1962b) notes that the variance of the mean serum enzyme responses after pancreozymin is significantly lower than after secretin in regard to amylase, and very significantly less after pancreozymin. When the t-test was applied to compare means of normal and pathological material, the t-value was invariably more significant in the post-pancreozymin samples. HOWAT's philosophy is that in the early phases of cancer of the pancreas or chronic pancreatitis, before significant acinar atrophy has taken place, that evocative tests are of value, but after continued ductal obstruction or glandular destruction, examination of the duodenal contents is preferable (HOWAT, 1964).

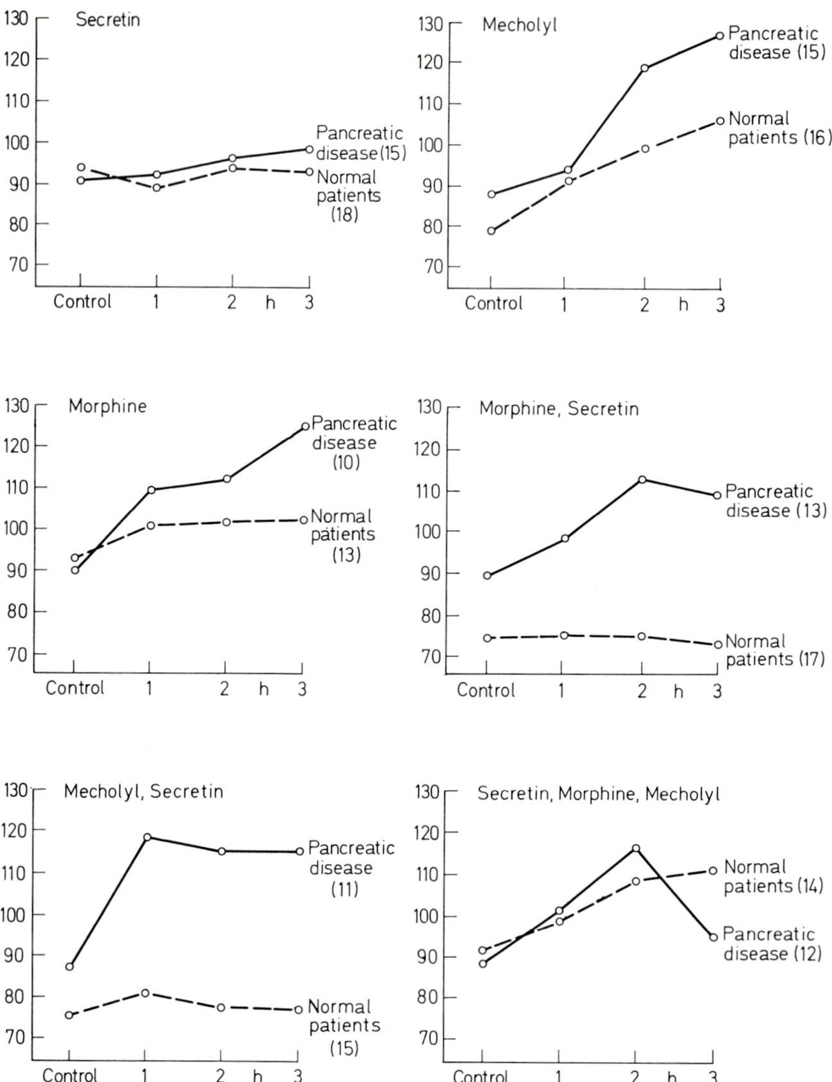

Fig. 7. Serial blood amylase concentrations (in milligrams per cent) before and after the administration of secretin, mecholyl, morphine, morphine-secretin, mecholyl-secretin, and secretin-morphine-mecholyl to patients with and without pancreatic disease (Dreiling et al., 1964)

Sun and Shay (1960) analyzed serum enzyme responses in the course of their pancreozymin-secretin test (see above). Serum enzymes were tested before injection of the pancreozymin and 1, 2, and 4 hours after secretin. Positive serum enzyme responses were observed in 9 of 18 patients with chronic pancreatitis, 3 of 3 patients with cancer of the ampulla of Vater and 1 of 5 patients with carcinoma of the pancreas. In a comparative study involving the use of secretin alone, the results were not felt to be as discriminatory. Of interest was the fact that 5 of 9 patients with chronic pancreatitis had positive serum enzyme tests, but normal findings on examination of the duodenal contents. On the other side of the coin, 9 patients with normal serum enzyme responses had low duodenal contents values. The authors feel that provocative enzyme tests be regarded as a screening device, and that abnormal or equivocal tests be confirmed by a test involving examination of the duodenal contents.

Our position remains as stated by DREILING (1962), that secretin-pancreozymin provocative tests are of little value in acute pancreatitis because of the great degree of overlap with normals. In chronic pancreatitis, there is too little a tendency for serum enzymes to rise because of parenchymal destruction. In cancer of the pancreas considered as a group the variability is too great. However, in cancer of the head of the pancreas, tremendous rises of serum enzymes are observed, and the responses can, to some extent, be considered diagnostic.

References

ÅGREN, G., LAGERLÖF, H.: The pancreatic secretion in man after intravenous administration of secretin. Acta med. scand. **90,** 1—29 (1936).

BANK, S., MARKS, I. N., MOSHAL, M. G., EFRON, G., SILBER, R.: The pancreatic function test method and normal values. S. Afr. med. J. **37,** 1061—1066 (1963).

BANWELL, J. G., NORTHAM, B. E., COOKE, W. T.: Secretory response of the human pancreas to continuous intravenous infusion of secretin. Gut **8,** 50—57 (1967).

BARON, J. H., PERRIER, C. V., JANOWITZ, H. D., DREILING, D. A.: Maximum alkaline (bicarbonate) output of the dog pancreas. Amer. J. Physiol. **204,** 251—256 (1963).

BAXTER, S. G.: Parallel concentration of enzymes in pancreatic secretion. Amer. J. dig. Dis. **2,** 108—111 (1935).

BAYLISS, W. M., STARLING, E. H.: The mechanism of pancreatic secretion. J. Physiol. (Lond.) **28,** 325—353 (1902).

BODANSZKY, A., ONDETTI, M. A., MUTT, V., BODANSZKY, M.: Synthesis of secretin. IV. Secondary structure in a miniature protein. J. Amer. chem. Soc. **91,** 944—949 (1969).

BURTON, P., EVANS, D. G., HARPER, A. A., HOWAT, H. T., OLEESKY, S., SCOTT, J. E., VARLEY, H.: A test of pancreatic function in man based on the analysis of duodenal contents after administration of secretin and pancreozymin. Gut **1,** 111—124 (1960a).

— HAMMOND, E. M., HARPER, A. A., HOWAT, H. T., SCOTT, J. E., VARLEY, H.: Serum amylase and serum lipase levels in man after administration of secretin and pancreozymin. Gut **1,** 125—139 (1960b).

CHIRAY, M., SALMON, A. R., MERCIER, A.: Action de la sécrétine purifiée; sur la sécrétion externe du pancréas de l'homme. Bull. Soc. Méd. Hôp. Paris. 3 ser. **50,** 1417—1426 (1926).

CHOI, H. J., GOLDSTEIN, F., WIRTS, C. W., MENDUKE, H.: Normal duodenal trypsin values in response to secretin. Pancreozymin stimulation with preliminary data in patients with pancreatic disease. Gastroenterology **53,** 397—402 (1967).

COMFORT, M. W., OSTERBERG, A. E.: Pancreatic secretion in man after stimulation with secretin and acetylbeta methylcholine chloride. A comparative study. Arch. intern. Med. **66,** 688—706 (1940).

DEBRAY, C., TOUR, J. de la, VAILLE, C., ROZE, C., SOUCHARD, M.: Contribution a l'étude de la sécrétion biliaire et pancréatique externe chez le Rat. J. Physiol. (Paris) **54,** 459—499 (1962).

DIAMOND, J. S., SIEGEL, S. A., GALL, M. B., KARLEN, S.: The use of secretin as a clinical test of pancreatic function. Amer. J. dig. Dis. **6,** 366—372 (1939).

— —: The secretin test in the diagnosis of pancreatic diseases with a report of one hundred thirty tests. Amer. J. dig. Dis. **7,** 435—442 (1940).

DREILING, D. A.: The technique of the secretin test. Normal ranges. J. Mt Sinai Hosp. **21,** 363—372 (1955).

—: Discussion. In Ciba Foundation Symposium: The Exocrine Pancreas (A.V.S. de REUCK, Ed.). Boston: Little, Brown 1962, pp. 253—254.

— HOLLANDER, F.: Studies in pancreatic function, preliminary series of clinical studies with secretin test. Gastroenterology **11,** 714—729 (1948).

— —: Studies in pancreatic function: II. A statistical study of pancreatic secretion following secretin in patients without pancreatic disease. Gastroenterology **15,** 620—627 (1950).

— NIEBURGS, H. E., JANOWITZ, H. D.: Combined secretin and cytology test in the diagnosis of pancreatic and biliary tract cancer. Med. Clin. N. Amer. **44,** 801—815 (1960).

— JANOWITZ, H. D.: The secretion of electrolytes by the human pancreas. Gastroenterology **30,** 382—390 (1956).

— —: The laboratory diagnosis of pancreatic disease: Secretin test. Amer. J. Gastroent. **28**, 268—275 (1957).
— —: The secretion of electrolytes by the human pancreas. The effect of Diamox, ACTH, and disease. Amer. J. dig. Dis. **4**, 137—144 (1959).
— —: The measurement of pancreatic secretory function. In Ciba Foundation Symposium: The Exocrine Pancreas (A.V.S. de Reuck, Ed.). Boston: Little, Brown 1962, pp. 225—252.
— Richman, A.: Evaluation of provocative blood enzyme tests employed in diagnosis of pancreatic disease. Arch. intern. Med. **94**, 197—212 (1954).
— Janowitz, H. D., Perrier, C. V.: Pancreatic Inflammatory Disease. A Physiologic Approach. New York: Harper & Row 1964.

Duncan, P. R., Harper, A. A., Howat, H. T., Oleesky, S., Varley, H.: The effect of pancreozymin in human subjects. J. Physiol. (Lond.) **111**, 63P (1950).

Go, V. L. W., Hoffman, A. F., Summerskill, W. H. J.: Pancreozymin: Sites of secretion and effects on pancreatic enzyme output in man. J. clin. Invest. **48**, 29a—30a (1969). (Abstract 94)

Goldstein, F., Wirts, C. W., Cozzolino, H. J., Menduke, H.: Secretin tests of pancreatic and biliary tract disease. Arch. intern. Med. **114**, 124—131 (1964).

Greenlee, H. B., Longhi, E H., Guerrero, J. D., Nelson, T. S., El-Bedri, A. L., Dragstedt, L. R.: Inhibitory effect of pancreatic secretin on gastric secretion. Amer. J. Physiol. **190**, 396—402 (1957).

Hanscom, D. H., Littman, A.: Dose-response relationships to pancreozymin in normal subjects and patients with chronic pancreatitis. Gastroenterology **45**, 209—214 (1963).

Hansky, J., Tiscornia, O. M., Dreiling, D. A., Janowitz, H. D.: Maximal secretory capacity of the canine pancreas in response to pancreozymin and secretin. Amer. J. Physiol. **206**, 351—356 (1964).

Grossman, M. I., Stability of secretin. Gastroenterology **57**, 767 (1969).

Harper, A. A., Raper, H. S.: Pancreozymin, a stimulant of the secretion of pancreatic enzymes in extracts of the small intestine. J. Physiol. (Lond.) **102**, 115—125 (1943).

Hartley, R. C., Gambill, E. E., Summerskill, W. H. J.: Pancreatic volume and bicarbonate output with augmented doses of secretin. Gastroenterology **48**, 312—317 (1965).

Howat, H. T.: Editorial. Usefulness of gastrointestinal hormones in diagnosis. Gastroenterology **42**, 72—76 (1962).
— Discussion. In Ciba Foundation Symposium: The Exocrine Pancreas (A.V.S. de Reuck, Ed.). Boston: Little, Brown 1962, p. 253.
— Evocative serum enzyme tests. In Pathogenese, Diagnostik, Klinik und Therapie der Erkrankungen des Exokreinen Pankreas (Henning, N., Heinkel, K., Schön, H., Eds.). Europäisches Pankreas-Symposion, 24. 5. bis 26. 5. 1963 in Erlangen. Stuttgart: F. K. Schattauer 1964, p. 163.

Isenberg, J. I., Grossman, M. I.: Comparison of subcutaneous and intravenous secretin in man. Gastroenterology **56**, 88—91 (1969).

Janowitz, H. D., Dreiling, D. A.: The pancreatic secretion of fluid and electrolytes. In Ciba Foundation Symposium: The Exocrine Pancreas (A.V.S. de Reuck, Ed.). Boston: Little, Brown 1962, pp. 115—133.
—: Pancreatic secretion of fluid and electrolytes. In Handbook of Physiology Section 6: Alimentary Canal. Vol. II, Secretion (C. F. Code, Ed.). Washington, D. C.: American Physiological Society 1967, pp. 925—933.

Johnston, C. G., Ball, E. G.: Variations in inorganic constituents of the pancreatic juice during constant drainage of the pancreatic ducts. J. biol. Chem. **86**, 643—653 (1930).

Jorpes, J. E.: The isolation and chemistry of secretin and cholecystokinin. Gastroenterology **55**, 157—164 (1968).
— Mutt, V.: On the biological activity and amino acid composition of secretin. Acta chem. scand. **15**, 1790—1791 (1961).
— —: The gastrointestinal hormones secretin and cholecystokinin. Ciba Foundation Symposium on The exocrine pancreas. London: Churchill Ltd. 1962, pp. 150—164.
— — Magnusson, S., Steele, B. B.: Amino acid composition and N-terminal amino acid sequence of porcine secretin. Biochem. biophys. Res. Commun. **9**, 275—279 (1962).

Kay, A. W.: Effect of large doses of histamine on gastric secretion of HCl; an augmented histamine test. Brit. med. J. **1953II**, 77—80.

Konturek, S. J.: Comparison of pancreatic responses to natural and synthetic secretins in conscious cats. Amer. J. dig. Dis. **14**, 557—565 (1969).

Lagerlöf, H. O.: Pancreatic secretion: Pathophysiology. In Handbook of Physiology Section 6: Alimentary Canal. Vol. II, Secretion (C. F. Code, Ed.). Washington, D.C.: American Physiological Society 1967, pp. 1027—1042.

— : Pancreatic function and pancreatic disease studied by means of secretin. Acta med. scand. **Suppl. 128,** 1—289 (1942).
— Schütz, H. B., Holmer, S.: A secretin test with high doses of secretin and correction for incomplete recovery of duodenal juice. Gastroenterology **52,** 67—77 (1967).
Lake, M.: Diagnostic value of secretin test, including report of 19 operated or autopsied cases with anatomical studies of pancreas. Amer. J. Med. **3,** 18—30 (1947).
Lemon, H. M., Byrnes, W. W.: Cancer of the biliary tract and pancreas: Diagnosis from cytology of duodenal aspiration. J. Amer. med. Ass. **141,** 254—257 (1949).
Lim, R. K. S., Matheson, A. R., Schlapp, W.: An improved method for investigating the secretory function of the stomach and duodenum in the human subject. Quart. J. exp. Physiol. **13,** 333—345 (1923).
McNeer, G., Ewing, J. H.: Exfoliated pancreatic cancer cells in duodenal drainage: A case report. Cancer **2,** 643—645 (1949).
Marks, I. N., Tompsett, S. L.: The diagnosis of pancreatic disease with special reference to a test of pancreatic secretion utilizing both secretin and pancreozymin stimulation. Quart. J. Med. **27,** 431—461 (1958).
Mellanby, J.: The isolation of secretin — its chemical and physiological properties. J. Physiol. (Lond.) **66,** 1—18 (1928).
Mutt, V., Jorpes, J. E.: Secretin, isolation and determination of structure. IUPAC Internat. Congress on Chemistry of Natural Products, Stockholm, June 26 — July 2, 1966. Section 2 C — I. p. 119.
— —: Isolation of aspartyl-phenylalanine amide from cholecystokinin-pancreozymin. Biochem. biophys. Res. Com. **26,** 392—397 (1967).
— —: Secretin, Cholecystokinin. Communicated at the International Symposium on the "Pharmacology of Hormonal Polypeptides and Proteins" at the University of Milan, Sept. 14—16, 1967, Plenum Press 1968a, pp. 569—580.
— —: Structure of porcine cholecystokinin-pancreozymin. 1. Cleavage with thrombin and with trypsin. Europ. J. Biochem. **6,** 156—162 (1968c).
— —: Chemistry and physiology of cholecystokinin-pancreozymin. Proc. Internat. Un. Physiol. Sciences Vol. VI, 14 Internat. Congr. Washington 1968b, p. 193.
Nieburgs, H. E., Dreiling, D. A., Rubio, C., Reisman, H.: The morphology of cells in duodenal drainage smears: Histologic origin and pathologic significance. Amer. J. dig. Dis. **7,** 489—505 (1962).
Ondetti, M. A., Rubin, B., Engel, S. L., Pluščec, J., Sheehan, J. T.: Cholecystokinin-pancreozymin: Recent developments. Amer. J. dig. Dis. **15,** 149—156 (1970).
Pascal, J. P., Sannou, N., Ribet, A.: Exploration of pancreatic exocrine function by continuous infusion of secretin. Amer. J. dig. Dis. **13,** 213—221 (1968).
Perrier, C. V.: La sécrétion hydrobicarbonatée du pancréas. Clinique. Stimulation maximale. Acta Gastro-ent. Belg. **29,** 163—172 (1966).
— Dreiling, D. A., Janowitz, H. D.: A stop flow analysis of pancreatic secretion. The effect of transient occlusion on the electrolyte composition of pancreatic juice. Gastroenterology **46,** 700—705 (1964).
Petersen, H.: The effect of pure natural secretin on the bicarbonate secretion into the duodenum in man. Scand. J. Gastroent. **5,** 105—111 (1970).
Popper, H. L., Necheles, H.: A new test for pancreatic function: Experimental observations. Gastroenterology **1,** 490—499 (1943).
Preshaw, R M., Grossman, M. I.: Comparison of subcutaneous and intravenous administration of pancreatic stimulants. Amer. J. Physiol. **209,** 803—810 (1965).
Raskin, H. F., Wenger, J., Sklar, M., Pleticka, S., Yarema, W.: Diagnosis of cancer of the pancreas, biliary tract and duodenum by combined cytologic and secretory methods. I. Exfoliative cytology and a description of a rapid method of duodenal intubation. Gastroenterology **34,** 996—1008 (1958).
Rosenberg, I. R., Friedland, N., Janowitz, H. D., Dreiling, D. A.: The effect of age and sex upon human pancreatic secretion of fluid and bicarbonate. Gastroenterology **50,** 191—194 (1966).
Rubin, C. E., Massey, B. W., Kirsner, J. B., Palmer, W. L., Stonecypher, D. D.: The clinical value of gastrointestinal cytologic diagnosis. Gastroenterology **25,** 119—138 (1953).
Sarles, H.: Editor. Pancreatitis. Symposium, Marseilles, April 25 and 26, 1963. Basel: S. Karger 1965.
Solomon, A. K.: Electrolyte secretion in the pancreas. Fed. Proc. **11,** 722—731 (1952).
Somogyi, M.: Diastatic activity of human blood. Arch. intern. Med. **51,** 665—679 (1941).
Stening, G. F., Vagne, M., Grossman, M. I.: Relative potency of commercial secretins. Gastroenterology **55,** 687—689 (1968).
Sun, D. C. H.: The use of pancreozymin-secretin test in the diagnosis of pancreatitis and tumors of the pancreas. Gastroenterology **45,** 203—208 (1963).

—: Normal values for pancreozymin-secretin test. Gastroenterology **44,** 602—606 (1963).
— Shay, H.: Pancreozymin-secretin test. The combined study of serum enzymes and duodenal contents in the diagnosis of pancreatic disease. Gastroenterology **38,** 570—581 (1960).
Vagne, M., Grossman, M. I.: Comparison of intravenous and subcutaneous secretin in dogs. Gastroenterology **54,** 907—912 (1968).
— Stening, G. F., Brooks, F. P., Grossman, M. I.: Synthetic secretin: Comparison with natural secretin for potency and spectrum of physiological actions. Gastroenterology **55,** 260—267 (1968).
Wenger, J., Raskin, H. F.: The diagnosis of cancer of the pancreas, biliary tract and duodenum by combined cytologic and secretory methods. II. The secretin test. Gastroenterology **34,** 1009—1017 (1958).
Werner, B., Mutt, V.: The pancreatic response in man to the injection of highly purified secretin and of pancreozymin. Scand. J. Clin. Lab. Invest. **6,** 228—236 (1954).
Wormsley, K. G.: Response to secretin in man. Gastroenterology **54,** 197—209 (1968).
—: The response to infusion of a combination of secretin and pancreozymin in health and disease. Scand. J. Gastroent. **4,** 623—632 (1969).
Zimmerman, M. J., Dreiling, D. A., Rosenberg, I. R., Janowitz, H. D.: Secretion of calcium by the canine pancreas. Gastroenterology **52,** 865—870 (1967).

On the Use of Cholecystokinin in the Roentgenological Examination of the Extrahepatic Biliary Tract and Intestines

A. Torsoli, M. L. Ramorino, and R. Carratù

With 17 Figures

Cholecystokinin (CCK) (Jorpes and Mutt, 1954) induces contraction and emptying of the human gall bladder. The active nature of the emptying is demonstrated by the increase in intravesicular pressure both before and during evacuation. The contraction induces emptying since the increase of the gall bladder pressure exceeds the resistance of the cholecysto-cystic junction. Cholecystokinin also relaxes Oddi's sphincter, and the sphincteric relaxation allows the lower bile and pancreatic ducts to empty. Finally, Cholecystokinin has certain motility effects on the small and large intestines.

These effects in man correspond to experimental findings and provide of a basis for using CCK in the radiologic examinations of the biliary tract (cholecystography, intravenous cholangiography, pre- and postoperative cholangiography). When compared with the conventional fatty meal (2 egg yolks), which is commonly used as a cholecystokinetic agent, CCK has the following advantages:

a) CCK may be given intravenously, and therefore does not involve gastro-duodenal transit. Subsequent radiologic examinations of the digestive tract are not influenced by the presence of a meal in the stomach and duodenum.

b) The dosage can be graduated according to the clinical purposes.

c) It gives a good visualization of the biliary ducts and of the choledocho-duodenal passage.

d) It reduces the duration of the cholecystokinetic test: 15—30 min, as opposed to 60 min of the conventional technique.

1. Gall Bladder and Cholecysto-Cystic Junction

Intraluminal pressure records show that the basal pressure in the human gall bladder ranges from 0 to 16 cm H_2O (Alessandrini, Palagi, Ramorino and Ribotta, 1960). The cholecysto-cystic junction offers a resistance to the passage of fluids, which averages 15 cm H_2O. The resistance to flow is lower in the opposite direction, i. e., from the cystic duct to the gall bladder (Caroli, Varay and Gilles, 1945). When CCK is given (Cassano, Torsoli and Alessandrini, 1959; Torsoli, Ramorino and de Maio, 1961), the gall bladder pressure increases after a short period of latency. It quickly equals, and then exceeds, the resistance of the junction, reaches its maximum level and returns slowly to the resting values. Intraluminal pressures as high as 20, 25, or 30 cm H_2O may be reached. In normal subjects, the maximum intraluminal pressure level of the gall bladder does not rise above the level of liver secretion (30 cm H_2O: Jordan, 1964). The pressure pattern is largely dependent on the dosage and the rate of administration of CCK (Fig. 1a, b). The effect of CCK is not altered by atropine (Naito, Iwata and Saito, 1963).

If the gall bladder is filled with contrast medium it can be seen that emptying begins as soon as the vesicular pressure exceeds the resistance of the junction, and continues as long as the pressure remains above the basal values. Cholecysto-cystic resistance, however, is not constant even in the same subject. Immediately after CCK it may exceed the basal values, whereas during emptying it may be found to be below these levels. Intravesicular pressure records show no evidence of phasic contraction or peristalsis (Torsoli, 1964).

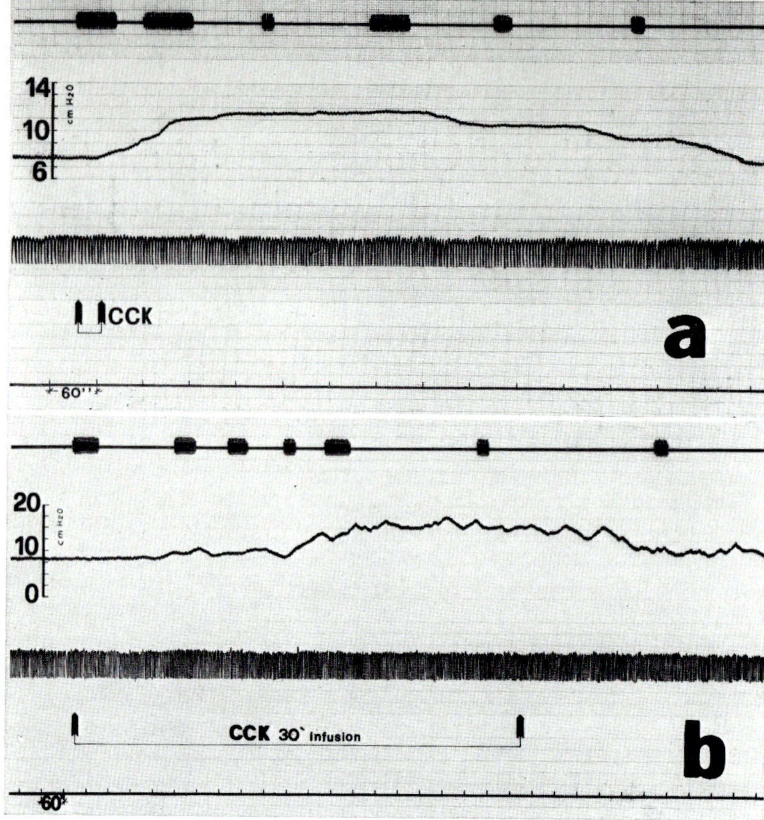

Fig. 1. Effect of CCK (75 IDU) on the intraluminal gall bladder pressure. Postoperative cholangiography. a: intravenous injection in 30 sec; b: intravenous infusion in 30 min. First tracing: synchronization with cinefluorography; third tracing: pneumograph; fourth tracing: time

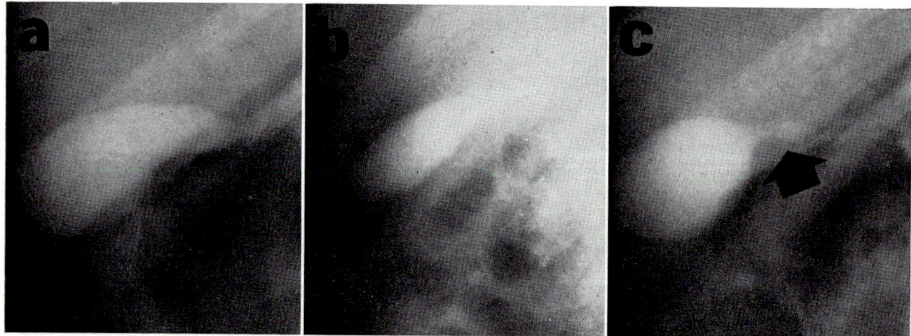

Fig. 2. Infundibular contraction (arrow) after CCK (75 IDU in 3 min). Cholecystography in a subject with apparently normal gall bladder. a: preliminary X-ray film; b: 30 min after fatty meal. Second examination 4 days later; c: 12 min after CCK. [From Acta Radiol. **55**, 193—206 (1961)]

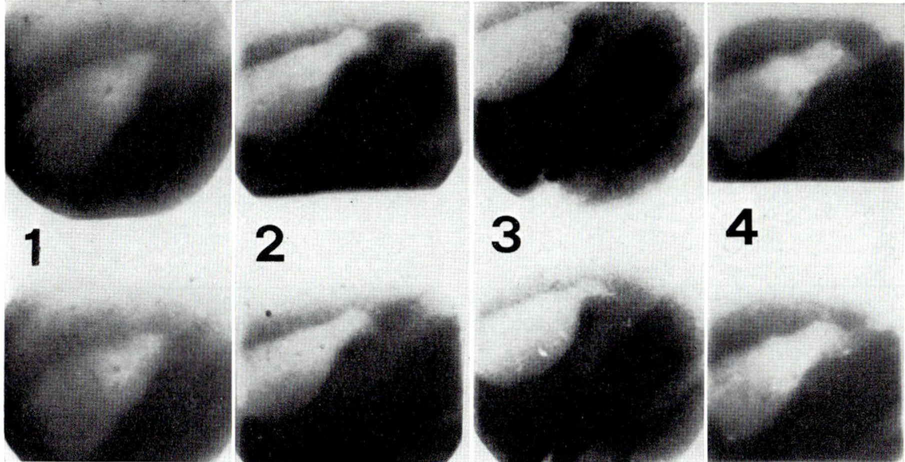

Fig. 3. Contraction and decontraction of the infundibulum after CCK (75 IDU in 3 min). Cholecystography in a subject with apparently normal gall bladder. Cinefluorographic sequences. 1: before CCK; 2, 3, 4: 5, 7, 15 min after CCK

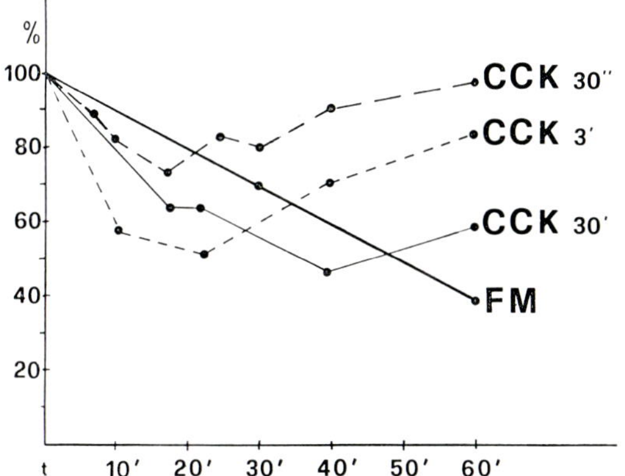

Fig. 4. Gall bladder emptying rates in 42 subjects, following conventional fatty meal (FM) and CCK (1 IDU per kg. body weight, in 30 sec or 3 min or 30 min)

Using CCK in standard dosage (1 IDU/kg in 3 min), changes in both size and shape of the gall bladder are often more evident at the infundibulum. The prevalence of the infundibular contraction is sometimes clearly visible (Fig. 2); very slow contractions and decontractions may also be seen on this site (Fig. 3). After the fatty meal the gall bladder emptying is usually more complete, but slower, the maximum evacuation taking about one hour. The reduction in size of the gall bladder is concentric, and the visibility of the bile ducts is neither complete nor constant.

Comparing various dosages of CCK (Fig. 4) it appears that intravenous infusion of 0.5 to 1 IDU per kg weight in normal saline, in 30 min, produces an effect more closely resembling that of the conventional fatty meal. If the same dose of CCK is injected intravenously in 30 sec, emptying of the gall bladder is very quick. Sometimes, however, despite gall bladder contraction only a partial emptying of short duration, or no emptying at all, can be observed. Some pain in the right hypochondrium may be experienced in these cases, and the failure of the gall

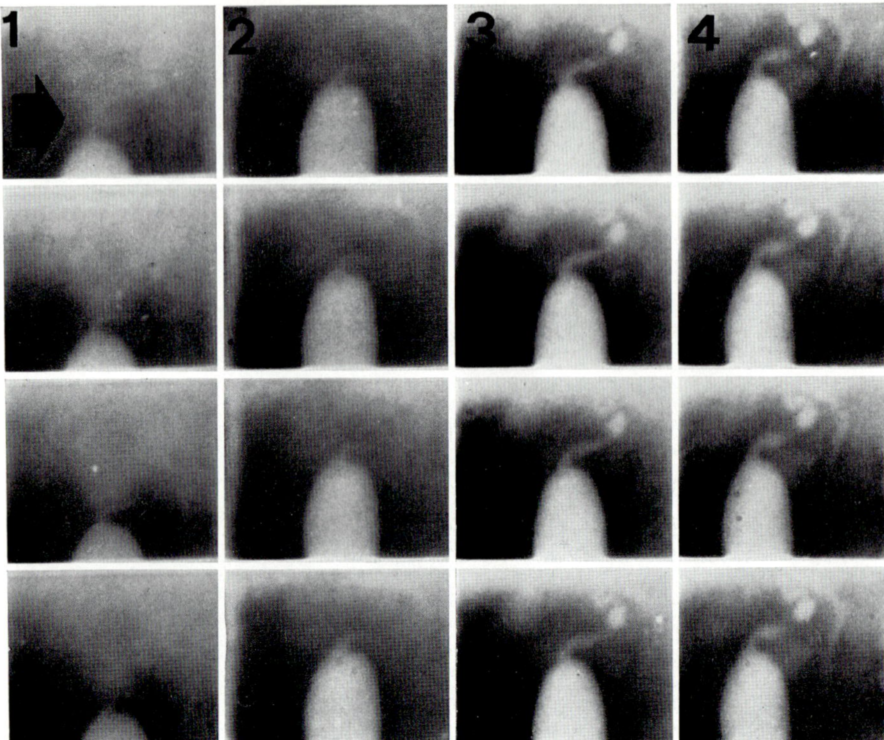

Fig. 5. Effect of amyl nitrite upon blockage of the cholecysto-cystic junction (arrow), produced by an overdose of CCK (75 IDU in 30 sec). Cholecystography in a subject with apparently normal gall bladder. Cinefluorographic sequences. 1: Blockage of the junction; 2, 3, 4: relaxing effect of amyl nitrite. [From Acta Radiol. **55**, 193—206 (1961)]

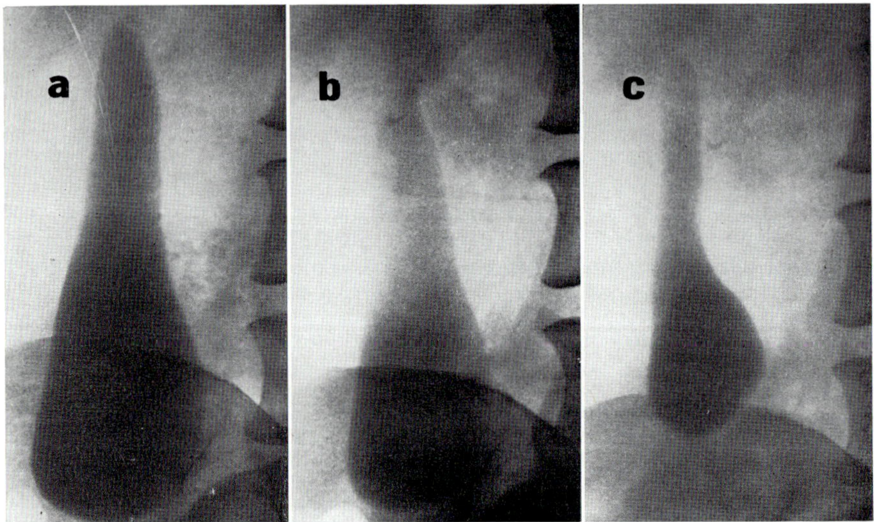

Fig. 6. Delayed gall bladder emptying after fatty meal, normal response to CCK (75 IDU in 3 min), indicating absence of organic or functional alterations at the cholecysto-cystic junction (primary hypotonicity of the gall bladder). Cholecystography: a: preliminary X-ray film; b: 30 min after fatty meal; second examination 5 days later; c: 15 min after CCK

bladder to empty appears to be due to a blockage of the cholecysto-cystic junction. This blockage can be temporarily abolished by amyl nitrite (Fig. 5). Larger amounts of CCK, as well as morphine (CAROLI et al., 1945) and the abrupt distension of the gall bladder (TORSOLI, 1964), definitely increase the resistance of the junction. The ability of amyl nitrite to reverse these effects is important evidence in favour of the sphincter-like role of the cholecysto-cystic junction.

Standard doses of CCK (1 IDU/kg weight in 3 min) may therefore be considered the test of choice in evaluating the muscular response of the gall bladder and cholecysto-cystic junction. When gall bladder emptying after the fatty meal is poor or absent, a normal emptying after CCK indicates impairment of vesicular contractility (Fig. 6); a blockage of the gall bladder evacuation after CCK suggests organic and/or functional alterations of the junction.

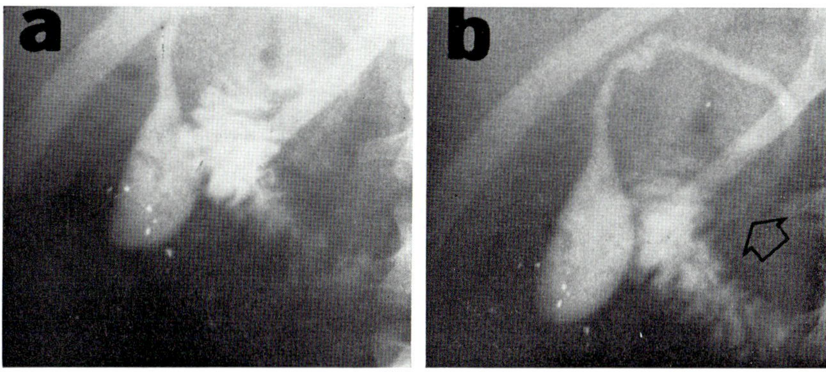

Fig. 7. Good filling of the bile ducts (a) and visibility of the choledocho-duodenal junction (a; b: arrow) (75 IDU in 3 min). Cholecystography in a subject with apparently normal gall bladder. [From Acta Radiol. **55**, 193—206 (1961)]

CCK is preferable to the conventional fatty meal when a good visualization of the bile ducts is required (Fig. 7), or when any variation in gastro-duodenal transit is suspected to interfere with the cholecystographic results (subjects with gastric resection or gastro-intestinal anastomoses: (COLAGRANDE, RAMORINO and SISTI, 1960).

2. Sphincter of Oddi

Standard doses of CCK decrease the resistance of the choledocho-duodenal junction, and increase both the frequency and duration of the opening phases of Oddi's sphincter (Fig. 8). After CCK, intraluminal pressure of the common bile duct decreases if the gall bladder is removed (Fig. 9), and increases if the gall bladder is functioning normally (Fig. 10).

The muscle surrounding the lower end of the bile and pancreatic ducts has both a tonic and a phasic activity. The former is measured by the choledocho-duodenal "passage pressure"; the latter consists of opening and closing movements.

The opening movement corresponds to a progressive relaxation of the various parts of the sphincter, from top to bottom; the closing movement consists of a half-way ring-like sphincteric contraction, followed by an upward contraction of the upper part of the muscle and a downward movement of the lower part and the ampulla. In subjects without anatomical or functional changes of the sphincter, these opening and closing movements last for 0.5 to 3 sec each (CASSANO et al., 1959; TORSOLI, 1964).

A relaxing effect of the sphincter may be observed 30 to 60 sec after the intravenous injection of a standard dose of CCK. This period of latency could cor-

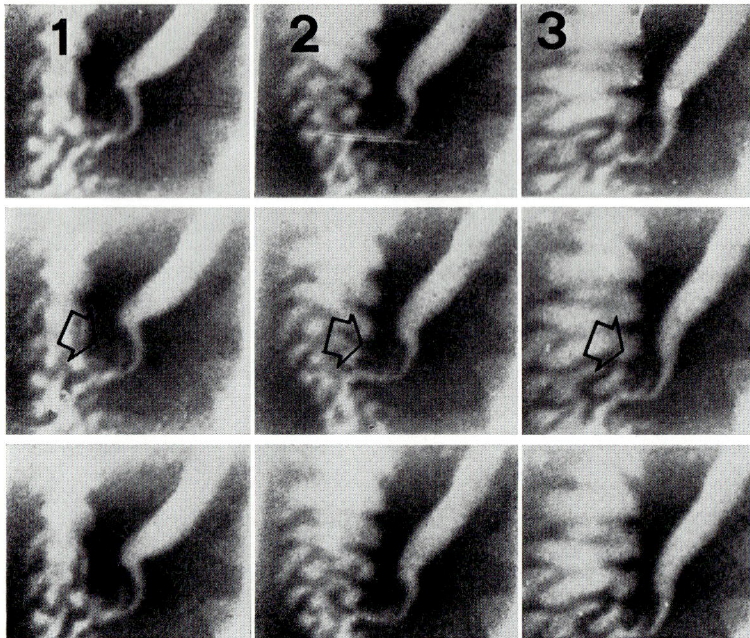

Fig. 8. Relaxing effect of CCK (75 IDU in 3 min) on Oddi's sphincter (arrows). Cinefluorographic sequences in a subject with apparently normal sphincter. [From Acta Radiol. **55,** 193—206 (1961)]

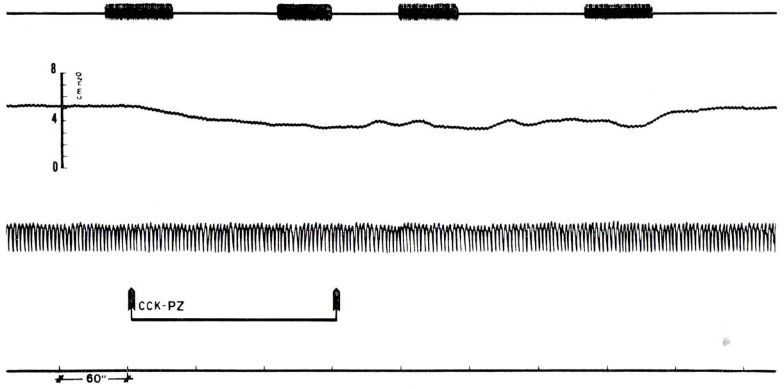

Fig. 9. Effect of CCK (75 IDU in 3 min) on intraluminal pressure of common bile duct. Postoperative cholangiography in a cholecystectomized patient with normal activity of Oddi's sphincter. First tracing: synchronization with cinefluorography; third tracing: pneumograph

respond to the first phase of the timed biliary drainage (after stimulation by oil or magnesium sulphate); duodenal contractions, which may in themselves cause the closing of the sphincter, are often detectable (Torsoli, 1964; Dahlgren, 1966).

Sphincteric relaxation after CCK is demonstrable even after morphine (Ramorino, Colagrande, Monti and Sisti, 1960; Jacobsson, 1965), suggesting that CCK is the most powerful physiologic oddian dilator. In fact, it can be successfully employed to drain the common duct in patients with biliary stasis

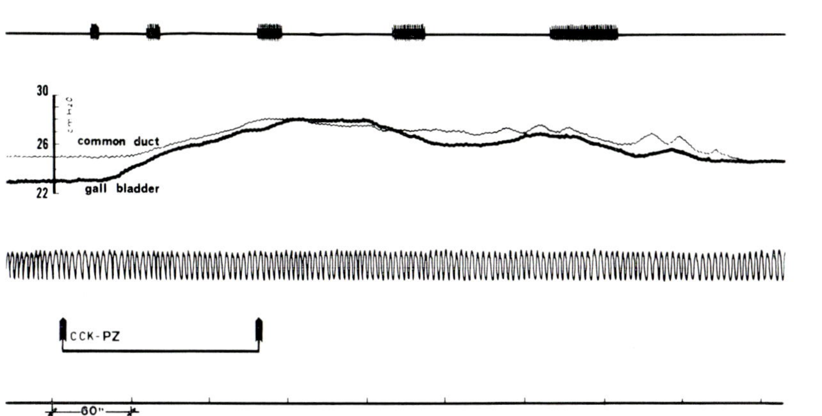

Fig. 10. Effect of CCK (75 IDU in 3 min) on intraluminal pressure of common bile duct and gall bladder. Postoperative cholangiography in a subject with apparently normal gall bladder and Oddi's sphincter activity. First tracing: synchronized cinefluorography; third tracing: pneumograph

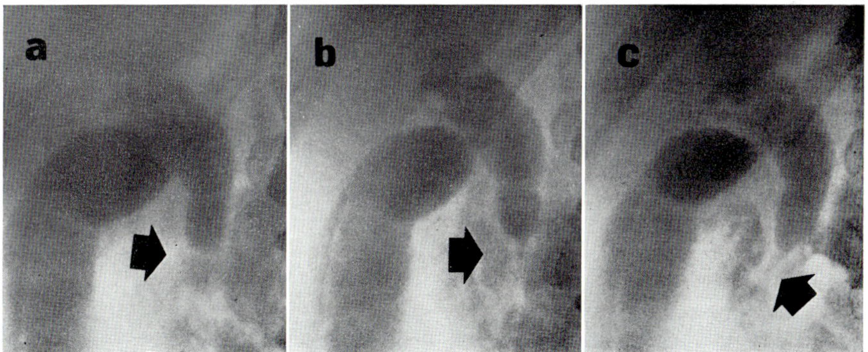

Fig. 11. Partial relaxing effect of CCK (75 IDU in 3 min) on a narrowed Oddi's sphincter (arrows) — odditis. Intravenous cholangiography: a: before CCK; b, c: after CCK

(Fig. 11, 12). In surgical and non-surgical cholangiography, it may contribute to the detection of the organic or functional nature of the oddian stenoses (Fig. 12, 13) (Colagrande et al., 1960; Grassberger and Seyss, 1963; Backlund, 1964).

3. Intestines

CCK increases the mechanical activity of the jejunum, the ileum (Fig. 14) and, to a lesser extent, the colon. The main effect of the increased activity is a reduction of the transit time of intestinal contents (Fig. 15). True peristaltic movements (mass movements) may sometimes be elicited in the colon.

The intestinal motility effect of CCK is demonstrable 2 to 5 min after the intravenous injection of a standard dose. It is independent of the gall bladder contraction and can be registered even in cholecystectomized subjects (Monod, 1964; Dahlgren, 1966). It is atropine-sensitive (Naito et al., 1963).

CCK has therefore been used as a time-saving technique in X-ray examinations of the small intestine. CCK is given intravenously when the barium meal is in the upper jejunum; the contrast medium usually reaches the caecum within 10

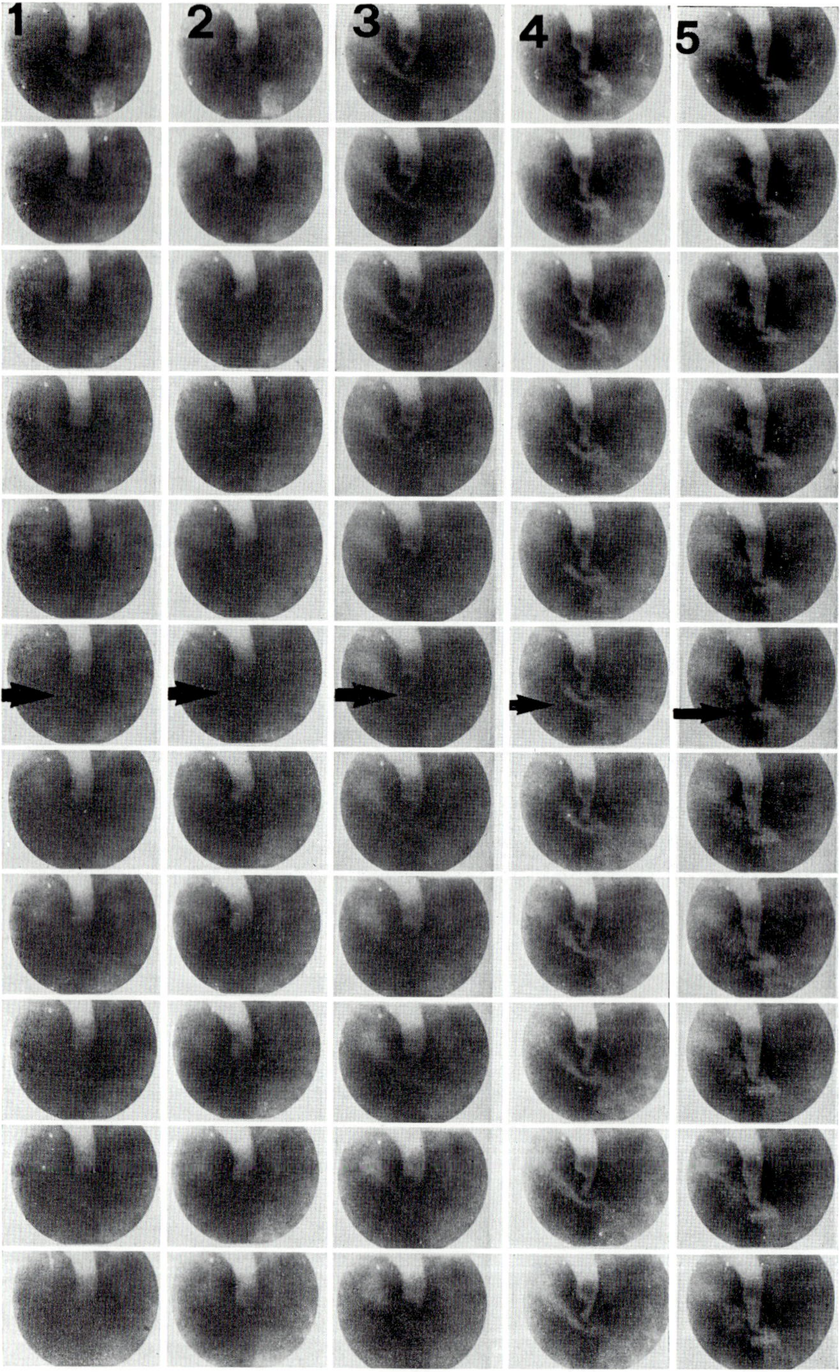

Fig. 12. Relaxing effect of CCK (75 IDU in 3 min) on Oddi's sphincter (arrows) in a patient with partial choledochal obstruction by a stone. Postoperative cholangiography. Cinefluorographic sequences: 1: before CCK; 2, 3, 4, 5: after CCK

to 20 min. In contrast with prostigmine, there is no hypersecretion or change in the mucosal folds. Good results have been obtained in segmental diseases of the small intestine as well as in non-tropical sprue (MONOD, 1964; MORIN, BESANÇON, GRALL, JOUVE and DEBRAY 1965; BACKLUND, 1964, 1967; BARAG and BOUDET, 1967; MORIN, GRALL, JOUVE, BELLIN and DEBRAY, 1968; PARKER and BENEVENTANO, 1968).

The motility effects of CCK on the duodenum have not yet been sufficiently elucidated. X-ray observations (TORSOLI et al., 1961) show that after CCK there is first an activation of duodenal motility, then a prolonged period of apparent inactivity, with distension of the viscus and prominence of the mucosal folds. Consequently the transit of contents is slowed down. These aspects correspond to the relaxation of Oddi's sphincter. It may be that they allow the duodenum to retain the biliopancreatic juices in order to favour the mixing and imbibition of contents.

Effects of Caerulein on the Extrahepatic Biliary Tree and Intestines

The effects of Caerulein (CRL) on the biliary system and intestines, in man, closely resemble those produced by CCK (BERTACCINI, BRAIBANTI and OLIVA, 1969; CARRATŬ, ARCANGELI and PALLONE, 1971). Preliminary results indicate that, when compared on a molar basis, the threshold dose in man accounds for the higher potency of CRL as a cholecystokinetic factor (CARRATŬ, ARCANGELI and PALLONE, 1971).

CRL (0.25 to 2 ng per kg weight in normal saline, intravenous infusion of 30 min) provokes contraction and emptying of the gall bladder (Fig. 16). In comparison with the conventional fatty meal, its action on the cholecysto-cystic junction is more marked. It relaxes the sphincter of Oddi, even after morphine (Fig. 17). CRL also produces an increase of jejuno-ileal motility with acceleration of transit, and sometimes colonic peristaltic movements. Studies are still in progress on the effect of CRL at the duodenal level.

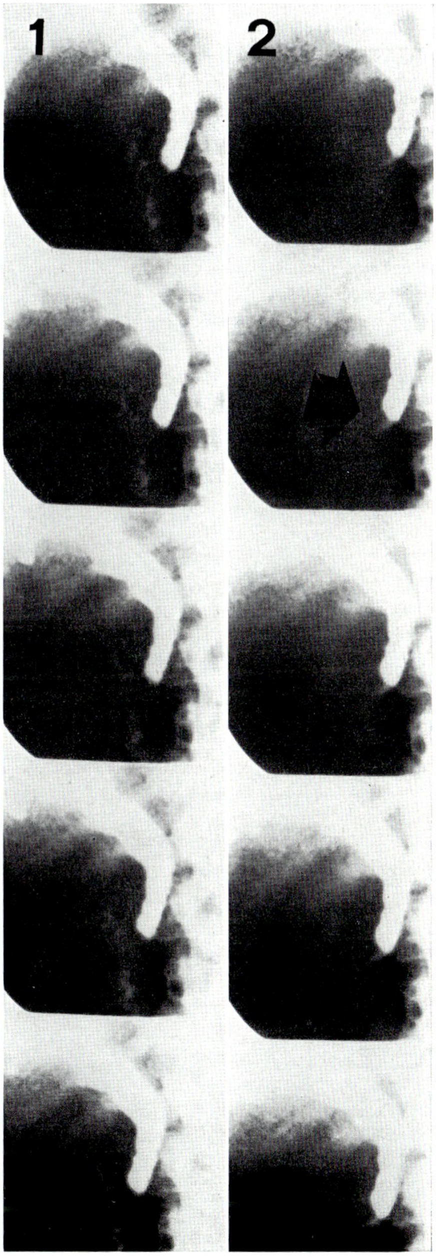

1 2

Fig. 13. Relaxing effect of CCK (75 IDU in 3 min) on the upper tract of Oddi's sphincter (arrow). Postoperative cholangiography in a subject with sclerosing odditis. Cinefluorographic sequences: 1: before CCK; 2: after CCK

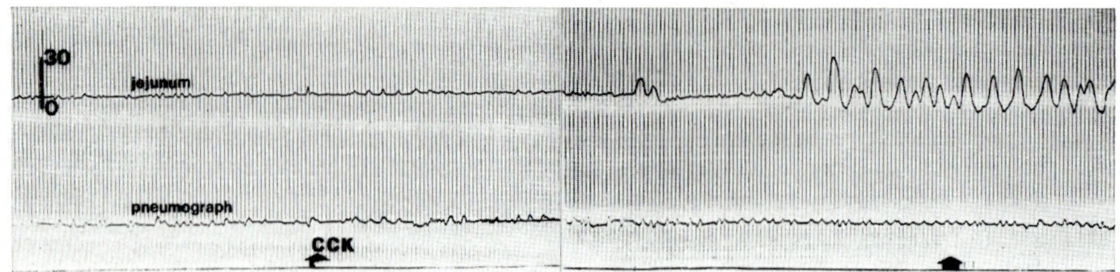

Fig. 14. Effect of CCK (75 IDU in 3 min) on intraluminal pressure activity of the jejunum, recorded by open-ended tip. Each space between vertical lines corresponds to 1 sec

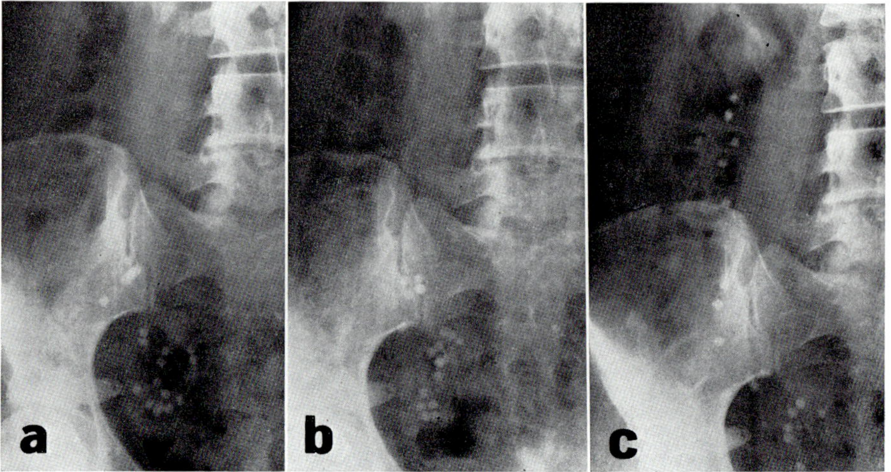

Fig. 15. Effect of CCK on radiopaque markers measuring intestinal transit time. a: preliminary X-ray film showing the majority of markers in the ileum; b: no significant change 30 min after infusion of normal saline; c: 50% of markers in the caecum and ascending colon 30 min after CCK (75 IDU in 30 min)

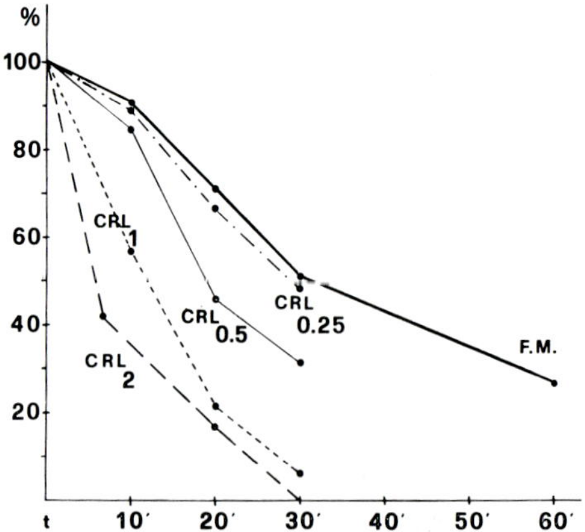

Fig. 16. Gall bladder emptying rates in 35 healthy subjects following fatty meal (FM) and Caerulein (CRL) at various doses (0.25 to 2 ng per kg weight per min, for 30 min). [From Rendic. R. Gastroenterol. 3, 28—33 (1971)]

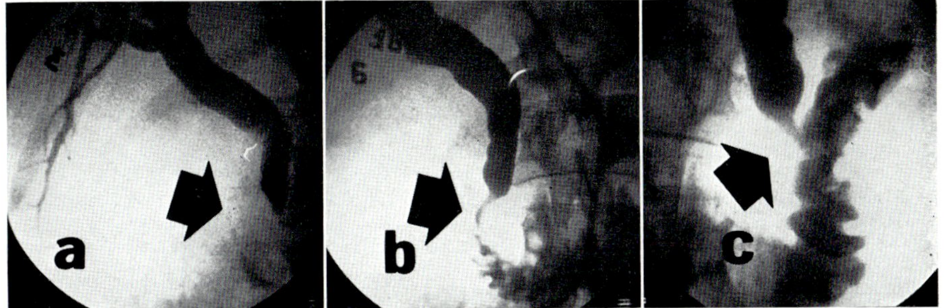

Fig. 17. Relaxing effect of CRL on the morphine-induced spasm of the sphincter (arrows). Postoperative photofluorocholangiography. a: spasm of the sphincter; b, c: 8 and 20 min after CRL (1 ng per kg weight per min, for 30 min). [From Rendic. R. Gastroenterol. **3**,28—33 (1971)[

References

ALESSANDRINI, A., PALAGI, L., RAMORINO, M. L., RIBOTTA, S.: "Contributo allo studio dell'attività motoria biliare. 1° Rilievi elettromanometrici in condizioni 'basali'". Arch. Ital. Mal. Appar. Dig. **27**, 529—547 (1960).

BACKLUND, V.: "Cholecystokinin vid cholangiografier". Svenska Läk.-Tidn. **61**, 3813—3819 (1964).

— "Cholecystokinin vid röntgenundersökningar". Svenska Läk.-Tidn. **64**, 2473—2476 (1967).

BARAG, N., BAUDET, Y.: "Technique de l'emploi de la cholécystokinine dans le transit accéléré du grêle". J. Radiol. **48**, 489—492 (1967).

BERTACCINI, G., BRAIBANTI, T., OLIVA, F.: "Cholecystokinetic activity of the new peptide caerulein in man". Gastroenterology, **56**, 862—867 (1969).

CAROLI, J., VARAY, A., GILLES, E.: "Le fonctionnement du sphincter vésiculaire chez l'homme: observation d'une double intubation". Arch. Mal. Appar. Dig. **34**, 350—356. (1945).

CARRATÚ, R., ARCANGELI, G.: PALLONE F.: "Effect of caerulein on the human biliary tract". Rendic. R. Gastroenterol. **3**, 28—33 (1971)

CASSANO, C., TORSOLI, A., ALESSANDRINI, A.: "Aspetti dinamici di fisiologia e fisiopatologia biliare". In: Atti XIII Congresso Soc. Ital. Gastroenterol. Bologna: CAPPELLI, 1959 pp. 107—142.

COLAGRANDE, C., RAMORINO, M. L., SISTI, P.: "Su l'impiego della colecistocinina negli esami radiologici dell'apparato biliare". Arch. Ital. Mal. Appar. Dig. **27**, 469—481 (1960).

DAHLGREN, S.: "Cholecystokinin: pharmacology and clinical use". Acta Chir. Scand. Suppl. **357**, 256—260 (1966).

GRASSBERGER, A., SEYSS, R.: "Die funktionelle intraoperative Cholangiographie". Wien. Klin. Wschr. **75**, 736—738 (1963).

JACOBSSON, B.: "The morphology of the choledocho-duodenal junction and the functional properties of the extra-hepatic biliary ducts in cholecystectomised patients". R. I. H. **15**, 939—953 (1965).

JORDAN, P. H.: "Physiology of bile secretion". Amer. J. Surg. **107**, 367—370 (1964).

JORPES, E., MUTT, V.: "On the action of highly purified preparations of secretin and of pancreozymin". Arkiv. Kemi. **7**, 553—559 (1954).

MONOD, E.: "Action entéro-kinétique de la cécékine". Arch. Mal. Appar. Dig. **53**, 607—608 (1964).

MORIN, G., BESANÇON, F., GRALL, A., JOUVE, R., DEBRAY, CH.: "Technique d'accélération du transit du grêle". Arch. Mal. Appar. Dig. **54**, 1285—1290 (1965).

— GRALL, A., JOUVE, R., BELLIN, A., DEBRAY, CH.: "La technique du grêle accélérée par la cécékine. Bilan de 250 examens". Arch. Mal. Appar. Dig. **57**, 956 (1968).

NAITO, S., IWATA, R., SAITO, T.: "Etudes sur la cholécystokinine: son mode d'action sur la contraction de la vésicule biliaire". Presse Méd. **71**, 2688—2689 (1963).

Parker, J. G., Beneventano, T. C.: "Cholecystokinin as an adjunct in small bowel contrast studies". Abstr. Amer. Gastroenterol. Ass. Meeting. In: Gastroenterology **54**, 1260 (1968).
Ramorino, M. L., Colagrande, C., Monti, G., Sisti, P.: "Effetti della colecistocinina su l'apparato biliare extraepatico e sul duodeno". Arch. Ital. Mal. Appar. Dig. **27**, 403—432 (1960).
Ramorino, M. L., Ammaturo, M. V., Anzini, F.: "Effect of Caerulein on Small and Large Bowel Motility in Man". Rendic. R. Gastroenterol. **2**, 172—175 (1970).
Torsoli, A.: "Studî su l'attività motoria biliare". Il Fegato **10**, 131—221 (1964).
— Ramorino, M. L., Colagrande, C., de Maio, G. P.: "Experiments with Cholecystokinin". Acta Radiol. **55**, 193—206 (1961).

Chapter VI

Gastrointestinal Hormones and Islet Function*

E. F. PFEIFFER, S. RAPTIS and R. FUSSGÄNGER

With 37 Figures

I. Introduction

The development of reliable, fast and precise methods for determining both insulin and glucagon in blood has initiated major progresses in clarifying the mechanisms operative in control of pancreatic islet function. Certainly, the action of nutrients, the so-called diabetogenic hormones and antidiabetic drugs had been elaborated first.

However, secondly, but quite apropos and perfectly fitting the picture came as a by-product of the work on insulin secretion the re-discovery and the revival of the old concept that glucose fed by mouth is having different influences on insulin (and glucagon) secretion as has the intravenous glucose administration. In consequence of these studies it has been established that the involvement and active participation of intestinal hormones, originally held to only affect exocrine pancreatic tissue in order to facilitate intestinal absorption, is also regulating islet cell functions, i.e. the endocrine pancreas.

This chapter is discussing in a compilatory fashion the various findings leading to that concept of a double function of the different gut hormones on both external and internal digestion, i.e. on absorption of food stuffs by the intestinal wall into lymphatic and peripheral blood circulation and on uptake by the cells of various tissues and intracellular metabolism. Obviously, the general meaning of these mechanisms is of higher significance than thought before. It directly points to the importance of the quality rather than of the quantity of food in influencing internal secretion and, via secretion of metabolically important hormones, body cell composition. In that sense, this chapter is only touching one of the most important problems in the industrialized world: The influence of food selection on the composition of the body and the prevention of disease.

II. Historical Review

The basic and most important finding to date which stimulates discussion about and active research on intestinal control of islet function, consists of the difference between the physiological response to oral and i.v. administration of nutrients. As early as 1896, BIEDL and KRAUS of Vienna, demonstrated that

* Supported by grants from Deutsche Forschungsgemeinschaft (Pf/38/28, SFB 87 11 and 12)

glycosuria readily follows the administration of small amounts of glucose given intravenously, whereas large quantities of glucose given orally are tolerated without the excretion of sugar in the urine (TAYLOR and HULTON, 1916).

For a considerable period of time two theories were applied to explain these divergent findings. The first one (WOODYATT et al., 1916) originated from the difficulties in producing glycosuria even when large amounts of glucose are taken orally, which drew particular attention to the fact that the intestines of normal human subjects cannot absorb glucose, taken orally, as readily as when it is administered intravenously. Even in the case of i.v. glucose administration, this is only followed by the excretion of glucose in the urine if more than 1.8 g/kg body weight per minute are given (WOODYATT et al.). However, even larger amounts of oral glucose did not cause glycosuria.

The second theory, widely accepted even today, concentrated on the role played by the liver after the ingestion of food, mediated by portal circulation (CLAUDE BERNARD, 1877). It was apparent that, during absorption of sugar from the intestines, considerable amounts were taken up by the liver even during the first circulation.

More than 50 years went by before any new theories were put forward for consideration, i.e. careful analysis of glucose assimilation showed that identical glycemias, following both oral and i.v. glucose administration, did not result in the same glucose disappearance rates. Only following oral glucose administration was it possible to establish the rapid fall of blood glucose concentrations (CONARD et al. 1953; SCOW and CORNFIELD, 1954; CONARD, 1955). Moreover, when oral glucose was followed by i.v. glucose loads, a much more rapid fall in blood sugar level was observed than without prior oral glucose administration (SOMERSALO, 1950). This revived the old theory of BAYLISS and STARLING (1902) that an intestinal factor (or factors) was participating in the utilization of glucose which, once released into the circulation, also acted upon i.v. glucose assimilation.

In 1902 BAYLISS and STARLING were coining the expression "hormone" for secretin. They were convinced that this hormone, secretin, affected both the endocrine and the exocrine portion of the pancreatic gland. Although insulin was not known at that time, its contribution in controlling carbohydrate metabolism had been suggested by von MERING and MINKOWSKI (1889). Hence, several attempts were made to treat diabetic subjects (both successfully and unsuccessfully) with both secretin and oral duodenal extracts (MOORE et al., 1906; BAINBRIDGE and BEDDARD, 1906; DAKIN and RANSOM, 1906; FOSTER, 1906 and CROFTON, 1909). In 1904 HENRY DALE, from Starling's laboratory, reported about hypertrophy and hyperplasia of the islets of Langerhans produced by injecting secretin.

In a number of experiments several authors measured glucose in blood, once a method for the determination of hexoses was available, following i.v. injection of intestinal extracts in animals and man (OEHME and WIMMERS, 1923; TROTTEANO, 1924; NOVOA SANTOS, 1925; IVY and FISHER, 1924). However, in some of these reports, the fall in blood sugar following the injection of intestinal extracts was also observed in pancreatectomized animals. Hence, the involvement of insulin seemed unlikely in this mechanism.

The most important of these experiments were carried out by ZUNZ and LA BARRE. In 1928 they attempted to demonstrate the direct release of insulin in response to secretin by the classical anastomosis experiment in dogs (Fig. 1). The pancreatic vein of a donor dog was anastomosed to the jugular vein of a recipient dog. Following the opening of the anastomosis, a crude secretin preparation given to the donor not only produced a fall in blood sugar level in the donor animal, but also a much more impressive fall in blood sugar in the recipient.

From this finding it was concluded that secretin was responsible for the fall in blood sugar by stimulation of insulin secretion.

While ZUNZ and LA BARRE, like BAYLISS and STARLING, were convinced that the secretory action of their crude secretin preparation upon the exocrine portion of the pancreatic gland was identical to the hypoglycemic effect of the same preparation, they nevertheless attempted to distinguish between the two actions. The fraction which, in their view, had an effect upon the exocrine pancreatic tissue alone, was called "Excretin". The fraction with hypoglycemic properties they called "Incretin". According to LA BARRE and LÉDRUT (1934) "Incretin" showed hypoglycemic properties even following oral administration. This revival of the old experiments, mentioned above (MOORE et al., 1906), initiated new attempts at

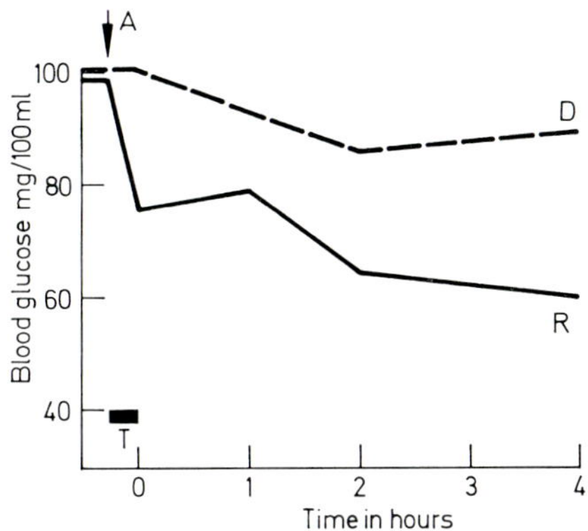

Fig. 1. Blood sugar response of donor dog (D) and recipient (R) to the intravenous injection of 19 mg of non hypotensive secretin into the donor at time A. During the time interval (T) the pancreatico-duodenal venous blood of the donor flowed into the jugular vein of the recipient. (From: LA BARRE, 1936; McINTYRE, 1967/69).

oral treatment of mild diabetics by intestinal extracts. Surprisingly, better control of the diabetic condition was obtained.

In the early thirties many papers appeared describing variable results and diverse findings as regards the theory of intestinal control of the endocrine pancreatic function (HELLER, 1931; LAUGHTON and MACALLUM, 1932; DUNCAN et al., 1935). However, a series of extremely critical papers from LOEW et al. (1939/40) overthrew all previous findings and, in particular, the idea of a close connection (via mutual humoral-hormonal regulations) between intestinal absorption of nutrients and intracellular uptake and metabolism, which belief was discarded. The gastrointestinal hormones fell into oblivion to such an extent that — according to the review of JORPES and MUTT — in 1960, pancreozymin-cholecystokinin was not even registered in the "Current List of Medical Literature".

However, the revival was already under way. It was initiated by the observations mentioned above, that in rats and in man, the rates at which glucose disappeared from the blood circulation were much more rapid in those cases in which the glucose was administered orally and not by the i.v. route (SCOW and CORNFIELD, 1954; CONARD et al., 1953; CONARD, 1955). The second step was possible after reliable methods for the determination of plasma and serum insulin had been developed. Following oral administration of glucose, insulin levels not only increased to much higher concentrations, but also remained elevated for a longer period of time than after i.v. glucose administration, irrespective of the higher glucose levels following i.v. injection (Fig. 2) (MCINTYRE et al., 1964;1965; ELRICK et al., 1964). In order to explain these differences satisfactorily, the existence of a specific factor of intestinal origin, stimulating the release of insulin, had to be taken into consideration.

This role was primarily ascribed to secretin as in the days of ZUNZ and LA BARRE when DUPRÉ (1964) showed that secretin was capable of improving the rate of glucose assimilation following i.v. administration, and PFEIFFER et al.

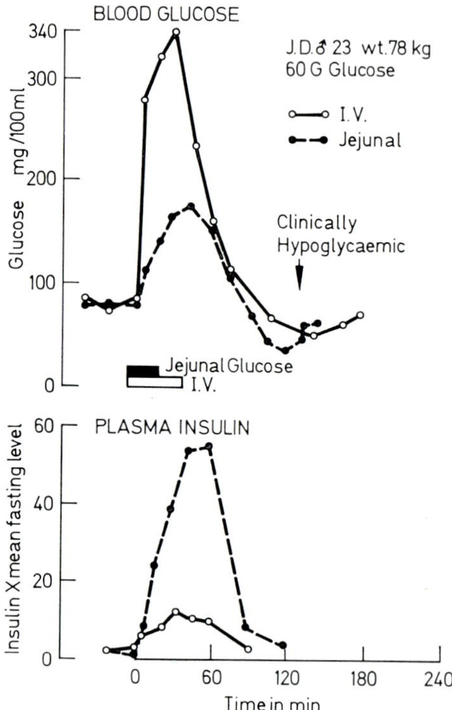

Fig. 2. Despite the much smaller rise in plasma glucose following its intrajejunal administration, compared with its intravenous administration, there is a far greater increment in the plasma insulin with the intrajejunal route. (From: MCINTYRE et al., 1965)

(1965) demonstrated the direct action of secretin on insulin release from pieces of pancreatic tissue in vitro even in the absence of glucose in the medium.

Eventually, the lower increase in blood insulin concentrations following parenteral rather than enteral glucose administration were also observed in subjects with porta-caval anastomosis (DUPRÉ, 1964; MCINTYRE et al., 1965). Hence, it was necessary to abandon the still highly esteemed theory (BASTENIE and CONARD, 1957) of primary liver perfusion of intestinal veinous blood being effectively related to these differences in the release of insulin in response to oral versus intravenous glucose administration.

In the following review we shall discuss these old as well as new observations in recent times. Glucose certainly is not the only food acting as a trigger for eliciting this intestinal-insular mechanism. Proteins and amino acids show similar activities. They all collaborate closely to link as closely as possible exocrine and endocrine digestion, i.e. extracellular and intracellular uptake of substrates. However, the final significance of this regulatory system under physiological and, in particular, under pathophysiological conditions, still remains to be elucidated.

III. Some Remarks on the Chemical Structure, Extra-insular Actions and Sites of Origin of the Gastrointestinal Hormones

According to the physiologists and, in particular, the noted representative of studies on both the mechanism of food ingestion and the conditioned reflexes (Pavlov, 1898), the absorption of nutrients into the digestive system induces the intestinal tract to release stimulants into the peripheral circulation affecting gastrointestinal function. Secretin, gastrin, pancreozymin-cholecystokinin, enteroglucagon and also serotonin, stimulate or inhibit the different phases of digestion.

Certain structural similarities initiated speculation as to phylogenetic relationships between the intestinal hormones gastrin and pancreozymin on the one hand, and the pancreatic hormones insulin and glucagon on the other hand, whereas secretin was held to maintain an intermediate position because of its chemical similarity to glucagon. Recently, Track (1969) had been investigating this subject. A protein similar to secretin was regarded as the common precursor.

1. Gastrin

The second intestinal hormone, gastrin, discovered by Edkins (1905) and isolated by Gregory and Tracy (1964), was the first substance of this group successfully synthesized (Anderson et al., 1964). Gastrin is found in various species, consistently in two forms, GI and GII, which differ only in that the tyrosyl residues in position 12, i.e. adjacent to the C-terminal pentapeptide, are sulfated, GII, or nonsulfated, GI, (Fig. 3). The molecular weight of human

Pig I — Pyr · Gly · Pro · Trp · Met · (Glu)$_5$ · Ala · Tyr · Gly · Trp · Met · Asp · Phe · NH_2
II (Tyr–SO_3H)

Human I — Pyr · Gly · Pro · Trp · Leu · (Glu)$_5$ · Ala · Tyr · Gly · Trp · Met · Asp · Phe · NH_2
II (Tyr–SO_3H)

Fig. 3. Structure of pig and human gastrin I und II.

Gastrin I amounts to 2.200, that of human gastrin II to 2.280. Methionine in position 5 of human gastrin is substituted by leucine in porcine gastrin (Fig. 3). The common C-terminal tetrapeptide-amide Try-Met-Asp-Phe-NH_2 represents the biologically active part of the molecule. Therefore, the C-terminal pentapeptide has been used successfully instead of the natural hormone (Morley et al., 1965). The tetra- and the pentapeptide, however, lose almost all activity following removel of the terminal amide group.

Argyrophilic cells in the antral parts of the stomach are considered to be the main producers of the hormone (SOLCIA and SAMPIETRO, 1965). Following examination by electron microscope (SOLCIA et al., 1967) the suggested site of origin was finally confirmed by means of the immunofluorescence technique (McGUIGAN, 1968). Whether the d-cells or the α1-cells of the pancreatic islets produce gastrin in a similar manner, remains open to question (BLOOM, 1931; THOMAS, 1937; HELLMANN et al., 1962; CAVALLERO et al., 1967). The antrum cells alone have been shown to do so, under physiological conditions. However, in the Zollinger-Ellison-syndrome, large amounts of gastrin have been recovered from blood (BERSON et al., 1970; BYRNES et al., 1970; McGUIGAN and TRUDEAU, 1970).

Physiologically, gastric secretion is stimulated by gastrin, which is released in response to the intake of nutrients into the antral parts of the stomach. Mechanical (*dilation*) and chemical (alcohol, amino acids, peptides) stimuli as well as stimulation of the vagus nerves and injections of acetylcholine induce gastrin secretion.

Gastrin increases the peristaltic movement of the stomach and actively influences enzyme production of the pancreas and the bile flow (SMITH and HOGG, 1966). In this respect its action is similar to that of cholecystokinin-pancreozymin (CCK-PZ). If acidic fluids come into contact with the pyloric region, gastric secretion is actively inhibited. Whether this diminution of gastric secretion is caused by direct effects of the acid or by a special inhibitory hormone is not yet clear (PENTHEIN and SCHOFIELD, 1959; DAVENPORT, 1967).

Hydrochloric acid acts as one of the most potent inhibitors of gastrin secretion (YALOW and BERSON, 1970). Accordingly, hypoacidity or total anacidity is ac-

Glucagon Mol. Wght. 3485
His-Ser-Gln-*Gly-Thr-Phe-Thr-Ser*-Asp-Tyr-*Ser*-Lys-Tyr-Leu-*Asp-Ser*-Arg-*Arg*-Ala-*Gln*-Asp-Phe-Val-*Gln*-Trp-*Leu*-Met-Asn-Thr

Secretin Mol. Wght. 3055
His-Ser-Asp-*Gly-Thr-Phe-Thr-Ser*-Glu-Leu-*Ser*-Arg-Leu-Arg-*Asp-Ser*-Ala-*Arg*-Leu-*Gln*-Arg-Leu-Leu-*Gln*-Gly-*Leu*-Val-NH_2

Cholecystokinin-Pancreozymin Mol. Wght. 3919 (CCK-PZ)
Lys-(Ala, Gly, Pro, Ser)-Arg-Val-(I leu, Met, Ser)-Lys, Asn-(Leu, Asp, Gln, His, Leu, Pro, Ser, Ser)-Arg-I leu-(Asp, Ser)-Arg-*Asp-Tyr-Met-Gly-Trp-Met-Asp-Phe-NH_2*
↓
SO_3H

Synthet. Octapeptide from CCK-PZ Mol. Wght. 1143 (ONDETTI, 1968)
Asp-Tyr-Met-Gly-Trp-Met-Asp-Phe-NH_2
↓
SO_3H

Gastrin I (Human) Mol. Wght. 2200
Pyr-Gly-Pro-Trp-Leu-Glu-Glu-Glu-Glu-Glu-Ala-Tyr-*Gly-Trp-Met-Asp-Phe-NH_2*
Gastrin II (Human) Mol. Wght. 2280
Pyr-Gly-Pro-Trp-Leu-Glu-Glu-Glu-Glu-Glu-Ala-Tyr-*Gly-Trp-Met-Asp-Phe-NH_2*
↓
SO_3H

Gastrin Pentapeptide Mol. Wght. 653
Gly-Trp-Met-Asp-Phe-NH_2
Caerulein Mol. Wght. 1258
Pyr-Gln-*Asp-Tyr*-Thr-Gly-Trp-Met-Asp-Phe-N*H*$_2$
↓
SO_3H

Fig. 4. Amino acid sequences of intestinal hormones (From: PFEIFFER et al., 1971).

companied by increased levels of gastrin in blood (YALOW and BERSON, 1970). Inhibition of gastric secretion by atropine does not prevent the secretion of gastrin following food intake. However, it does reduce the hydrochloric acid secretion rate and causes rises in the gastrin concentrations in blood (BERSON et al., 1970). Hypoglycemia caused by i.v. insulin administration does not always induce a rise in plasma gastrin, whereas i.v. calcium administration consistently stimulates gastrin secretion (BERSON et al., 1970). At the same time, obviously due to gastrin release, gastric secretion of acids is increased (PASSARO, BASSO and GORDON, 1970).

Under pathological conditions, in patients suffering from duodenal ulcer, pernicious anemia, Zollinger-Ellison-syndrome as well as after the administering of histamine, elevated levels of gastrin were determined (BERSON et al., 1970; BYRNES et al., 1970; MCGUIGAN and TRUDEAU, 1970). Increases in the gastral G-cells and signs of intensified secretion of gastrin were indicated from immunofluorescence findings in patients suffering from pernicious anemia (PEARSE, 1970). Some controversial findings regarding gastrin concentrations in patients with duodenal and stomach ulcers may be reconciled on the basis that an inverse relationship exists between secretion of HCl by the stomach and gastrin release (TRUDEAU and MCGUIGAN, 1971).

It is of interest to note that cholecystokinin-pancreozymin (CCK-PZ), as will be shown subsequently, not only demonstrates certain physiological actions similar to gastrin, but also shares its 5 terminal amino acids (MUTT and JORPES, 1967) (Fig. 4). In spite of the chemical relationship, cross reactions in the immunoassay are only rarely observed when CCK-PZ and gastrin are measured.

2. Cholecystokinin-Pancreozymin (CCK-PZ)

As early as 1902 BAYLISS and STARLING suggested that, not only was the pancreatic gland being affected by secretin, but that this was also producing an effect on the secretion of bile. Other laboratories observed the positive action of secretin on gallbladder contraction. It seems likely that impurities in the first secretin preparations with more specific substances affecting gallbladder action, called cholecystokinin (CCK) (IVY and OLDBERG, 1928) or pancreozymin (PZ) (HARPER and RAPER, 1943), were responsible for this action.

Clarification of somewhat confused situation, where at least two separate hormones should have an effect on both the pancreatic secretion and on the bile and the gallbladder function, came, when JORPES and MUTT (1966; 1970) and MUTT and JORPES (1968) noted that the pancreozymin and the cholecystokinin activities accompany one another in a quantitative manner during the course of successive purification procedures. After having isolated 20 mg of the pure CCK-PZ from 20 km of pig's intestines, the chemical structure was revealed. CCK-PZ is a single-chain polypeptide of 33 amino acids with a molecular weight of 3919 and, as mentioned above, it has a C-terminal end which is similar to that of gastrin and, as will be shown below, to that of caerulein (Fig. 4).

The biologically active part of the molecule resides in the C-terminal portion, as with gastrin. The C-terminal octapeptide was synthesized (ONDETTI et al., 1968), and displayed biological activities ten times that of the normal CCK-PZ on a weight basis (ONDETTI et al., 1970). The molecular weight of this synthetic peptide amounts to 1143. Moreover, it was found that the activity of the octapeptide with a sulfated tyrosyl residue was 700 times as high as that of the corresponding non-sulfated octapeptide.

As to the natural CCK-PZ preparation, 1 mg of pure substance is equivalent to 3,000 Ivy dog units for the CCK-activity and to 12,000 Crick-Harper-Raper-units for the PZ-activity. The synthetic octapeptide displays biological activity in the range of 30 Ivy dog units/μg (ONDETTI et al., 1968; 1970).

3. Secretin

Secretin was the first gastrointestinal hormone discovered (BAYLISS and STARLING, 1902). BAYLISS and STARLING called secretin a "hormone" under which name they pioneered to designate all substances with hormonal activity. It was isolated in pure form in 1961 (JORPES and MUTT, 1961). Its structure was determined (JORPES et al., 1962; MUTT and JORPES, 1966). Porcine secretin has 27 amino acid residues, a molecular weight of 3055, and does not contain any sulfur containing amino acids. In 1966 the polypeptide was synthesized (BODANSZKY et al., 1966). No fragments or synthetic peptides with partial structure of the original hormone are known to posses secretin type activity. However, as indicated in Fig. 5, 14 of the amino acid residues, counting from the N-terminal end,

Glucagon	*Secretin*	*Glucagon*	*Secretin*
His	*His*	*Ser*	*Ser*
Ser	*Ser*	Arg	Ala
Gln	Asp	*Arg*	*Arg*
Gly	*Gly*	Ala	Leu
Thr	*Thr*	*Gln*	*Gln*
Phe	*Phe*	Asp	Arg
Thr	*Thr*	Phe	Leu
Ser	*Ser*	Val	Leu
Asp	Glu	*Gln*	*Gln*
Tyr	Leu	Trp	Gly
Ser	*Ser*	*Leu*	Leu
Lys	Arg	Met	Val NH_2
Tyr	Leu	Asn	
Leu	Arg	Thr	
Asp	*Asp*		

Fig. 5. Amino acid sequences of glucagon and secretin (14 identical amino acids). (From: PFEIFFER et al., 1971)

are found at corresponding positions in glucagon (MUTT et al., 1965). Despite the striking similarity between secretin and glucagon, cross reactions in the immunoassay do not occur.

The pure natural secretin isolated by JORPES and MUTT contains 4000 clinical units/mg (JORPES and MUTT, 1970). 1 mg of the synthetic hormone supplied by Squibb Pharmaceuticals, New Brunswick/USA, displays an activity comparable to 4000—5000 clinical units (ONDETTI et al., 1968).

The biological activity is determined in animal experiments. The release of secretin is stimulated physiologically by acidification of the duodenum. It increases the blood circulation of the pancreas, and it induces excretion of water and bicarbonate in the pancreatic juice (SARLES et al., 1963; HARTLEY et al. 1965; WORMSLEY, 1968). Secretin stimulates water and bicarbonate secretion with the bile (WAITMAN and JANOWITZ, 1967). However, large amounts of secretin do not increase bile secretion by more than twice the initial quantity per time period. The release of secretin is elicited on a purely humoral basis. Conversely, secretin increases pancreatic secretion without any involvement of the autonomous nervous system. This has been demonstrated in cross-transfusion experiments in dogs as well as by transplantation of the pancreatic gland to other vascular regions of the body (BAYLISS and STARLING, 1902; FARRELL and IVY, 1926; STILL et al., 1933).

The slightest contact of the epithelial tissue in the upper intestine with hydrochloric acid is sufficient to release secretin into the peripheral circulation and to the pancreas. The half-life of secretin is extremely short, i.e. 3.2 minutes (LEHNERT et al., 1969). Secretin as well as glucagon inhibit gastric acid secretion and motility (GREENLEE et al., 1957; PETERSEN, BERSTAD and MYREN, 1970; DOTEVALL et al., 1970). This adverse effect may be related to the similarity in the structure of glucagon and secretin, and so may other effects which the two peptides have in common. Both hormones stimulate the release of insulin from the pancreas in vivo and in vitro, both hormones induce an increase in the volume of bile secretion, and both stimulate lipolysis in adipose tissue in vitro (RAPTIS et al., 1969a). However, despite the structural similarities, glucagon appears to have no effect on the exocrine secretion in the resting pancreas. Nevertheless, the administration of glucagon exerts a marked inhibitory effect on the output when pancreas is stimulated with exogenous secretin (DYCK et al., 1969; ZAYTZUK et al., 1967).

4. Caerulein

It is of interest to note that a decapeptide, caerulein, which was extracted from the skin of the Australian frog (Hyla caerulea) by ERSPAMER et al. (1966) has biological and chemical properties similar to those of PZ-CCK. It also contains the C-terminal pentapeptide amide of gastrin and CCK-PZ with a closely adjacent sulfated tyrosyl residue (Fig. 4). The structural similarity between the carboxyl terminal of caerulein and that of cholecystokinin-pancreozymin (CCK-PZ) and gastrin might account for the similarity in the action spectrum of caerulein, CCK-PZ and gastrin. A few nanograms of caerulein provoke a contraction of the gallbladder in vitro as well as in vivo and a relaxation of the sphincter of Oddi. On a molar basis, caerulein is 16-times as potent as CCK-PZ and 170-times as potent as gastrin I and II (VAGNE and GROSSMAN, 1968). In man, caerulein increases the peristaltic activity of the duodenum as well as the peristaltic activity and the tonus of the jejunum; it also stimulates the secretion of gastric acid. In addition, caerulein influences the exocrine function of the pancreas, increasing the volume excreted, the bicarbonate content, and the enzyme concentration (GROSSMAN, 1969).

5. Enteroglucagon

A substance having the same immunological properties as glucagon but manifesting different biochemical functions, has recently been extracted from the intestine (UNGER et al., 1968). This substance was first extracted with acid ethanol from gastric and duodenal mucosa of the dog (SUTHERLAND and DE DUVE, 1948; KENNY and SAY, 1962). Later on preparations from human stomach, duodenum and colon, were shown to exert glucagon like activity. This activity was demonstrated by the activation of liver adenyl cyclase (MAKMAN and SUTHERLAND, 1964). Fig. 6 shows the distribution of the glucagon like immunoreactivity in the upper gastrointestinal tract of a dog (UNGER and EISENTRAUT, 1967).

Cells having an appearance similar to that of pancreatic alpha-cells have been discovered in the intestinal mucosa of the rat by ORCI et al., (1968) with the help of the electron microscope. These cells are likely to secrete enteroglucagon. The intestinal alpha-cells as well as the chromaffine cells and the gastrin-producing cells are unlike each other even in the embryonic tissue of the rat and show typical secretion granules indicating their ability to function (DALDRUP and FORSSMANN, 1970).

The physiological role of enteroglucagon is still unknown. In an attempt to further identify enteroglucagon SAMOLS and MARKS (1967) demonstrated that pancreatic glucagon primarily stimulates insulin secretion and, secondarily, causes an increase in blood sugar, whereas the primary action of enteroglucagon was hyperglycemia and lipolysis. LÉFÈBVRE et al. (1969) isolated enteroglucagon from

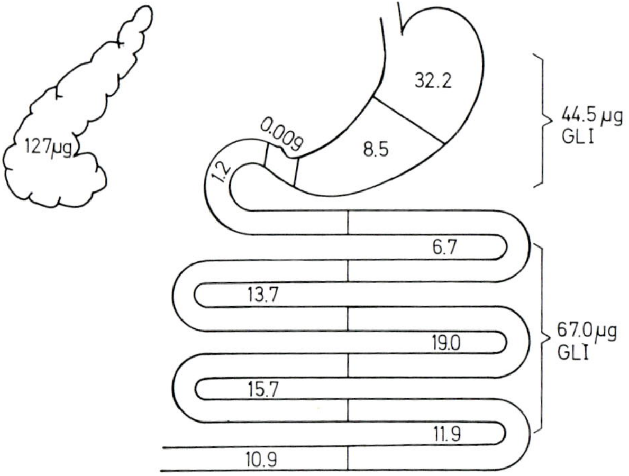

Fig. 6. The distribution of glucagon-like immunoreactivity of acid-alcohol extracts of the tissues of the upper gastrointestinal tract of a dog. (From: UNGER and EISENTRAUT, 1967)

an acid-ethanol extract of rabbit intestine; this could be separated into two fractions by electrophoresis. Both of these fractions showed strong lipolytic activity on the epididymal fat pad of the rat.

The glucagon type activity of the intestine, ascertained by immunological determination, has been described by UNGER et al. (1968). Comparing acid-ethanol extracts from the jejunum of the dog with a similar extract from the pancreas, they found that the volume of the eluate of the jejunal product on a Sephadex G-25 column was smaller than that of the pancreatic extract. They concluded that the molecular size of enteroglucagon was at least twice that of pancreatic glucagon.

After intraportal injection in dogs, the jejunal material confirmed hyperglycemic activity. In experiments with the isolated perfused liver of the rat, enteroglucagon showed no glycogenolytic activity, and consequently, did not increase cyclic-3'5' AMP of the liver.

The influence of enteroglucagon on islet cell function and nutritional aspects of its secretion will be discussed later (see p. 293).

IV. The Pharmaco-Chemical (or Pharmaco-Dynamic) Approach to the Intestinal Factor in Question

If, for the sake of clarifying the matter, we take it for granted that some factor (or factors) of intestinal origin is (or are) responsible for the remarkable action of the nutrients ingested by natural routes upon the pancreatic endocrine secretion, we should still keep the fact in mind that extracellular concentrations of glucose and amino acids per se affect the release of hormone from the islets. Pieces of pancreas and islets isolated from rabbits, rats and all other species of animals, examined in vitro, responded directly, and in relation to the concentrations of the nutrients employed, to the incubations in the various media (Fig. 7

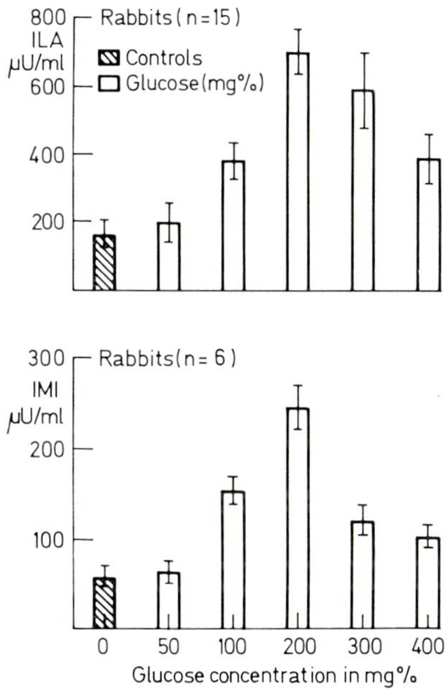

Fig. 7. In vitro secretion of insulin. Stimulation of insulin release (insulin-like activity (ILA) and immunologically measured insulin (IMI), μU/ml) from tissue slices of rabbit pancreas after an incubation of 150 min in 4 ml of Krebs-Ringer-phosphate buffer containing 50 to 400 mg-% of glucose in increasing concentrations. Maximum insulin release occurred at a concentration of 200 mg-% of glucose. (From: Pfeiffer et al., 1965)

and 8). Therefore, even under the stringent conditions of in vitro preparation, the action of each of the factors regulating exocrine as well as endocrine pancreatic secretion, i.e. secretin, pancreozymin-cholecystokinin, glucagon, gastrin, serotonin and some unidentified mucosal factor (s), has to be carefully evaluated when considering the nutritive action as such.

Some examples will be given to illustrate the results obtained; these findings may give us a better understanding of the controversies still existing. Pieces of pancreas from cultured fetal rat did not respond either to glucose or to glucagon alone but did so readily to the combination of both (Fig. 9) (Lambert et al., 1967). Secretin, on the other hand, was active on pieces of dog and rabbit pancreas,

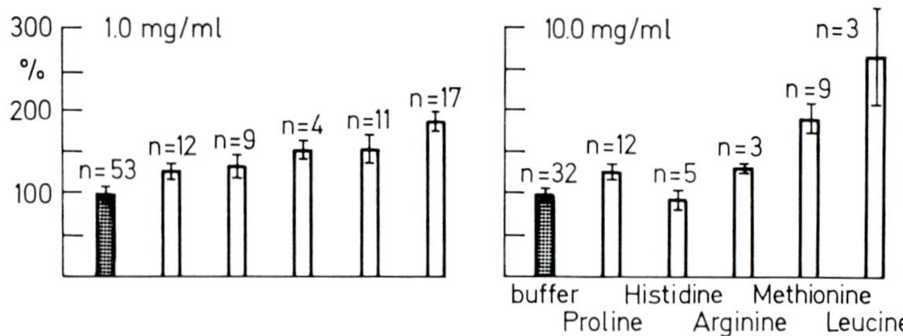

Fig. 8. Insulin secretion in vitro: Insulin release from pieces of rat pancreas effected by different amino acids. Most effective stimulation induced by L-leucine, least effective by histidine. (From: PFEIFFER, 1968)

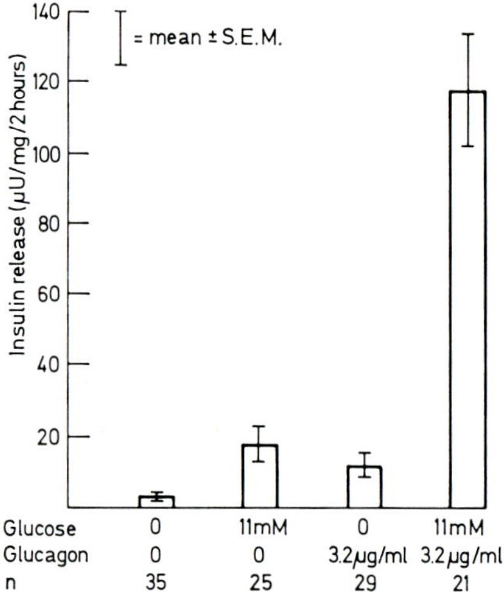

Fig. 9. Insulin release by organ cultures of fetal rat pancreas in the presence or absence of glucose and/or glucagon (cultured 4 days, then transferred to bicarbonate buffer with 0.5% albumin). (From: LAMBERT et al., 1967)

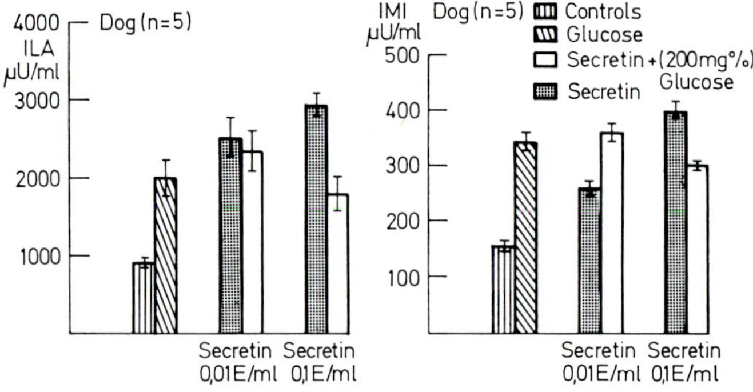

Fig. 10. In vitro secretion of insulin: stimulation of insulin release (ILA and IMI) from pieces of dog pancreas. No statistically significant changes of ILA to be observed after the addition of glucose to 0.01 U of secretin per ml; significant increase of IMI. Statistically significant inhibition of ILA and IMI release after the addition of 200 mg-% of glucose to 0.1 U of secretin per ml. (From: PFEIFFER et al., 1965)

alone, without glucose being added to the medium; moreover, secretin induced the release of ILA and IMI which was not potentiated by the presence of glucose in the incubation fluids (Fig. 10) (PFEIFFER et al., 1965).

These experiments were carried out on *pieces* of pancreas. Isolated rat *islets* incubated in the presence of various intestinal hormones with and without glucose

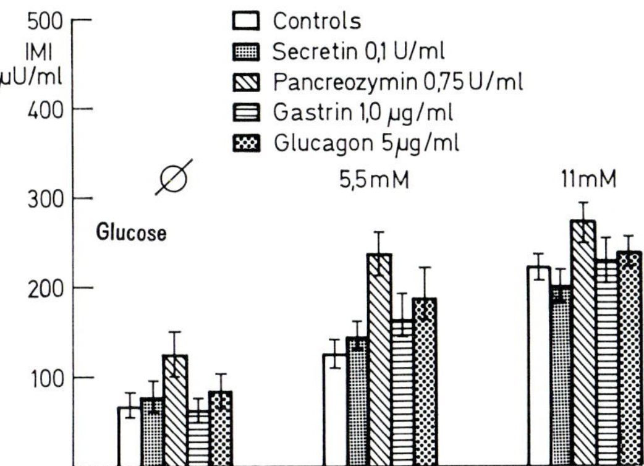

Fig. 11a. Influence of intestinal hormones on the insulin secretion of isolated Langerhans islets of the rat. Released insulin in μU/3 islets over 60 min ($n = 9$). (From: PFEIFFER, 1969; HINZ, RAPTIS and PFEIFFER, 1970)

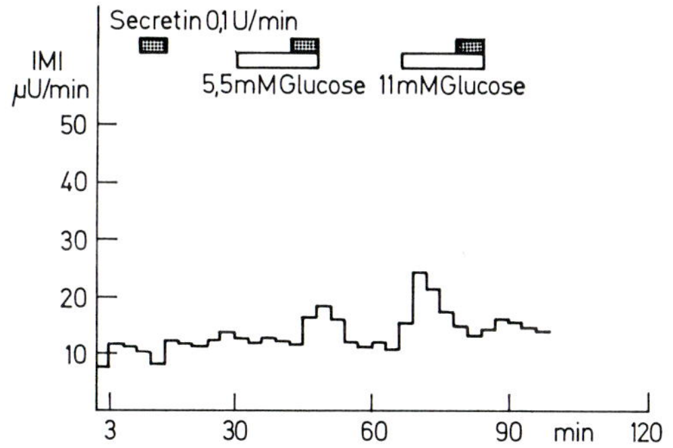

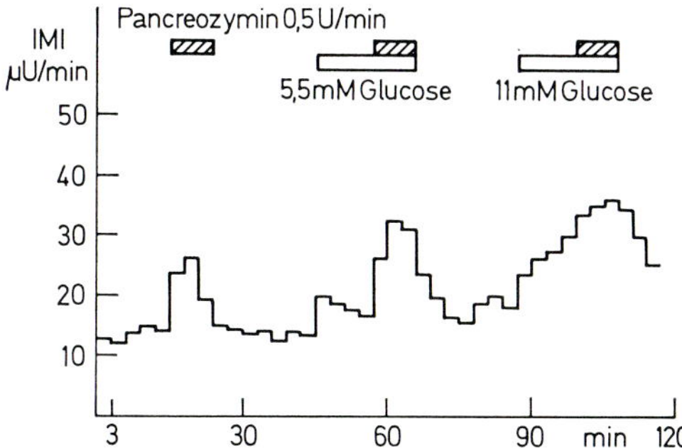

Fig. 11b. Effect of secretin and of pancreozymin on insulin secretion of isolated perifused islets without and with addition of variable glucose concentration in the perifusion medium. (From: HINZ et al., 1970; PFEIFFER et al., 1972)

in the medium, reacted differently again (HINZ et al., 1970): None of the hormones except pancreozymin elicited any insulin responses either in the presence or in the absence of glucose, while pancreozymin was active under any condition (Fig. 11a). This observation, to which we shall refer later, was corroborated by a slightly different approach. The islets were continuously perifused in an apparatus suggested by JUNOD et al. (1969), permitting dynamic studies of insulin secretion. Once more, without glucose being present in the perifusion fluid, secretin effected no insulin secretion while pancreozymin did (Fig. 11a); furthermore, various concentrations of glucose stimulated insulin release per se without showing any additional activity of secretin, while the effect of pancreozymin was significantly enhanced.

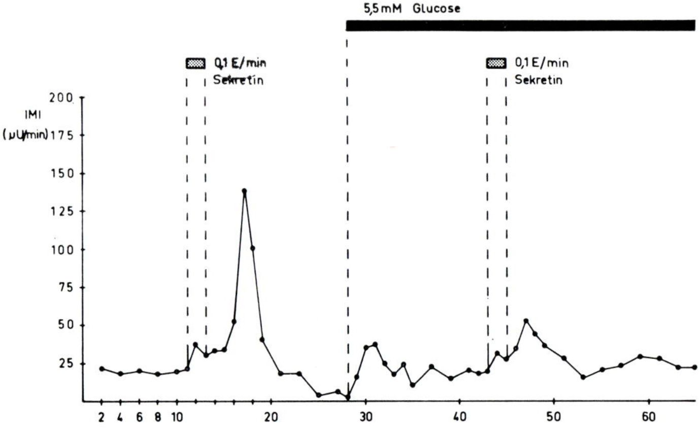

Fig. 12. The effect of secretin (0.1 U/min) on the glucose independent and glucose (5.5 mM) induced insulin secretion of the isolated perfused pancreas of the rat ($n = 2$). (From: PFEIFFER, 1969)

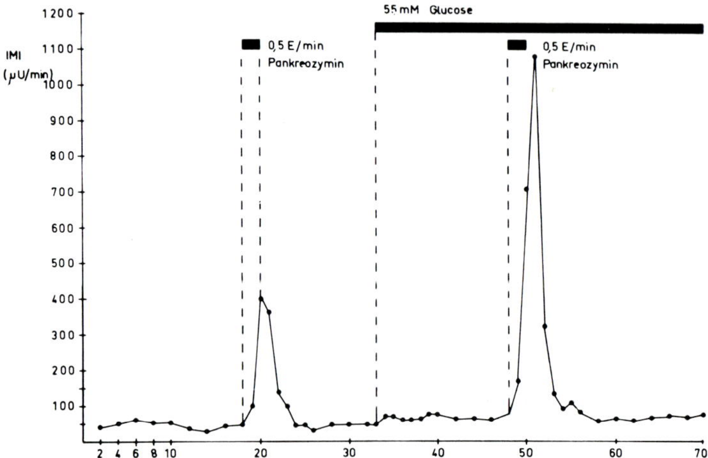

Fig. 13. The effect of pancreozymin (0.5 U/min) on the glucose independent and glucose (5.5 mM) induced insulin secretion of the isolated perfused pancreas of the rat ($n = 2$). (From: PFEIFFER, 1969)

Table 1. *Intestinal hormones influencing the in-vitro secretion of insulin*

Substance	Mode of Action	Species		Authors
Glucagon	+	IP	Dc	Candela et al. (1960)
	∅	IP	Rt	Coore and Randle (1964)
	(+)	IP	Rt	Turner and McIntyre (1966)
	+ (+)	CP	Rtf	Vecchio et al. (1966)
	+ (+)	IP	Rt	Devrim and Recant (1966)
	+ (+)	P	Rt	Grodsky and Bennett (1966)
	+	P	Rt	Sussman and Vaughan (1967)
	∅ (+)	II	Rt	Malaisse et al. (1967)
	∅ (+)	CP	Rtf	Lambert et al. (1967)
	+	IP	Rt	Milner and Hales (1967)
	+ (+)	IP	Rt	Hinz et al. (1969)
	∅	II	Rt	Buchanan et al. (1969)
	(+)	II	Rt	Montague and Taylor (1969)
	(+)	P	Rt	Curry (1970)
	(+)	II a P	Rt	Moody et al. (1970)
	∅ (+)	P	Dg	Iversen (1970)
	+ (+)	P	Rt	Basabe et al. (1971)
	(+)	CI	Rtf	Marliss et al. (1972)
	+ (+)	IT	SH	Sherman et al. (1971)
	+ (+)	II	Rt	Hinz et al. (1971)
	+ (+)	IP	Hf	Schaeffer et al. (1971)
Secretin	+	IP	Rt	Pfeiffer et al. (1965)
	+	IP	Rt	Telib et al. (1967)
	+	IP	Rt	Curtis et al. (1968)
	+	IP	Rb	Turner et al. (1968)
	∅	IP a I	Rtd	Guidoux-Grassi et al. (1968)
	(+)	II	Rt	Malaisse et al. (1968)
	∅	II	Rt	Lazarus et al. (1968)
	∅	II	Rt	Buchanan et al. (1969)
	+	P	Rt	Fussgänger et al. (1969)
	+	II	Rt	Meissner et al. (1969)
	+	IP	Rb	Turner (1970)
	∅	IP a I	Rt	Moody et al. (1970)
	(+)	P	Dg	Iversen (1972)
	+ (−)	P	Rt	Fussgänger et al. (1971)
	∅	II	Rt	Hinz et al. (1971)
		PI		
Pancreozymin	+	IP	Rt	Schröder et al. (1967)
	+	IP	Rt	Curtis et al. (1968)
	(+)	IP	Rb	Turner (1968)
	+ (+)	II	Rt	Malaisse et al. (1968)
	∅	II	Rt	Lazarus et al. (1968)
	∅	II	Rt	Buchanan et al. (1969)
	+	IP	Rb	Turner (1969)
	+ (+)	P	Rt	Fussgänger et al. (1969)
	+ (+)	II	Rt	Hinz et al. (1969)
	+ (+)	II	Rt	Meissner et al. (1969)
	+ (−)	II	Rt	Moody et al. (1970)
	+ (+)	P	Dg	Iversen (1972)
	+ (+)	II	Rt	Hinz et al. (1971)
		PI		
Gastrin	+	IP	Rb	Schröder et al. (1967)
	+	IP	R	Curtis et al. (1968)
	+ (−)	II	M	Lernmark and Hellman (1969)
	∅	II	Rt	Buchanan et al. (1969)
	+	II	Rt	Meissner et al. (1969)

Table 1. *(Continued)*

Substance	Mode of Action	Species		Authors
	∅	II	Rt	HINZ et al. (1969)
	∅	II	Rt	LAZARUS et al. (1968)
	+	P	Dg	IVERSEN (1972)
Serotonin	+	IP	Rb	TELIB et al. (1968)
	—	IP	H	FELDMANN et al. (1970)
	±	II	Rt	MALAISSE (1969)
Gut-extracts	+	IP	Dc	CANDELA et al. (1967)
	+ (+)	II	Rt	MALAISSE et al. (1968)
	+ (+)	IP	Rb	TURNER et al. (1970)
	(+)	II	Rt	MOODY et al. (1970)
A_1-cell extract	(—)	II	M	HELLMAN and LERNMARK (1969)

+ direct stimulation
— inhibition
(+) stimulation in combination with glucose, amino acids or sulfonylureas
(—) inhibition in combination with high glucose
∅ without effect
IT incubated tumor slices
IP incubated pieces
CP cultured pieces
P perfused
II incubated islets
PI perifused islets
CI cultured islet cell-monolayers
Dc duck
Rb rabbit
Rt rat
Rtf fetal rat
Hf fetal human
Dg dog
SH syrian hamster
Rtd duct ligated rat
M obese hyperglycemic mice
Mo monkeys
H hamster

Once again, slightly different although partially confirmative information was provided by examining the whole perfused rat pancreas with solutions containing the enteral hormones under consideration. If glucose is present in the perfusate the two- (GRODSKY et al., 1967) or rather, multi-compartmental release of insulin in response to the nutrient alone, should be noted.

As shown in Fig. 12 and in confirmation of the results obtained previously with pancreatic slices, secretin alone acts on that preparation containing both the exocrine and the endocrine pancreatic tissue to the extent that the following perfusion with 5.5 mM of glucose results in only minor insulin releases; later pulses of secretin are not potentiated by the presence of glucose in the perfusion medium. Again, and also confirming former observations with pieces of islets, pancreozymin stimulates the liberation of insulin from the isolated rat pancreas, but without glucose being more effective than secretin (Fig. 13), and, in addition, it is subject to potentiation by glucose. A similar increase in the action of glucose by glucagon and vice versa, was found when studying the isolated rat pancreas by GRODSKY et al. (1967).

Table 2. *Intestinal hormones influencing the in-vivo secretion of insulin as tested in experiments on animals*

Substance	Effects	Species	Authors
Glucagon	+	Dg	Campbell and Rastogi (1966)
	+	Dg	Léfèbvre and Luyckx (1966)
	+	Dg	Ketterer et al. (1967)
	+	Dg	Colwell et al. (1970)
Secretin	+	Dg	Dupré et al. (1966)
	+	Dg	Unger et al. (1966)
	+	Dg	Raptis et al. (1967)
	∅	Dg	Buchanan et al. (1968)
	+	Rt	Raptis et al. (1969)
	+/∅	Rt/Rtd	Goberna et al. (1971)
	+/∅	Mo/Rt	Glick et al. (1970)
	(−)	Dg	Chisholm (1971)
Pancreozymin	+	Dg	Unger et al. (1967)
	+	Dg	Meade et al. (1967)
	+	Dg	Buchanan et al. (1968)
	+	Rt	Raptis et al. (1969)
	+/+	Rt/Rtd	Goberna et al. (1971)
	+/+	Mo/Rt	Glick et al. (1970)
Gastrin	+	Dg	Unger et al. (1967)
	+	Dg	Kaneto et al. (1969)
Serotonin	∅	Dg	Raptis et al. (1967)
	+	Rt	Gagliardino et al. (1970)
Gut-extracts	+	Dg	Valverde et al. (1968)
	+	Rt	Fasel et al. (1970)
Caerulein	+	Dg/Rt	Erspamer (1971)

\+ stimulation
∅ without effect
Dg dog
Rt rat
Rtd rat duct ligated
Mo monkeys
(−) inhibition

Thus, many of the conflicting reports concerning the in vitro pharmacological studies on the pieces and in islets, as well as in the isolated pancreas (Table 1), were to be reconciled with ease when considering the different experimental conditions. A special subchapter in this review will be devoted to the role of glucose concentrations determining the stimulatory actions of some of the intestinal hormones upon both pancreatic insulin and glucagon secretion (see p. 289; subchapter VII).

Nevertheless, a number of similar, if not identical, observations were made, citing different actions, e.g. of pancreozymin and secretin, despite mutual stimulation of insulin secretion.

These findings already controvert ideas held elsewhere, that pharmaco-chemical effects *of* rather than physiological responses *to* the intestinal secretagogues have been demonstrated by the in vitro studies. It might well be that, in some cases,

Table 3. *Intestinal hormones influencing the insulin secretion in man*

Substance		Effects	Authors
Glucagon		+	Yalow et al. (1960)
		+	Weinges (1962) ***
		+	Dupré et al. (1966)
		+	Langs and Friedberg (1966)
	D	+	Melani et al. (1966/67)
		+ (+)	Samols et al. (1966)
		+	Karam et al. (1966)
		+	Lawrence (1966)
		+ (+)	Ryan et al. (1967)
	D	+	Simpson et al. (1966)
		+	Jarrett and Cohen (1967)
		+ (+)	Benedetti et al. (1968)
		+	Kaess et al. (1968)
	D	+	Weber et al. (1968)
	D	+	Kahil et al. (1970)
Secretin		+ (+)	Dupré et al. (1964/66)
		+	Dupré and Beck (1966) **
		+	Jarrett and Cohen (1967)
		(+) —	Bottermann et al. (1967)
		+ (+)	Boyns et al. (1967)
		+ (+)	Raptis et al. (1967)
		+	Dupré et al. (1968)
	D	+	Deckert (1968)
		—	Mahler and Weisberg (1968)
	D	+ (+)	Raptis et al. (1968)
		+ (+)	White and Dupré (1968)
		+	Chisholm et al. (1969)
		+ (+)	Dupré et al. (1969)
		+	Kaess et al. (1969)
	D	+ (+)	Raptis et al. (1969)
	D	+	Hindberg et al. (1970)
		+	Kahil et al. (1970)
		+	Kraegen et al. (1970)
		+	Lerner and Porte (1970)
Pancreozymin		—	Boyns et al. (1967)
		+	Mahler and Weisberg (1968)
		+ (+)	Schröder et al. (1968)
		+ (+)	Dupré et al. (1969)
	D	—	Schröder et al. (1969/70)
Gastrin		—	Jarrett and Cohen (1967)
		—	Pfeiffer and Raptis (1968)
		—	Kaes et al. (1968)
		— (+)	Dupré et al. (1969)
		+	Ohgawara et al. (1969)
		+	Rehfeld (1971)
Serotonin		—	Raptis (1967)
Duodenal extracts		+	Vanotti (1967)
		+	Dupré and Beck (1966)
		+	Fasel et al. (1970)
Caerulein		—	Falucca et al. (1969)

\+ stimulation
(+) stimulation in combination with glucose, amino acids, sulfonylureas
— without effect
** crude-secretin
*** ILA
D Diabetics

higher than physiological doses of the hormones were applied to the isolated cells, tissues and organs. However, the *synergistic* action of several hormones of intestinal origin must be considered (DUPRÉ, 1970) which might well simulate the activity of one hormone given in a higher than physiological dose.

A number of studies were performed, mainly in dogs, to examine insulin secretion *in vivo* in the pancreatic vein in response to different intestinal hormones (Table II). The results obtained were, in the majority of cases, in close agreement with those obtained from other experiments. The most interesting information to come to light was the extremely short interval which elapsed between injection of the insulin stimulating intestinal hormones, and the rise of insulin levels in serum or plasma as well as the transitory nature of the period when insulin levels were increased. Both phenomena may explain the negative observations reported by competent authors (BUCHANAN et al., 1968). Similarily, in human beings also, changes in insulin levels induced by injections of intestinal hormones, escaped notice (BOTTERMANN et al., 1967; BOYNS et al., 1967a, b). Other attempts to achieve insulin release in man in response to injections of intestinal hormones with or without the assistance of glucose, amino acids or sulfonylureas, are listed in Table III. Since more positive than negative results were obtained, it is probably correct to assume the accuracy of the former results.

Summing up, secretin, pancreozymin-cholecystokinin, gastrin, glucagon, serotonin and some mucosal extracts did display, partially in synergism with glucose or amino acids, insulin stimulating capacities in animals and in man.

V. Reaction of the Intestinal Hormones in Response to Ingestion of Food

Undoubtedly, a major step forward in solving the problem of intestinal control of food ingestion by influencing the exocrine *and* the endocrine portions of the pancreas, depends to a large extent upon the development of reliable methods for measuring these hormones in body fluids. A wealth of information regarding intestinal influence upon islet function was provided by the use of radioimmunoassay for insulin. The development of a new radioimmunoassay for glucagon might be regarded as another step forward in this direction.

It was therefore concluded that this glucagon was the *so-called* enteroglucagon which differed from pancreatic glucagon and which showed particular immunological and physical properties (EISENTRAUT et al., 1968). Thus, HEDING (1971) was able to demonstrate in a recent publication, using a differentiating antibody system, that enteroglucagon increases in the blood after an oral glucose load of 1.75 g per kg of body weight.

Confirming the original belief of SAMOLS et al. (1965) as well as of LAWRENCE (1966), UNGER et al. (1968) demonstrated that, in dogs, intraduodenal application of glucose, but not the i.v. injection, resulted in an increase of glucagon-like-immunoreactivity (GLI) in the caval vein (Fig. 14). Moreover, following intraduodenal glucose infusion, rises in GLI were recorded much earlier in the mesenteric vein than in the caval or pancreatico-duodenal vein (Fig. 14). Hence, another glucagon of intestinal origin, with specific response to the application of enteric glucose, had to be taken into consideration.

This rather unusual observation was supported by the anatomical, ultrastructural, bio-histo-and immunochemical demonstration showing the distribution of an immunoreactive GLA over the upper gastrointestinal tract. This theory had to be accepted when Samols and Marks (1967) recorded increases in plasma-GLI in response to intrajejunal glucose infusion in a totally pancreatectomized human subject (Fig. 15). Eventually, by means of specific antibodies differentiating between pancreatic and extrapancreatic glucagon, Heding (1968) found only

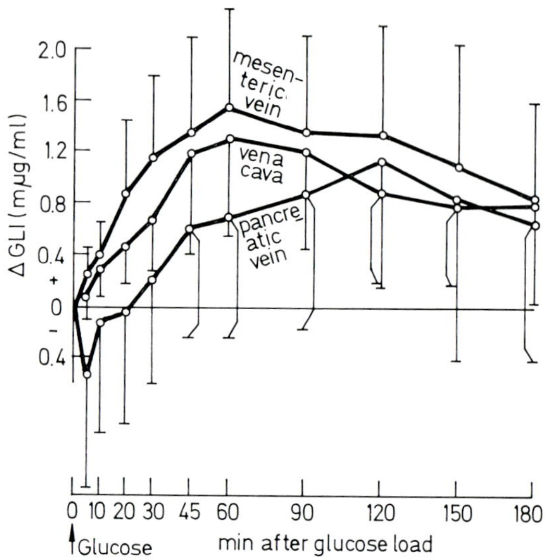

Fig. 14. Mean increments and standard deviations of glucagon-like immunoreactivity in the mesenteric vein, vena cava, and pancreaticoduodenal vein after intraduodenal glucose administration of 2 g/kg in a group of 12 dogs. (From: Unger et al., 1968)

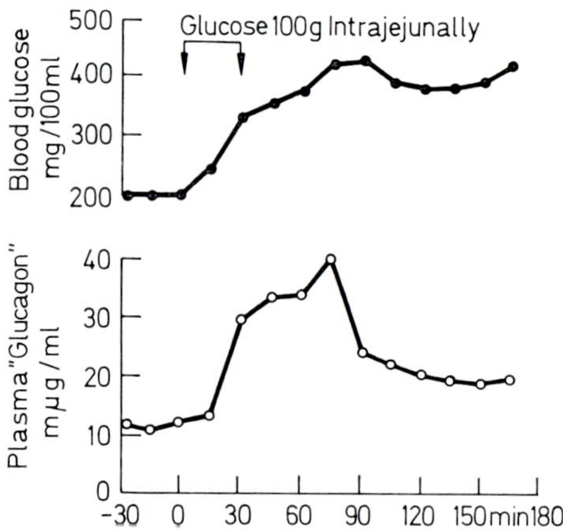

Fig. 15. Changes in blood glucose and immunoreactive glucagon in a totally pancreatectomised subject after the intrajenunal infusion of 100 g glucose. 36 hours after his usual injection of 40 U lente insulin. (From: Samols and Marks, 1967)

intestinal glucagon increases following oral glucose loads, and no changes in the levels of pancreatic glucagon.

It is assumed that this hormone is liberated during glucose absorption; consequently, it was called enteroglucagon (Samols et al., 1965; Samols et al., 1966).

Its insulin stimulating activity seems to be similar to that of pancreatic glucagon. Enteroglucagon activated insulin secretion in isolated islets and in in-vivo experiments (MOODY et al., 1970). Enteroglucagon, together with the other intestinal hormones, seems to be responsible for the difference in insulin secretion after an oral and an intravenous glucose load (UNGER and EISENTRAUT, 1967; PFEIFFER and RAPTIS, 1968).

REHFELD and HEDING (1970) recently demonstrated a highly increased level of enteroglucagon in blood following the administration of 100 g of glucose to a patient who experienced repeated hypoglycemic spells three to five hours after the ingestion of a heavy meal. This increase in enteroglucagon was observed prior to the increase in plasma insulin and lasted for about 30 minutes. The pancreatic glucagon fell below baseline after the glucose load.

Like the gastrointestinal hormones, caerulein also influences the endocrine function of the pancreas. In the dog, it stimulates insulin and glucagon secretion

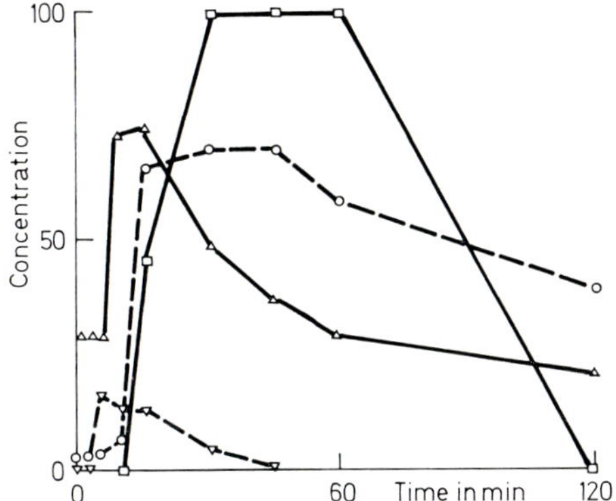

Fig. 16. Secretin, insulin, and pancreozymin levels after a 200 g glucose load showing positive responses in serum-I.R.G. □ = Pancreozymin (ng. per ml). △ = I.R.G. (ng. per ml). ○ = Insulin (microunits per ml). ▽ = Secretin (ng. per ml). (From: YOUNG et al., 1968)

(BERTACCINI et al., 1970). Contrary to expectations, caerulein neither increased insulin levels nor caused the glucose effect in metabolically normal human subjects to be increased (FALLUCA et al., 1969; GNUDI et al., 1970). In patients with islet cell tumors, however, caerulein caused a significant rise in plasma insulin, so that FALLUCA et al (1971) considered the intravenous injection of caerulein as a specific supplement to the diagnosis of insulinoma. The intravenous injection of caerulein performed on rats or dogs resulted in a significant increase of plasma insulin and increased the effect of glucose (GNUDI et al., 1970).

BERTACCINI et al. (1970) recently observed an increase in the secretion of insulin, of up to 250% of the base-line level, within 10 minutes after administering an intravenous injection of caerulein in dogs. Repeated injections of caerulein at short intervals brought about, on each occasion, a further increase in immunologically measurable insulin (IMI). It is therefore assumed that caerulein stimulates not only the secretion but also the synthesis of insulin. Moreover, caerulein also induces an elevation of glucagon levels in the blood of the pancreatico-duodenal vein of the dog (BERTACCINI et al., 1970).

Meanwhile, a gifted young biochemist, JOHN YOUNG, from Sidney/Australia, together with his colleagues, CHISHOLM et al. (1968a, b; 1969) overcame the difficulties which, for a long time, prevented the isotope labelling of the tyrosine-lacking secretin, and also suggested a technique for measuring pancreozymin by radioimmunoassay. By a tragic coincidence, JOHN YOUNG died very recently. However, one of the most brilliant contributions which he left us, demonstrated the successive increases in plasma of three intestinal hormones (secretin, pancreozymin and glucagon) in response to a 200 g oral glucose load (Fig. 16). Following smaller amounts of glucose taken orally, or after glucose and hydrochloric acid administered intraduodenally, secretin always increased in blood, not only before the other entero-hormones, but also before oral glucose had entered the upper intestinal tract. Since injection of pentagastrin also stimulated secretin secretion, a chain of reactions of the following order was postulated by the Australian

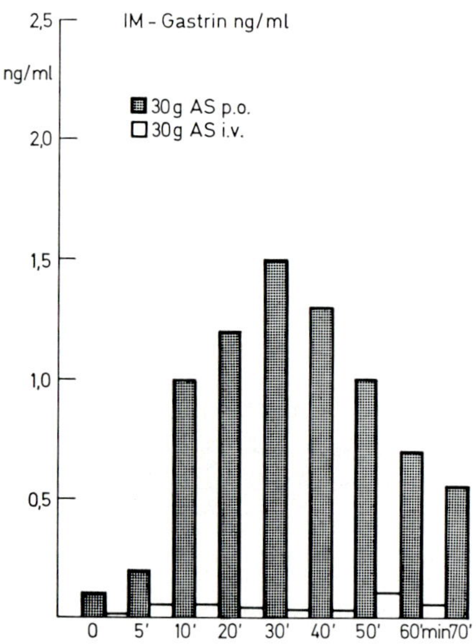

Fig. 17. Radioimmunologically measurable gastrin in human plasma after oral or intravenous administration of 30 g of amino acids. (From: RAPTIS et al., 1971)

investigators: glucose contacting the gastric mucosa cells — liberation of gastrin resulting in a stimulation of the release of secretin — release of insulin. As it happens, evidence for gastrin release of the antrum cells following glucose and alcohol ingestion were provided by the electron microscope (FORSSMANN et al., 1968), while RAPTIS et al. (1971) following amino acid application, measured serum gastrin increases in response to oral administration alone, and not to i.v. injection (Fig. 17). Here again, contact of nutrients as such, and not just of glucose with the upper intestinal tract, might be regarded as indispensable for eliciting the intestino-insular mechanism.

Needless to say, the reaction of the intestinal hormones in response to ingestion of food, and in relation to the subsequent changes in the blood concentrations of the islet hormones, will be the main subjects for research in the near future.

After intestinal absorption, amino acids stimulate glucagon secretion from the pancreatic alpha-cells, either directly or via pancreozymin.

VI. Chemical Configuration and Endocrine Action of the Intestinal Hormones. The Role of the Exocrine Pancreas in the Regulation of Islet Function by Intestinal Hormones

Attempts to correlate the endocrine effects of the intestinal hormones with their chemical configuration, and to study some of these actions, under pathological conditions, represent another important aspect of the matter. As shown previously by examination of the isolated pancreas, secretin effects rapid release of insulin but, without glucose in the perfusate, its action not being potentiated by

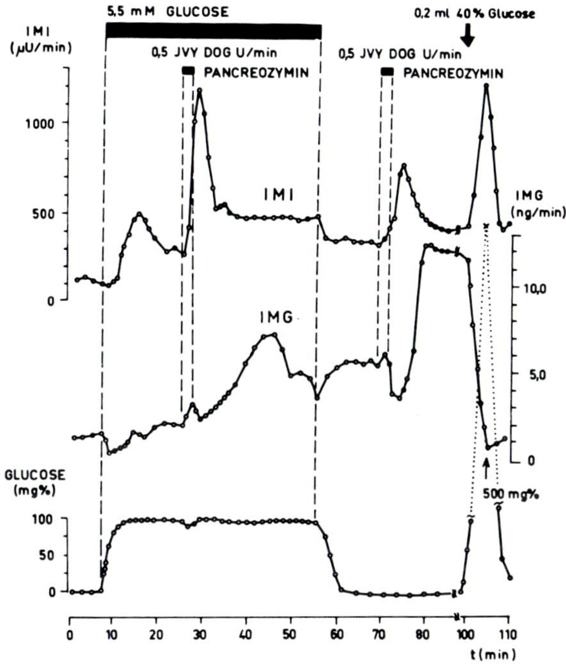

Fig. 18. Release of insulin (IMI) and glucagon (IMG) from the isolated perfused rat pancreas induced by pancreozymin. (From: FUSSGÄNGER et al., 1969)

the addition of glucose. Pancreozymin, on the other hand, was also effective with or without glucose in the perfusate, but was strikingly potentiated when glucose was present in the medium. Moreover, whereas secretin had been completely ineffective in stimulating *pancreatic glucagon* secretion, pancreozymin did induce glucagon secretion (Fig. 18) (FUSSGÄNGER et al., 1969). However, unlike the effects shown by studies performed in dogs (UNGER et al., 1967), pancreozymin always stimulated the liberation of glucagon *after* the insulin secretion. It should be noted that both the insulin and the glucagon responses are inversely influenced by the concentration of glucose in the medium.

As mentioned previously, progress in chemistry of protein hormones has permitted the further examination of synthetic fragments of the natural hormones with respect to their insulin and/or glucagon stimulating capacities. The C-terminal portion of pancreozymin and, of course, the synthetic octapeptide of pancreozymin share 5 amino acids of the C-terminal with human gastrin I and, as is self-evident, with the gastrin-pentapeptide (provided by ICI) and the decapeptide caerulein.

Significant increases in the secretion of insulin are effected, in the presence or absence of glucose, by the gastrin-pentapeptide, although no potentiating action

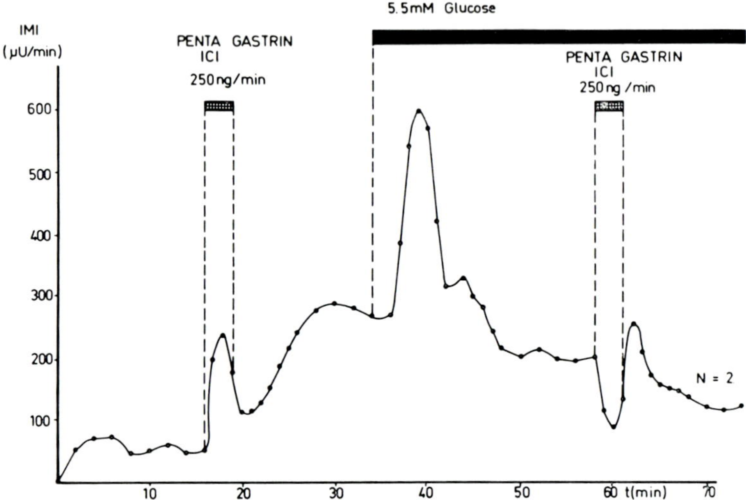

Fig. 19. Release of insulin (IMI) from the isolated perfused rat pancreas induced by pentagastrin ICI (250 ng/min) without and with glucose (5.5 mM). (From: Pfeiffer et al., 1971; Fussgänger et al., 1972)

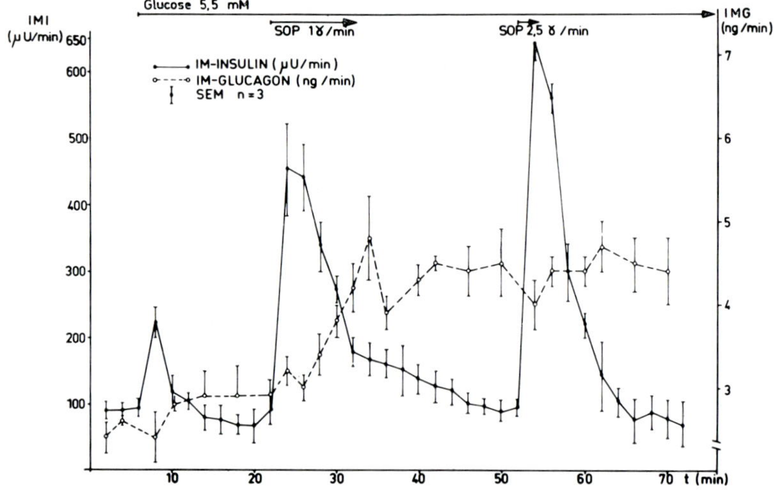

Fig. 20. Release of insulin (IMI) and glucagon (IMG) from the isolated perfused rat pancreas induced by synthetic octapeptide of pancreozymin (SOP) (0.34 and $0.85 \cdot 10^{-6}$ M) with glucose (5.5 mM). (From: Pfeiffer et al., 1971; Fussgänger et al., 1972)

should be attributed to the gastrin-glucose combination (FUSSGÄNGER et al., 1972) (Fig. 19). On the other hand, the pancreozymin-octapeptide demonstrates the same potentiation of the glucose-induced insulin secretion as the natural hormone; again glucagon rises *after* insulin in the perfusate (FUSSGÄNGER et al., 1972) (Fig. 20).

Glucagon and secretin also show structural similarities; they have 14 amino acids in common (Fig. 5). They both share the advantage of being able to promote the release of insulin from the pancreas of human diabetics otherwise not responsive to either glucose and/or tolbutamide (MELANI et al., 1967; RAPTIS et al., 1968;

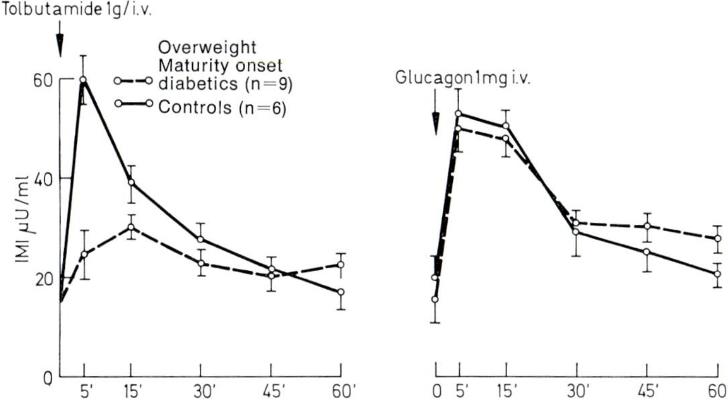

Fig. 21. Immunologically measurable insulin (IMI) in metabolically normal subjects ($n = 6$) and obese adult-onset diabetics ($n = 9$) after intravenous injection of tolbutamide and glucagon. (From: MELANI et al., 1967/68).

DECKERT, 1968) (Figs. 21; 22). Pancreozymin, on the other hand, is quite ineffective in diabetics (SCHRÖDER et al., 1970) (Fig. 23).

In the diabetic pancreas, the intestinal hormones secretin and glucagon had a marked effect on the impaired endocrine portion of the gland in the case of intact surrounding exocrine tissue. What is the effect of intestinal hormones on the intact endocrine portion in case of impaired function of the exocrine part of the gland? This will be our next subject for discussion.

Thus, in non-diabetics with clinical evidence of chronic insufficiency of the exocrine pancreas due to chronic pancreatitis, during the usual secretin — (2 Units/kg body weight) and pancreozymin — (CCK-PZ 1 Unit/kg body weight)

Table 4. *Changes in the volume, bicarbonate content, and enzyme content (amylase, trypsin and lipase) of pancreatic fluid following injection of secretin and pancreozymin respectively, in 30 normal human subjects and in 13 patients suffering from chronic pancreatic insufficiency (Mean ± SEM).* (From: RAPTIS et al., 1971)

60 min after 2 U/kg B.W. secretin i.v.

	$n = 30$ Controls	$n = 13$ Pancreat. ins.
Bicarbonate m Eq	26.4 ± 2.7	9.2 ± 2.1
Volume ml/kg	4.9 ± 0.9	2.7 ± 1.0

10 min after 1 U/kg CCK-PZ i.v.

	$n = 30$ Controls	$n = 13$ Pancreat. ins.
Amylase SE	65000 ± 6400	10000 ± 6700
Trypsin mU	42000 ± 3140	8400 ± 1680
Lipase m Eq	459 ± 30,2	151,7 ± 31,2

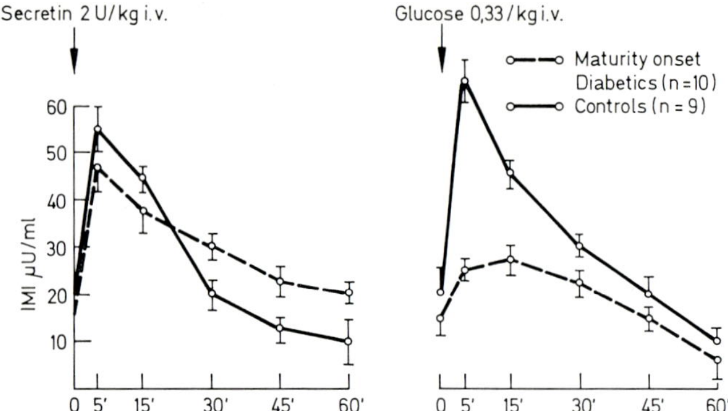

Fig. 22. The effect of secretin (2 U/kg i.v.) and of glucose (0.33 g/kg i.v.) on serum insulin levels (IMI) of metabolically normal subjects ($n = 9$) and adult-onset diabetics with normal body weight ($n = 10$). (From: Raptis et al., 1968; Pfeiffer and Raptis, 1970)

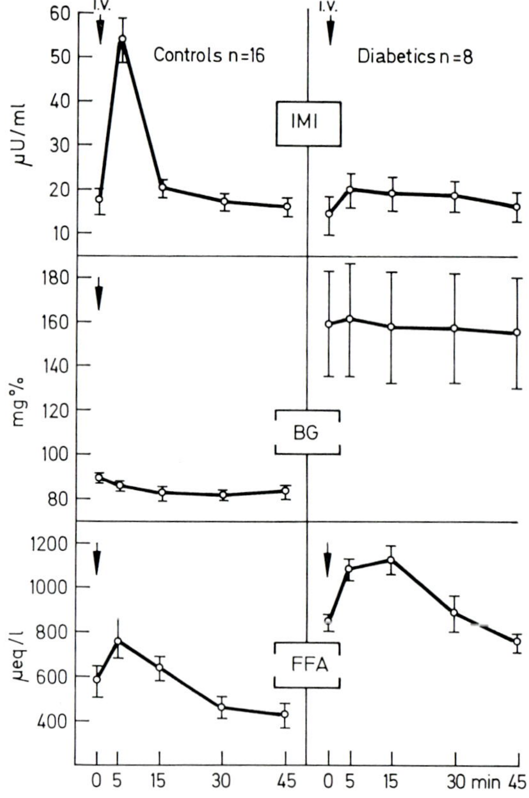

Fig. 23. Changes of immunologically measurable insulin (IMI), blood glucose (BG) and free fatty acids (FFA) after intravenous injection of pancreozymin (CCK-PZ "Vitrum", 2 U/kg) in metabolically normal subjects and adult-onset diabetics. (From: Schröder et al., 1970)

response tests for examining volume, bicarbonate and enzyme production of the exocrine pancreas, blood was also provided for determination of blood glucose and immunologically measurable insulin (IMI) (RAPTIS et al., 1970; RAPTIS et al., 1971).

Significant differences were established between the responses of controls and patients, with respect to the parameters of pancreatic exocrine function (Table 4). Fig. 24 shows the insulin responses of 11 of these patients and of the 30 normal controls to secretin and pancreozymin, respectively. The brief but strikingly significant increases in the plasma insulin initiated by the intestinal hormones in

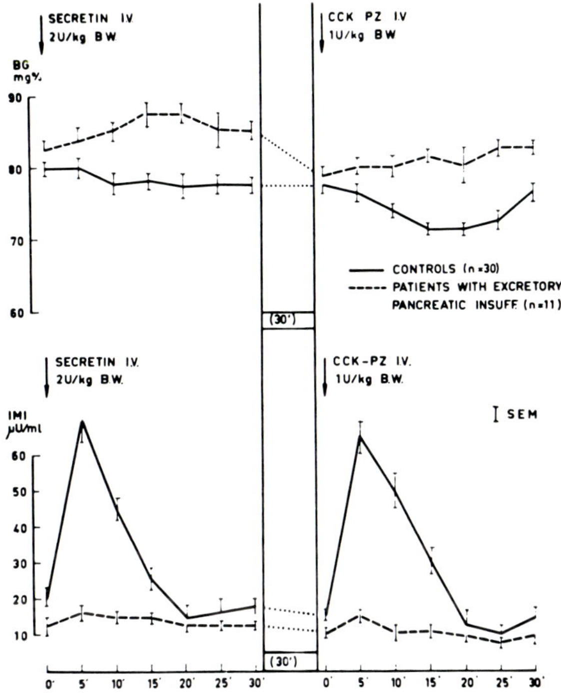

Fig. 24. Blood glucose (BG) and immunologically measurable insulin (IMI) following i.v. injection of secretin and pancreozymin (CCK-PZ) in plasma of patients suffering from excretory pancreatic insufficiency ($n = 11$) and in normal controls ($n = 30$) (Mean $\pm$ SEM). (From: RAPTIS et al., 1971)

the normal subjects were completely absent in the patients. When the same patients were subjected to oral and i.v. glucose tolerance tests, the much higher increases in blood insulin, normally observed following oral glucose administration as opposed to i.v. glucose administration, were lacking in this case; on the other hand, the increase of insulin in blood following the administration of glucose i.v. rose to levels comparable with those noted in the controls; in both the patients and the controls, identical rates of glucose disappearance were noted (Fig. 25).

Similarily, in patients suffering from *cystic fibrosis* of the pancreas, with intact "glucose tolerance", the insulin responses to oral and i.v. glucose loads, respectively, amounted to the same levels (HANDWERGER et al., 1969). On the other hand, DECKERT and WORNING (1970) measured little or no rise in the serum insulin following secretin, in patients suffering from severe pancreatic exocrine insufficiency.

From these findings it was inferred that the insulin stimulating action of the intestinal hormones is abolished when normal exocrine pancreatic tissue is absent, i.e. that the exocrine pancreatic tissue is essential for insulin stimulating action of the intestinal hormones. Moreover, since the specific effect of oral glucose, when compared to i.v. glucose administration, with respect to insulin secretion, had disappeared in the same patients, it seems likely that, in man, secretin and/or pancreozymin are involved in the mechanisms mediating gastrointestinal regulation of insulin liberation.

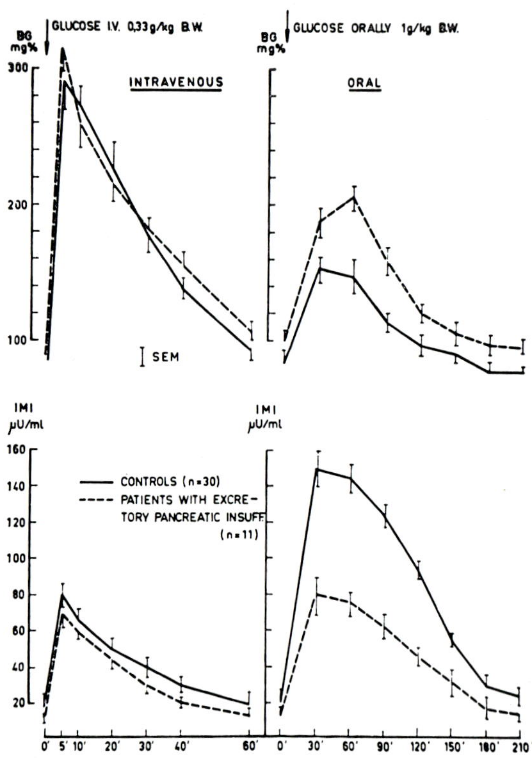

Fig. 25. Blood glucose (BG) and blood insulin (IMI) concentrations in patients with excretory pancreatic insufficiency ($n = 11$) and in normal controls ($n = 30$) (Mean $\pm$ SEM) following i.v. and oral glucose loads. (From: RAPTIS et al., 1971)

These conclusions were partially supported, as mentioned before in subchapter IV of this paper, by experiments performed on rat islets in vitro (GUIDOUX-GRASSI and FELBER, 1969; HINZ et al., 1970, 1971). In the in vivo laboratory studies (GOBERNA et al., 1970; GOBERNA et al., 1971), exocrine insufficiency was established by ligation of the two main ducts of the pancreas and the 6—8 accessory ducts merging into the common bile duct. Six weeks later involution of the ligated pancreas corresponded to about 80% loss of the original weight of the gland (Fig. 26). In spite of this remarkable diminution of exocrine tissue, the insulin responses to glucose were unaffected in the ligated rats, as compared to the controls; pancreozymin also elicited rises in insulin and slight but significant falls in glucose in both the ligated animals and the controls (Fig. 27). On the other

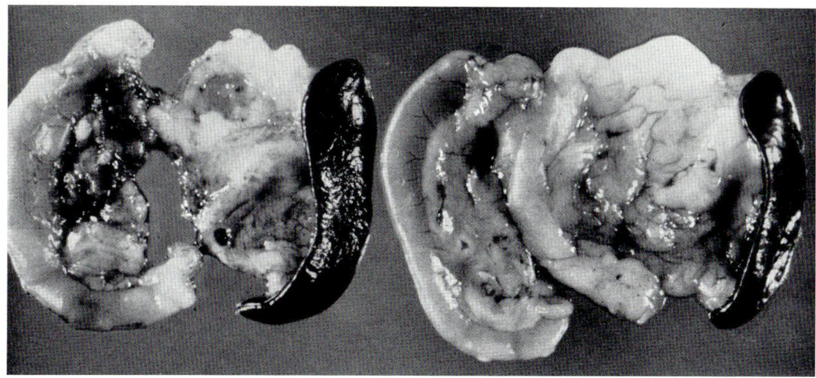

Fig. 26. Pancreas of rat before (right part of Fig.) and 6 weeks after (left part of Fig.) ligation of ductuli pancreatici. (From: GOBERNA et al., (1971)

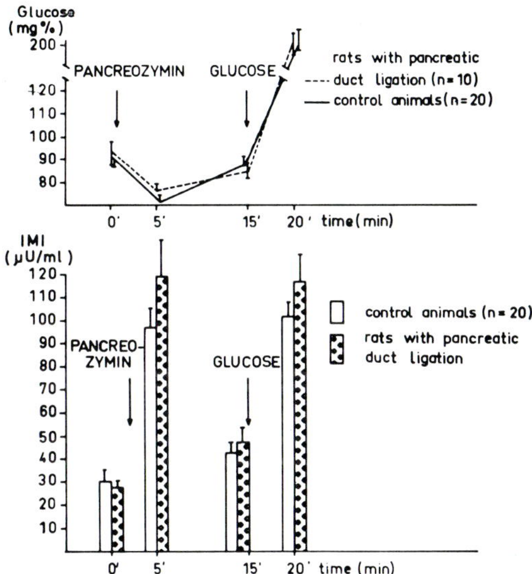

Fig. 27. Effect of i.v. injection of pancreozymin and glucose on blood glucose and insulin release in rats with ligated pancreatic duct ($n = 10$) and in control animals ($n = 20$). (From: GOBERNA et al., 1971)

hand, in the animals with experimentally induced atrophy of the pancreas, insulin responses to secretin were absent, while glucose injected 15 min. after the hormone was still effective (Fig. 28).

Hence, it seems likely that, in rats, secretin acts on the β-cells partially via the exocrine tissue of the pancreas (as originally suggested by GUIDOUX-GRASSI and FELBER (1969), while pancreozymin affects insulin release independently of the exocrine cells. Also the isolated islets of Langerhans, completely stripped of all exocrine tissue, did not respond to secretin, gastrin and glucagon, but only to pancreozymin. Hence, the singularly positive action of pancreozymin on insulin release of the rat islets adds another specific feature to the differences between the biological actions of pancreozymin and secretin on the pancreas: the different influences on the exocrine pancreatic function (WANG and GROSSMANN, 1951), the stimulation of glucagon release from the dog and the rat pancreas (UNGER et al., 1967; FUSSGÄNGER et al., 1969; GOBERNA et al., 1970), and the potentiation of glucose induced insulin liberation from the isolated perfused rat pancreas confined to pancreozymin (FUSSGÄNGER et al., 1969, 1971; HINZ et al., 1970).

Consequently, classification of the insulin releasing actions of the intestinal hormones, according to whether or not they are dependent on the presence of intact exocrine pancreatic tissue has, so far, only been possible with regard to the rat pancreas. In human subjects, suffering from chronic insufficiency of the

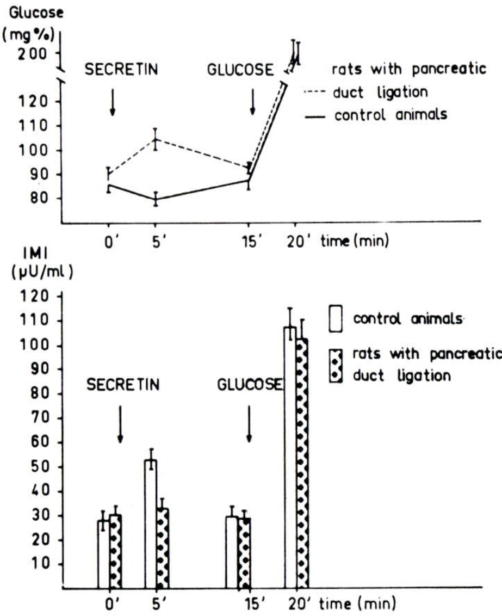

Fig. 28. Effect of i.v. injection of secretin and glucose on blood glucose and insulin release in rats with ligated pancreatic duct ($n = 18$) and in control animals ($n = 19$). (From: GOBERNA et al., 1971)

pancreas, even pancreozymin was ineffective. However, in human patients, the experimental animals and the isolated islets, all three examples of islets, not surrounded or supported by normal exocrine tissue, normal insulin responses to glucose were found. This means that the hypothetical "Glucose Receptor" of the β-cell or its surface works more or less independently of both the exocrine pancreatic tissue and the intestinal hormones. Diabetes is certainly not the primary sequence ensuing from the deterioration of either the gastrointestinal influences on insulin secretion or the alteration of the exocrine portion of the pancreas.

On the other hand, the also hypothetical "Entero-Receptor" of the β-cell, responding to the insulin releasing action of intestinal hormones as secretin and pancreozymin in man, and gastrin, secretin and glucagon in rats, is probably entirely dependent upon sufficient amounts of exocrine pancreatic tissue. It may be that the receptor is limited in its action on exocrine cells which might mediate gastrointestinal control of insulin secretion by special, not yet established intrapancreatic exocrine-endocrine channels.

VII. Reestablishment of the Primary Role of Non-Physiological Glucose Levels in Regulating Insulin and Glucagon Secretion, Irrespective of Cholecystokinin-Pancreozymin and Secretin Action

Involvement of gastrointestinal hormones in the regulation of glucose homeostasis has to be considered in relation to several features previously shown to occur in some in vivo and in vitro experiments, concerning the release of insulin and glucagon from the pancreas of laboratory animals.

1. It has been demonstrated that glucose is one of the major factors regulating insulin secretion and glucagon release.
2. The extent of the response of insulin and glucagon is altered by gastrointestinal hormones, liberated into the circulation following oral ingestion of food, i.e. glucose.
3. Blood glucose in turn limits the effectiveness of certain gastrointestinal hormones, i.e. cholecystokinin-pancreozymin and secretin.
4. On account of the immediate vicinity of glucagon producing α_2-cells and insulin secreting β-cells within the islets of Langerhans, a mutual interaction of both hormones should be taken into consideration.

An integral role in the regulation of insulin and glucagon secretion is exerted by glucose. Whereas increasing glucose concentrations stimulate insulin secretion, as has been demonstrated in detail by several groups, i.e. GRODSKY et al. (1967), GRODSKY et al. (1970) and MALAISSE (1969), glucagon is suppressed (UNGER et al. (1968), OHNEDA et al. (1969), VANCE et al. (1968), BUCHANAN et al. (1969b), CHESNEY and SCHOFIELD (1969), FUSSGÄNGER et al. (1969), IVERSEN (1971)). On the other hand, it is well established that hypoglycemia is one of the main signals for glucagon secretion, whether induced by fasting, (UNGER et al. (1963), LAWRENCE (1966), ASSAN et al. (1966), AGUILAR-PARADA et al. (1969a)), insulin treatment, (UNGER et al. (1962), OHNEDA et al. (1969), BUCHANAN et al. (1969)), sulfonylureas, (AGUILAR-PARADA et al. (1969b)), or inhibition of glucose metabolism by constant treatment with phlorizin (UNGER et al. (1962)).

Since variations in the actual glucose concentration, occurring naturally in vivo, are of little consequence, the importance of glucose in regulating glucagon secretion has been questioned by VANCE et al. (1968), and according to in vitro experiments with guinea-pig islets, by EDWARDS et al. (1970). LUYCKX and LÉFÈBVRE (1969) instead suggested the importance of free fatty acids (FFA) and their ability to inhibit glucagon secretion in dogs, as well as in rats (LUYCKX et al., 1971). EDWARDS et al. (1969) also produced evidence supporting the primary role of FFA in regulating glucagon secretion. Moreover, MÜLLER et al. (1971a) clearly demonstrated the occurrence of an alanine-glucose-shuttle as being involved in the regulation of glucagon secretion.

Nevertheless, glucagon secretion, in response to different glucose concentrations, is well documented by in vitro experiments with rats as performed by FUSSGÄNGER et al. (1971). Fig. 29 indicates dose-response relationship of glucose at various concentrations and the mean secretion rates of insulin and glucagon in the isolated perfused rat pancreas.

Be this as it may, glucose seems to regulate both hormones much more efficiently by the oral route of application: it stimulates insulin secretion and suppresses glucagon secretion (SANTEUSIANO et al., 1971). The possible implication that gastrointestinal hormones increase the secretion of insulin (PFEIFFER and RAPTIS, 1968; MARKS and SAMOLS, 1970) induced by glucose, has been confirmed previously by the cavo-portal-shunt experiments in rats, of ASSAL et al. (1971) and, similarily, with the combined isolated perfused rat intestine together with the pancreas by PENHOS et al. (1969).

In contrast, significance of the intestinal modulation of insulin secretion initiated by oral glucose in dogs, has been questioned by SELTZER and McNEFF (1967) and UNGER et al. (1968). Increase in the secretion of insulin by combined stimulation with glucose and pancreozymin has, however, been reported in dogs

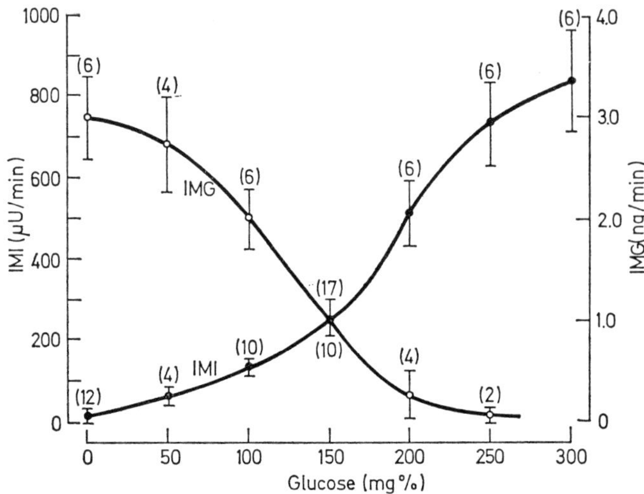

Fig. 29. Dose response relationship between glucose and the mean secretion rate of insulin (IMI) and glucagon (IMG) of the isolated perfused rat pancreas. (From: FUSSGÄNGER et al., 1971)

by MEADE et al. (1967) and in vitro withthe isolated perfused rat pancreas by FUSSGÄNGER et al. (1969).

By using a similar mechanism, it has been suggested that glucagon suppression is greatly increased by secretin (SANTEUSIANO et al., 1971) in dogs. The effect of various concentrations of glucose and secretin on glucagon secretion has been studied in perfusion experiments with rat pancreas, but here, secretin was at variance with that of dogs and showed differences whether administered with or without glucose. Whereas inhibition of the rise in glucagon due to the abundance of glucose was observed, in combination with glucose, 5.5 mM. secretin actually stimulated glucagon secretion (FUSSGÄNGER 1972) (Fig. 30). Moreover, cholecystokinin-pancreozymin (CCK-PZ) is distinguished by its ability to stimulate both insulin and glucagon secretion (UNGER et al., 1967). Similar results have been obtained by IVERSEN (1972) in vitro with the isolated perfused dog pancreas. An identical increase of both hormones, within seconds, has been demonstrated. With the isolated perfused rat pancreas (FUSSGÄNGER et al., 1969), there was instantaneous response of insulin, but a delayed secretion of glucagon following CCK-PZ.

Glucose modifies this response significantly; Fig. 31 indicates the range within which CCK-PZ will potentiate glucose induced insulin secretion. Comparing the

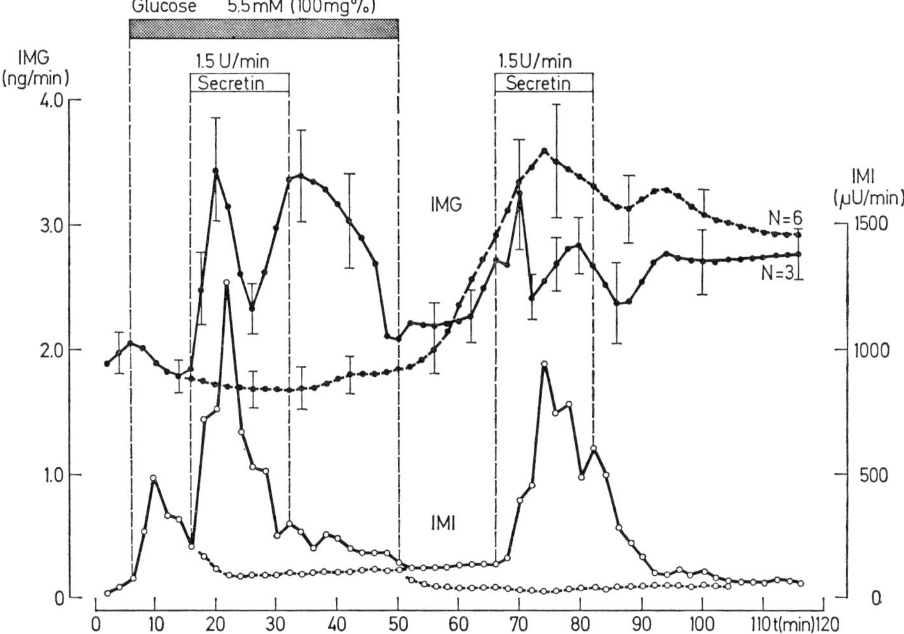

Fig. 30. Secretion of insulin (IMI) and glucagon (IMG) in response to secretin at 5.5 mM glucose and without glucose of the isolated perfused rat pancreas ($n = 6$); o—o IMI (Secretin), o—o IMI (Controls), •—• IMG (Secretin), •—• IMG (Controls) (From: Fussgänger et al.; 1972)

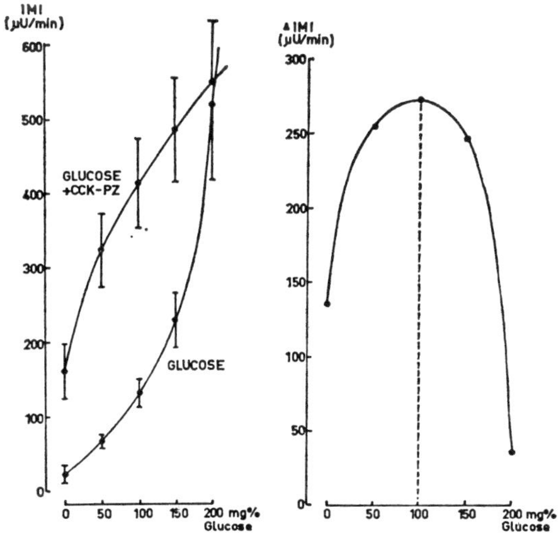

Fig. 31. Dose response relationship between glucose and glucose together with cholecystokinin and the mean insulin secretion rate of the perfused rat pancreas (left part of the Fig.). Mean increase of insulin secretion of the isolated perfused rat pancreas following cholecystokinin at different concentrations of glucose (right part of the Fig.). (From: Fussgänger et al., 1971)

effect of glucose at various concentrations with the combined effect of glucose together with CCK-PZ, we observed an increased response of insulin well within the range of physiological glucose levels of 5.5 mM (100 mg-%) (FUSSGÄNGER et al., 1972). On the other hand, secretin did not potentiate glucose induced insulin secretion in experiments similar to those conducted with CCK-PZ. Only short-lived responses of similar extent, whether administered with or without glucose, have been observed (Fig. 30). Moreover, at high glucose concentrations, 11 mM (200 mg-%) there was evidence of an inhibition of glucose induced insulin secretion (Fig. 32) (FUSSGÄNGER et al, 1971), which is in accordance with experiments in dogs (CHISHOLM, 1971) but at variance with those in man (CHISHOLM et al.,

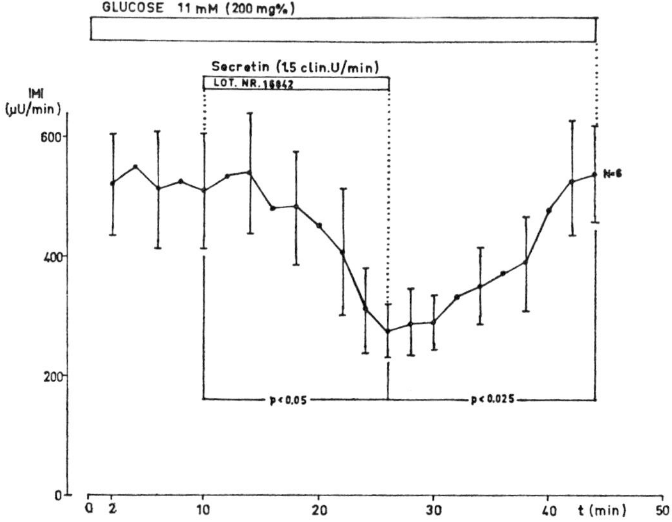

Fig. 32. Inhibition of the glucose induced insulin secretion of the isolated perfused rat pancreas by secretin (From: FUSSGÄNGER et al.; 1971)

1969; KRAEGEN et al., 1970), where inhibitory effects of secretin on insulin secretion have never been observed.

It is interesting to note, at this point, that secretin induced insulin response in vivo is not accompanied by a subsequent fall of glucose in blood, either in rats, dogs or man. CCK-PZ, in contrast, affects glucose levels quite differently in dogs and rats. Hence, consistent with the observed similar response of glucagon and insulin, it increases the blood glucose in dogs, but decreases the blood glucose in rats, where glucagon will rise within a certain interval following stimulation with CCK-PZ. CCK was demonstrated as having hypoglycemic effects even in totally pancreatectomized rats (RAPTIS et al., 1969). Further studies are necessary to evaluate whether this observation was due to an insulin secretion of intestinal origin, as has been shown to occur in the duodenum of rats by HÅKANSON and LUNDQUIST (1971) or whether it is the result of a direct hypoglycemic action of CCK-PZ.

On account of some in vitro experiments with isolated islets, the significance of the well known gastrointestinal hormones secretin and pancreozymin as the specific enteral messengers has been questioned by MALAISSE and MALAISSE-LAGAE (1968), TURNER (1970) and MOODY et al. (1970) in favor of an intestinal factor of duodeno-jejunal origin (DJE) (TURNER, 1970) or of jejunal-ileal origin (TOT) (MOODY, 1970) increasing glucose induced insulin release more effectively. The original suggestion by UNGER et al. (1968) and VALVERDE et al. (1970) that glucagon-like immunological activity of enteral origin (GLI), later called enteroglucagon, liberated in response to oral glucose (UNGER et al., 1961; HANSON et al., 1967; BUCHANAN et al., 1967; VALVERDE et *al.*, 1968; LUYCKX and LÉFÈBVRE, 1969) might share the ability of insulin stimulating activity with the well known effects of glucagon of pancreatic origin (CURRY, 1970), has nevertheless been disproved by MARCO et al. (1970, 1971) and MARCO et al. (1972). Yet the insulin stimulating activity isolated by MOODY et al. (1970) exhibits properties which could, in fact, be an alternative with glucose potentiating properties. However, significant stimulation of insulin secretion, tested with isolated rat islets, in combination with glucose, has not been observed unless glucose concentrations have been raised to 8.3 mM (150 mg-%) or even higher. Unfortunately, all further purifications of their TOT fraction II were evaluated at very high glucose concentrations of 16.5 mM (300 mg-%). Certainly, such levels will never occur in the postprandial phase of ingestion under normal conditions. We wish, once again, to draw particular attention to the differences observed with combined stimulation of glucose and gastrointestinal hormones: glucagon will increase insulin secretion all over the range of various glucose concentrations, the same applies to the GI-factor tested by MALAISSE and MALAISSE-LAGAE (1968); secretin does not potentiate at any concentration, TOT displays significant effects at moderately increased and high glucose levels, but pancreozymin remains close to the physiological range of fasting glucose levels. A significant conclusion might be contained in this fact if one tentatively speculates on the necessity of spot-insulin in the absorptive phase of ingestion when circulating glucose levels are still low or, depending on the nature of nutrient absorbed, may not rise at all.

As has been outlined above, glucose concentrations of more than 200 mg-% are of crucial significance since secretin and cholecystokinin-pancreozymin, at this concentration, might act in an inhibitory rather than in a stimulatory fashion on insulin secretion.

Concerning studies in vitro, especially with isolated islets, there is one other problem which it is necessary to consider when carrying out those studies. Since glucagon is known to affect glucose induced insulin release in a positive manner and is, itself, stimulated by gastrointestinal hormones, i.e. pancreozymin, any conditions which might undermine appropriate glucagon secretion, might give unsatisfactory results, provided that endogenous glucagon, on account of its proximity to the β-cell, stimulates insulin secretion as suggested by SAMOLS et al. (1966). The presence of specific glucagon receptors, aline β-cell membranes, has been demonstrated previously by GOLDFINE et al. (1972), bringing glucagon effects, or at least stimulation of the membrane bound "messenger enzyme" adenyl cyclase, well within the range of physiological glucagon levels, 10^{-10} M. Damage of the outer islet cell core, which in the rat comprises mostly α-cells, quite reasonably explains the failure of BUCHANAN et al. (1969a) to demonstrate either glucagon or marked insulin release following CCK-PZ.

Furthermore, the technique applied by MALAISSE et al. (1967) using the addition of guinea-pig anti-insulin serum in the incubation medium even though not influencing insulin secretion directly, might exhaust the α-cells of glucagon (see MÜLLER et al., 1970b). Secondary effects of substances like CCK-PZ on insulin secretion, i.e. by endogenous glucagon, might consequently vanish. Hitherto, however, insulin release has never been analyzed convincingly in the absence of endogenous glucagon. So far, every effort to destroy the α-cells selectively, has failed (PERINGS et al., 1969). Hence the original suggestion of HAIST (1965) which led him, according to electron microscopic studies, to demonstrate the very thin line separating α-cells and β-cells and to speculate that "the juxtaposition of these different cell types provides the possibility for some intrinsic regulation of interrelated function" remains speculative.

It is suggested that glucagon secretion is controlled by endogenous insulin. This recent concept is supported by several findings in spontaneous and experimental diabetes mellitus. ASSAN et al. (1969), AGUILAR-PARADA et al. (1969c), UNGER et al. (1970) and MÜLLER et al. (1970) observed inappropriately high glucagon levels in contrast to the hyperglycemia in diabetic men. Induction of

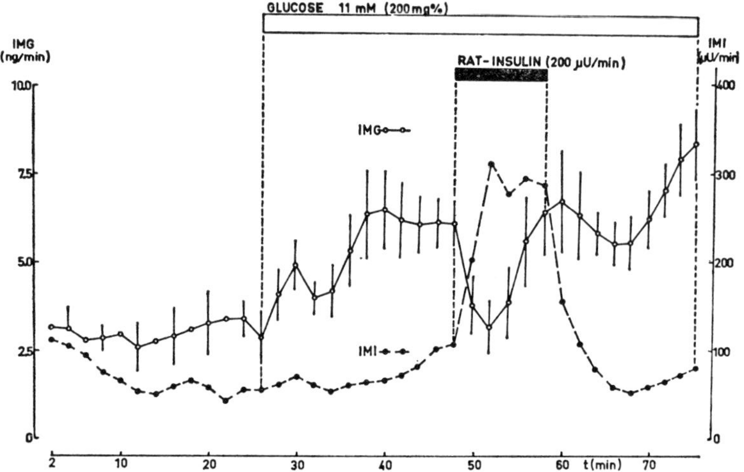

Fig. 33. Stimulation of glucagon (IMG) secretion by 11 mM glucose and suppression of this response following exogenous rat insulin of the isolated perfused pancreas of streptozotocin diabetic rats. (From: FUSSGÄNGER et al., 1971)

diabetes mellitus by streptozotocin in rats showed the same results (KATSILAMBROS et al., 1970). As outlined by MÜLLER et al. (1971b) impaired metabolism of glucose within the α-cells due to the lack of insulin was the suggested cause of the defective glucagon suppression. Infusion of insulin reversed the observed glucagon hyperresponsiveness. Since in vivo changes in the actual insulin levels are always correlated with changes in the glucose concentration, the question as to whether insulin or the accompanying fall of glucose level caused the restoration of normal glucagon levels, remained unresolved.

To compare the response of the normal and the diabetic pancreas to glucagon stimulators, CCK-PZ, and inhibitors, glucose, or the combined effect, the role of endogenous insulin was studied (FUSSGÄNGER et al., 1971). The isolated perfused rat pancreas, according to the method of SUSSMAN et al. (1966), was used in these experiments. Two groups of animals were employed: Normal fasting rats deprived of food for 12 hours before preparation of the isolated organ, and rats pretreated with streptozotocin 65 mg/kg i.v. 48 hours prior to the experiment. The results in part confirmed the suggestions of MÜLLER et al. (1971b). The diabetic organ is capable of releasing high amounts of glucagon under diabetic conditions: i.e. when glucose levels are high, Fig. 33; insulin partially suppressed this response. Moreover, comparing the dose response relationship of glucose and glucagon secretion, some unexpected features have been observed: Fig. 34 compares the mean glucagon secretion rate of normal (N) and diabetic (D) pancreases at various glucose concentrations. The complete reversal of the glucose effect is obvious. As can be seen from the point of intersection of both curves, at 100 mg-% glucagon response was identical in both groups, whereas, at glucose levels below 100 mg-%, glucagon secretion diminished in comparison with the normal organ. It was a noticable fact that increasing glucose levels, beyond the physiological range, resulted in considerable stimulation of glucagon secretion in the diabetic organ. The differences in the CCK-PZ effect of the normal and the diabetic pancreas is indicated in the next Fig. 35. The lack of endogenous insulin secretion causes decreased

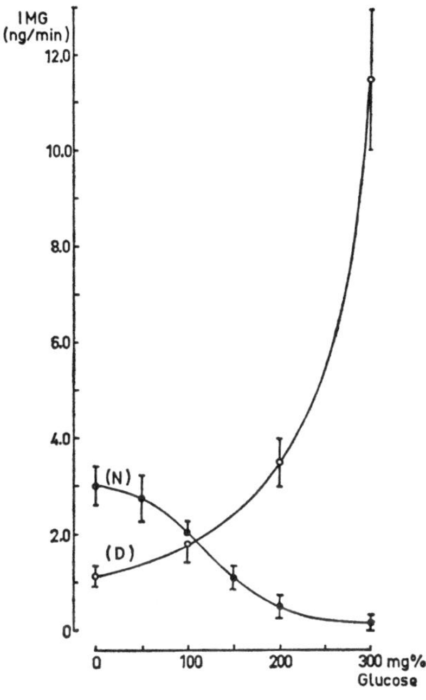

Fig. 34. Dose-response-relationship between glucose and the mean secretion rate of glucagon of the isolated perfused pancreas of normal (N) and streptozotocin diabetic rats (D). (From: Fussgänger et al., 1971)

response of glucagon at low glucose levels, again glucagon secretion seems to be unaffected within the normal fasting range of glucose, according to the point of intersection of both curves, whereas, at glucose levels above 100 mg-%, glucagon secretion is higher in the diabetic organ. In fact, the endogenous insulin secretion induced by CCK-PZ in the normal organ seems to correlate with a potentiating effect upon glucagon secretion at glucose levels below 100 mg-%. Endogenous insulin however, suppresses the glucagon secretion at glucose levels above 100 mg-%.

Exogenous insulin has been shown to stimulate glucagon secretion at glucose levels below 100 mg-% (Fig. 36), is ineffective at 100 mg-% of glucose, but suppresses glucagon secretion induced by the lack of endogenous insulin with high glucose levels (Fussgänger et al., 1971; Buchanan, 1971). The differences shown by secretin and insulin when stimulating or inhibiting either insulin or glucagon secretion, whether glucose is high or low, calls for some studies concerning the

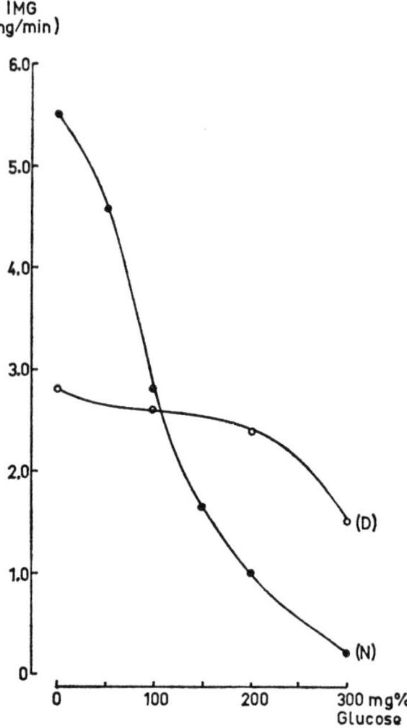

Fig. 35. Mean increase of glucagon secretion rates of the isolated perfused pancreas of normal (N) and diabetic rats (D) following cholecystokinin at different glucose concentrations. (From: FUSSGÄNGER et al., 1971)

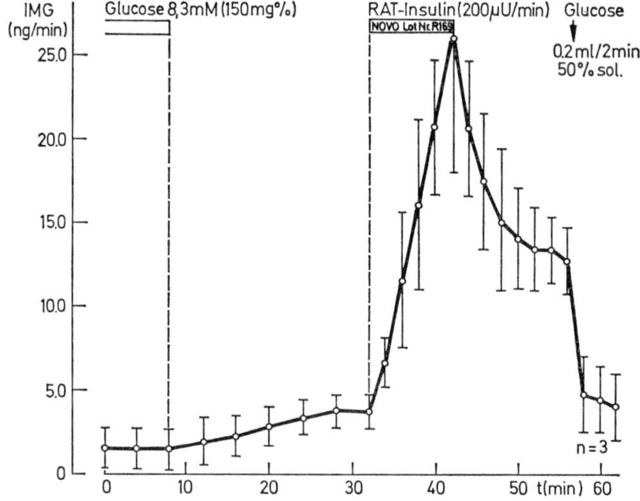

Fig. 36. Stimulation of glucagon (IMG) following exogenous rat insulin of the isolated perfused rat pancreas induced by omission of glucose. (From: FUSSGÄNGER et al., 1971)

release of insulin in response to gastrin by LERNMARK et al. (1969), demonstrating stimulation of insulin secretion at low (60 mg-%) glucose but inhibition at high (300 mg-%) levels.

It has been suggested that gastrin occurs within the islets of Langerhans (LOMSKY et al., 1969) and extracts of pancreatic α_1-cells of pigeons were shown to inhibit insulin secretion (HELLMAN and LERNMARK, 1969). Based on these findings the authors speculated on the role of α_1-cells and of gastrin, in the regulation of insulin release by local mechanisms. Regarding the reverse observations on insulin and glucagon modifying response of gastrin of gastric origin, both hormones might influence the pancreatic α_1-cell in the same way. Hence, a mutual interaction of three hormones might be anticipated to control each other. While interrelationships have not been defined and gastrin never has been convincingly demonstrated as being extracted or secreted from the α_1-cells of pancreatic origin we will disregard its existence in the concluding considerations.

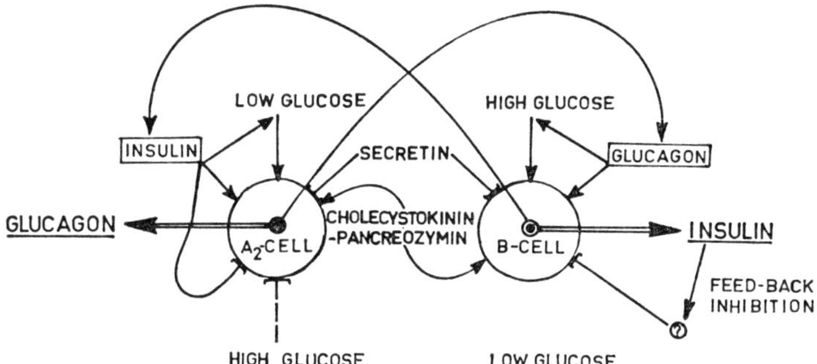

Fig. 37. Regulation of insulin and glucagon secretion at different glucose concentrations. Mutual interactions of the islet hormones. $\rightarrow$ = stimulation, $\dashv$ = inhibition low $\leqq$ 5.5 mM < high glucose (From: FUSSGÄNGER et al.; 1972)

We have tried to outline the mutual interaction of the islet hormones and the regulatory role which secretin and pancreozymin might play at different glucose concentrations. Fig. 37 indicates schematically the β-cell and the α_2-cell of the islets of Langerhans. Arrows indicate stimulatory and inhibitory functions.

The β-cell responds to high glucose concentrations with an insulin output; the response is increased by glucagon of endogenous origin. Glucagon itself, in turn, provides stimulatory conditions by its well-known hyperglycemic effects, activating glycogenolysis and gluconeogenesis within the liver. The α_2-cell responds to low glucose levels with glucagon output. Insulin, by its own action of lowering glucose within the circulation, potentiates glucagon release at low glucose levels. Both hormones maintain their effectiveness by a feed-forward type mechanism. In turn, glucose is regulated by the α-β-cell couple in a feed-back inhibitory mode of progression.

The gastrointestinal hormones secretin and pancreozymin serve as modulating discriminators: CCK-PZ induces insulin release mainly at low glucose concentrations around the fasting level, supporting glucagon secretion at the same time. Secretin causes a parallel response in the same way, but in contrast to CCK-PZ, will suppress insulin at high glucose levels and vice versa: inhibits glucagon secretion at low glucose levels. It might be stated, conclusively, that secretin, at first triggering secretion, consecutively prevents inappropriate high insulin output with increasing glucose concentrations, and, in turn, it prevents an overshooting of glucagon response under any hypoglycemic condition. CCK-PZ potentiates the effectiveness of glucose on insulin release but diminishes glucagon suppression by glucose. It is suggested that both hormones take care of the moment to moment regulation of the α-β-cell couple in response to glucose or other fuels.

VIII. The Significance of Intestinal Modulation of Islet Function

Irrespective of the probable mediatory role played by the exocrine pancreatic portion, the question arises as to whether the entero-hormones act on *their* receptor in a competitive or non-competitive, in a synergistic, or antagonistic fashion (Grossman, 1969). Combination of several insulin secretagogues presumably affecting the glucose- *and* the entero-receptor, such as tolbutamide and pancreozymin, or glucose, tolbutamide and secretin, induces the same islets or pancreas pieces, subjected to multiple incubations, to release more and more insulin (Telib and Pfeiffer, 1970). However, systematic studies of the combined action of several intestinal hormones have not yet been carried out.

All of the pharmalogical effects of the enteric hormones described up to now on the islets of Langerhans were of the rapid and short-lived type. Since all the intestinal hormones, but gastrin, were added to the list of hormones stimulating lipolysis in isolated fat cells through cyclic AMP-production (Raptis et al., 1969a; Rodbell et al., 1970) involvement of the second and third messenger system may be assumed.

However, the feeding of isocaloric diets containing carbohydrates of different insulin stimulating capacities, i.e. starch and sucrose, to rats, resulted in an exaggerated response of both insulin and pancreatic glucagon to the arginine stimulation in the latter group (Laube et al., 1970).

Since the glucagon responses are in complete contrast to the effect of the nutrients as such, activation of the hormone synthesizing apparatus of both the α- and the β-cells, i.e. of the biosynthesis of the whole Langerhans islets, mediated by pancreozymin, seems likely.

In Table 5 are listed, in a form of summary, some questions related to the physiological and pathophysiological significance of an intestinal, hormonally mediated influence on islet function.

Table 5. *Physiological and pathophysiological meaning of effective or ineffective control of insulin secretion via enteric hormone(s)*

1. Providing information of the β-cells *before* increase in blood glucose following intestinal resorption is stimulating release of pancreatic insulin?
2. Providing acute and maximal stimulation of insulin secretion by the *combined* effect of several β-cytotrophins acting on different compartments of the β-cells?
3. *Preventing hypoglycemia* following protein ingestion because of activation of the pancreozymin-glucagon-lipolysis-insulin-lipogenesis-mechanisms?
4. Being causative related to the *delayed rise in plasma insulin* in many early and elderly diabetics following glucose by virtue of a defective intestinal hormone response to glucose?
5. Being causative related to the *hypoglycemic attacks* encountered in a) the dumping and b) the carzinoid-syndromes?

Some of these questions might be answered positively on grounds of the presently available findings (i.e. 1, 2 and 3), some might be flatly rejected (i.e. 4). Time and further development of reliable radioimmunoassays for the intestinal hormones will allow a deeper understanding of this presumably onto- and phylogenetically based regulatory system.

At any event, complex interactions and interdependencies between the endocrine and the exocrine glands, between the incretory and the excretory cells of the pancreas and certain parts of the intestine, may play a role in regulating the basic responses of the pancreatic islets to food intake, and of the following metabolic and hormonal sequences.

IX. Summary and Conclusions

Revival of the old concept of BAYLISS, STARLING and DALE resulted from the demonstration of the insulin stimulating capacities of secretin, pancreozymin, gastrin, enteroglucagon, serotonin and of an unidentified mucosal factor of the intestine both in vitro and in vivo. In addition, pancreozymin caused glucagon releases, and potentiated the insulin stimulating action of amino acids and glucose. In elderly diabetics, both secretin and glucagon markedly improved the unsatisfactory insulin responses to glucose or tolbutamide given i.v. In exocrine pancreatic insufficiency due to chronic pancreatitis, neither secretin nor pancreozymin elicited the slightest insulin responses. Furthermore, the normally greater insulin responses to orally administered glucose than to glucose given i.v. were abolished in those patients as well. The same unresponsiveness of the β-cells to secretin was observed in rats suffering from experimentally induced insufficiency of the exocrine pancreas, and, with respect to secretin, gastrin and glucagon, in isolated rat islets exposed to the insulin stimulating action of these enteric hormones. Hence, the exocrine pancreatic tissue might be essential for the insulin stimulating action of the intestinal hormones *and* sufficient amounts of intact exocrine pancreatic tissue are thought to mediate the specific action of orally administered nutrients on an Entero-Receptor of the β-cells. Its role might have been decisive in former times, and still may be in some species, when food supply mainly consists of proteins and fat, i.e. substrates from animal sources. The actions of these nutrients alone, and, in particular, when source of supply does not effect considerable increases in blood, providing sufficiently high extracellular concentrations of the substrates to initiate insulin releases per se, requires support by additional stimuli of insulin secretion. This additional support is given by the intestinal hormones via the Entero-Receptor.

Similar receptors might exist on the α-cell surface to respond to some of the intestinal hormones, as well. Release of pancreatic glucagon by virtue of the lipolytic and glycogenolytic actions of this second pancreatic hormone should add to the mechanism preventing hypoglycemia following non-carbohydrate containing meals.

In the course of evolution, and in particular at the present time, when human beings and domesticated animals are fed mainly on carbohydrates, activation of this mechanism only adds to the stimulation of the Glucose-Receptor of the β-cells sensitive to the carbohydrates to secrete further quantities of rapidly released insulin. This process might facilitate development and frequency of hyperinsulinism in obesity in animals and in man, i.e. establishment of one of the major causes in the pathogenesis of diabetes. Time will show whether further insight into the complex interactions and interdependencies between endocrine and exocrine glands, between incretory and excretory cells of the pancreas and certain parts of the intestine may, and the ensuing metabolic and hormonal sequences will, lead us to therapeutic approaches of this mechanism for the prophylaxis of obesity and diabetes.

References

Aguilar-Parada, E., Eisentraut, A. M., Unger, R. H.: Pancreatic Glucagon Secretion in Normal and Diabetic Subjects. Amer. J. med. Sci. **257**, 415—419 (1969).

— — — Effects of Starvation on Plasma Pancreatic Glucagon Levels in Normal Men. Metabolism **18**, 155—162 (1969 a)

— — — Effect of HB 419 Induced Hypoglycemia on Pancreatic Glucagon Secretion. Horm. Met. Res. Suppl. **1**, 48 (1969 b).

— — — Pancreatic Glucagon Secretion in Normal and Diabetic Subjects. Amer. J. med. Sci. **275**, 415 (1969 c).

Anderson, J. C., Barton, M. A., Gregory, R. A., Hardy, P. M., Kenner, G. W., McLeod, J. K., Preston, J., Sheppard ,R. C., Morley, J. S.: The Antral Hormone Gastrin. II. Synthesis of Gastrin. Nature (Lond.) **204**, 933—934 (1964).

Assal, J. P., Levrat, R., Stauffacher, W., Renold, A. E.: Metabolic Consequences of Portocaval Shunting in the Rat. Effects of Glucose Tolerance and Serum Immunoreactive Insulin Response. Metabolism **20**, 850—858 (1971).

Assan, R., Hautecouverture, G., Guillemant, S., Dauchy, F., Protin, P., Derot, M.: Evolution de paramétres hormonaux et energétiques dans 10 acido-cetoses diabètiques graves. Path. et Biol. **17**, 1095 (1969).

— Rosselin, G., Drouet, I., Dolais, I., Tchobroutsky, G., Dérot, M.: Dosage radio-immunologique du glucagon plasmatique chez l'homme. Résultats Préliminaires. Ann. Endocr. (Paris) **27**, 690—695 (1966).

Bainbridge, F. A., Beddard, A. P.: Secretin in Relation to Diabetes Mellitus. Biochem. J. **1**, 429—438 (1906).

Basabe, J. C., Lopez, N. L., Viktora, J. K., Wolff, F. W.: Insulin Secretion Studied in the Perfused Rat Pancreas II. Effect of Glucose, Glucagon, 3′—5′ Adenosine Monophosphate, Theophylline, Imidazole and Phenoxybenzamine. Diabetes **20**, 457—466 (1971).

Basténie, P. A., Conard, V.: Essai d'interprétation des épreuves d'hyperglycémie provoquée. Rev. franç. Étud. clin. biol. **2**, 223, 229 (1957).

Bayliss, W. M., Starling, E. H.: Mechanism of Pancreatic Secretion. J. Physiol. (Lond.) **28**, 325—353 (1902).

Benedetti, A., Simpson, R. C., Grodsky, G. M., Forsham, P. H.: Serum Insulin Response to Glucagon as an Index of Insulin Reserve. In: Pharmacology of Horm. Polypeptides and Proteins. Proc. Inter. Symp. on the Pharmac. of Hormonal Polyp. Milan 1967. New York: Plenum Press 1968, p. 304—312.

Bernard, C.: Lécons sur le Diabète. Baillière, J. B., Paris (1877).

Berson, S. A., Walsh, I. H., Yalow, R. S.: Radioimmunoassay of Gastrin in Human Plasma and Regulation of Gastrin Secretion. XVI. Nobel Symposium Frontiers in Gastrointestinal Hormone Research, July 20—21, 1970. Almqvist and Wiksell, Stockholm (in press).

Bertaccini, G., de Caro, G., Melchiorri, P.: The Effects of Caerulein on Insulin Secretion in Anaesthetized Dogs. Brit. J. Parmacology **40**, 78—85, (1970).

Biedl, A., Kraus, R.: Über intravenöse Traubenzuckerinfusionen am Menschen. Wien. klin. Wschr. **9**, 55—58 (1896).

Bloom, E.: A New Type of Granular Cell in the Islets of Langerhans of Man. Anat. Rec. **49**, 363—374 (1931).

Bodanszky, M., Ondetti, M. A., Levine, S. D., Narayanan, V. L., Saltza von, M., Sheehan, J. T., Williams, N. J., Sabo, E. F.: Synthesis of a Heptacosapeptide Amide with the Hormonal Activity of Secretin. Chemistry and Industry **42**, 1757—1758 (1966).

Bottermann, P., Souvatzoglou, A., Schwarz, K., Stimulierung der Beta-Cytotropen-Wirkung von Tolbutamid durch Secretin beim Menschen. Wien. klin. Wschr. **45**, 549—550 (1967).

Boyns, D. R., Jarrett, R. J., Keen, H.: Intestinal Hormones and Plasma Insulin. Lancet **1966 I**, 409—410. Diabetologia (Abstr.) **3**, 52 (1967).

— — — Intestinal Hormones and Plasma Insulin. An Insulinotropic Action of Secretin. Brit. med. J. II., 676—678 (1967).

Buchanan, K. D.: Insulin and Glucose Control of Pancreatic Glucagon Release. 7th Annual Meeting of the European Soc. f. the Study of Diabetes, Southhampton 15. 9. 1971, Abstr. 31.

BUCHANAN, K. D., VANCE, J. E., AOKI, T., WILLIAMS, R. H.: Rise in Serum Immunoreactive Glucagon after Intrajejunal Glucose in Pancreatectomized Dogs. Proc. Soc. exp. Biol. (N.Y.) **126**, 813 (1967).
— — — DINSTL, K., WILLIAMS, R. H.: Effect of Blood Glucose on Glucagon Secretion in Anesthetized Dogs. Diabetes **18**, 627—632 (1969).
— — MORGAN, A., WILLIAMS, R. H.: Effect of Pancreozymin on Insulin and Glucagon Levels in Blood and Bile. Amer. J. Physiol. **6**, 1293—1298, (1968).
— — WILLIAMS, R. H.: Insulin and Glucagon Release from Isolated Islets of Langerhans. Effect of Enteric Factors. Diabetes **18**, 381—386 (1969 a).
— — — Effects of Starvation on Insulin and Glucagon Release from Isolated Islets of Langerhans of the Rat. Metabolism **18**, 155—162 (1969 b).
BYRNES, D. J., YOUNG, J. D., CHISHOLM, D. J., LAZARUS, L.: Serum Gastrin in Patients with Peptic Ulceration. Brit. med. J. **2**, 626—629 (1970).
CAMPBELL, J., RASTOGI, K. S.: Effects of Glucagon and Epinephrine on Serum Insulin and Insulin Secretion in Dogs. Endocrinology **79**, 830—835 (1966).
CANDELA, R. R.: Effect of the Glucagon on the Plasma Insulin-Activity after Hypophysectomy. Experientia **16**, 320—322 (1960).
— NGOMA, J. M., MBENSA, L.: Duodenal Insulin-Stimulating Factor. Lancet **1967 I**, 568—570.
CAVALLERO, C., SOLCIA, E., SAMPIETRO, R.: Cytology of Islets Tumors and Hyperplasias Associated with the Zollinger-Ellison Syndrome. Gut **8**, 172—178 (1967).
CHESNEY, T. McC., SCHOFIELD, I. G.: Studies on the Secretion of Pancreatic Glucagon. Diabetes **18**, 627—632 (1969).
CHISHOLM, D. J., YOUNG, J. D., LAZARUS, L.: The Gastrointestinal Stimulus to Insulin Release. I Secretin. J. clin. Invest. **48**, 1453—1460 (1969).
— KRAEGEN, E. W., YOUNG, J. D., LAZARUS, L.: Comparison of Secretin Response to Oral, Intraduodenal or Intravenous Glucose Administration. Horm. Metab. Res. **3**, 180—183 (1971).
COLWELL, A. R., ZUCKERMAN, L.: Regulation of Insulin Release by Pancreatic Glucagon. Diabetes **19**, 429—737 (1970).
COORE, H. G., RANDLE, P. J.: Regulation of Insulin Secretion Studied with Pieces of Rabbit Pancreas Incubated *in vitro*. Biochemistry **93**, 66—78 (1964).
CONARD, V.: Mésure de l'assimilation du glucose base théorique et applications cliniques. Acta gastro-ent. belg. **18**, 803—813 (1955).
— FRANCKSON, R. I. M., BASTÉNIE, P. A., KESTENS, I. C., KOVACS, L.: Études critiques du triangle d'hyperglycémie intravaineux chez l'homme normal et détermination d'un coéfficient d'assimilation glucidique. Arch. int. Pharmacodyn. **93**, 277—284 (1953).
CROCKFORD, P. M., HAZZARD, W. R., WILLIAMS, R. H.: Insulin Response to Glucagon. The Opposing Effects of Diabetes and Obesity. Diabetes **18**, 216—224 (1969).
CROFTON, W. M.: Pancreatic Secretion in the Treatment of Diabetes. Lancet **1909 I**, 607—611.
CURTIS, J. D., DUPRÉ, J., BECK, J. C.: Effects of Secretin, Pancreozymin and Gastrin on Insulin Release *in vitro*. Clin. Res. **16**, 521 (1968).
CURRY, D. L.: Glucagon Potentiation of Insulin Secretion by the Perfused Rat-Pancreas. Diabetes **19**, 420 (1970).
DALDRUP, J., FORSSMANN, W. G.: Elektronenmikroskopie zur Entwicklung der intestinalen endokrinen Zellen im Rattenmagen. In: Endokrinologie der Entwicklung und Reifung 16. Symp. Dtsch. Ges. Endokrin. Ulm, Februar 1970. Springer-Verlag, Berlin, Heidelberg, New York, p. 256—257.
DAKIN, H. D., RANSOM, C. C.: Note on the Treatment of a Case of Diabetes Mellitus with Secretin. J. biol. Chem. **2**, 305—314 (1906).
DALE, H.: In the Islets of Langerhans in the Pancreas. Phil. Trans. B **197**, 25—36 (1904).
DAVENPORT, H. W.: Physiology of the Digestive Tract 3. Edit. Year Book Med. Publ. Chicago 1967, p. 150.
DECKERT, T.: Insulin Secretion Following Administration of Secretin in Patients with Diabetes Mellitus. Acta endocr. (Kbh.) **59**, 150—158 (1968).
— WORNING, H.: Insulin Secretion after Administration of Secretin to Normal and Diabetic Subjects and Patients with Chronic Pancreatitis. 5th Ann. Meeting Europ. Ass. for the Study of Diabetes. Montpellier 1969 (Abstr. p. 99). Diabetologia (Abstr.) **6**, 42 (1970).
DEVRIM, S., RECANT, L.: Effect of Glucagon on Insulin Release in Vitro. Lancet **1966 II**, 1227.
DOTEVALL, G., GILLBERG, R., KOCH, N. G., WALAN, A.: Stimulatory and Inhibitory Effects on Gastric Secretion in Man by Glucagon Infusion in Small Doses. 4th World Congress of Gastroenterology, Copenhagen 1970. Advances Abstr. Edited by Dan. Gastroent. Ass. p. 145.

Duncan, G. G., Shumway, N. P., Williams, T. L., Fetter, F.: The Clinical Application of Duodenal Extract in Diabetes Mellitus. Amer. J. Med. Sci. **189**, 403—407 (1935).

Dupré, J., An Intestinal Hormone Affecting Glucose Disposal in Man. Lancet **1964 a** II, 672—673.

— Effect of Route of Administration on Disposal of Glucose Loads. Amer. J. Physiol. **175**, 58—64 (1964 b).

— Regulation of the Secretions of the Pancreas. Ann. Rev. Med. **21**, 299—314 (1970).

— Beck, J. C.: Stimulation of Release of Insulin by an Extract of Intestinal Mucosa. Diabetes **15**, 555—559 (1966).

— Curtis, J. D., Unger, R. H., Waddell, R. W., Beck, J. C.: Effects of Secretin, Pancreozymin or Gastrin on the Response of the Endocrine Pancreas to Administration of Glucose or Arginine in Man. J. clin. Invest. **48**, 745—757 (1969).

— — Waddell, R. W., Beck, J. C.: Regulation of Pancreatic Endocrine Function by Gastrointestinal Hormones. Proc. Roy. Soc. Med. 8, 815—816 (1968).

— Rojas, L., White, J. J., Unger, R. H., Beck, J. C.: Effects of Secretin on Insulin and Glucagon in Portal and Peripheral Blood in Man. Lancet II, 26—27 (1966).

Dyck, W. P., Rudick, J., Hoexter, B., Janowitz, H. D.: Influence of Glucagon on Pancreatic Exocrine Secretion. Gastroenterology **56**, 531—537 (1969).

Edkins, J. S. On the Chemical Mechanism of Gastric Secretion. Proc. roy. Soc. **76**, 376—379 (1905).

Edwards, J. C., Howell, S. L., Taylor, K. W.: Fatty Acids as Regulators of Glucagon Secretion. Nature (Lond.) **224**, 80—88 (1969).

— — — Fatty Acids and the Release of Glucagon From Isolated Guinea-pig Islets Incubated in Vitro. Biochem. biophys. Res. Commun. **215**, 310—315 (1970).

Eisentraut, A. M., Ohneda, A., Aguilar-Parada, E., Unger, R. H.: Immunologic Discrimination between Pancreatic Glucagon and Enteric Glucagon Like Immunoreactivity (GLI) in Tissues and Plasma. Diabetes (Abstr.) **17**, Suppl. 1, 321 (1968).

Elrick, H., Stimmler, C., Hlad C. J., Jr., Arai, Y.: Plasma Insulin Response to Oral and Intravenous Glucose Administration. J. clin. Endocr. **24**, 1076—1082 (1964).

Erspamer, V.: Biogenic Amines and Active Polypeptides of the Amphibian Skin. Pharmacol. Rev. **3**, 327—350 (1971).

— Roseghini, M., Endean, R., Anastasi, A.: Biogenic Amines and Active Polypeptides in the Skin of Australian Amphibians. Nature (Lond.) **212**, 204—206 (1966).

Fallucca, F., Carratu, R., Tamburrano, G., Javicoli, M., Menzinger, G.: Effecto della caeruleina somministrata per via venosa rapida nell'uomo, sui livelli plasmatici die glucagone, insulina e glucosio. Folia endocr. (Roma) **22**, 524—531 (1969).

— — — — — Andreani, D.: Effects of Caerulein and Pancreozymin on Insulin Secretion in Normal Subjects and in Patients with Insuloma. Horm. Met. Res. Suppl. 1971 (In print).

Farrell, J. I., Ivy, A. C.: Contributions to the Physiology of the Pancreas II. The Proof of a Humoral Mechanism for External Pancreatic Secretion. Amer. J. Physiol. **78**, 325—338 (1926).

Fasel, J., Hadjikhani, H., Felber, J. P.: The Insulin Secretory Effect of the Human Duodenal Mucosa. Gastroenterology **59**, 109—113 (1970).

Feldman, J. M., Lebowitz, H. E.: Specificity of Serotonin Inhibition of Insulin Release from Golden Hamster Pancreas. Diabetes **19**, 475—479 (1970).

Forsmann, W. G., Orci, L., Rouiller, Ch.: Glukagon-bildende und andere endokrine Zellen im Magendarmepithel und ihre Ultrastruktur. 14. Symp. Dtsch. Ges. Endokr., Heidelberg 7.—9. März 1968. Springer-Verlag, Berlin, Heidelberg, New York 1968, p. 252—256.

Foster, N. B.: Cases of Diabetes Treated with Secretin. J. biol. Chem. **2**, 297—303 (1906).

— unpublished results (1972).

Fussgänger, R. D., Goberna, R., Laube, H., Schröder, K. E., Straub, K., Pfeiffer, E. F.: Glucagon Secretion from the Isolated Perfused Rat Pancreas, Influenced by the Glucose-, Tolbutamide-, and Pancreozymin-Mediated Release of Pancreatic Insulin. Israel J. med. Sci. 8, 2—3 (1972).

— Goberna, R., Schröder, K. E., Laube, H., Pfeiffer, E. F.: Abnormally High Glucagon Secretion of the Streptozotocin Diabetic Isolated Perfused Rat Pancreas. Evidence for a Lack of Suppression Due to the Deprivation of Endogenous Insulin Release. 7th Annual Meeting of the European Soc. f. the Study of Diabetes, Southampton, 15. 9. 1971. Abstr. 67.

— Straub, K., Goberna, R., Jaros, P., Schröder, K. E., Raptis, S., Pfeiffer, E. F.: Primary Secretion of Insulin and Secondary Release of Glucagon from the Isolated Perfused Rat Pancreas Following Stimulation with Pancreozymin. Horm. Met. Res. Suppl. **1**, 224 to 227 (1969).

GAGLIARDINO, J. J., ZIEHER, L. M., ITURRIZA, F. C., HERNANDEZ, R. E., RODRIGUEZ, R. R.: Serotonin-Mediated Hypoglycemia. Congress of the Intern. Diabetes Federation Buenos Aires, August 23.—28., 1970 (Abstr. Nr. 103). Excerpta Medica Foundation ICS, 209.

GLICK, Z., BAILE, C. A., MAYER, J.: Insulinotropic and Possible Insulin Like Effects of Secretin and Cholecystokinin-Pancreozymin. Endocrinology **86**, 927 (1970).

GNUDI, A., BERTACCINI, G., COSCELLI, C., AGOSTI, V., PALAMRI, V.: The Action of Caerulein, a New Extractive Peptide, on Insulin Levels and Glucose Metabolism. 5. Ann. Meeting of Europ. Ass. of Diabetes Montpellier 16—18 Sept. 69. Diabetologia (Abstr.) **6**, 46 (1970).

GOBERNA, R., RAPTIS, S., FUSSGÄNGER, R. D., PFEIFFER, E. F.: Effect of Secretin and Pancreozymin on Insulin Secretion in Exocrine Pancreatic Insufficiency in Rat. 5th Ann. Meeting Europ. Ass. for the Study of Diabetes, Montpellier 1969 (Abst. p. 110). Diabetologia (Abstr.) **6**, 46 (1970).

— FUSSGÄNGER, R. D., RAPTIS, S., TELIB, M., PFEIFFER, E. F.: The Role of the Exocrine Pancreas in the Stimulation of Insulin-Secretion by Intestinal Hormones. II. Insulin Responses to Secretin and Pancreozymin in Experimental Insufficiency of the Exocrine Pancreas. Diabetologia **7**, 68—72 (1971).

GOLDFINE, J. D., BIRNBAUMER, L., ROTH, J.: Glucagon Receptor in Islet Cells: Binding of J-125-Glucagon and Activation of Adenyl Cyclase. Diabetes **20**, Suppl. 1, 341 (1971).

— ROTH, J., BIRNBAUMER, L.: Glucagon Receptors in Beta-Cells. J. Biol. Chem. **247**, 1211—1213 (1972).

GREENLEE, H. B., LONGHI, E. H., GUERRERO, J. D., NELSON, T. S., EL-BEDRI, A. L., DRAGSTEDT, L. R.: Inhibitory Effect of Pancreatic Secretin on Gastric Secretion. Amer. J. Physiol. **190**, 396—402 (1957).

GREGORY, R. A., TRACY, H. J.: The Constitution and Properties of Two Gastrins Extracted from Hog Antral Mucosa. Gut **5**, 103—117 (1964).

GRODSKY, G. M., BENNETT, L. L.: Effect of Glucose "Pulse", Glucagon and Cations Ca^{++}, Mg^{++} und K^{+} on Insulin Secretion *in vitro*. J. clin. Invest. **45**, 1018 (1966).

— BENNETT, C. C., SMITH, D. F., SCHMID, F. C.: Effect of "Pulse" Administration of Glucose or Glucagon on Insulin Secretion in Vitro. Metabolism **16**, 222—228 (1967).

— LANDAHL, H., CURRY, D., BENNETT, L.: A Two-Compartmental Model For Insulin Secretion. Advanc. Metab. Disord. Suppl. **1**, 45—50 (1970).

GROSSMAN, M. I.: In Proceedings of the Symposium on the Exocrine Pancreas, Queen's University Kingston, Ontario, Canada, 5.—7. Juni 1969 (in print).

GUIDOUX-GRASSI, L., FELBER, J. P.: Effect of Secretin on Insulin Release by Rat Pancreas. 4th Ann. Meeting Europ. Ass. of the Study of Diab. Louvain, 1968. Diabetologia (Abstr.) **4**, 386 (1969).

HAIST, R. E.: Effects of Changes in Stimulation in the Structure and Function of Islet Cells. In "On the Nature and Treatment of Diabetes Mellitus". Excerpta Medica Found. ICS 84, Amsterdam 1965, p. 12—30.

HÅKANSON, R., LUNDQUIST, I.: Occurrance of Insulin in Rat Duodenum and its Depletion with Alloxan. Experimentia **27**, 1220 (1971).

HANDWERGER, S., ROTH, J., GORDEN, P., SANT'AGNESE, P. D., CARPENTER, D. F., PETER, G.: Glucose intolerance in cystic fibrosis. New Engl. J. Med. **281**, 451—461 (1969).

HANSON, J., OHNEDA, A., EISENTRAUT, A. M., UNGER, R. H.: Characterization of Gut "glucagon". Clin. Res. **15**, 43 (1967). (Abstr.)

HARPER, A. A., RAPER, H. S.: Pancreozymin, a Stimulant of the Secretion of Pancreatic Enzymes in Extracts of the Small Intestine. J. Physiol. (Lond.) **102**, 115—125 (1943).

HARTLEY, R. C., GAMBILL, E. E., SUMMERSKILL, W. H. J.: Pancreatic Volume and Bicarbonate Output with Augmented Dose of Secretin. Gastroenterology **48**, 312—317 (1965).

HEDING, L. G.: Glucagon Antibodies for the Radioimmunoassay of Pancreatic and Gut Glucagon. 4th Meeting Europ. Diab. Ass. Louvain, 22.—24. July 1968. Diabetologia (Abstr.) **4**, 388 (1968).

— Radioimmunological Determination of Pancreatic and Gut Glucagon in Plasma. Diabetologia **7**, 10—19 (1971).

HELLER, H.: Über das blutzuckersenkende Hormon der Darmschleimhaut (Duodenin). Wien. klin. Wschr. **44**, 476—480 (1931).

HELLMAN, B., LERNMARK, A.: Inhibition of the *in vitro* Secretion of Insulin by an Extract of Pancreatic α_1-cells. Endocrinology **84**, 1484 (1969).

— ROTHMAN, U., HELLERSTRÖM, C.: Identification of a Specific Type of a Cell Located in the Central Part of the Pancreatic Islets of Horse. Gen. comp. Endocr. **2**, 558—567 (1962).

HINDBERG, I., ENK, B., PERSON, I.: Insulin-Stimulation by Secretin in Diabetics. Effect of Repeated and of Varied Doses. Horm. Met. Res. Suppl. **2**, 131—134 (1970).

HINZ, M., KATSILAMBROS, N., SCHWEIZER, B., RAPTIS, S., PFEIFFER, E. F.: The Role of the Exocrine Pancreas in the Stimulation of Insulin Secretion by Intestinal Hormones. I. The Effect of Pancreozymin, Secretin, Gastrin and of Glucagon upon Insulin Secretion of Isolated Islets of Rat Pancreas. Diabetologia **7**, 1—5 (1971).
HINZ, M., RAPTIS, S., PFEIFFER, E. F.: Comparative Studies on the Effects of Intestinal Hormones on Insulin Secretion by Fragments of Pancreas and Isolated Islets of Langerhans of Rat. 5. Kongr. Europ. Diab. Ges. Montpellier 16.—18. September, 1969. Diabetologia (Apstr.) **6**, 49 (1970).
IVERSEN, J.: Secretion of Immunoreactive Insulin and Glucagon from the Perfused Canine Pancreas Following Stimulation with Adenosine 3′—5′-monophosphate (cyclic AMP), Glucagon and Theophylline. VII. Intern. Cong. Diab. Fed. Buenos Aires 1970 Excerpta Medica Found. ICS 209 Abstr. 98.
— Secretion of Glucagon from the Isolated Perfused Canine Pancreas. J. clin. Invest. **50**, 123 (1971).
— Gastrointestinal Hormones and the Secretion of Glucagon and Insulin from the Isolated, Perfused Canine Pancreas. Diabetologia **7**, 399 (1971) Abstr.
— Gastrointestinal Hormones and the Secretion of Glucagon and Insulin from the Isolated, Perfused Canine. Pancreas. Israel J. med. Sci. 8, 57 (1972).
IVY, A. C., FISCHER, N F.: The Presence of an Insulin-Like Substance in Gastric and Duodenal Mucosa and its Relation to Gastric Secretion. Amer. J. Physiol. **67**, 445—453 (1924).
— OLDBERG, E.: Hormone Mechanism for Gallbladder Contraction and Evacuation. Amer. J. Physiol. **86**, 599—613 (1928).
JARRETT, R. J., COHEN, N. M.: Intestinal Hormones and Plasma-Insulin. Lancet II, 861—863 (1967); — Diabetologia (Abstr.) **4**, 175 (1968).
JORPES, J. E., MAGNUSSON, S., STEELE, B.: Amino Acid Composition and N-Terminal Amino Acid Sequence of Porcine Secretin. Biochem. biophys. Res. Commun. **9**, 275—279 (1962).
— MUTT, V.: Sécrétine, Pancréozymine et Cholécystokinine, les hormones silencieuses. Path. et Biol. **8**, 1177—1192 (1960).
— — On the Biological Activity and Amino Acid Composition of Secretin. Acta chem. scand. **15**, 1790—1791 (1961).
— — Cholecystokinin and Pancreozymin One Single Hormone? Acta physiol. scand. **66**, 196—202 (1966).
— — Cholecystokinin (CCK). Klin. Wschr. **48**, 65—71 (1970).
— — Secretin. 3rd Symp. European Pancreatic Club, Prag, 2.—4. July, 1968. Czech. Med. Press, Praha 1970, p. 16—20.
JUNOD, A. J., LETARTE, S., LAMBERT, A. E., STAUFFACHER, W.: Study in Spiny Mices (Acomys Cahirnus): Metabolic State and Pancreatic Insulin Release *in vitro*. Horm. Met. Res. Suppl. **1**, 45—52 (1969).
KAESS, H., BRECH, W., SCHLIERF, G.: Der Einfluß von Glukagon auf die exokrine und endokrine Pankreasfunktion. Klin. Wschr. **46**, 1314—1315 (1968).
— SCHLIERF, G., VON MIKULICZ-RADECKI: Die Wirkung gastrointestinaler Hormone auf den Kohlenhydratstoffwechsel bei Patienten mit portocavalem Shunt. 75. Kongreß Dtsch. Ges. Inn. Med. Wiesbaden, 1969. Bergmann-Verlag München, 1969, p. 647—650.
KAHIL, M. E., MCILHANEY, G. R., JORDAN, P. H.: Effect of Enteric Hormones on Insulin Secretion. Metabolism **19**, 50—57 (1970).
KANETO, A., TASAKA, Y., KOSAKA, K., NAKAO, K.: Stimulation of Insulin Secretion by the c-Terminal Tetrapeptide Amide of Gastrin. Endocrinology **84**, 1098—1106 (1969).
KARAM, J. H., GRASSO, S. G., WEGIENKA, L. C., GRODSKY, G. M., FORSHAM, P. H.: Effect of Selected Hexoses of Epinephrine and of Glucagon on Insulin Secretion in Man. Diabetes **15**, 571—578 (1966).
KATSILAMBROS, N., ABD EL RAHMAN, J., HINZ, M., FUSSGÄNGER, R. D., SCHRÖDER, K. E., STRAUB, K., PFEIFFER, E. F.: Action of Streptozotocin on Insulin and Glucagon Responses of Rat Islets. Horm. Met. Res. **2**, 268—270 (1970).
KENNY, A. J., SAY, R. R.: Glucagon-Like Activity Extractable from the Gastro-Intestinal Tract of Man and other Animals. J. Endocr. **25**, 1—7 (1962).
KETTERER, H., EISENTRAUT, A. M., UNGER, R. H.: Effect upon Insulin Secretion of Physiologic Doses of Glucagon Administered Via the Portal Vein. Diabetes **5**, 283—288 (1967)
KRAEGEN, E. W., CHISHOLM, D. J., YOUNG, J. D., LAZARUS, L.: The Gastrointestinal Stimulus to Insulin Release. II. A Dual Action of Secretin. J. clin. Invest. **49**, 524—529 (1970).
LA BARRE, J., LÉDRUT, J.: A propos de l'action hypoglycémiante des extraits duodénaux. C. R. Soc. Biol. (Paris) **115**, 750—759 (1934).
LAMBERT, A. E., VECCHIO, D., GONET, A., JEANRENAUD, J. B., RENOLD, A.: Organ Culture of Fetal Rat Pancreas: Effect of Tolbutamide, Glucagon and other substances. In: Tolbutamide After Ten Years. Brook Lodge Symp., Augusta., Mich., March 6.—7. 1967 ICS **149** Excerpta Medica Foundation p. **11**.

LANGS, H. M., FRIEDBERG, D.: Effectiveness of Glucose Admistered Orally in Overcoming the Epinephrine Block of Insulin Secretion. Clin. Res. (Abstr.) **14**, 283 (1966).

LAUBE, H., FUSSGÄNGER, R. D., GOBERNA, R., SCHRÖDER, K. E., HINZ, M., STRAUB, K., PFEIFFER, E. F.: Arginin-induzierte Sekretion von Insulin und Glukagon bei verschiedenen Diätformen. 16. Symp. Dtsch. Ges. f. Endokrinologie, Ulm 1970, Springer-Verlag 1970, p. 352.

LAUGHTON, N. B., MACALLUM, A. B.: The Relation of the Duodenal Mucosa to the Internal Secretion of the Pancreas. Proc. roy. Soc. B **111**, 37—46 (1932).

LAWRENCE, A. W.: Radioimmunoassayable Glucagon Levels in Man: Effects of Starvation, Hypoglycemia and Glucose Administration. Proc. nat. Acad. Sci. (Wash.) **55**, 316 (1966).

LAZARUS, N. R., VOYLES, N. R., TANESE T., DEVRIM, S., RECANT, L.: Extra Gastrointestinal Effects of Secretin, Gastrin and Pancreozymin. Lancet II, 248—250 (1968).

LÉFÈBVRE, P. J., LUYCKX, A.: Glucagon Stimulated Insulin Release. Lancet I, 1040 (1966).

— UNGER, R. H., VALVERDE, I., RIGOPOULOU, D., LUYCKX, A. S., EISENTRAUT, A. M.: Effect of Dog Jejunum "Glucagon-Like Immunoreactive Material" on Adipose Tissue Metabolism. Horm. Met. Res. Suppl. **1**, 143—144 (1969).

LEHNERT, P., STAHLHEBER, H., FORELL, M. M., DOST, F. H., FRITZ, H., HUTZEL, M., WERLE E.: Bestimmung der Halbwertszeit von Sekretin. Klin. Wschr. **47**, 1200—1204 (1969).

LERNER, R. L., PORTE, D., Jr.: Uniphasic insulin responses to secretin stimulation in man. J. clin. Invest. **49**, 2276—2280 (1970).

LERNMARK, A., HELLMAN, B., COORE, H. G.: Effects of Gastrin on the Release of Insulin *in vitro*. J. Endocr. **43**, 371—375 (1969).

LOEW, E. R., GRAY, J. S., IVY, A. C.: The Effect of Duodenal Instillation of Hydrochloric Acid upon the Fasting Blood Sugar of Dogs. Amer. J. Physiol. **126**, 270—276 (1939).

— — — The Effect of Acid Stimulation of the Duodenum upon Experimental Hyperglycaemia and Utilization of Glucose. Amer. J. Physiol. **128**, 298—306 (1940).

LOMSKY, R., LANGER, F., VORTEL, V.: Immunohistochemical Demonstration of Gastrin in Mammalian Islets of Langerhans. Nature (Lond.) **223**, 618—619 (1969).

LUYCKX, A. S., LÉFÈBVRE, P. J.: Release of Glucagon or a Glucagon Like Immunoreactive Material by Rat Jejunum Incubated *in vitro*. In: M. Margoulies (Ed.): Protein and Polypeptide Hormones. Part III. Amsterdam, Excerpta Medica Found. 1969, p. 884—887.

— — Arguments for Regulation of Pancreatic Glucagon Secretion by Circulating plasma Free Fatty Acids. Proc. Soc. exp. Biol. **133**, 524 (1970).

— MASSI-BENEDETTI, F., LÉFÈBVRE, P. J.: Glucagon Response to Hypoglycemia in Isolated Perfused Rat Pancres and its Modification by Circulating Levels of Free Fatty Acids. 7th Ann. Meeting of the Europ. Soc. f. the Study of Diabetes. Southampton, 15.—17.9.1971 Abstr. 115.

MAHLER, R. J., WEISBERG, H.: Failure of Endogenous Stimulation of Secretin and Pancreozymin Release to Influence Serum-Insulin. Lancet **1968 I**, 448—451.

MALAISSE, W.: Etude de la Sécrétion Insulinique *in vitro*. Edit. Arsacia S.A. Bruxelles 1969.

— MALAISSE-LAGAE, F.: Insulin Secretion by Isolated Islets of Langerhans. Effects of Pancreatic and Intestinal Hormones. Acta diab. lat. **5**, 64 (1968).

— — MAYHEW, D. A.: A Possible Role for the Adenylcyclase System in Insulin Secretion. J. clin. Invest. **46**, 1724 (1967).

— — LACY, P. E., WRIGHT, P. M.: Insulin Secretion by Isolated Islets in the Presence of Glucose, Insulin and Anti-Insulin Serum. Proc. Soc. exp. Biol. **124**, 497 (1967).

MARCO, J., BAROJA, I. M., DIAZ-FIERROS, M., VILLANUEVA, M. C., VALVERDE, I.: Relationship between Insulin and Gut Glucagon Like Immunoreactivity (GLI) Secretion in Normal and Gastrectomized Subjects. J. clin. Endocrin. (1972) (in print).

— FALOONA, G. R., UNGER, R. H.: Effects of Gut Glucagon Like Immunoreactivity on Insulin Secretion. Diabetes **19**, 366 (1970).

— — — The Effect of Endogenous Intestinal Glucagon Like Immunoreactivity (GLI) on Insulin Secretion and Glucose Concentration in Dogs. J. clin. Endocrin. Metab. **33**, 318 (1971).

MARKS, U., SAMOLS, E.: Intestinal Factors in the Regulation of Insulin Secretion. Advanc. Metab. Disord. **4**, 1—38 (1970).

MARLISS, E. B., BLONDEL, B., LAMBERT, A. E., STAUFFACHER, W.: Insulin Release from Monolayer Cultures of Rat Pancreas Cells. Israel J. med. Sci. 8, 23 (1972).

MCGUIGAN, J. E.: Gastric Mucosal Intracellular Localization of Gastrin by Immunofluorescence. Gastroenterology **55**, 315—317 (1968 a).

— Immunochemical Studies with Synthetic Human Gastrin. Gastroenterology **54**, 1005—1011 (1968 b).

— TRUDEAU, W. L.: Studies with Antibodies to Gastrin, Radioimmunoassay in Human Serum and Physiological Studies. Gastroenterology **58**, 139—150 (1970).

McIntyre, N.: The Intestinal Control of Insulin Secretion. An Historical Introduction. IDF Congress Stockholm 1967 Excerpta Medica Foundation ICS 172, p. 425—432.

— Holdsworth, C. D., Turner, D. S.: New Interpretation of Oral Glucose Tolerance. Lancet **1964 II**, 20—21.

— — — Intestinal Factors in the Control of Insulin Secretion. J. clin. Endocr. **25**, 1317—1324 (1965).

Meade, R. C., Kneubuhler, H. A., Schulte, W. J., Barboriak, J. J.: Stimulation of Insulin Secretion by Pancreozymin. Diabetes **16**, 141—144 (1967).

Meissner, H. P., Biro, G., Kettl, G., Mizumo, H., Weinges, K. F.: Vergleichende Untersuchungen über die insulinstimulierende Wirkung verschiedener sog. „intestinaler Hormone" on isolierten Inseln der Ratte in vitro. 75. Tagung Dtsch. Ges. Inn. Med., Wiesbaden 14.—17. 4. 1969 Abstr. Nr. 164, p. 89, Bergmann-Verlag München 1969.

Melani, F., Lawecki, J., Bartelt, K. M., Pfeiffer, E. F.: Insulinspiegel bei stoffwechselgesunden Fettsüchtigen und Diabetikern nach intravenöser Gabe von Glukose, Tolbutamid und Glucagon. Diabetologia (Abstr. 115) **2**, 210 (1966); **3**, 422—426 (1967).

Mering, J. von, Minkowski, O.: Diabetes Mellitus and Pancreasextirpation. Arch. exp. Path. Pharmak. **26**, 371—390 (1889).

Millner, R. D. G., Hales, C. N.: The Role of Calcium and Magnesium in Insulin Secretion from Rabbit Pancreas Studied *in vitro*. Diabetologia **3**, 47—49 (1967).

Montague, W., Taylor, K. W.: Islet Cell Metabolism During Insulin Release; Effect of Glucose, Citrate, Octanoate, Tolbutamide, Glucagon and Theophylline. Biochem. J. **115**, 257 (1969).

Moody, A. J., Heding, L. G., Markussen, J., Steenstrup, C., Sundby, F.: The connection between Gut GLI and Insulin Releasing Activity. In: Origin, Chemistry, Physiology and Pathophysiology of the Gastrointestinal Hormones. Schattauer-Verlag, Stuttgart-New York 1970, p. 184—198.

— Markussen, J., Schaich Fries, A., Steenstrup, C., Sundby, F.: The Insulin Releasing Activities of Extracts of Pork Intestine. Diabetologia **6**, 135—140 (1970).

Moore, B., Edie, E. S., Abram, J. H.: On the Treatment of Diabetes Mellitus by Acid Extract of Duodenal Mucous Membrane. Biochem. J. **1**, 28—36 (1906).

Morley, J. S., Tracy, H. J., Gregory, R. A.: Function Relationships in the Active C-Terminal Tetrapeptide Sequence of Gastrin. Nature (Lond.) **207**, 1356—1359 (1965).

Müller, W. A., Faloona, G. R., Aguilar-Parada, E., Unger, R. H.: Abnormal Alpha-Cell Function in Diabetes Response to Carbohydrate and Protein Ingestion. New Engl. J. Med. **283**, 109—115 (1970).

— — Unger, R. H.: The Effect of Experimental Insulin Deficiency on Glucagon Secretion. J. clin. Invest. **50**, 1992—1999 (1971 b).

— — — The Effect of Alanine on Glucagon Secretion. J. clin. Invest. **50**, 2215 (1971 a).

Mutt, V., Jorpes, J. E.: Secretin: Isolation and Determination of Structure (abstr.). Proc. I.U.P.A.C. Fourth International Congress on the Chemistry of Natural Products, June 26—July 2, 1966, Stockholm, Sweden. Section 2C-3.

— Jorpes, J. E.: Contemporary Developments in the Biochemistry of the Gastrointestinal Hormones. Recent Progr. Hormone Res. **23**, 483—491 (1967).

— — Structure of Porcine Cholecystokinin-Pancreozymin I Cleavage with Thrombin and with Trypsin. Europ. J. Biochem. **6**, 156—162 (1968).

— — Cholecystokinin-Pancreozymin. Proc. of the 3. Symp. of Europ. Pancr. Club 2.—4. July 1968. Czech. Med. Press, Praha, 1970, p. 21—24.

— Magnusson, S., Jorpes, J. E., Dahl, E.: Structure of Porcine Secretin I. The Degradation with Trypsin and Thrombin. Sequence of the Tryptic Peptides. The C-Terminal Residue. Biochemistry **4**, 2358—2371 (1965).

Novoa Santos, R.: L'action hypoglycémiante de la sécrétine duodénale. Bull. Soc. Chim. biol. (Paris) **7**, 1151—1162 (1925).

Oehme, C., Wimmers, K.: Wirkung von Duodenalschleimhautextrakten (Sekretin) auf den Blutzucker mit Bemerkungen zur Bewertung der Blutzuckerkurve bei alimentärer Hyperglykämie. Z. ges. exp. Med. **38**, 1—12 (1923).

Ohgawara, H., Mizuno, Y., Tasaka, Y., Kosaka, K.: Effect of the C-Terminal Tetrapeptide Amide of Gastrin on Insulin Secretion in Man. J. clin. Endocr. **29**, 1261—1262 (1969).

Ohneda, A., Aguilar-Parada, E., Eisentraut, A. M., Unger, R. H.: Control of Pancreatic Glucagon Secretion by Glucose. Diabetes **18**, 1—10 (1969).

Ondetti, M. A., Sheehan, J. T., Bodansky, M.: Synthesis of Gastrointestinal Hormones. In: Intern. Symp. on the Pharmacology of Hormonal Polypeptides and Proteins. Milan, Italy, Sept. 14—16, 1967, New York, Plenum Publ. Corp. 1968, p. 18—31.

ONDETTI, M. A., SHEEHAN, J. T., PLUŠČEC, J.: Recent Advances in the Synthesis of Gastrointestinal Hormones. In: Peptides: Chemistryand Biochemistry (Proc. First Amer. Peptide Symposium, Yale Univ., 1968), edit. by B. WEINSTEIN and S. LANDE, p. 181—190. New York: Marcel Dekker, Inc., 1970.

ORCI, L., PICTET, R., FORSSMANN, W. C., RENOLD, A. E., ROUILLER, CH.: Structural Evidence of Glucagon Producing Cells in the Intestinal Mucosa of the Rat. Diabetologia **4**, 56—67 (1968).

PASSARO, E., Jr., BASSO, N., GORDON, E.: Calcium Stimulation of Gastric Secretion. 4th World Congress of Gastroenterology, Copenhagen 1970. Advances Abstr. Edited by Dan. Gastroent. Ass. p. 147.

PAWLOW, I. P.: Die Arbeit der Verdauungsdrüsen. München: I. F. Bergmann 1898.

PEARSE, A. G. E.: Persönliche Mitteilung. II. European Gastric Club, Erlangen 1970.

PENHOS, J., WU, CH. H., BASABE, J. C., LOPEZ, N., WOLFF, F. W.: A Rat Pancreas-Small Gut Preparation for the Study of Intestinal Factors and Insulin Release. Diabetes **18**, 733 (1969).

PENTHEIN, M., SCHOFIELD, B.: Release of Gastrin from the Pyloric Antrum Following Vagal Stimulation by Sham Feeding in Dogs. J. Physiol. (Lond.) **148**, 291—305 (1959).

PERINGS, E., ROHR VON, S., CREUTZFELDT, W.: Untersuchungen über die Wirkung von Neutralrot-Injektionen auf den Kohlehydratstoffwechsel und die A-Zellen von Ratten und Meerschweinchen. 14. Symp. Dtsch. Ges. Endokrinol. Springer-Verlag, Berlin 1969.

PETERSEN, H., BERSTAD, A., MYREN, J.: Effect of Secretin on Histamine and Pentagastrin Stimulated Secretion of Acid in Man. 4th World Congress of Gastroenterology, Copenhagen 1970, Adv. Abstr. Edited by Dan. Gastr. Ass. p. 137.

PFEIFFER, E. F.: Insulin Secretion *in vitro*: Comparative Aspects and Comparisons with Studies on Release of Insulin *in vitro*. Pharmacology of Hormonal Polyp. and Proteins, Milan,Italy, 14—16 Sept. 1967, Adv. in Exp. Med. and Biology, Plenum Press, New York, 1968, p. 317—335.

— Intestinal Factors Controlling Insulin Secretion. VI Congr. IDF, Stockholm 1967, Exc. Med. Found. ICS **172** 419—424 (1969).

— Intestinale Hormone und Insulinsekretion. Verh. Dtsch. Ges. Inn. Med. 75 Band. Verlag J. F. Bergmann 1969, München, p. 296—315.

— FRANK, M., FUSSGÄNGER, R., GOBERNA, R., HINZ, M., RAPTIS, S.: Gastrointestinal Hormones and Islet Function. XVI Nobel Symp. Frontiers in Gastrointestinal Hormone Research, July 20—21, 1970, Almquist and Wiksell Stockholm (in press) 1973.

— — RAPTIS, S.: Gastrointestinal Hormones and Islet Function. 6th Capri Conf., March 29—30, 1972. Acta Diabetologica Latina, Vol. IX, Suppl. 1, 1972, 231—273.

— RAPTIS, S.: Intestinale Hormone und Insulinsekretion. Klin. Wschr. **46**, 337—342 (1968a).

— — Direkte und indirekte Einflüsse intestinaler Hormone auf die Insulinsekretion. Symp. Dtsch. Ges. für Ernährung. Klin. Ernährungslehre III, München 1968 b. Steinkopf Verlag Darmstadt, 1970, p. 34—48.

— TELIB, M., AMMON, J., MELANI, F., DITSCHUNEIT, H.: Direkte Stimulierung der Insulinsekretion in vitro durch Sekretin. Dtsch. med. Wschr. **90**, 1663—1669 (1965); — Diabetologia **1**, 131—132 (1965).

RAPTIS, S.: Enterohormone und endokrimes Pankreas. Serie Gastroenterologie und Stoffwechsel. Stuttgart: Thieme 1973.

— FAULHABER, J. D., SCHRÖDER, K. E.: The Effect of Intestinal Hormones upon Lipolysis of Isolated Human Fat Cells. Horm. Met. Res. Suppl. **1**, 249—250 (1969 a).

— Intestinale Hormone und Inselfunktion der gesunden und kranken menschlichen Bauchspeicheldrüse. Habilitationsschrift Ulm 1971. Thieme Verlag Stuttgart (in press).

— GOBERNA, R., SCHRÖDER, K. E., DITSCHUNEIT, H. H., PFEIFFER, E. F.: Die Wirkung der intestinalen Hormone Sekretion und Pankreozymin bei der totalpankreatektomierten Ratte. 75. Kongreß Dtsch. Ges. Inn. Med. Bergmann-Verlag, München 1969, p. 650—653.

— RAU, R. M., HARTMANN, W., CLODI, P. H., PFEIFFER, E. F.: Effect of Secretin and Pancreozymin on Insulin Secretion in Patients with Exocrine Pancreatic Insufficiency. 5th Ann. Meeting Europ. Ass. Diab. Montpellier 1969. Diabetologia (Abstr.) **6**, 61 (1970).

— — SCHRÖDER, K. E., HARTMANN, W., FAULHABER, J. D., CLODI, P. H., PFEIFFER, E. F.: The Role of the Exocrine Pancreas in the Stimulation of Insulin Secretion by Intestinal Hormones. III. Insulin Responses to Secretin and Pancreozymin and to Oral and Intra-Venous Glucose, in Patients Suffering From Chronic Insufficiency of the Exocrine Pancreas. Diabetologia **7**, 160—167 (1971).

— ROTHENBUCHNER, G., SCHRÖDER, K. E., STRAUB, K., BIRK, J., PFEIFFER, E. F.: Radioimmunologische Bestimmung von Gastrin im menschlichen Serum. Acta endocr. (Kbh.) Suppl. **152**, 10 (1971).

Raptis, S., Schröder, K. E., Faulhaber, J. D., Pfeiffer, E. F.: Stimulierung der Insulinsekretion durch Sekretin bei Diabetikern. Dtsch. med. Wschr. **93**, 2420—2424 (1968).
— — — — Antagonistische Wirkungen von intestinalen Hormonen und Diazoxid auf die Insulinsekretion beim Menschen. Horm. Met. Res. Suppl. **1**, 116—121 (1969).
— — Melani, F., Beyer, J., Pfeiffer, E. F.: Die Beeinflussung der Insulinsekretion durch Sekretin in vivo. Panel discussion "Intestinal Function in Relation to Insulin Secretion". 6th Congr. I.D.F., Stockholm, Aug. 1967. In: E. F. Pfeiffer; Intestinal factors controlling insulin secretion. 6th Congr. I.D.F., Stockholm 1967. Exc. Med. Found. ICS 172/1969, p. 419—424.
— — Pfeiffer, E. F.: Insulin Stimulating Action of Secretin in Maturity Onset Diabetics. Horm. Met. Res. Suppl. **1**, 91—92 (1969).
Rehfeld, J. F.: Effect of Gastrin and its Terminal Tetrapeptide on Insulin Secretion in Man. Acta endocrinologica **66**, 169—176 (1971).
— Heding, L. G.: Increased Release of Gut Glucagon in Reactive Hypoglycaemia. Brit. med. J. **2**, 706—707 (1970).
Rodbell, M., Birnbaumer, L., Pohl, S. L.: Adenyl Cyclase in Fat Cells. III ,Stimulation by Secretin and the Effects of Trypsin on the Receptors for Lipolytic Hormones. J. biol. Chem. **245**, 718—722 (1970).
Ryan, W. G., Nibbe, A., Schwartz, T. B.: Beta-Cytotropic Effects of Glucose, Glucagon and Tolbutamide in Man. Lancet **1967 I**, 1255—1256.
Samols, E., Marks, V.: Nouvelles conceptions sur la signification fonctionelle du glucagon (pancréatique et extrapancréatique). Journée Ann. de Diab, Hotel-Dieu, Flammarion 1967, p. 43—66.
— Marri, G., Marks, V.: Interrelationship of Glucagon, Insulin and Glucose: The Insulinogenic Effect of Glucagon. Diabetes **15**, 855—866 (1966).
— Tyler, J., Marri, G., Marks, V.: Stimulation of Glucagon Secretion by Oral Glucose. Lancet **1965 II**, 1257—1259.
— — Megyesi, C., Marks, V.: Immunochemical Glucagon in Human Pancreas, Gut and Plasma. Lancet **1966 II**, 727—729.
Santeusiano, F., Faloona, G. R., Unger, R. H.: Glucagon Suppressing Action of Secretin. Diabetes **20**, Suppl. 1, 339, Abstr. 49 (1971).
Sarles, H., Pastor, J., Pauli, A. M., Barthelemy, M.: Determination of Pancreatic Function. Gastroenterologia (Basel) **99**, 279—300 (1963).
Schaeffer, L. D., Wilder, M. W., Williams, R. H.: Insulin and Glucagon Release from Human Fetal Pancreas Slices *in vitro*. Diabetes Suppl. **20**, 326 (1971).
Schröder, K. E., Raptis, S., Faulhaber, J. D., Pfeiffer, E. F.: Die Wirkung von Pankreozymin auf Blutzucker, immunologisch meßbarem Insulin, freien Fettsäuren und Glycerin beim Menschen. 14. Symp. Dtsch. Ges. Endokrinologie, Heidelberg 7.—9. März 1968, Springer-Verlag, p. 170—171.
— — — I. D. Fussgänger, R. D., Straub, K., Pfeiffer, E. F.: Differences in the Alpha- and Beta-Cytotropic Effect of Pancreozymin in Normal and Diabetic Subjects. 4. Kongr. Dtsch.Diab. Ges., Ulm 1969. Diabetologia (Abstr.) **6**, 81 (1970).
— — Telib, M., Pfeiffer, E. F.: Intestinal Hormones Affecting Insulin Secretion *in vitro*: Secretin, Pancreozymin, Gastrin. 6th Congr. Intern. Diabetes Federation. In: E. F. Pfeiffer: Intestinal Factors Controlling Insulin Secretion. 6th Congr. I.D.F. Stockholm 1967. Exc. Med. Found. ICS 172/1969, p. 419—424.
Scow, R. P., Cornfield, J.: Quantitative Relations Between the Oral and Intravenous Glucose Tolerance Curves. Amer. J. Physiol. **179**, 435—438 (1954).
Seltzer, H. S., McNeff, J.: Similar Insulin Secretory Response to Oral and Intraveneous Glucose Loads in Dogs. Clin. Res. (Abstr.) **15**, 138 (1967).
Sherman, B., Gordon, P., Roth, J.: Stimulation of Insulin Secretion of Slices of a Transplantable Beta-Cell Tumor of Syrian Hamsters *in vitro*. J. clin. Invest. in press. (1971).
Simpson, R. G., Benedetti, A., Grodsky, G. M., Karam, J. H., Forsham, P. H.: Stimulation of Insulin Release by Glucagon in Non-Insulin Dependent Diabetics. Metabolism **15**, 1046—1049 (1966).
Smith, A. N., Hogg, D.: Effect of Gastrin II on the Motility of the Gastrointestinal Tract. Lancet **1966 I**, 403—404.
Solcia, E., Sampietro, R.: Cytologic Observations on Pancreatic Islets with Reference to Some Endocrine-Like Cells of the Gastrointestinal Mucosa. Z. Zellforsch. **68**, 689—698 (1965).
— Vassallo, G., Sampietro, R.: Endocrine Cells in the Antro-Pyloric Mucosa of the Stomach. Z. Zellforsch. **81**, 474—486 (1967).
Somersalo, O.: Staub Effect in Children. Acta paediat. (Helsinki) (Suppl. 78) 1950.

Still, E. U., Bennett, A. L., Scott, V. B.: A Study of the Metabolic Activity of the Pancreas. Amer. J. Physiol. **106**, 509—523 (1933).

Sussman, K. E., Vaughan, G. D.: Insulin Release After ACTH, Glucagon, and Adenosine-3′-5′-phosphate (cyclic AMP) in the Perfused Isolated Rat Pancreas. Diabetes **16**, 449—454, (1967).

— — Timmer, R. F.: An in vitro Methode for Studying Insulin Secretion in the Perfused Isolated Rat Pancreas. Metabolism **15**, 466 (1966).

Sutherland, E. W., de Duve, Ch.: Origin and Distribution of the Hyperglycemic-Glycogenolytic Factor of the Pancreas. J. biol. Chem. **175**, 663—674 (1948).

Taylor, A. E., Hulton, F.: Limit of Assimilation of Glucose. J. biol. Chem. **25**, 173—179 (1916).

Telib, M.: Der Einfluß von Monosacchariden und Hormonen auf die Insulin-Sekretion verschiedener Wirbeltiere. Inaug.-Diss. Frankfurt 1967.

— Vergleichende Untersuchungen über den Einfluß von Monosacchariden und Hormonen auf die Insulinsekretion des isolierten Pankreasgewebes einiger Säugetiere und des Frosches. Z. ges. exp. Med. **147**, 316—332 (1968).

— Pfeiffer, E. F.: Dynamics of Insulin Secretion *in vitro*: Effects of Repeated Induction of Insulin Release by Single and Multiple Stimulants. Endokrinologie **56**, 2 (1970).

— Raptis, S., Schröder, K. E., Pfeiffer, E. F.: Serotonin and Insulin Release *in vitro*. Diabetologia **4**, 253—256 (1968).

Thomas, T.: Cellular Components of the Mammalian Islets of Langerhans. Amer. J. Anat. **62**, 31—39 (1937).

Track, N. S.: Possible Evolution of the Endodermal Polypeptide Hormones Insulin, Glucagon, Secretin and Gastrin. Diabetologia (Abstr.) **5**, 56 (1969).

Troteano, V. C.: Recherches experimentales sur les variations de la glycémie determinée par la sécrétine. C. R. Soc. Biol. (Paris) **91**, 1368 (1924).

Trudeau, W. L., McGuigan, J. E.: Relations between Serum Gastrin Levels and Rates of Gastric Hydrochloric Acid Secretion. Gastroenterology **284**, 408—412 (1971).

Turner, D. S.: Incretin — an Insulinotrophic Hormone? (Abstract) Program Brit. Diabetes Assoc. Meeting London, 1967, p. 1010. Diabetol. **4**, 177 (1968).

— Intestinal Hormones and Insulin Release: *In vitro* Studies using Rabbit Pancreas. Horm. Metab. Res. **1**, 168 (1969).

— Gastrointestinal Hormones and Insulin Secretion *in vitro*. In: Origin, Chemistry, Physiology and Pathophysiology of the Gastrointestinal Hormones. Schattauer-Verlag, Stuttgart-New York 1970 p. 171—184.

— McIntyre, N.: Stimulation by Glucagon of Insulin Release from Rabbit Pancreas *in vitro*. Lancet **1966 I**, 351—352.

Unger, R. H., Aguilar-Parada, E., Müller, W. A., Eisentraut, A. M.: Studies of Pancreatic Alpha-Cell Function in Normal and Diabetic Subjects. J. clin. Invest. **45**, 387 (1970).

— Eisentraut, A. M.: Études récentes sur la physiologie du glucagon. Journées de Diabet. Hôtel-Dieu, Vol. I Flammarion, Paris 1967 a, p. 1—18.

— — Glucagon. In: Hormones in Blood. (Gray, C. H., Bacharach, A. L., eds.) Vol. I Academic Press London and New York 1967 b, p. 83—128.

— — Madison, L. L.: The Effect of Total Starvation upon the Levels of Circulating Glucagon and Insulin in Men. J. clin. Invest. **42**, 1031,—1034 (1963).

— — McCall, M. S., Madison, L. L.: Measurement of Endogenous Glucagon in Plasma and the Influence of Blood Glucose Concentration upon its Secretion. J. clin. Invest. **41**, 682 (1962).

— — Sims, M., McCall, M. S., Madison, L. L.: Sites of Origin of Glucagon in Dogs and Humans. Clin. Res. **9**, 53 (1961).

— Ketterer, H., Dupré, J., Eisentraut, A. M.: The Effects of Secretin, Pancreozymin and Gastrin on Insulin and Glucagon Secretion in Anesthetized Dogs. J. clin. Invest. **46**, 630—645 (1967).

— — Eisentraut, A., Dupré, J.: Effect of Secretin on Insulin Secretion. Lancet **1966 II**, 24—26.

— Ohneda, A., Valverde, I., Eisentraut, A. M., Exton, J.: Characterization of the Responses of Circulating Glucagon-Like Immunoreactivity to Intraduodenal and Intravenous Administration of Glucose. J. clin. Invest. **47**, 48—65 (1968).

Vagne, M., Grossman, M. I.: Cholecystokinetic Potency of Gastrointestinal Hormones and Related Peptides. Amer. J. Physiol. **215** 881—884 (1968).

Valverde, I., Rigopoulou, D., Exton, J., Ohneda, A., Eisentraut, A. M., Unger, R. H.: Demonstration and Characterization of a Second Fraction by Glucagon Like Immunoreactivity in Jejunal Extracts. Amer. J. med. Sci. **255**, 6 (1968).

VALVERDE, I., RIGOPOULOU, MARCO, J., FALOONA, G. R., UNGER, R. H.: Characterization of Glucagon Like Immunoreactivity (GLI). Diabetes **19**, 614 and 624 (1970).

VANCE, J. E., BUCHANAN, K. D., CHALLONER, D. R., WILLIAMS, R. H.: The Effect of Glucose Concentration on Insulin and Glucagon Released from Isolated Islets of Langerhans of the Rat. Diabetes **17**, 187—193 (1968).

— — WILLIAMS, R. H.: Effect of Starvation and Refeeding on Serum Immunoreactive Insulin and Glucagon Levels. J. Lab. Clin. Med. **72**, 290 (1968).

VANOTTI, A.: HADJIKHANI, H., FASEL, J., GUIDOUX, L., FELBER, J. P.: The Endocrine Function of the Intestinal Mucosa. Amer. J. Proctol. **20**, 68—71 (1969).

VECCHIO, D., LUYCKX, A., ZAHND, G. R., RENOLD, A. E.: Insulin Release Induced by Glucagon in Organ Cultures of Fetal Rat Pancreas. Metabolism **15**, 577—581 (1966).

WAITMAN, A. M., JANOWITZ, H. D.: The Effect of Secretin and Acetazolamide on the Volume and Electrolyte Composition of Hepatic Bile in Man. J. clin. Invest. (Abstr.) **46**, 1127 (1967).

WANG, C. C., GROSSMAN, M. I.: Physiological Determination of Release of Secretin and Pancreozymin from Intestine of Dogs with Transplanted Pancreas. Amer. J. Physiol. **164**, 527—545 (1951).

WEBER, B., QUABBE, H. J., HELGE, H.: Glucagoninduzierte Insulinsekretion bei adipösen und juvenilen Diabetikern 14. Symp. Dtsch. Ges. Endokr., Heidelberg 1968, Springer-Verlag, Berlin-Heidelberg-New York 1968, p. 272—281.

WEINGES, K. F.: Das Verhalten der insulinähnlichen Aktivität (ILA) und der Glukoseverwertung (GA) im peripheren Blut nach intravenösen oder oralen Glukosegaben und nach Glukagonbelastung beim Menschen. 1. Symp. d. Dtsch. Diabetes-Komitee, 26. bis 27. 10. 1962, p. 53—56, Düsseldorf, Thieme-Verlag.

WHITE, J. J., DUPRÉ, J.: Regulation of Insulin Secretion by the Intestinal Hormone Secretin: Studies in Man Via Transumbilical Portal Vein Catheterization. Surgery **64**, 204—213 (1968).

WOODYATT, R. T., SANSUM, W. D., WILDER, R. M.: Prolonged and Accurately Timed Intravenous Injections of Sugar. J. Amer. med. Ass. **65**, 2067—2081 (1916).

WORMSLEY, K. G.: Response to Secretin in Man. Gastroenterology **54**, 197—209 (1968).

YALOW, R. S., BERSON, S. A.: Immunoassay of Plasma Insulin Concentrations in Normal and Diabetic Man: Insulin SecretoryResponse to Glucose and other Agents. J. Clin. Invest. **39**, 1041—1052 (1960).

— — Radioimmunoassay of Gastrin. Gastroenterology **58**, 1—14 (1970).

YOUNG, J. D., LAZARUS, L., CHISHOLM, D. J.: Secretin and Pancreozymin-Cholecystokinin After Glucose (Letter to the Editor). Lancet **1968 a II**, 914.

— — — ATKINSON, F. F. V.: Radioimmunoassay of Secretin in Human Serum. J. nucl. Med. **9**, 641—642 (1968 b).

— — — — Radioimmunoassay of Pancreozymin Cholecystokinin in Human Serum. J. nucl. Med. **10**, 743—745 (1969).

ZAYTZUCK, R., AMATO, J. J., PALOYAN, E., BAKER, R. J.: Inhibition of Pancreatic Exocrine Secretion by Glucagon. Surg. Forum **18**, 410—411 (1967).

ZUNZ, E., LA BARRE, J.: Hyperinsulinémie consécutive après l'injection de solution de sécrétine non-hypotensive. C. R. Soc. Biol. (Paris) **98**, 1435—1438 (1928).

Chapter VII

The Use of Cholecystokinin in the Roentgenological Examination

II. Clinical Aspects

JACQUES PLESSIER

With 10 Figures

I. Introduction. Early History

Like the bladder, which can be distended by urine, the gallbladder is often distended by bile in consequence of obstruction or atony of its expulsive power (GALEN).

1800 years after GALEN, IVY and coworkers (IVY and OLDBERG 1928; IVY et al., 1928, 1930) described a method enabling us by means of an extract of the intestinal mucosa to influence the contractibility of the gallbladder. Contraction of the gallbladder, following the administration of 25—30 mg dry powder of the mucosal extract every 10 min in 5 healthy persons and 3 patients, was visualized roentgenologically. IVY (1947, 1955) envisaged the use of the active component, named cholecystokinin (CCK), in the diagnosis of biliary dyskinesia. After a dose of 11 mg in 5 persons and 23 mg in 3 subjects DENTON, GERSHBEIN and IVY (1950) observed on some occasions a complete absence of contraction or a very strong evacuation.

British authors (DUNCAN, HARPER, HOWAT, OLEESKY and VARLEY, 1950, 1952; DUNCAN et al., 1953; BURTON et al., 1960) suggested the use of "pancreozymin", as discovered by HARPER and RAPER (1943) in the extract of intestinal mucosa, for the study of the function of the gallbladder. The bile was collected with a duodenal tube and the reduction in volume of the gallbladder was measured in the cholecystographic picture. The large amounts of the highly impure preparation needed for an injection, 150—200 mg, was an obstacle limiting the use of the technique. Not more successful was an attempt by MORIN, BUSSON and BLANCHET (1955) to use a poorly purified cholecystokinin preparation.

When a cholecystokinin preparation with 20 IVY dog units per mg, as purified by JORPES and MUTT (1954, 1956, 1959), was obtained, its applicability as an adjuvant in cholecystography was demonstrated by JÖNSSON (1955), BRODÉN (1956), WERNER (1956) and BERK and FEIGELSON (1957). Except for a mild flush reaction in the face in some cases, the product was well tolerated, if injected 1 U/kg i.v. during the course of ½ min. In the 14 normal cases of the series of BRODÉN there was a contraction of the gallbladder and filling of the common duct within one minute and in some cases a spontaneous reflux into the hepatic ducts, irrespective of whether morphine was given. The picture was the same irrespective of the presence of bile stones. GUNNARSSON (1956) recommended the use of CCK in cases not responding to the fat meal or where a deficient release of endogenous CCK was suspected. In October 1956 ADLERCREUTZ, JORPES, MUTT and WEGELIUS (1957) communicated in the Société Nationale Française de Gastro-entérologie on a series of 30 normal subjects with radiographs taken every minute during the first 10 min and then 15, 20 and 60 min after injection. After 1 min there was a distinct contraction of the gallbladder followed by a visualization of the common duct which reached its maximum within 5 to 10 min. The authors observed rhythmic contractions alternating with relaxations of the gallbladder.

The following discussion deals with the experiences of the large number of authors who thereafter used cholecystokinin with a strength of 250—300 U/mg, as purified by JORPES and MUTT (1961, 1962) and here called CCK J. M., in their studies on the evacuation of the gallbladder, the filling of the common duct and of the intrahepatic biliary ducts and the behavior of the sphincter of Oddi. Oral cholecystography with single or serial uptakes, radiomanometry, cinematography and scintigraphy were applied, the dose or the variable doses of CCK being administered either as a single i.v. injection lasting ½ up to 5 min, as repeated injections or as an i.v. infusion.

The extrabiliary action of CCK on the *motility* of the duodenum and particularly of the *jejuno-ileum* has allowed the development of a technique with a highly reduced transit time in the radiologic examination of the small intestine.

The *vasomotor effect* in the splanchnic area obtained by intra-celiac injection of CCK is quite considerable. It is, however, much more pronounced after the *intra-arterial injection of secretin.*

Cholecystokinin is furthermore a valuable adjuvant in the pharmaco-scintigraphy of the bile ducts and the pancreas.

II. Cholecystokinin and the Evacuation of the Gallbladder

1. In Healthy Subjects

JORPES, MUTT, TOMENIUS and BACKLUND (1957, 1958) made, using oral cholecystograms in 59 patients (35 normal subjects, 16 with biliary lithiasis and 8 with an atonic gallbladder), a comparison between CCK and the egg-yolk meal. Radiographs were taken before the fat meal and every 5 min during the first ½ h, then every 15 min during the first hour and then hourly until 3 h. Two to five days later a similar analysis was made before and after i.v. injection of 40 or 75 units of CCK. Four cases, refractive to the egg-yolk meal, did react to CCK. In 14 cases the reaction after CCK was stronger than occurred after the egg-yolk meal, in 16 cases equal and in 5 cases weaker. A similar distribution was found among the 15 cases with biliary lithiasis. In all cases the reaction to CCK was faster, within 1—2 min, than with the fat meal, the maximum being reached within 10—20 min. The response was also more regular.

The experiences of several Swedish authors have been presented in a series of communications and summarizing articles dealing with the chemistry, biological activities and clinical applications of CCK (JORPES and MUTT, 1959, 1967, 1969; JORPES, MUTT and TOCZKO, 1964; JORPES, MUTT, TOMENIUS and BACKLUND, 1957, 1958; MUTT and JORPES, 1968a, b).

In studying the behavior of the gallbladder and the sphincter of Lutkens of the dog towards CCK, ALLEGRI, BALDRIGHI and MONTEMARTINI (1957) found a response to CCK within 60 sec after injection, predominantly located in the neck region. BRODÉN (1958), still working with the old preparation of CCK with 22 units per mg, found side reactions to be minimal if the i.v. injection was administered slowly during the course of 20—30 sec. 60—75 units was found to be a suitable dose.

MEINARDUS (1959), in a series of 25 patients, observed a less satisfactory contraction of the gallbladder in only 3 of the cases. A similar frequency, 3 out of 30 cases, was reported by BRÜNNER and GUDBJERG (1959) and by HAEX and LIMBURG (1960) (3 out of 27 patients).

In a preliminary series of cholecystograms starting in 1959 in cooperation with P. PORCHER, J. CAROLI and coworkers we used 75 units of CCK, J. M. (250 U/mg) and duodenal intubation (PLESSIER, 1960), oral cholecystography with pictures taken in frontal and lateral positions (PLESSIER and MARSICO, 1960) or chronoradiocinematography (GILLES and PLESSIER, unpublished). The volume of the gallbladder was calculated according to the method of J. TOULET (1953). In a series of 40 patients, studied by means of duodenal intubation and cholecystography, 15 min after the i.v. injection, the volume was reduced by more than 50% in 85% of the cases (Fig. 1). In 15% of the cases the reduction was less than 20%. It seemed unnecessary to follow the effect for a longer period than 20 min. The chronoradiocinematography produced a picture every two seconds (PORCHER et al., 1967) whereby the intermittent evacuation of the gallbladder following the single injections of CCK could be demonstrated. The appearance in the duodenum of bile, enriched with pigments, followed the same course.

EDHOLM (1958) examined 102 patients with biliary pathology, including 60 cases with biliary calculi. Five cases were examined in the prone position and 97 in the supine right anterior oblique position (15 to 20 degrees). In all but 10 cases the CCK was given in i.v. infusion. The volume of the gallbladder was reduced to more than half apart from 2 cases who showed a resistance to even a double dose of CCK. Here the wall of the gallbladder seemed to be altered. No hindrance to the flow of bile was experienced in the 70 lithiasis cases. Some patients complained of pain or discomfort which disappeared, when the infusion of CCK was stopped.

In a cholecystographic study on 69 patients, women during the menopause, DUX and THURN (1960) obtained films 2, 5 and 15 min after injection in 35 of the cases, made rapid seriography with an Odelka camera in 19 cases and Roentgen-cinematography in 15 cases. The contraction of the infundibulum followed immediately after the i.v. injection. The expulsion of bile, marked with contrast medium, as seen in the cineradiography, was rhythmic with a short periodicity (2 to 3 sec). This type of evacuation had no similarity to the passive and continuous evacuation as found in a water pump system. The fundic and the corpuscular parts of the shadow disappeared quickly and symmetrically.

After a latent period of 10—30 sec following the injection of CCK TORSOLI, RAMORINO, COLAGRANDE and DEMAIO (1961) observed a period of tonic contraction, lasting for 15 to 60 sec, with closure of the infundibulum-cystic duct junction, followed by an expulsion period lasting 5 to 30 min when the junction was open. During the tonic contraction the transverse diameter of the infundibulum is reduced and its demarcation lines usually unrecognisable. During the first 10 min the contraction of the infundibular part of the gallbladder predominates. In some cases the response to CCK is excessive with a disappearance of the infundibular cavity and reclosure of the cystic canal more or less obstructing the bile flow. Such a picture with the specific action on the infundibulum, is typical of the action of CCK. After the egg-yolk meal it is seen at first at the end of the evacuation period. In its action on the gallbladder CCK is a quite specific agent, its action on the infundibulum being almost proportional to the dose and the rapidity of its administration.

Bossi (1961) gave 75 units of CCK either as an infusion dissolved in 250 ml physiological saline solution during 20 min or as a single injection lasting 30 sec. 2—3 exposures were made during the first 5 min and a single exposure 10 min after injection. He insisted on the importance of the side view in order to distinguish between the contraction and evacuation. The maximal evacuation was 75% of the initial volume at the same time as the surface reduction was 50%. A reduction in volume of less than 25% is considered to be abnormal.

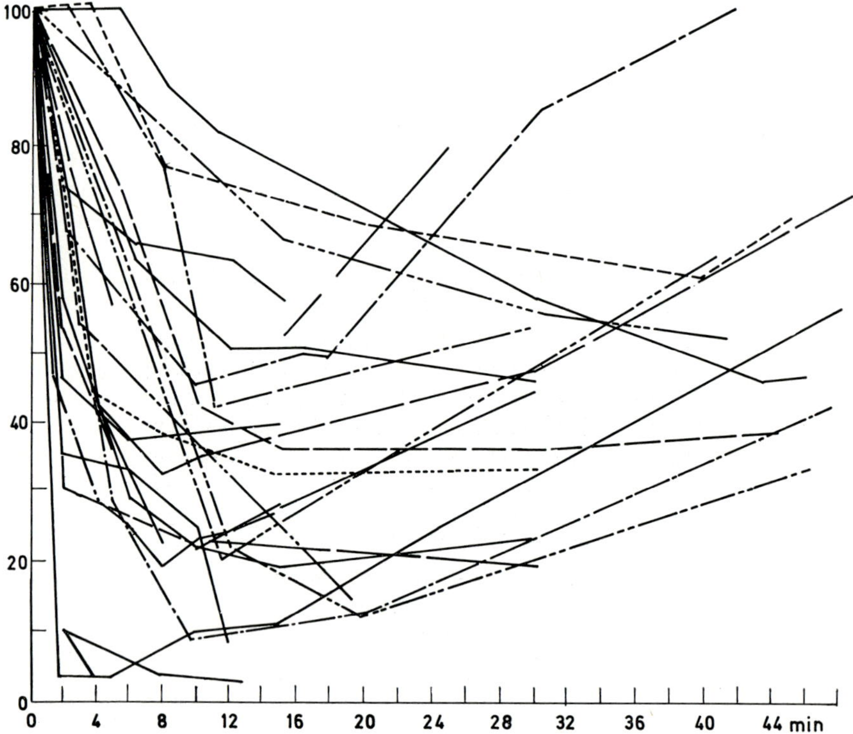

Fig. 1. Duodenal intubation and cholecystographies showed in 85% of the 40 subjects studied a more than 50% reduction in volume of the gallbladder as calculated according to Toulet

Mamie and Kleinert (1962) injected 75 units i.v. during the course of 4—5 min and took films at 2, 10, 20 and 30 min thereafter. They measured the transverse diameter of the gallbladder at its highest value. In 40 cases out of 72 the mean reduction of the gallbladder shadow was 2/3 of the initial value. In most cases the response developed in 2—10 min and lasted for 20 min. Sometimes the effect slowed down considerably after the first 10 min. In 21 of the cases there was a weaker reaction, but strong enough to provoke an evacuation of the gallbladder; in 11 cases no reduction of the dimensions was seen. The authors found a "fighting" gallbladder in 16 cases out of 72 observations, and were impressed by the sudden contraction of the infundibulum.

We recommend the thesis of LESCUT of Lille (1963) who studied, in different groups, the effect of the time of injection on function. In 91 cases, he injected 25 units per min during *three min* and in 27 cases 15 units per min in *five min*. In 17 cases a comparative study of the two methods was made. In the first group, there was no vesicular contraction in three cases (3.3%); it was moderate (less than 50% in ten minutes) in 67% of the cases and important (more than 50%) in 29.7% of the cases. If the injections were made over five min time, the percentage was 11.1; 40.7; 48.2; respectively. An elective contraction of the

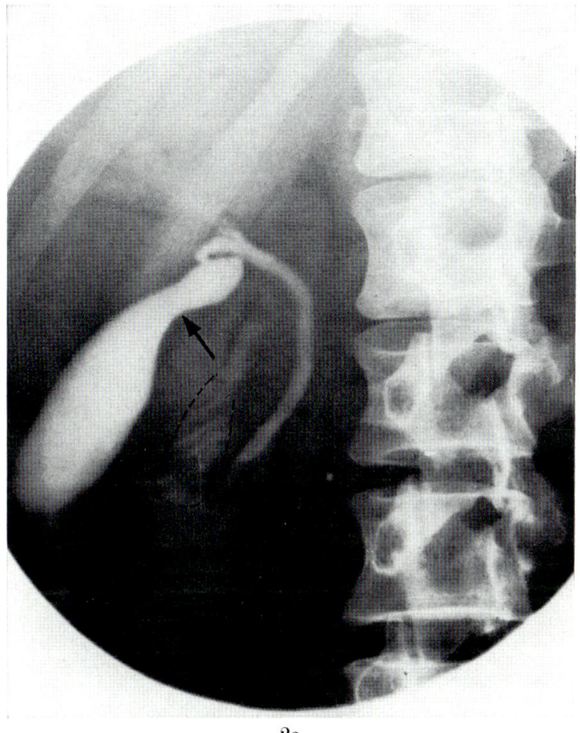

2a

Fig. 2a–c. The action of CCK is predominant in the infundibular region. The common bile duct is visible. Within 1 min the duodenum begins to be filled and thereafter follows during 5 — 10 min a continuous dilatation

infundibulum was noted in 25% of the cases and according to the intensity and the time of the beginning of the contraction, it may, or may not cause evacuation. The lithiasic gallbladder reacted in almost the same way as a non lithiasic gallbladder. In chronic pancreatitis, the percentage of strong responses is much higher.

COZZOLINO, GOLDSTEIN, GREENING and WIRTS in 1963 measured the contraction and the volume of the gallbladder, according to the method of SIFFERT (1949) in 17 control cases and 7 patients having a cystic duct syndrome. Pictures were taken 2, 3, 5, 8, 10, 15 and 20 min after injection. The graphic representation of normal subjects was similar to that which we have described before (Fig. 1). But all the patients with a cystic duct syndrome had a residual vesicular volume more than 50%; usually the gallbladder became spherical.

Later on, we shall come back to the excessive and predominant action of cholecystokinin on the infundibulum and the cystic duct.

DAHLGREN (1966), studying the evacuation of the gallbladder, found that a variation of dose between 0.3 U/kg and 1 U/kg body weight has no influence upon the results.

GRILL, PICHLMAIER, NEFF and STUHLFAUTH (1963) likewise paid particular attention to the regulatory mechanism for the emptying of the gallbladder and to the importance of the cervix region.

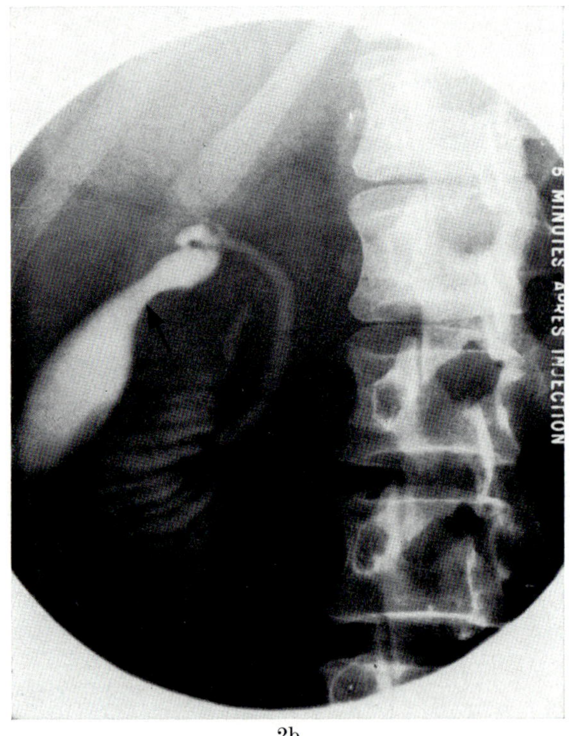

2b

NATHAN, NEWMAN, MACFARLAND and MURRAY (1969) found a reduction of less than 35% of the initial volume in only 19 out of 50 cases. The contraction of the gallbladder proceeded in a regular manner. A prolonged contraction of the cystic duct was interpreted as pathological. The diameter of the duct, varying between 1 and 4 mm, was difficult to measure due to the Heisterian valves.

WESTBROOK (1970) injected CCK in a series of 22 patients during the course of 3 min and took pictures after 1, 3, 5, 8, 10 and 20 min. After 10—15 min the residual volume after contraction of the gallbladder was considerably below 50% of the initial volume, in all but 2 cases.

BACKLUND (1970) found that CCK in 15% of his patients increased the tone of the vesicular wall without provoking an evacuation of the gallbladder. In his material of 400 pathological cases, half of the cases had a normal reaction to CCK, whereas in the other half the symptoms were aggravated with progressive alterations of the vesicular wall resulting in an inability to concentrate the contrast medium. The disturbed motility of the gallbladder, thus observed under the action of CCK, has according to BACKLUND a prognostic value in evaluating the future course of the illness. His experience extended from 1957 to 1970 (Jorpes, et al., 1957, 1958; Backlund and Peterson, 1962, 1965; Backlund, 1964, 1967, 1968, 1970).

To this we can add a series of 1500 cholecystograms of our own performed during the years 1962—1970 using the purified CCK with 250 Ivy dog units per mg (Plessier et al., 1966).

We have modified our previous technique to some extent. The right anterior oblique position is, with few exceptions, the best. The time of injection is also

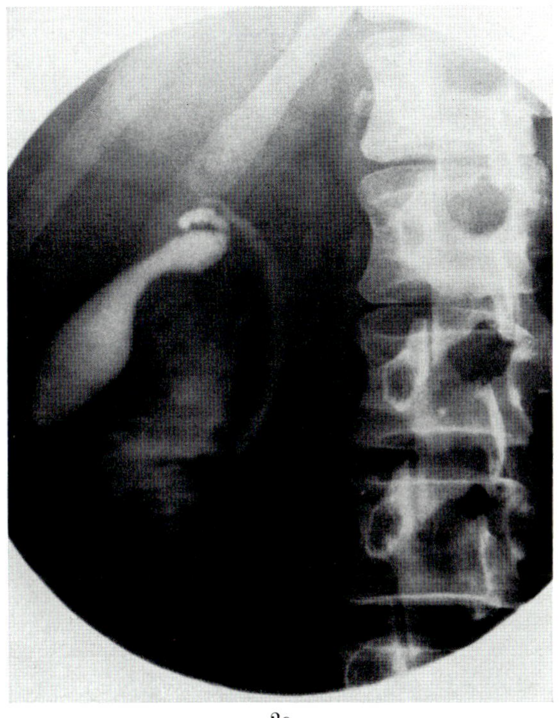

2c

shortened. After dissolving 75 units of CCK in 7.5 ml physiological saline solution, 1 U/kg is injected intravenously during the course of 30 sec. Films are taken after 1, 3, 5 and 10 min, counting from middle of the injection time (Fig. 2a, b, c). In about half of the number of cases the evacuation of the gallbladder was followed on the television screen. In reviewing the series of 100 normal subjects and a series of lithiasis cases, where the gallbladder still retained the capacity to concentrate the contrast medium, we could only confirm our previous findings from 1959 and 1960 concerning the sudden onset of the evacuation after the CCK injection. From the first minute the infundibular region was clearly visualized. When the fundus began to contract, the diverticulae of Luschka were more distinctly recognized. The gallstones moved freely. Only once did we see a microcalculus retained in the cystic duct. This tiny stone was invisible in the previous pictures taken after a fatty meal. In our lithiasis material the evacuation of the gallbladder after CCK proceeded normally except in a few cases, where the swollen mucosa partly occluded the cystic duct. Lithiasis and dyskinesia are two quite different pathological phenomena.

2. The Pathology of Gallbladder Evacuation

By combining duodenal intubation with cholecystography using CCK GARBSCH, MÜLLNER and TRETENKAHN (1961) were able to divide their dyskinesia material in three groups: hyperkinetic, hypokinetic and hypertonic (16, 15 and 6 cases respectively). They measured the maximum diameter of the gallbladder and the bilirubin concentration, paying particular attention to dyskinesias of the infundibulo-ductal region. Radiography after CCK was a prerequisite for the differential diagnosis.

American colleagues COZZOLINO, GOLDSTEIN, GREENING and WIRTS (1963) have, since cholecystokinin became available reanimated the discussion of *the cystic duct syndrome* previously studied by a number of authors like SCHMIDEN (1920), BERG (1922), ALBOT et al., (1957), CAROLI (1949), POILLEUX (1947) and DEBRAY et al. (1958). The authors made the remarkable observation that the filling and the evacuation of the gallbladder after the fat meal proceeded as in healthy subjects in the 7 cases studied by them. The use of CCK in the oral cholecystographies and duodenal intubation allowed them in every case to demonstrate a partial obstruction of the cystic duct. The CCK injection elicited an abdominal pain, which was ameliorated by nitroglycerine. Cholecystectomy was performed in all cases with disappearance of the symptoms. Attention had been paid by the authors to the subjective symptoms and to the results of the duodenal intubation, the pancreatic secretion test, the cholecystogram, to the peroperative findings and to the histological examination.

FARRAR (1966) called attention to the relative frequency, 10%, of faulty diagnosis, with negative cholecystographic findings, usually hidden calculi or dyskinesia of the infundibular-cystic duct region, which can be visualized after an i.v. CCK injection.

MACFARLAND and CURRIN (1969) likewise found the pain provoked by CCK, and ameliorated by nitroglycerine, in combination with the spasm in the infundibular region, as visualized in cholecystography, to be satisfactory diagnostic criteria justifying an operation. One of the patients, considered to be a mental case, experienced 20 sec after the CCK injection a violent pain, lasting for one hour, which was ameliorated by nitroglycerine. After cholecystectomy the cystic duct was found to be fibrotic. The long term course was uneventful as in 2 other cases operated upon

WESTBROOK (1970) studied 9 cases, in which the *residual volume* of the gallbladder was high, 70 to 90% of the initial volume. In 3 of his patients he found a "fighting" gallbladder. The pain developed after CCK, lasting for 3 to 8 min after injection, was almost identical to the spontaneous pain. In 8 of his cases the symptoms disappeared after cholecystectomy.

Among our 700 cases of biliary dyskinesia the majority belong to the group characterized as vesicular *hypertony* with prolonged spasm of the infundibular region. In this syndrome the gallbladder really deserves the epithet "fighting". The attempts at evacuation can be seen on the television screen. By means of CCK the cause of the subjective symptoms, most frequently occurring in female patients, can be objectively demonstrated within a few minutes (Fig. 3a, b, c, d, e, f). It is no longer necessary to repeat the side examination in order to measure the angle of erection of the gallbladder as described by ALBOT et al., (1951).

Likewise preoperative transparietal radiomanometry as developed by KAPANDJI (1959) is superfluous. In all our patients the radiological observations were supplemented by duodenal intubation.

In a number of cases, about 100, the gallbladder seemed to be asystolic in response to the resistance in the duct.

If the behavior of the gallbladder is analyzed closely after a viral hepatitis, the whole accessory biliary system is in an atonic state, the mucosa of the gallbladder being unable to concentrate the contrast medium.

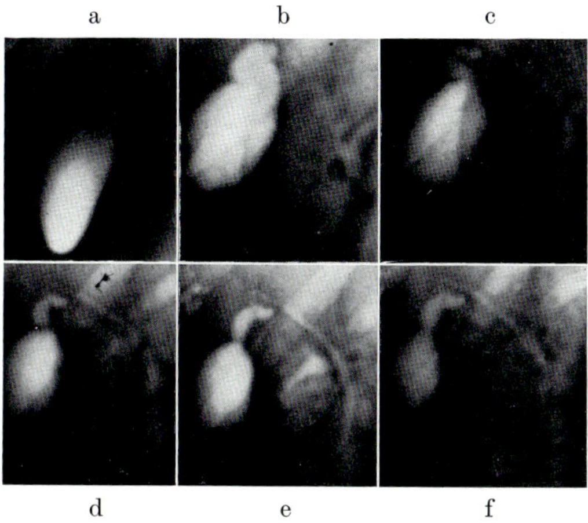

Fig. 3. The severe pain, developing one minute after the CCK-injection and lasting for more than 10 min, was identical with the spontaneous attacks, experienced by the patient, and coincided with an infundibular spasm, which lasted for 15 min

A *hypertonic state*, with almost complete emptying of the gallbladder within 1 to 3 min after the i.v. injection, was observed in about 40 cases presenting allergic symptoms or with parietal alterations of the ASCHOFF sinuses (Fig. 4a, b, c, d). Bacteriological analysis of the bile from the patients with a hypertonic gallbladder most often showed an infection with enterococci or E. coli and sometimes pathogenic staphylococci, in no case due to side contamination from the duodenal tube.

Cases of typhic cholecystitis with reduced motility of the gallbladder and a deficient capacity to concentrate were rare in our series. The bile collected with the duodenal tube, after CCK was concentrated and rich in pigment and salmonellae, visible on direct inspection. VEJBORA, SVATOS and DVORACKOVA (1967) observed a permanent reduction in the contractibility of the gallbladder in guinea pigs sensitized to E. coli and in normal guinea pigs treated with a dose of Endotoxine S and paratyphoid B.

Genuine atony of the gallbladder as described by KEHR, HENSCHEN and particularly by CHIRAY and LOMON of Paris, PAVEL of Bucarest and MILOCHEVITCH of Belgrad are rare. These atonic states are characterized by a deficient contractility of the gallbladder both before and after a fatty meal. The bile collected by the duodenal tube is of increased volume and rich in pigments. Repeated stimulation with warmed olive oil or with magnesium sulfate is often needed to produce an evacuation. Usually no bacteria or leucocytes are seen in the bile.

A series like this may possibly include patients with a *deficient capacity to release endogenous CCK*. In normal persons, the bile collected after CCK is always rich in pigments. In our series we looked for and found very few cases with a genuine atonic state of the gallbladder. In these cases CCK did not produce any contraction in any part of the gallbladder. Attempts to stimulate the bile flow into the duodenum resulted only in an increased choleresis but never in a

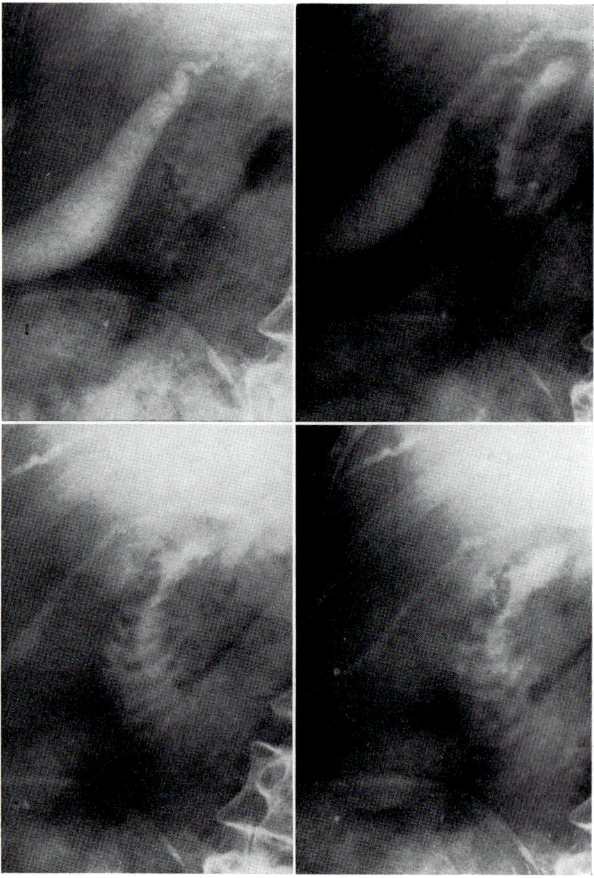

Fig. 4. A patient with general allergic symptoms and a hypertonic early response to CCK. After 3 min the gallbladder was emptied. Due to the hypotonic sphincter of Oddi the duodenum was immediately filled

contraction of the gallbladder. In this connection we have determined the level of CCK in the blood before and after CCK stimulation, according to the method of SVATOS (1957, 1959) (Fig. 5) in which serum or urine of the patient is injected into a guinea pig and the increase in the intravesicular pressure measured manometrically. There was no rise in the CCK level of the plasma or in the "urocholecystokinin" content of the urine following the duodenal stimulation. On the contrary the content of an *anticholecystokinetic factor*, as determined according to the method of CAROLI, PLESSIER and PLESSIER (1960), was constantly increased after the duodenal stimulation. In contradistinction to normal cases and cases with an infundibular dyskinesia, in which the level of the anticholecystokinetic factor is lowered after duodenal stimulation, the level is not lowered in a normal way (Fig. 6a, b).

The CCK injected into the two patients (Fig. 6a, b) seems to have been inactivated. In fact we found that CCK, incubated with slices of gallbladder mucosa, in particular with slices of the neck area loses its capacity to contract the guinea pig gallbladder in situ. Since slices of other tissues, not even of the

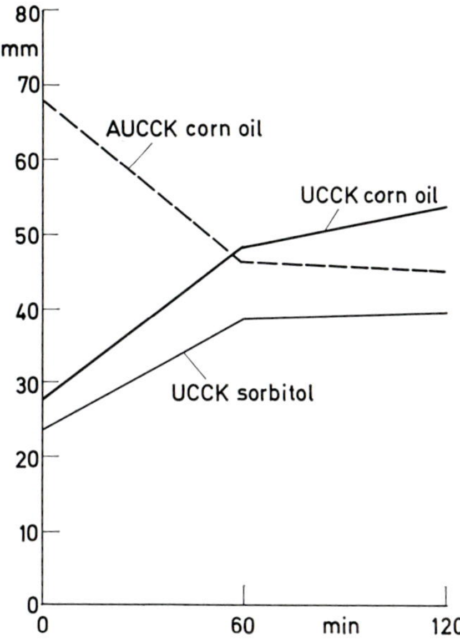

Fig. 5. A control group. After absorption of sorbitol or corn oil there is an increase in the urocholecystokinin concentration of the urine at the same time as there is a drop in the "anti-CCK" activity

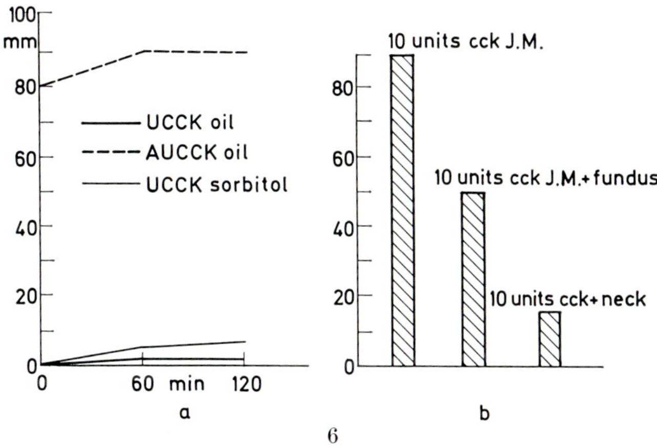

Fig. 6. An authentic atonic state of the gallbladder. Sorbitol and oil do not provoke a release of urocholecystokinin and the "anti-CCK" remains on a high level (a). 10 U of CCK incubated with mucosal extract of the collum region were completely inactivated (b)

duodeno-jejunum, did not possess this capacity we concluded that this anti-cholecystokinetic factor is secreted mainly from the mucosa of the gallbladder. *After cholecystectomy* the patient regained a normal level of endogenous CCK and anticholecystokinetic factor in the serum. I.v. injection of CCK in the female patient now resulted in an opening of the sphincter of Oddi and an acceleration of intestinal peristalsis, evidently due to the action of the CCK injected.

A number of authors have pointed out the similarity existing between *migraine and biliary dyskinesias*. Without entering a discussion about the neural and digestive factors which evoke a crisis, the author will shortly refer to some observations made during a crisis in persons known to suffer from migraine. The number of cases is relatively small, since it is ethically and technically impossible deliberately to evoke a crisis in a patient, not even by instilling into the duodenum the most badly tolerated food-stuffs like chocolate, cacao butter or fried ham (PLESSIER, 1960).

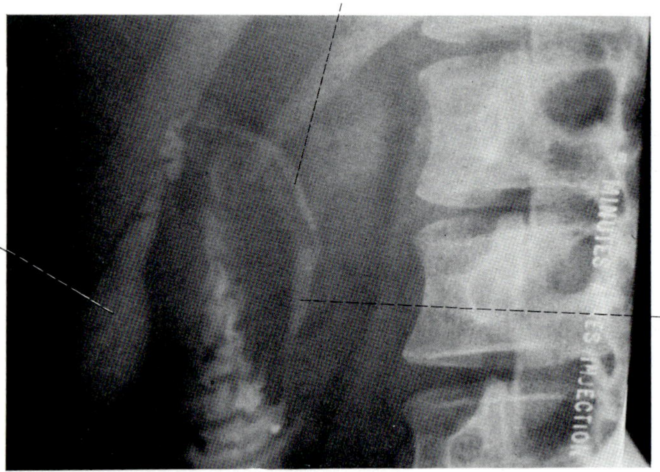

Fig. 6 c. It is impossible to visualize the upper 2/3 of the common bile duct, because of a very low implantation of the cystic duct

Cholecystography performed on the day of a severe crisis showed a prolonged effect of CCK, sometimes lasting for one hour. All the changes following a CCK injection are aggravated. The periods of contraction and evacuation last for several minutes instead of seconds under normal conditions and the infundibular spasm is almost permanent. In the case, in which a crisis starts during the course of duodenal intubation, the periodical ejaculations of dark bile follow every tenth minute continuing for $1\frac{1}{2}$ to 2 h after the CCK injection. In between the crises the same subjects react normally to CCK, full restoration being observed during the following days.

In another situation, during pregnancy, cholecystography is avoided. During the course of a Caesarean section, as observed by POTTER (1936), the gallbladder does not contract after pituitrine, whereas the uterus does, evidently due to a deficient muscular function since the shape of the gallbladder and the composition of the bile are normal.

In studying the cholecystokinetic effect of a fat meal in young women during the course of their pregnancy some authors found that the evacuation of the gallbladder becomes more and more slow and incomplete only returning to normal several days after delivery, a phenomenon not always combined with a gastric hypokinesia (Boyden and Rigler, 1944).

We have tried to avoid cholecystography in pregnant women and determine instead the urocholecystokinin content of the urine after a fat meal. The level of urocholecystokinin showed no variation. Cholecystokinin almost completely loses its activity when injected into pregnant guinea pigs. The same happens when CCK is incubated with slices of uterus and placenta from pregnant guinea pigs and subsequently injected into non-pregnant animals.

We also studied the influence of chorionic gonadotrophine, oestradiol, progesterone and oestrone injected in progressively increasing doses in guinea pigs, prepared according to the technique of Svatos (1957, 1959), followed by 5 units of CCK. Only progesterone and oestrone seemed to exert an inhibitory action, proportional to the dose injected.

We also tried, in 40 patients, to study by means of duodenal intubation the functional response of the gallbladder to CCK during the different phases of the menstrual cycle (Plessier et al., 1961). During the premenstrual period the appearance of bile was delayed, the volume was reduced and the period of collection was prolonged. The individual variations in the findings, however, did not allow any definite conclusions with exclusion of other etiological factors.

The drug Norethindrone, taken in an anti-mitotic dose of 40—80 mg, aggravates an infundibulo-ductal dyskinesia and blocks completely the vesicular response to 1 U/kg of CCK. Morphine does not act on the corpus and its action on the neck is weaker than that of the fatty meal. After an injection of more than 20 mg of morphine ½ h in advance, CCK loses its cholecystokinetic activity. During the action of morphine it is even in chronic addicts practically impossible to provoke an evacuation of the gallbladder.

When injected in doses up to 0.16 mg in guinea pigs, weighing 400 g, before or simultaneously with CCK, morphine behaved similarly. Besides CCK a number of drugs, e.g. morphine and pethidine® evoke a contraction of the *isolated* guinea pig gallbladder (Paris, Robelet, Salembier and DuBois, 1962). An incomplete reaction to the morphinicals is supplemented by the action of CCK. In their studies of the action of CCK on the extrahepatic biliary tree after morphine administration the authors obtained the most variable results, contractions without evacuation or any appreciable reduction of the X-ray shadow. Bizard and Paris (1960a, b) considered that the analgesic effect of morphine in the painful attacks of biliary distension is due to the combined action on the bile ducts and the central nervous system.

Dextromoramide has an inhibitory action when given in large doses (Plessier and Plessier, 1963). Danhof (1966, 1967) studied the action of a benzomorphine derivative, Pentazocine®. In 30 male subjects, 20 to 45 years of age, the volume and the concentration of bile obtained at duodenal intubation after CCK were the same with or without Pentazocine.

3. Side Reactions

The CCK J. M., of 10% purity with 250—300 Ivy dog units per mg is very well tolerated. The flush reaction with a facial feeling of heat observed in using the early preparations of the Swedish CCK with 22 U/mg does not occur any longer. In rare single cases the patient has a feeling of nausea and increased jejunal peristalsis and, in cases with an organo-functional resistance in the bile passage, a spontaneous pain, developing within 2 min and usually disappearing within 3—5 min. Similar symptoms arise after intraduodenal stimulation with Sorbitol, arachis oil or corn oil, when the outflow of bile is hindered and the contractility is normal. In similar cases we found that the symptoms are elicited also by smaller doses of CCK, even with $^1/_{10}$ of the ordinary dose, and that a prolongation of the injection time does not change the outcome.

III. Cholecystokinin and the Common Bile Duct

The findings of CASSANO et al. (1959), COLAGRANDE et al. (1960), TORSOLI et al. (1961 a, b; 1970) and of ALESSANDRINI et al. (1961) on this topic are dealt with in a separate chapter of this volume.

1. Retrograde Visualization of the Bile Ducts

EDHOLM (1958) compared the influence of the dorsal decubitus position and backward inclination on reversed filling into the common hepatic duct and the intrahepatic biliary tree after injection of CCK. In the horizontal position the visualisation of the common hepatic canal can be obtained in 48% of the cases. In cases examined in the Trendelenburg position, this visualization is obtained in 74% of the cases. Hepatic reflux does not indicate biliary disease. In the experiments of TOMENIUS and BACKLUND (1958, 1959) and JORPES et al. (1957, 1958) the common hepatic duct and even the beginning of the intrahepatic ducts were visualized. LESCUT (1963) observed reflux into the hepatic duct in 21 cases out of 100 and in 11 cases out of 17 with chronic pancreatitis. There was in these cases no correlation between the reduction in volume of the gallbladder and the intrahepatic reflux. The same percentage with reflux was observed, when CCK was given by infusion during 5 min, in 8 out of 21 cases amongst which 3 suffered from chronic pancreatitis.

In looking over our 1500 cholecystographies, and those from the literature, we got the impression that intrahepatic reflux is due not only to the state of the sphincter of Oddi but in normal subjects to the radiological technique used, the site of implantation of the cystic duct. As an example of this we were unable to visualize the upper $^2/_3$ of the common bile duct due to a very low implantation of the cystic duct (Fig. 6 c).

2. Cholecystokinin and Visualization of the Common Bile Duct

In comparing the cholecystographic picture after a fat meal and after CCK in their 59 cases JORPES et al. (1957, 1958) demonstrated the superiority of CCK for the visualization of the common duct with respect to the rapidity of obtaining the pictures and to their constant quality. In all the cases without lithiasis both the common and the cystic ducts were visible after CCK; after the fat meal they failed to appear in 7 cases. The same regularity was observed after CCK in the 16 lithiasis cases, whereas after the fat meal the choledochus failed to appear in 4 of them. An explanation for the failure of MEINARDUS (1959) to obtain a good opacification of the bile may well have been that he injected the CCK during the course of two minutes and took his pictures between 5 and 7 min. We have resorted since 1960 (PLESSIER and MARSICO, 1960) to a fairly rapid injection and the high quality of the pictures taken 2 to 3 min after injection. In 30 out of 40 cases the full extent of the main duct was visible with a clear delineation of the lower common duct and the sphincter of Oddi. In the 6 cases, where only the upper common duct was visible, the poor visualization was mostly due to a prolonged spasm in the sphincter of LUTKENS, in 4 cases there was a deficient evacuation of the gallbladder.

GROS and WEILL (1960), Strasburg, obtained a good visualization of the common duct in 9 out of 11 cases, the two failures being a case with dyskinesia and one with lithiasis. The diameter of the choledochus was greater after CCK than after the fat meal.

In comparing the efficiency of different means for visualization of the biliary ducts FEIGELSON, BERK, JOYRICH, GAGLIARDI and SHUFRO (1960) found satisfactory visualization in 57.4%, when using Cholex (1053 cases), 62% with olive oil (102 cases), 74.4% with 60 ml of a 33% solution of sorbitol in water (15 cases), 71% with safflower oil (33 cases) and 81.7% with CCK (49 cases). The common duct was visualized within one minute, the optimal visibility lasting as far as to the eighth minute.

MAMIE and KLEINERT (1962) took only one picture 2 and 10 min after injection and obtained good visualization of the choledochus in 28 out of 40 cases with normal gallbladders. In addition to the high percentage of successful choledochographies the authors pointed out the quality of the choledochography with a massive filling of the common duct even as far as the papilla, which in most cases could be easily localized. The pictures of the lower common duct were even superior to those obtained by cholangiography. Only in three cases was choledochography poor or useless.

LESCUT (1963) divided his material in three categories; no visualization of the choledochus (15 cases), a poor one (11 cases) and a good one (65 cases), 71.4%. In the 65 cases the choledochus was often visible in the first films. Sometimes the visualization was satisfactory at first in the films taken at 5 min, justifying repeated exposures from the first to the tenth min. Administration of CCK during the course of 5 min does not improve the visibility. GLEASON (1965) obtained within the first 5 min after the i.v. injection a good visualization of the common duct in 85% of the cases.

As to the diameter of the common duct NATHAN et al. (1969) found it to be 2—5 mm or 6 mm in 2 out of 50 normal persons. In order to demonstrate an eventual obstruction the authors paid attention to infundibulo-ductal region and also to the persistance of contrast material in the choledochus.

A number of authors have described progressive movements of the choledochus under the influence of CCK, with variations in the diameter and the tonicity of the wall under the influence of CCK and the secondary hypercholeresis (GRILL et al., 1963). This topic has been dealt with by TORSOLI et al. (1961a, b) and by MAGEE (1965).

IV. Cholecystokinin, the Sphincter of Oddi and Duodenal Motility

The relaxing effect of CCK on the sphincter of Oddi is prompt, strong and prolonged and is specific for CCK as compared with other agents eliciting a contraction of the gallbladder. SANDBLOM, VOEGTLIN and IVY (1935) registered simultaneously the intramural resistance and the duodenal motility in the anesthetized dog. After injection of 5 to 10 mg of a crude CCK preparation the intramural resistance rose from 70 to 320 mm of water and then returned to normal within 15—30 sec. After cholecystectomy the increase in the intramural resistance was not constant and diminished slowly. The phenomenon seemed to be independent of the gallbladder and duodenal motility, which increased in 87% of the cases.

The relaxing action of CCK on the sphincter of Oddi was demonstrated by FRIEDMAN and SNAPE (1945). The mechanism of the relaxation was studied by HONG, MAGEE and CREWDSON (1956) by means of procaine and hexamethonium. After eliminating the influence of choleresis by ligating the hepatic ducts, ALLEGRI et al. (1957) perfused the lower part of the choledochus under constant pressure and measured the output of bile and the intraduodenal and intravesicular pressures. After an i.v. injection of CCK the rate of flow of bile through the sphincter of Oddi did not increase immediately but 10 to 30 sec later, whereas the sphincter relaxation was of a much longer duration, 8 to 10 min. This relaxation, which can be observed also after cholecystectomy, is independent of the variations in tone of the duodenal wall which is of short duration and not influenced by the rate of perfusion of the fluid. The movements of the sphincter are consequently independent of the duodenal musculature. In order to distinguish the phases of the sphincter contraction and the influence of drugs, particularly of CCK upon them, single exposures are not sufficient. For this purpose a number of pictures are taken quickly or a radio-television or still better cine is used. The individual pictures can then be analyzed in a viewer one after another. In normal subjects duodenal filling as seen on radio-television, begins between 30 and 90 sec after the injection of CCK. Likewise LESCUT (1963) often found the iodinated bile appearing in the duodenum within one minute.

We use the technique developed by PORCHER, CAROLI, PEGUIGNOT and DELATTRE (1956, 1957) for the study of the different types of contractions in the Oddi region by means of cineradiomanometry. "Pyloric" contractions are not the most frequent observed. More frequently one can see a tranquilization of an antiperistaltic type, i.e. closure of the sphincter progresses from below, resulting in an extinction of its structure and a horizontal amputation of common duct. Under the action of CCK formations simulating biliary calculi disappear as occurred following atropine.

Under normal conditions one can see before the injection of CCK a permanent movement going on with alternating opening and closing of the sphincter of Oddi, both of equal duration, about 3 sec. It is striking to note the contrast existing between a higher frequency and a longer duration of the opening times of the sphincter of Oddi after the injection of CCK, and the longer time to reach the residual pressure in the case where CCK is injected at the very moment when the "residual time" starts. This time to reach the residual pressure can be increased by 3 to 4 minutes.

After CCK injection there always exists a great decrease in the level of this residual pressure. According to our observations (PLESSIER and MARSICO, 1960) using CCK, the pressure fell to 7 cm, instead of 14 cm if no CCK is administered.

Likewise GRANSER, HERTING, RISSEL and WEWALKA (1956) found the action of CCK to be the most reliable and the most prolonged in a series consisting of 30 cats.

GRASSBERGER and SEYSS (1963) recommended per-operative cholangiography for the study of the sphincter of Oddi. Particular emphasis was laid on an exposure during the i.v. injection of 75 units of CCK and 1, 2 and 3 min thereafter. In a series of 53 patients they distinguished 3 types: one with a normal cholangiogram without papillary changes, a second with functional modifications, and a third with anatomical changes. According to the authors the state of the papilla and its reaction to CCK facilitates the decision, whether cholecystectomy alone or an incision of the papilla should be performed. The method rendered a particular service in icteric patients, making in some cases a major surgical intervention superfluous.

In the third group with anatomical changes, no reaction can be observed. The pathological processes in the muscularis propria of the bile duct are so pronounced that no dilatation is obtained. Sometimes a paradoxal response with a narrowing of the papillary canal can be seen.

In experimental material GRANSER et al. (1956) observed similar abnormal reactions in pregnant animals, probably caused by severe pathological processes. The test has its limitations because it measures only the function of the papillary canal, with no information about the underlaying histological changes. In two cases, one with a carcinoma of the bile duct and one with a cancer pancreatis, no dilatation of the papillary canal was observed. In 24 patients of the first type good dilatation took place, likewise in 10 out of 15 patients of the second type, the dyskinesia group. In 5 there were slight alterations of the papilla but no reaction. In the 14 patients of the third type with pronounced anatomical alterations there was no reaction from the side of the papillary canal.

BLASBERG, EDMUNDS and FINBY (1964) investigated the size of the common duct in a series of 34 asymptomatic post cholecystectomy patients. At the time of optimal visualization of the biliary tract, 25 units of CCK were injected i.v. Roentgenograms were exposed 5 and 10 min after the injection. Only 4 patients, with an average duct size of 8 mm, failed to show evidence of change either in width or density after cholecystokinin. In 4 patients there was complete emptying from the common duct of the contrast material. One patient with a common duct of 11 mm diameter showed a decrease of 5 mm; in 3 other cases there was a decrease of 3 mm. Almost half of the total (15 patients) showed a difference of 1 mm. Slight decrease of density was seen in practically all patients. The authors were not certain whether the effect of CCK is contraction of the duct wall or relaxation of the sphincter of Oddi.

Working with cholecystectomized dogs, with a cannula in the common duct and the stump of the gallbladder for the registration of the pressure, STASSA and GRAFE (1968) perfused the biliary ducts with a 50% solution of Cholegrafin, 15 drops/min. Since the results with the fat meal varied too much, the authors used CCK, 1 U/kg, followed by film exposures 1, 2, 5, 10 and 15 min after injection. On two separate days they studied the effect of morphine, 0.15 mg/kg, probanthine, 10 ml, and of CCK. The same series were repeated after a sphincterotomy followed by vagotomy. Previous to the cholecystectomy the contrast medium passed directly into the duodenum in intermittent portions without any peristalsis in the common bile duct and with an open sphincter of Oddi. Morphine had no effect on the gallbladder. Two minutes after injection the common duct was dilated and the intrahepatic bile ducts filled. The passage of contrast material to the duodenum ceased and the sphincter of Oddi contracted. The effect of morphine was abolished by CCK and by probanthine with an immediate reappearance of contrast medium in the duodenum and a narrowing of the calibre of the intrahepatic bile ducts. The gallbladder, which contracted vigorously after CCK, did not react to probanthine.

After sphincterotomy the "jet" effect during the passage of contrast material into the duodenum is lost. Likewise the response to morphine and probanthine if the sphincterotomy has been complete.

The response of the biliary ducts to morphine, probanthine and CCK is not altered by cholecystectomy nor by vagotomy. Cholecystectomy, alone or with vagotomy, does not cause any dilatation of the bile ducts and does not modify any of the many effects of CCK. The authors enumerated three different effects of CCK: contraction of the gallbladder, relaxation of the sphincter of Oddi and acceleration of the peristalsis of the small bowel. They recommended the use of CCK and probanthine for the elimination of spasm in the sphincter of Oddi and found it likely that by these means small residual stones in the bile ducts could be removed without operation.

On the 10th Congress of the Argentine Gastro-enterological Society LONGO, HUARTE, DAGOSTINO and MANNAMA (1969) reported on the different drugs used in the analysis of the functional and morphological state of the sphincter of Oddi: magnesium sulfate, novocaine, xylocaine, hydrochloric acid in the duodenum or Buscopan and prostigmine intravenously. They outlined the difficulties encountered in the analysis of the behavior of the sphincter of Oddi under the influence of CCK during the pre- and postoperative cholangiograms. They reported on 20 cases where the use of CCK in the pre-operative cholangiography enabled them to differentiate between functional and pathologic states of the sphincter. Thereby an unnecessary papillotomy could be avoided and adequate therapy instituted.

In spite of careful performance of cholangiography there are situations where the interpretation of the films is difficult, e.g. after medication or in cases of oedema or clots in the ducts.

In an investigation of 296 patients subjected to choledochotomy for cholelithiasis NYLANDER (1970) made pre-explorative, postexplorative, and postoperative cholangiography. Stones had escaped detection in 9% of the 132 cases with contrast-medium passage to the duodenum both pre- and post-exploratively, in 16% of the 76 cases with passage pre- but not post-exploratively, in 5% of the 57 cases with passage only post-exploratively, and in no less than 65% of the 31 cases with passage neither pre- nor post-exploratively.

It appears obvious that the passages must be given as much attention as possible, and that we must use pharmacological agents capable of improving the opacification of the Oddian area on premedicated and narcotized patients.

Cholecystokinin and the Postoperative Choledochus

a) The cystic duct stump syndrome

The pain provoked by injection of CCK after cholecystectomy is not necessarily due to a dyskinesia of the sphincter of Oddi. It can be a question of a stump syndrome as it was the case in a patient, a female, 53 years of age, following cholecystectomy 10 years earlier, observed by MACFARLAND and CURRIN (1969). Because of pain of biliary type an i.v. cholangiogram was made. An electrocardiographic examination made simultaneously with the CCK injection showed an inversion of the T wave. In addition the patient experienced an acute pain, simulating cardiac angina. On reexploration of the operation field the authors discovered a 5 cm stump of the cystic duct free of concrements. After its removal the subsequent course was uneventful.

b) Transhepatic percutaneous cholangiography

By means of transhepatic percutaneous cholangiography as performed in 5 cases WIECHEL (1964) found 5 calculi larger than the size of a pea in the choledochus. Two of them could be removed by means of CCK. 1—2 U/kg seemed to be the optimal dose.

c) Oil-ether infusion into the common duct

There seems to be a method, by means of CCK, to ameliorate the drawbacks of the method of washing out the common duct as described already by WALKER (1891) and FONTAN (1892). The technique consists of an instillation of olive oil and ether into the common duct in order to induce an evacuation of small calculi. In 1964 ROSENQVIST described two cases in which an otherwise obligatory choledochotomy could be avoided. During the course of 5 days he infused in the morning through a cannula 50 ml of physiological saline solution mixed with 20 ml soy bean oil and 2—3 ml of ether into the common duct. DAHLGREN (1966) usually infused through a T-tube a mixture of 5 ml of sterile olive oil and 5 ml ether 3 min after the i.v. injection of 1 U/kg of CCK.

This flushing of the common bile duct was repeated on three consecutive days. The expulsive effect of CCK was controlled by subsequent cholangiography. DAHLGREN uses the technique regularly since 1965.

Likewise AGUIRRE, HALABI, GIFFONIELLO, DIAZ and AREAL (1969) used the technique for the expulsion of small biliary calculi. They regularly found that the injection of 75 units of CCK over 3 min was followed within one minute by a hypotonic state of the duodenum with opening of the papilla and a reduced motility and pressure in the biliary ducts. The effect lasted for 5 to 8 min. During this time they instilled a mixture of equal parts ether and olive oil in 1 ml portions, adjusting the speed in order to avoid pain due to dilatation of the common duct on the evaporation of the ether. The authors reported on two successful cases, in which the dilatation of the sphincter of Oddi after CCK was of a considerable size.

d) Cholecystokinin and other compounds acting on the sphincter of Oddi

Atropine and N-butyl hyoscine do not interfere with the action of CCK on the sphincter of Oddi. A 1% solution of lignocaine introduced into the duodenum shortens the time of closure of the sphincter, in particular if it is abnormally prolonged (PLESSIER and PLESSIER, 1963). The spasmogenic effect of morphine is counteracted by CCK (BRODÉN, 1958; PLESSIER, 1960; STASSA and GRAFE, 1968). It is not possible to improve the visualization of the intrahepatic bile ducts by combining the morphine with CCK. One can, however, by means of rapid seriographs or radiocinematography analyze the sphincter region in spite of the morphine blockage, if CCK is injected and exposures made simultaneously (Fig. 7a, b). Using the technique of Kehr to perform an infusion into the duodenum under pressure PARIS, ROBELET, SALEMBRIER and DUBOIS (1962) studied the effect of morphine drugs and CCK in a group of cholecystectomized patients submitted to choledochotomy and in a group of normal patients. When a small dose of morphine, 5 mg, was used, and films were taken at short intervals during 10 min, it was possible by means of CCK to follow the emptying of the gallbladder and the common duct.

V. The Use of Cholecystokinin in Endoscopy

a) Duodenoscopy

On the fourth International Congress of Gastroenterology Oi et al. (1970) reported on the use of duodenoscopy sometimes combined with catheterization of the Wirsungian duct in order to study the papilla and to collect the secretions after pancreatic stimulation with secretin and CCK. Other Japanese authors (Takagi, 1970) used duodenoscopy for the visualization of the Wirsungian duct and for retrograde cholangiographies. Probably the visualization of the papilla and its relaxation would have been facilitated if the authors had used CCK.

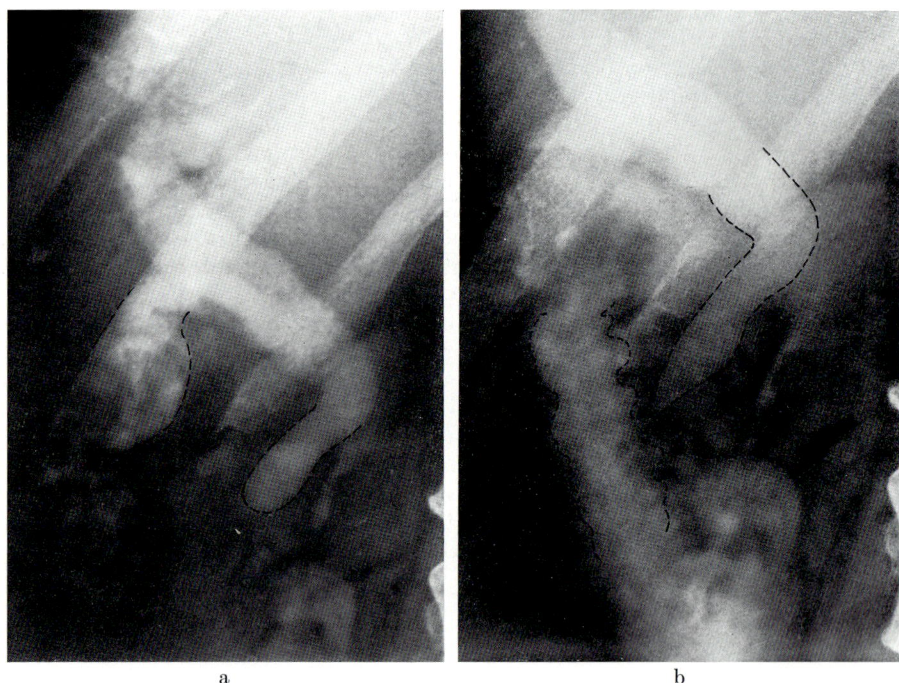

Fig. 7. Morphine aggravates the spasm in the sphincter of Oddi and blocks the passage through the duodenum (a). 20 min later the patient had an attack of severe pain which was ameliorated by $1\frac{1}{2}$ U/kg of CCK at the same time as the sphincter opened (b)

b) Cholecystokinin in laparoscopy

Ricordeau and Plessier (unpublished) used CCK on different occasions for the diagnosis of an intrahepatic ectopic gallbladder. The gallbladder emerging from the surface of the liver can easily be taken for an hydatid cyst. The contraction of the "cyst" under the action of CCK gives in a few minutes the right diagnosis (Fig. 8).

c) Cholecystokinin and transvesicular cholangiography (Royer camera)

Together with Foures (Foures and Plessier, 1959, unpublished) we had an opportunity to follow the opacification of the bile ducts under laparoscopy and to take films before and after the injection of CCK with a good view of the infundibulo-canal region and the sphincter of Oddi.

d) Cholecystokinin and pancreatography

In 1856 Claude Bernard called attention to the congestion of the pancreas which takes place during digestion. That such congestion can be provoked in the anesthetized cat by acetyl choline, histamine, secretin and cholecystokinin was shown by Holton and Jones (1960). The congestion caused by secretin or CCK was not inhibited by atropine or mepyramine. Working with the isolated dog pancreas Hermon-Taylor (1968) found the vasodilatation to precede the secretory response after secretin. A similar effect on the pancreatic arterial flow is, according to Dorigotti and Glässer (1968), exerted by CCK and caerulein.

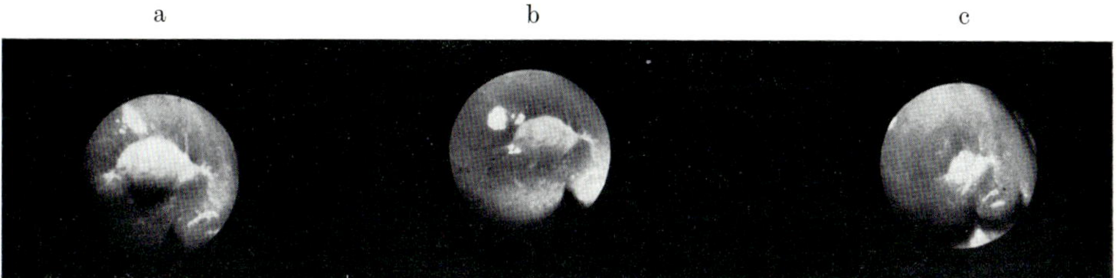

Fig. 8. A case of ectopic intrahepatic gallbladder. The gradual disappearance of this false "intrahepatic cyst" in the minutes, b after 1 min and c after 5 min, following injection of CCK makes obvious the diagnosis of intrahepatic ectopic gallbladder (patient of Prof. Caroli — Laparoscopy by Dr Ricourdeau)

Taylor, Macken and Fiore (1966) were the first to inject secretin in man directly into the trunk of the celiac artery. Since 1967 we have tried, in cooperation with a group of coworkers from the departments of Professor Caroli and Professor Cherigie to compare the response to secretin of the endocrine and the exocrine pancreas with the parenchymatographic pictures after intraceliac injection of secretin and lately even of CCK (Plessier et al., 1967; Plessier, 1971). The insulin response was measured from the level of plasma insulin as determined by Rosselin. The plasma glucagon was likewise determined by Assan. After intraarterial injection of secretin, 1 U/kg, and of contrast medium, after 1½ min we obtained a good pancreatographic picture in 22 out of 24 subjects with a normal exocrine pancreas (Fig. 9a, b).

In *acute pancreatitis* the parenchymatographic picture after intraarterial secretin injection is normal as well as the secretory response to secretin.

Pancreatic cysts following an acute pancreatitis are visible as lacunae.

The extensive *parenchymatous changes* seen in chronic pancreatitis and in carcinoma result in a *complete absence* of a parenchymatographic picture. This occurred in 47 cases of our own out of 50 cases.

Analysis of the duodenal content has shown that there is a high correlation between the bicarbonate and enzyme content and the parenchymatographic picture. A total lack of enzymes and bicarbonate secretion can be observed when the pancreatic duct is blocked by a cyst, in spite of which a normal parenchymatography is possible. This occured in 1% of our analyses in combination with increased values for blood amylase and lipase after secretin- and CCK stimulation.

Without making such a comparison between the parenchymatographic picture and the secretory response to secretin Udén (1969) analyzed 20 patients suspected for carcinoma, 5 of which had carcinoma and 2 with a pseudocyst. Arteriography with and without secretin were made in each patient. He found a 3.8 to 4.8 mm increase in the diameter of the gastroduodenal vessels. The blood flow to the pancreas was increased facilitating the cancer diagnosis in the 5 cases. The pathological vascularization was particularly well visualized. The test was well tolerated by the patients, as was found in our series as well.

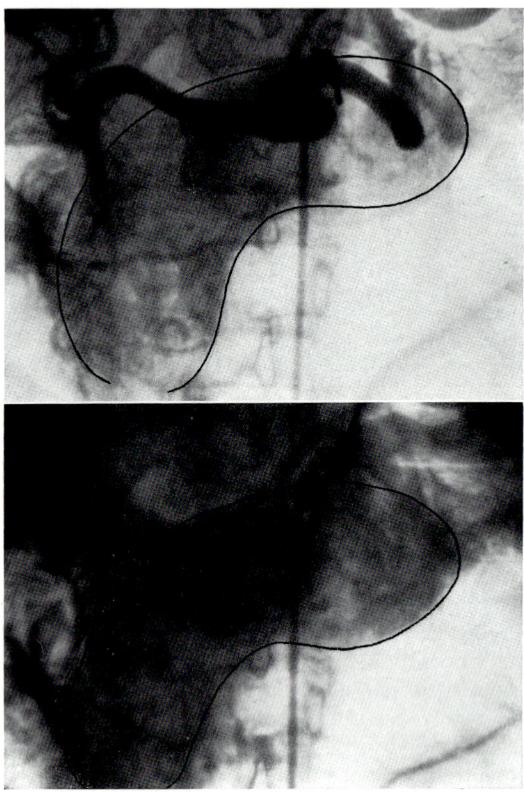

Fig. 9. Arterial and venous parenchymatography after 1 U/kg of secretin in the celiac artery in persons with normal external pancreatic secretion and after an acute pancreatitis

Cen, Rosenbusch, Frik and Kalf (1969) performed the intraarterial injection of crude secretin during the course of 20—30 sec and took the film $1\frac{1}{2}$ min later. They performed 50 celiac angiograms and found, like the previous authors, the technique very useful. They supplemented their series with a number of celiac angiograms using epinephrine, 5 to 8 μg, injected during 2 sec. Films were taken after 3 sec and with a smaller amount of contrast medium.

Our experience with CCK is not so favorable. We did not find the same correlation between the parenchymatographic picture and the external secretory capacity of the gland, nor could we with CCK improve the vascularization of tumors as obtained after secretin. As to the endocrine system, secretin injected into the celiac artery, produces up to 500% increase in the insulin concentration of the plasma both in normal subjects and in pathological cases. The stimulation of the beta-cells by secretin seems to be independent of the arterial vasodilatation (PLESSIER et al., 1971). On the other hand we found secretin to be a poor stimulator of the alfa-cells. The glucagon secretion after secretin was inconstant in contradistinction to the effect after CCK, which seems to be a specific stimulant of the alfa-cells.

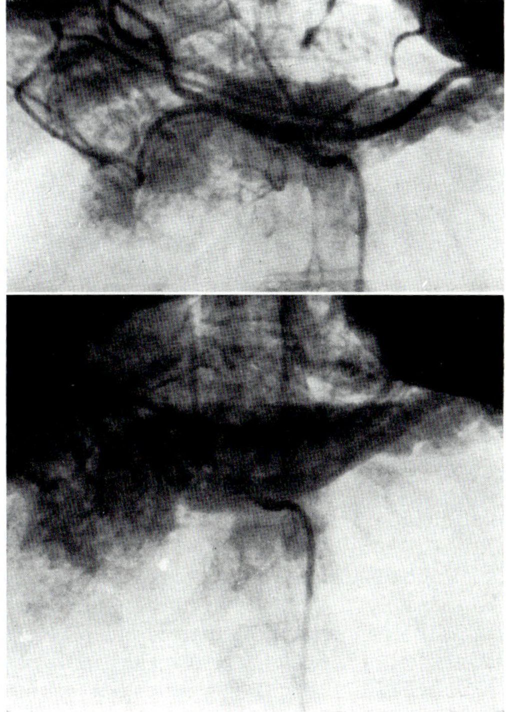

Fig. 10

VI. Cholecystokinin in the Scintigraphy of the Gallbladder and Pancreas

a) Scintigraphy of the gallbladder

NORDYKE (1965) tried by means of liver function tests and radioisotope scintigraphy of the choledocho-duodenal junction to differentiate between surgical and non-surgical patients in severe icteric cases. ^{131}I-labelled Rose bengal was used for measuring the hepatic function. The rate of disappearance of Rose bengal in the blood was measured on the lateral surface of the head.

The function of the bile ducts was indicated by the appearance of radioactivity in the duodenum after stimulation with CCK. 30 min after the i.v.

injection of 15 to 30 μC of ^{131}I-labelled Rose bengal; a contraction of the gall-bladder and opening of the sphincter of Oddi were provoked by means of 20 units of CCK. The increase in radioactivity in the intestine occurred even in cholecystectomized patients. CCK eliminates the drawbacks in using the fat meal, the prolonged contraction of the pyloric region and the slow passage of the contrast medium. The bile ducts were considered to be normal when the radioactivity in the intestine returned to the basal level within 15 min. If no increase in radioactivity occurred another CCK injection was given. No increase in the radioactivity within 20 min indicated a complete obstruction. Among the 69 non-surgical icteric cases 15 were considered to be particularly severe. 4 cases with cholangiolithic hepatitis, 3 cases with methyl-testosterone hepatitis, 2 with icterus due to chloropromazine or as a complication of a pancreatitis, 1 with liver metastases, 1 with an amoebic abscess and one with biliary cirrhosis. When the author applied the Rose bengal test in combination with CCK 13 of these cases were correctly classified as non-surgical. Englert Jr and Chiu (1966) have suggested to replace the instrumental parasurgical methods by a radioisotopic technique of more physiological value for the quantitative analysis of bile evacuation. The night before, 8 male subjects ingested 5 to 20 microcuries of ^{131}I-labelled iopanoic acid and 6 g of the same acid but not labelled. The activities were registered continuously. These subjects received either a fatty meal or a continuous infusion of impure CCK (Boots) at the rate of 11.7 mU/kg/min (Ivy dog units) during 86 min; 4 subjects received only one injection of CCK each. They studied the reproducibility of the method in repeating the test 3 times at intervals of one week in some patients. The efficiency of the evacuation and its importance can be measured by the rate of radioactivity before and after evacuation. The percentages of evacuation could be reproduced in each individual case. The physiological stimulation due to the fatty meal or continuous infusion of CCK gave similar results. A single and rapid intravenous injection of CCK produced a short and incomplete evacuation. The average of the total duration of evacuation would be respectively, for the fatty meal and the continuous infusion of CCK, 54 and 46 min, the percentage evacuation being 84% and 78%. It seems that for the study of residual radioactivity, the authors did not take into consideration the filling process which follows almost immediately the evacuation period as we have noticed during introduction of a duodenal tube accompanied with cholecystography face and side views, after CCK single injections. We must also point out that these incomplete results, following single injection, are obtained with *non purified CCK* preparations, giving variable percentage evacuation in the ordinary cholecystographies.

b) Cholecystokinin in pancreatic scintigraphy

A number of authors have tried to improve the quality of the pictures of the pancreas obtained after an injection of selenomethionine by giving a fat meal or an i.v. injection of CCK. The results reported during the last years are somewhat discouraging. Leger, Roucayrol, Lenriot (1971) found in chronic pancreatitis that 5 scintigraphies were non-interpretable, 10 normal, 20 of poor or heterogenous fixation, 6 with lacunar formations simulating pseudocysts of pancreas, and 39 were absolutely blank (49.2%). The percentage of anomalies, reaching 94.2% in the cases of pancreatitis with calcification, was 57.1% of the cases without calcification, where the diagnosis is most difficult. These percentages correlated well with the concentrations of bicarbonate and enzymes found in the secretin and CCK tests.

We tried, in cooperation with DE SAINT LAURENT, TROUPEL and DEL SALLO (unpublished), to improve the pharmacoscintigraphy of the pancreas and to correlate the radioactivity of the duodenal contents with the bicarbonate and lipase values found after secretin and CCK. The radioactivity recovered after secretin and in particular after CCK is in normal subjects 100 to 200 times higher than the basal concentration. We also tried to find out whether cases with chronic pancreatitis and those with a cancer pancreatis show a difference in the radioactivity of the separately collected duodenal and jejunal contents. The question is still open whether stimulation of the acinar cells with secretin or CCK will improve the scintigraphic picture.

The only method available for the differentiation between cancer and chronic pancreatitis is cytological examination of the duodenal contents as collected with the duodenal tube or by punctioning or catheterization of the Wirsungian duct (HENNING, WITTE and BRESSEL, 1960; DREILING, NIEBURGS and JANOWITZ, 1960; RASKIN, WENGER, SKLAR, PLETICKA and YAREMA, 1958; WENGER and RASKIN, 1958). The residual fluorescence due to tetracycline is considered to be normal after injection of CCK. It indicates whether the patients have really been subjected to tetracycline. This widespread fluorescence spot of post CCK smears in ultraviolet light is obvious, due to the concentration of tetracycline in bile by the gallbladder mucosa. It is totally different from the pin-point fluorescent spot of post secretin smears of pancreatic juice, considered to be abnormal (PLESSIER, ECONOMOPOULOS, PLESSIER, 1965).

VII. Cholecystokinin and Duodenal and Ileal Peristalsis

During recent years this topic has been dealt with by a number of authors (FRANZEN, 1961; GRILL et al., 1963; DAHLGREN, 1964, 1966; GLEASON, 1965; MONOD, 1964; GRALL, 1967; MORIN et al., 1965, 1966; PLESSIER, 1969; PLESSIER et al., 1969; BACKLUND, 1967, 1968, 1970).

a) Cholecystokinin and duodenal peristalsis

Working with anesthetized dogs SANDBLOM, VOEGTLIN and IVY (1935) noted an increased duodenal motility after CCK injections in 87% of their animals, followed by a reduced motility. This duodenal effect is abolished if CCK is destroyed by alkalies, enzymes or heating.

ADLERCREUTZ et al. (1957, 1960) registered the duodenal pressure with a Miller-Abbott tube and the peristaltic movements before, during and after the i.v. injection of 75 units of CCK in man. 45 sec after the start of the injection there was a drop in the pressure. Peristaltic movements stop and tone decreases 45 sec after the start of the injection; it is only after the arrival of the bile into the duodenum that a sudden increase in the duodenal pressure is noted and followed by a reduction in the 7th minute. The results are the same but more pronounced in cholecystectomized patients. DAHLGREN (1966) observed after the i.v. injection of 1 U/kg of CCK both in man and in the dog an increased peristaltic activity of the duodenum lasting for 3 to 5 min. If the influence of the bile is excluded through catheterization of the common bile duct and the cystic duct according to the technique of Svatos, the duodenal movements are unchanged or reduced while the ileal peristalsis is accelerated (PLESSIER, 1969).

TORSOLI, RAMORINO, COLAGRANDE and DEMAIO (1961a) observed after CCK relaxation of duodenal tone sometimes alternating with increased peristalsis. The upper and lower sphincters of the duodenum sometimes seem to be in a hypertonic state, with the duodenal contents in some way enclosed. According to our experience CCK induces an exaggeration of this physiological phenomenon resulting in nausea and general symptoms simulating the functional subjective troubles elicited by endogenous CCK.

In contradistinction DAHLGREN (1964) stated that the injection of secretin does not provoke any increase in the duodenal peristalsis. CCK, however, augmented the motility of the efferent loop. The duration of the phenomenon was prolonged when the afferent loop in the dog was occluded, creating an afferent loop syndrome (ALS). DAHLGREN considered the CCK test in man to be positive, when the injection elicited a flow of bile and vomiting similar to the postprandial reaction. These symptoms occur after injection of secretin and CCK in the sitting position and become significant when the discomfort and epigastric strain last at least 10 mins.

In utilizing the same technique we collect the liquid from the afferent loop before and after the CCK injection for a qualitative and quantitative analysis of the bile acids and the bacterial population.

b) Cholecystokinin and the ileal peristalsis

In the years 1959 to 1961 we prepared more than 3000 guinea pigs according to the technique of Svatos. After injecting 1 to 5 units of CCK there was an increased intestinal peristalsis accelerating the passage of the fecal material. We considered at that time that the phenomenon was due to impurities in the CCK preparation. In the meantime DAHLGREN (1966) demonstrated that the accelerating action on the intestinal peristalsis increased in proportion to the degree of purity, from 20 to 250 and 3000 Ivy dog units per mg in the pure CCK.

The first application of CCK in the radiological examination of the small intestine in man was made by FRANZEN (1961). He demonstrated that the barium contrast was transported down to the valvula Bauhini in 10 min, when the i.v. CCK injection was made three hours after taking the barium meal. GRILL et al. (1963) observed in 5 cholecystectomized patients a similar increase in motility in the whole intestine, likewise ascribed by them to impurities in the CCK preparation. GLEASON (1965) insisted that the increase in intestinal motility is due to CCK, the barium reaching the caecum within 15 min after the CCK injection in 70% of the cases studied.

In 1964 MONOD found the enterokinetic action of CCK to be much superior to that of prostigmine, because it was not accompanied by any considerable alteration in the delineation of the mucosa nor by any hypersecretion. The action lasted for only 15 to 20 min, and therefore one has to wait for the opacification of the jejunum before injecting the CCK, which furthermore sometimes provokes a momentaneous atonic state in the duodenum. The effect is the same even after cholecystectomy, but when the effect on the gallbladder is poor the effect on the intestine is also very weak. CCK and prostigmine evidently act on different receptors, since one of them can show full activity when the other one fails.

MORIN et al. (1969) reported on 5 years' experience comprising 251 cases, in which the state of the small intestine was studied by means of CCK. Ten minutes after injection of an emulsion of 150 g barium and 150 ml of water they injected 75 units of CCK intravenously and followed the passage of the barium contrast as far as to cecum. This took place in 5 to 10 min, in which time cinematographic pictures were taken. The authors insist upon the necessity to wait for the barium column to reach the jejunum: they propose to wait for 10 up to 30 or 40 min so that 5 or 6 loops of the small intestine instead of 2 or 3 loops become filled, as CCK acts on the *whole of the small intestine*. Under these conditions the barium contrast in practically every case reached the cecum. When the passage was delayed the authors gave metoopramide intravenously or a new CCK injection. Out of 251 subjects there were only two „resistant“ cases. Among their 99 pathological cases there were 38 cases with bands and adhesions, 16 cases with Crohn's disease, 9 cases with unspecific fibrosis and 6 cases of ileo-cecal tuberculosis.

We have fully confirmed their findings and we likewise insist upon a 15 min interval between the barium intake and the injection of CCK in order not to miss the enterokinetic effect. We also tried to accelerate the ileal passage of our instruments for multiple biopsies so that biopsies of the lower ileal region could be done. Unfortunately it is in the most severe pathological cases, like severe glutenenteropathy or in badly treated diabetes that CCK fails to act. The sound loaded with mercury may in these cases need several days to proceed, as confirmed by several controlfilms before and after repeated intravenous injections of CCK.

BACKLUND (1970) also pointed out that failure of the test can be due to a too rapid injection and to the distension of the duodenum under the action of CCK. The author uses, either cineradiology, or films of small size 70 × 70 mm or 100 × 100 mm. The patient lies for 15 min on his right side before the CCK, 40 units, is injected. If the passage is slow one has to look for biliary disturbances or cholecystopathies of some kind necessitating a cholecystographic examination. In a normal series of 50 men and 50 females the barium contrast reached the cecum in 5 to 15 min.

The work of DAHLGREN (1966) with the pure CCK, 3000 U/mg, and the stimulation through endogenous CCK after a fat meal (FRANZEN, 1961) or after Sorbitol (PORCHER and CAROLI, 1957) allow the conclusion that the enterokinetic action observed is elicited by the pure gastrointestinal hormone and not due to impurities acting on the intestinal musculature. The action is also independent of the bile flow because it is elicited after cholecystectomy and after ligation or a total pathological obstruction of the bile ducts. Furthermore it differs pharmacologically from the action on the gallbladder and on the spincter of Oddi. It is completely blocked by atropine (NAITO et al., 1963; HEDNER et al., 1967).

DAHLGREN used CCK in experimental duodenal and ileal obstructions.

MATUCHANSKY et al. (1970) studied the correlation in man between the speed of propulsion through the small intestine and the absorption under the influence of CCK and metoclopramide. The two drugs provoked in every case a considerable acceleration of the propulsion through the small intestine. At the same time the transverse diameter of the intestine was reduced to the half, whereas the rate of flow, as measured in situ, did not vary significantly. The secretion of water, sodium and chloride into the lumen was increased. Hypersecretion of sodium was the result of a significant reduction in reabsorption. The potassium and bicarbonate balance did not show any variation.

VIII. Conclusions

The dual action of CCK, the contraction of the gallbladder and the relaxation of the sphincter of Oddi, makes the hormone a useful tool for the diagnosis of different types of functional and organic anomalies in the biliary system. Both effects are visible in films taken after 1 to 2 min. It is usually at that early phase that choledochography is best. The i.v. injection of 0.5 to 1 U/kg of CCK gives, in normal cases, within 10 min a more than 50% reduction in the volume of the gallbladder and a satisfactory choledochography in 85% of the subjects.

The stimulating action of CCK on the infundibular region has made a renewed study of dyskinesia originating from the infundibulo-cystic duct region and from the sphincter of Oddi possible. The use of CCK facilitates the differentiation of gallbladder disorders into dyskinesias, atonic states due to deficient endogenous release of CCK, which react normally to exogenous CCK, and asystolic states due to a permanent or an intermittent obstruction in the cystic duct. We can now interprete the functional megacholedochus as being due to a longer duration and more pronounced initial tonic phase of the Oddian action of CCK before the relaxation period sets in.

Other biological actions of CCK make it useful in clinical radiology. Its accelerating action on intestinal peristalsis in more than 80% of the cases enables us to follow the passage of barium contrast through the small intestine in less than 15 min. Furthermore its dilating action on the pancreatico-duodenal vessels facilitates the interpretation in selective angiography.

The action of CCK on the gallbladder and the sphincter of Oddi is not influenced by atropine. Its accelerating action on intestinal peristalsis, however, is blocked by atropine. Morphine reduces or blocks the action of CCK on the gallbladder but the spasm it provokes on the sphincter of Oddi, is resolved by CCK.

References

ADLERCREUTZ, E., JORPES, J. E., MUTT, V., WEGELIUS, C.: L'emploi de la cholécystokinine dans la cholécystographie. Arch. Mal. Appar. dig. **46**, 414—418 (1957).

— PETTERSSON, T., ADLERCREUTZ, H., GRIBBE, P., WEGELIUS, C.: Effect of cholecystokinin on duodenal tonus and motility. Acta med. scand. **167**, 339—342 (1960).

AGUIRRE, C., GIFFONIELLO HALABIM, A., DIAZ, A., AREAL, R. M.: Tratamiento de la litiasis residual del coledoco por medio de la colecistoquinina asociada a la instilacion local de éter-aceite. Pren. méd. argent. **56**, 726—758 (1969).

ALBOT, G., POILLEUX, F., KAPANDJI, M., CALVET, E.: Rôle des spasmes cystiques et des dysplasies endocriniennes non obliterantes de la region cervico-cystique. Dans l'apparition des lithiases vesiculaires. Presse méd. **65**, 1525—1527 (1957).

— TOULET, J., BONNET, G. F.: Essais de cholécystographie de face et de profil: Arch. Mal. Appar. dig. **40**, 1187—1191 (1951).

ALESSANDRINI, A., PALAGI, L., RAMORINO, M. L., COLAGRANDE, C.: Contributo alla studio dell'attivita motoria biliare. Rass. Fisiopat. clin. ter. **33**, 1160—1188 (1961).

ALLEGRI, A., BALDRIGHI, V., MONTEMARTINI, C.: Effetti della colecistochinina sulla dinamica della vie biliari con particolare riguardo al comportamento degli sfinteri colecistico e choledocio. Arch. Sci. med. **104**, 656—675 (1957).

BACKLUND, V.: Cholecystokinin vid cholangiografier. Svenska Läk.-Tidn. **61**, 3813—3819 (1964).

— Cholecystokinin vid röntgenundersökningar. Svenska Läk.-Tidn. **64**, 2473—2476 (1967).

— Cholecystokinin-pankreozymin (CCK-PZ) vid tunntarmsundersökningar. Nord. Congr. Radiol., Copenhagen 29. 5.—1. 6. 1968.

— Die Verwendung des Cholecystokinins in der Röntgendiagnostik. Der Radiologe **10**, 36—39 (1970).

— PETERSON, H. J.: Erfarenheter av cholecystokinin vid gallvägskirurgi. Opusc. med. (Stockh.) **7**, 292—293 (1962).

— — Die Verwendung des Cholecystokinins in der Chirurgie der Gallengänge. Der Radiologe **5**, 100—104 (1965).

BERG, J.: Studien über die Funktion der Gallenwege unter normalen und gewissen abnormen Verhältnissen. Acta chir. scand. **2**, 1—3 (1922).
BERGERET, A., CAROLI, J.: Doit-on enlever parfois des vésicules histologîquement saines? Contribution à l'étude des atrésies congénitales du cystique. Arch. Mal. Appar. dig. **36**, 433—440 (1947).
BERK, J. E., FEIGELSON, H. H.: Preliminary observations on the use of cholecystokinin in cholecysto-cholangiography and on simultaneous cholecystoangiography and pyelography using Duografin. Bull. Sinai Hospital Detroit **5**, 2—7 (1957).
BIZARD, G., PARIS, J.: La cholécystokinine. Lille méd. **5**, 850—857 (1960a).
— — Actions pharmacologiques sur les voies biliaires. Actualités pharmacol. I. Paris: Masson et Cie 1960b.
BLASBERG ,G., EDMUNDS, R. T., FINBY, N.: Effect of cholecystokinin on the normal common duct after cholecystectomy. Surg. Forum **15**, 375—377 (1964).
BOSSI, R.: La prova colecistocinina. Minerva med. **52**, 1109—1114 (1961).
BOYDEN, E. A., RIGLER, L. G.: Initial emptying of the stomach in primigravidae as related to evacuation of the biliary tract. Proc. Soc. exp. Biol. (N.Y.) **56**, 200—201 (1944)
BRODÉN, B.: Försök med cholecystokinin vid cholecystografi. Nord. Med. **56**, 1182 (1956).
— Experiments with cholecystokinin in cholecystography. Acta Radiol. (Stockh.) **49**, 25—30 (1958).
BRUENNER, S., GUDBJERG, C. E.: Cholecystokinin, ein neues Gallenblasenkontraktionsmittel. Fortschr. Röntgenstr. **91**, 84—86 (1959).
BURTON, P., HARPER, A. A., HOWAT, H. T., SCOTT, J. E., VARLEY, .H: The use of cholecystokinin to test gall bladder function in man. Gut **1**, 193—204 (1960).
CAROLI, J.: In: DEBOUVRY, J.: Radiomanométrie contribution à la physiopathologie des voies biliaires. Presses Universitaires. Thèse de Paris 1941.
— Etude des dyskinésies biliaires. In: Les Acquisitions Médicales Récentes. I, Edit.: Paris, Editions médicales Flammarion 1949.
— PEQUIGNOT, G., DELATTRE, M.: Contribution du radiocinéma à l'étude du fonctionnement des voies biliaires de l'homme. Sem. Hôp. Paris **6**, 975—1000 (1956).
— PLESSIER, J., PLESSIER, B.: L'hormone inhibitrice de la cholécystokinine; son rôle en pathologie biliaire et pancréatique. Rev. franc. Étud. clin. biol. **6**, 545—557 (1960).
CASSANO, C., TORSOLI, A., ALESSANDRINI, A.: Aspetti dinamici di fisiologica e fisiopatologica biliare. Atti XIII Congresso Soc. Ital. Gastroenterol. (Bologna) 1959 pp. 107—142.
CEN, M., ROSENBUSCH, G., FRIK, W., KALFF, G.: Pharmakoangiographie des Pankreas mit Sekretin und Adrenalin. Dtsch. med. Wschr. **39**, 1970—1971 (1969).
COLAGRANDE, S., RAMORINO, M. L., SISTI, P.: Sul impiego della "colecistocinina" negli esami radiologicali dell'apparato biliare. Arch. ital. Mal. Appar. dig. **27**, 469—481 (1960).
COZZOLINO, H. J., GOLDSTEIN, F., GREENING, R. R., WIRTS, C. W.: The cystic duct syndrome. J. Amer. med. Ass. **185**, 920—924 (1963).
DAHLGREN, S.: The afferent loop syndrome. Acta chir. scand. Suppl. **327** (1964).
— Cholecystokinin: pharmacology and clinical use. Acta chir. scand. Suppl. **357**, 256—260 (1966).
— THORÉN, L.: Intestinal motility in low small bowel obstruction. Acta chir. scand. **133**, 417—421 (1967).
DANHOF, I. E.: Mechanism of action of cholecystokinin in the dog. The Physiologist **9**, 164 (1966).
— Pentazocine effects on gastrointestinal motor functions in man. Amer. J. Gastroent. **48**, 295—310 (1967).
DEBRAY, C., ROUX, M., LE CANUET, R., LAUMONIER, R.: Diseases of the gallbladder siphon. In: World Congress Gastroenterology, Washington 1958, pp. 324—331.
DENTON, R. W., GERSHBEIN, L. L., IVY, A. C.: Response of human and canine gallbladder to cholecystokinin. J. appl. Physiol. **2**, 671—679 (1950).
DORIGOTTI, L., GLÄSSER, A. H.: Comparative effects of caerulein, pancreozymin and secretin on pancreatic blood flow. Experientia **24**, 806—807 (1968).
DREILING, D. A., NIEBURGS, H. E., JANOWITZ, H. D.: The combined secretin and cytology test in the diagnosis of pancreatic and biliary tract cancer. Med. Clin. N. Amer. **44**, 810—815 (1960).
DUNCAN, P. R., HARPER, A. A., HOWAT, H. T., OLEESKY, S., VARLEY, H.: The effects of pancreozymin on human subjects. J. Physiol. (Lond.) **111**, 63P (1950).
— — — — — Tests of gallbladder function in man. Gastroenterologia **78**, 349—353 (1952).
— — — — — SCOTT, J. E.: The use of a cholecystokinetic agent in preparations of pancreozymin to study gallbladder function in man. J. Physiol. (Lond.) **121**, 19—20P (1953).
DUX, A., THURN, P.: Zum Entleerungsmechanismus der Gallenblase. Fortschr. Röntgenstr. **92**, 630—644 (1960).

EDHOLM, P.: Emptying of the human gallbladder under the stimulus of cholecystokinin. Acta Radiol. (Stockh.) **50**, 521—532 (1958).
ENGLERT, E. Jr., CHIU, V.: Quantitative analysis of human biliary evacuation with a radioisotopic technique. Gastroenterology **50**, 506—518 (1966).
FARRAR, J. T.: Underdiagnosis of biliary tract disorders. Gastroenterology **51**, 1074—1075 (1966).
FEIGELSON, H. H., BERK, J. E., JOYRICH, H. M., GAGLIARDI, R. A., SHUFRO, A. S.: The effectiveness of oral cholecystagogues and intravenous cholecystokinin in producing bile duct visualization during oral cholecystography. Radiology **75**, 268—271 (1960).
FRANZEN, J.: Beziehungen des Gallenflusses zur Ileozökalregion. Fortschr. Röntgenstr. **95**, 769—781 (1961).
FRIEDMAN, M. H. F., SNAPE, W. J.: Comparative effectiveness of extracts of intestinal mucosa in stimulating the external secretions of the pancreas and liver. Fed. Proc. **4**, II, 21—22 (1945).
GARBSCH, H.: Zur Röntgenuntersuchung der Gallenwegsdyskinesien. Radiol. Austria **12**, 157—166 (1961).
— MÜLLNER, TH., NEUMAYR, A., TRETENHAHN, W.: Zur Differenzierung der Gallenwegsdyskinesien. Wien. Z. inn. Med. **42**, 41—54 (1961).
GLEASON, P. G.: Cholecystokinin in oral cholecystography and cholangiography N.Y. Med. J. **65**, 252—257 (1965).
GRALL, A.: Le radiocinéma accéléré de l'intestin grêle. Technique d'utilisation de la cholécystokinine. Etude de 170 cas. Dissertation. Service d'électroradiologie, Central-Bichat. Fac. Med. Université de Paris, 1967.
GRANSER, G., HERTTING, G., RISSEL, E., WEWALKA, F.: Untersuchungen über die Beeinflussung des Sphinkter Oddi. Arch. int. Pharmacodyn. Ther. **105**, 389—402 (1956).
GRASSBERGER, A., SEYSS, R.: Die funktionelle intraoperative Cholangiographie. Wien klin. Wschr. **75**, 736—738 (1963).
GRILL, W., PICHLMAIER, H., NEFF, V., STUHLFAUTH, K.: Beitrag zur Motilität der Gallenwege. Münch. med. Wschr. **105**, 130—136 (1963).
GROS, C., WEILL, F.: A propos de l'emploi en radiographie biliaire d'un nouvel agent cholécystokinétique. La "Cholécystokinine" Strasbourg Médical **11**, 429—435 (1960).
GUNNARSON, E.: Discussion. Nord. med. **16**, 1956.
HAEX, A. J. CH., LIMBURG, D.: Cholecysto-cholangiografie met behulp van cholecystokinine. Ned. T. Geneesk. **11**, 1445—1447 (1960).
HARPER, A. A., RAPER, H. S.: Pancreozymin, a stimulant of the secretion of pancreatic enzymes in extracts of the small intestine. J. Physiol. (Lond.) **102**, 115—125 (1943).
HEDNER, P., PERSSON, H., RORSMAN, G.: Effect of cholecystokinin on small intestine. Acta physiol. scand. **70**, 250—254 (1967).
HENNING, N., WITTE, S., BRESSEL, D.: Über den Befund von Leberzellen im Duodenalinhalt und seinen diagnostischen Wert. Med. Klin. **55**, 692—694 (1960).
HERMON-TAYLOR, J.: A technique for perfusion of the isolated canine pancreas. Response to secretin and gastrin. Gastroenterology **55**, 488—501 (1968).
HOLTON, P., JONES, M.: Some observations on changes in the blood content of the cat's pancreas during activity. J. Physiol. (Lond.) **150**, 479—488 (1960).
HONG, S. S., MAGEE, D. F., CREWDSON, F.: The physiologic regulation of gallbladder evacuation. Gastroenterology **30**, 625—630 (1956).
IVY, A. C.: Motor dysfunction of the biliary tract. Amer. J. Röntgenol. **57**, 1—11 (1947).
— Cholecystokinin. In: Polypeptides which stimulate plain muscle, Ed.: J. H. GADDUM. The WILLIAMS & WILKINS COMPANY, Baltimore, 1955, pp. 115—119.
— DREWYER, G. E., ORNDOFF, B. H.: Effect of cholecystokinin on human gallbladder. Endocrinology **14**, 343—348 (1930).
— KLOSTER, G., LUETH, H. C., DREWYER, G. E.: On the preparation of "cholecystokinin". Amer. J. Physiol. **91**, 336—344 (1928).
— OLDBERG, E.: Hormone mechanism for gallbladder contraction and evacuation. Amer. J. Physiol. **86**, 599 (1928).
JÖNSSON, G.: Short communication delivered at Karolinska Sjukhuset, Stockholm, August 6, 1955.
JORPES, J. E., MUTT, V.: On the action of highly purified preparations of secretin and of pancreozymin. Arkiv f. Kemi **7**, 553—559 (1954).
— — Swed. pat. No 156013 (1956).
— — Secretin, pancreozymin and cholecystokinin. Gastroenterology **36**, 377—383 (1959).
— — The gastrointestinal hormones, secretin and cholecystokinin-pancreozymin. Ann. intern. Med. **55**, 395—405 (1961).
— — Secretin, pancreozymin and cholecystokinin. Acta Gastro-ent. belg. **36**, 377—383 (1959).

Jorpes, J. E. Mutt, V.: The gastrointestinal hormones secretin and cholecystokinin. In: Ciba Foundation Symposium on "The exocrine pancreas". Ed.: A. V. S. de Reuck and M. P. Cameron Churchill Ltd, London, 1962, pp. 150—164.
— — Cholecystokinin pancreozymin (CCK-PZ). Nord. med. 8, 237—268 (1967).
— — Clinical aspects of the gastrointestinal hormones secretin and cholecystokinin. Scand. J. Gastroent. **4**, I, 49—57 (1969).
— — Toczko, K.: Further purification of cholecystokinin and pancreozymin. Acta chem. scand. **18**, 2408—2410 (1964).
— — Tomenius, J., Backlund, V.: Cholecystokinin vid röntgenundersökning av gallvägarna. Svenska Läk.-Tidn. **54**, 2736—2741 (1957).
— — Tomenius, J., Backlund, V.: Cholecystokinin in roentgenologic examination of the biliary tract. Röntgenblätter **11**, 145—157 (1958).

Kapandji, M.: Les syndromes radiomanométriques de profil des dyskinésics par hypotonie généralisée des voies biliaires et par hypertonie du sphincter d'Oddi décelés par la radiomanométrie par ponction transpariéto-hépatique pré-opératoire. Rev. int. Hépat. **2**, 661—706 (1952).

Leger, L., Roucayrol, J. C., Lenriot, J. P.: Scintigraphie à la sélénométhionine dans les pancréatites aigues et chroniques. Communication orale. Acta gastro-ent. belg. — à paraître 1971.

Lescut, J. Ch.: Sur l'emploi de la cholécystokinine dans le radiodiagnostic des affections des voies biliaires. Thesis. Clin. Mal. Appar. dig. Lille, France. 1963.

Longo, O., Huarte, C., d'Agostino, J., Mammana, L.: Colecistoquinina y colangiografia per y post operatoria. Xe congreso argentino de Gastro-enterologica. Mar del Plata 1969.

MacFarland, J., Currin, J.: Cholecystokinin and the cystic duct syndrome clinical experience in a community hospital. Amer. J. Gastroent. **52**, 515—522 (1969).

Magee, D. F.: Physiology of gallbladder emptying. In: The biliary system, Symposium Nato Advanced Study Institute. Ed.: W. Taylor, Oxford. Blackwell Scientif. Publ. 1965, pp. 233—247.

Mamie, M., Kleinert, R.: Cholécystokinine et cholécystographie. Praxis Rev. Suisse Méd. **51**, 279—283 (1962).

Matuchansky, C., Huet, J., Rambaud, J. Cl., Bernier, J. J.: Effets chez l'homme de l'accélération du transit intestinal provoquée par la cholécystokinine sur l'absorption jéjunale de l'eau et des électrolytes. In: Biologie et Gastroentérologie Tome II 1970, pp. 195—196. Suppl. 2. Arch. Mal. Appar. dig. 1970.

Meinardus, K.: Cholecystokinin bei der Cholecystographie. Schweiz. med. Wschr. **89**, 407—408 (1959).

Monod, E.: Action entéro-kinétique de la Cécékine. Arch. Mal. Appar. dig. **53**, 607—608 (1964).

Morin, G., Besancon, F., Grall, A., Debray, Ch., Jouve, R., Garat, J.-P.: La cholécystokinine appliquée au radiodiagnostic de l'intestin grêle: nouvelle technique de radiocinématographie complète en quelques minutes avec 62 observations. Entretiens de Bichat. Radiologie 247—250 (1966).
— — — Jouve, R., Debray, Ch.: Technique d'accélération du transit du grêle. Arch. Mal. Appar. dig. **54**, 1285—1290 (1965).
— Busson, A., Blanchet: Discussion orale. Arch. Mal. Appar. dig. **46**, 418 (1957).
— Grall, A., Jouve, R., Bellin, A., Besancon, F., Debray, Ch.: La technique du grêle accélérée par la cholécystokinine. Bilan de 251 examens. Arch. Mal. Appar. dig. **58**, 483 à 485 (1969).

Mutt, V., Jorpes, J. E.: Secretin, Cholecystokinin, In: Internat. Symp. on the Pharmacol. of Hormonal Polypeptides and Proteins. (Milan, Italy, Sept. 14—16, 1967.) New York. Plenum Press, 1968, pp. 569—580.
— — Structure of porcine cholecystokinin-pancreozymin. I. Cleavage with thrombin and with trypsin. Europ. J. Biochem. **6**, 156—162 (1968).

Naito, S., Sivata, R., Taito, T.: Etude sur la cholécystokinine, son mode d'action sur la contraction de la vésicule biliaire. Presse méd. **71**, 2688—2689 (1963).

Nathan, M. H., Newman, A., MacFarland, J., Murray, J.: Cholecystokinin in cholecystography. Radiology **93**, 1—8 (1969).

Nordyke, R. A.: Surgical vs. nonsurgical jaundice: differentiation by combination of Rose Bengal-131 J and standard liver function test. J. Amer. med. Ass. **194**, 949—953 (1965).

Nylander, G.: Vid koledokotomi kvarlämnade gallvägskonkrement. Nord. Med. **83**, 116—117 (1970).

Oi, I., Kobayashi, S., Kondo, T.: Endoscopic pancreato-cholangiography. Diagnosis of cancer of the pancreas. In: Abstr. 4th World Congr. Gastroenter. Copenhagen, July 1970. Edit. P. Riis, P. Anthonisen and H. Baden, Copenhagen, 1970, p. 493.

PARIS, J., ROBELET, A., SALEMBIER, Y., DU BOIS, R.: Etude expérimentale des effets de la cholécystokinine sur les voies biliaires soumises à l'action des substances morphiniques. Rev. int. Hépat. **12**, 1071–1091 (1962).

PLESSIER, J.: Confrontation des actions cholécystokinétiques et cholérétiques de la cholécystokinine, du sorbitol, de l'huile d'olive et du sulfate de magnésie. Path. Biol. **8**, 1201 à 1210 (1960).

— Communication orale sur l'accélération du transit du grêle par la cholécystokinine. Arch. Mal. Appar. dig. **58**, 486 (1969).

— Confrontations entre la valeur de la parenchymatographie, la capacité exocrine du pancréas, l'insulinémie, la glucagonémie obtenues par injection intra-coeliaque de secrétine purifiée. Acta gastro-ent. belg. — à paraître 1971.

— ASSAN, R., BENNET, J., BIGOT, P., CHENARD, A., DOYON, D., ECONOMOPOULOS, P., MONNIER, J., MUSSY, F., ROSSELIN, P.: Confrontations entre les réponses secrétoires externes et internes (insuline et glucagon plasmatiques) et la valeur de la parenchymatographie, obtenues après injection de secrétine intracoeliaque. Acta gastro-ent. belg. (A paraître, 1971).

— DOYON, D., BENETT, J., STOOPEN, M., ECONOMOPOULOS, P., CHERIGIE, E., CAROLI, J.: Effets de la secrétine intra-artérielle en angiographie coeliaque (artériographie souplée avec le tubage duodénal). Arch. Mal. Appar. dig. **57**, 307–315 (1967).

— ECONOMOPOULOS, P., PLESSIER, B.: Premiers résultats des tests de fluorescence (Tétracycline) au cours de la double épreuve secrétine-pancréozymine. Acta gastro-ent. belg. **29**, 179–182 (1966).

— GRALL, A., JOUVE, R., BELLIN, A., BESANCON, F., DEBRAY, CH.: La technique du grêle accélérée par la cholécystokinine. Bilan de 251 examens. Arch. Mal. Appar. dig. **58**, 483–485 (1969).

— MARSICO, G.: La cholécystokinine. Son emploi en cholécystographie, radiomanométrie et cinématographie biliaire. Ann. Radiol. (Paris) **3**, 801–810 (1960).

— PLESSIER, B.: Réponse de la vésicule biliaire in situ du cobaye aux stimulations successives ou simultanées de cholécystokinine et de morphine ou de dextromoramide. Rev. int. Hépat. XIII, **4**, 283–288 (1963).

— — Un accélérateur inattendu du transit intestinal (grêle et colon) Sem. des Hôp. **29**, 1890 (1957).

— WETTENDORFF, P., PLESSIER, B., COHEN, J.: L'atonie vésiculaire chez la femme et le cobaye gravides. Essai d'explication par le dosage biologique des hormones digestives. Ann. Biol. clin. **19**, 843–850 (1961).

POILLEUX, F.: Les dystonies biliaires: Dystonies du system vesiculaire. In: Rapport au 50 ème Congrès de Chirurgie, Paris, Octobre 1947.

PORCHER, P., CAROLI, J., PEQUIGNOT, G., DELATTRE, M.: Contribution du radiocinéma à l'étude physiologique des voies biliaires. Acta gastro-ent. belg. **20**, 7–18 (1957).

POTTER, M. S.: Observations of the gallbladder and bile during pregnancy at term. J. Amer. med. Ass. **106**, 1070–1074 (1936).

RAMORINO, M. L., COLAGRANDE, C., MONTI, G., SISTI, P.: Effetti della colecistocinina su l'apparato biliare extraepatico e sul duodeno. Arch. ital. Mal. Appar. dig. **27**, 403–432 (1960).

RASKIN, H. F., WENGER, J., SKLAR, M., PLETICKA, S., YAREMA, W.: The diagnosis of cancer of the pancreas, biliary tract, and duodenum by combined cytologic and secretory methods. I. Exfoliative duodenal intubation. Gastroenterology **34**, 996–1008 (1958).

ROSENQVIST, H.: Cholecystokinin as an adjuvant in biliary surgery. Opusc. med. (Stockh.) **9**, 3–8 (1964).

SANDBLOM, P., VOEGTLIN, W. L., IVY, A. C.: The effect of cholecystokinin on the choledochoduodenal mechanism (sphincter of Oddi). Amer. J. Physiol. **113**, 175–180 (1935).

SCHMIEDEN, V.: Über die Stauungsgallenblase. Zentralbl. Chir. **47**, 257–258 (1920).

SIFFERT DE PAULA E SILVA, G.: Calculo do volume da vesicula biliar. Brasil-méd. **62**, 45, 46, 4, 11 (1948).

— — Simple method for computing the volume of the human gallbladder. Radiology **52**, 94–102 (1949).

STASSA, G., GRAFE, W.: The cineradiographic evaluation of the biliary tract after drug therapy following colecystectomy, sphincterotomy and vagotomy. Radiology **91**, 297–230 (1968).

SVATOS, A.: Pancreozymin activity of urine. Naturwissenschaften, **45**, 523–524 (1957).

— Cholecystokinin activity of urine. Science **129**, 566–567 (1959).

TAKAGI, K. Retrograde pancreatography and cholangiography with fiberduodenoscopy. In: Abstr. 4th World Congr. Gastroenterol. Copenhagen, July 1970, p. 500. Edit.: P. RIIS, P. ANTHONISEN and H. BADEN, Copenhagen, 1970.

TAYLOR, D. A., MACKEN, K. L., FIORE, A. S.: Angiographic visualization of the secretin-stimulated pancreas. Radiology **87**, 525—526 (1966).
TOMENIUS, J., BACKLUND, V.: Cholecystokinin vid röntgenundersökning av gallvägarna. Nord. Med. **61**, 46—47 (1959).
TORSOLI, A., RAMORINO, M. L., ALESSANDRINI, A.: Motility of the biliary tract. Rendic. R. Gastroenterol. **2**, 67—80 (1970).
— — COLAGRANDE, C., DEMAIO, G.: Experiments with cholecystokinin. Acta Radiol. (Stockh.) **55**, 193—206 (1961a).
— — PALAGI, L., COLAGRANDE, C., BASCHIERI, I., RIBOTTA, S., MARINOSCI, M.: Observations roentgencinématographiques et électronmanométriques sur la motilité des voies biliaires. Sem. Hôp. Paris **37**, 790—802 (1961b).
TOULET, J.: Méthode pratique du calcul du volume vésiculaire et du pourcentage volumétrique d'évacuation. Rev. Int. Hépat. **111**, 169—212 (1953).
UDÉN, R.: Effect of secretin in celiac and superior mesenteric angiography. Acta Radiol. Diagnosis **8**, 497—513 (1969).
VEJBORA, O., SVATOS, A., DVORACKOVA, I.: Influence of sensitization of the organism with E. coli and S. paratyphi endotoxin on the contractile capacity of the gallbladder. Cas. Lék. ces. **106**, 16, 424—429 (1967).
WENGER, J., RASKIN, H. F.: The diagnosis of cancer of the pancreas, biliary tract and duodenum by combined cytologic and secretory methods. II. The secretin test. Gastroenterology **34**, 1009—1019 (1958).
WERNER, B.: Invärtesmedicinska synpunkter på pankreasfunktionen. Nord. Med. **55**, 169—170 (1956).
— MUTT, V.: The pancreatic response in man to the injection of highly purified secretin and of pancreozymin. Scand. J. clin. Lab. Invest. **6**, 228—236 (1954).
WESTBROOK, R. I.: The value of cholecystokinin cholecystography in evaluating gallbladder disease. Neb. St. med. J. **55**, 4, 245—250 (1970).
WIECHEL, K. L.: Percutaneous transhepatic cholangiography. Acta chir. scand. Suppl. **330** (1964).

Author Index

Page numbers in *italics* refer to the bibliography

Subject Index*

* Prepared by E. Jorpes.